**Medical Imaging**
Edited by Okechukwu Felix Erondu

**Published by InTech**
Janeza Trdine 9, 51000 Rijeka, Croatia



**Publishing Process Manager** Marija Radja

**Technical Editor** Teodora Smiljanic

**Cover Designer** InTech Design Team

Additional hard copies can be obtained from orders@intechopen.com

Medical Imaging, Edited by Okechukwu Felix Erondu
p. cm.
ISBN 978-953-307-774-1

For EU product safety concerns:
IN TECH d.o.o., Prolaz Marije Krucifikse Kozulić 3, 51000 Rijeka, Croatia,
info@intechopen.com or visit our website at intechopen.com.

# Meet the editor

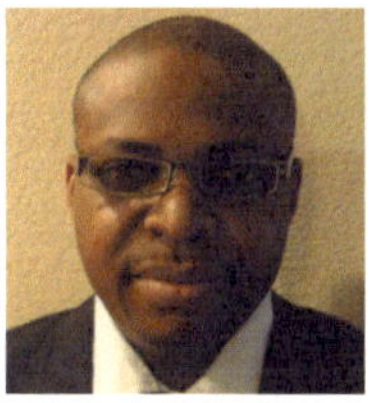

Dr. Felix Okechukwu Erondu is a practicing medical imaging consultant with clinical experience spanning over nineteen years. He is an Adjunct senior lecturer in the Department of Medical Radiography and Radiological sciences in the University of Nigeria, Enugu campus and senior research fellow with over 40 scientific publications in renown international journals. Dr Erondu also holds the post of the Medical director of Image Diagnostics Ltd, Nigeria, a chain of ultramodern diagnostic facilities engaged in medical imaging and clinical support services. He has served as a board member of Nnamdi Azikiwe University Teaching Hospital and chairman of Radiographers Registration Board of Nigeria. He holds a masters degree in Medical Imaging and a doctorate in Medical Physics.

# Contents

# Preface

Medical imaging was primarily seen as the use of non-invasive techniques to create internal images of the human body for clinical or medical purposes. This rapidly evolving field of medicine originated in the first decade of the $19^{th}$ century, when Wilhelm Röntgen, a professor of physics at Würzburg University in Germany, discovered electromagnetic radiation. After the World War Two, the development of computer technology has triggered an amazing revolution in medical imaging techniques.

What we know about and do with medical imaging has changed tremendously over the past decade, beginning with the basics, following with the breakthroughs, and moving on to the abstract.

There is a continuous drive not only to improve the diagnostic yield of medical imaging techniques for clinical use, but also the management of the huge amount of digital information available to medical imaging departments. Today there is an increasing interest to harness medical imaging processes to improve research in the biophysical domain.

Medical imaging has experienced tremendous progress during the past decade. Continuous innovations have been fueled by the need to improve diagnostic yield and achieve fast turnaround through robust information management, which should ultimately improve patient outcome. The rapid changes in digital technology have also created opportunities for the development of high-tech equipment employed in medical imaging practice.

Incidentally, these changes tend to revolve around key modalities such as radiography, computed tomography, scintigraphy, magnetic resonance imaging and ultrasound. In many instances, one modality tends to augment the limitations associated with others. This book approaches the concept of medical imaging from a wider perspective not considered by many authors in this area. It consists of four sections and eighteen chapters and topics.

The first section deals with basic concepts such as identification of structures in medical images, 3D image segmentation, image analysis, texture analysis, radiation protection and simulations.

Section two concentrates on the image processing techniques, quality metrics as well as tools required to optimize patient processes.

Section three deals with applications of medical techniques in clinical settings, while the last section explores the advances made in this area including PET/CT hybrid technique, optical imaging thermography, mitosis detection, phase contrast microscopy and use in image-guided surgery.

It is hoped that this book bridges the gap between the core clinical books reserved for medical diagnosis and the wide ranging possibilities in the field of biological research. It is a must-read for all practitioners and researchers interested in medical imaging.

This book is an attempt to present the old, understand the current and appreciate the great advancements into the future of medical imaging. It will be an invaluable resource to those interested in history, clinical applications and unlimited horizons presented by medical imaging science.

My acknowledgement goes to all the authors, who have made scholarly contributions to the book from diverse backgrounds. I am also grateful and indebted to the publishing process managers Bojana Zelenika and Marija Radja for carefully directing the editorial process and for their patience even when I couldn't meet the scheduled timeline.

**Felix Okechukwu Erondu Ph.D**
Adjunct Senior Lecturer in Radiography and Medical Imaging
University of Nigeria
Nigeria

# Part 1

## Basic Concepts in Medical Imaging

# 1

# Identification of Structures in Medical Images[1]

Marina de Sá Rebelo[1], Sérgio Shiguemi Furuie[2], Lincoln de Assis Moura Jr[2], Eduardo Tavares Costa[3,4] and Marco Antonio Gutierrez[1]

[1]*Heart Institute (InCor) - University of São Paulo Medical School*
[2]*Polytechnic School – University of São Paulo*
[3]*School of Electrical and Computer Engineering- University of Campinas*
[4]*Center for Biomedical Engineering - University of Campinas*
*Brazil*

## 1. Introduction

The development of automatic systems for medical image processing, which can effectively act as an agent to aid medical diagnosis, is a goal that has been pursued by researchers since the first works on the field of medical image processing in the 80´s. The automation of image analysis tasks can produce very interesting results such as less time spent by specialists, decrease of intra-and inter-observer differences, second opinions to non-specialists and in educational systems. Any automatic system deployed for analysis and visualization of images involves the identification of objects and often the relationships among them. The automatic identification of structures is a research area of image processing that still has great challenges. In tasks that involve primarily activities of calculation, the computer's processing power is incomparably higher than the humans. However, in recognition and analysis tasks, the human brain possesses a strong ability that is not obtained by any computational system. For a given scene, humans possess a unique ability to distinguish the objects that are significant and, among them, those that represent the focus of interest for a particular situation.

In the routine of medical image analysis, doctors often deal with images in which the visual perception is not sufficient for identification of some particular structure under study. They need, therefore, conceptual hypotheses so as to perform this task. At each new image analyzed a doctor uses a huge amount of knowledge accumulated over the years of clinical practice. This is a typical feedback and a case base reasoning system, as each new image analyzed gives the doctor more knowledge about a specific problem. A system of medical aid for identification and analysis of structures should also be able to incorporate and use knowledge about the problem domain.

## 2. Identification of structures in digital images

### 2.1 Problem statement

Automatic recognition and identification of structures are fields of Computer Vision. The recognition of structures is a difficult task because many factors influence its computation.

---

[1] Portions adapted, with permission, from *Computers in Biology and Medicine* 37 (2007) 1183 - 1193

These can include restrictions on permissible forms, the semantics of the context of the scene and the information present in the image itself (Suetens et al, 1992). After recognizing the set of objects in the scene, the next step in the interpretation process is the identification of one or more objects of particular interest in the recognized set. There is a distinction between the concepts of recognition and identification of structures. There are many definitions in the literature for recognition (or discovery) of structures. We use here a simple definition, given by Suetens et al (1992):

> *"The recognition (or detection) of structures is the task of finding and labeling parts of a digital image that correspond to objects in the scene."*

Once the recognition step has been performed, the next step is to identify one or all instances of a particular structure. The definition of object identification is not precise and, depending on the application, may be mistaken for recognition. In this text, identification is defined by the authors as:

> *The identification of a particular set of structures is to set apart from the recognized structures the one or ones that correspond to the object under study.*

The term segmentation is sometimes used by researchers as a synonym to identification as defined above. The canonical definition of segmentation is the subdivision of the image into its components (Gonzales & Woods, 2000; Jain, 1989). Strictly speaking, segmentation corresponds only to the first step of the recognition process.

### 2.2 Automatic identification

The steps involved in the automatic identification of structures are usually divided into different levels. Some authors have proposed a division into two levels: low and high (Ballard & Brown, 1982; Sonka et al, 1998) while others use three processing levels: low, medium and high (Gonzales & Woods, 2000; Niessen, 1997).

The low processing level deals with functions similar to automated human visual reactions that normally require little or no knowledge about the content of the image (Gonzalez & Woods, 2000; Sonka, 1998). It is mainly or almost entirely based on intrinsic image data, without inclusion of *a priori* information. It includes activities such as the basic process of image formation, filtering for noise reduction and correction of acquisition artifacts. In addition, there are processes to decrease the huge amount of data present in the original image to obtain parametric images describing relevant information. Examples of relevant parameters are local contrast, texture, curvature and movement. At the intermediate processing level the tasks are performed by extraction and characterization of components in the images resulting from the low level process. This stage includes activities such as identification, representation and description of the image information through models. For authors who do not use this classification, these functions are usually defined as low-level processing (Ballard & Brown, 1982; Sonka, 1998). The authors that include the intermediate level point out that the difference to the low level processing is that, based on some restrictions, it is possible to select - or highlight - relevant information to a particular application and formalize this information using models that include some information *a priori* about the application domain, thus making it easier the subsequent high-level tasks (Niessen, 1997). Moreover, the result of this processing step generates no more pictures, but representation of objects in the picture. The high processing level is based on knowledge, goals and strategies on how to achieve those goals more efficiently. Using knowledge about the image structure, image data is systematically evaluated. Hypotheses are confirmed or rejected by the data. Routines for processing high-level information should be organized to produce rapid searches. The difference between high-level and intermediate level processing is the explicit use of knowledge about the context of the image under analysis.

## 3. Automatic identification in medical images

In medical applications, the ultimate goal of automatic image analysis is to obtain not only qualitative results, but also quantitative data for assessing objectively the changes in relation to normal standards. To obtain such results it is necessary first to identify the object of interest and then carefully analyze it. Among the applications for which identification of structures is an important step are: visualization and surgical planning, planning for radiotherapy procedures, identification of tumors, malformations and dysfunctions, classification of organs, tissues and cells, and retrieval of similar cases in image content based databases.

In the case of image volumes, or 3D image data, automatic identification involves a large number of operations starting from the original acquired data: they must be processed so that object slices are formed by applying filters and reconstruction algorithms. Once the slices have been obtained, further transformations in the image are needed in order to make the data more suitable for identification. Such transformations may include processes as edge detection algorithms and structure recognition. Then high level procedures involving the use of *a priori* knowledge to determine the searched structure are used and, specific analysis of the found structures can be performed

The results of methods for identification of structures in medical images can be affected by image artifacts. Images contain noise that can alter the intensity of a pixel such that its classification becomes uncertain. They also have finite pixel size and, for this reason, are subject to partial volume averaging effect where individual pixel volumes contain a mixture of tissue classes so that the intensity of a pixel in the image may not be consistent with any one structure. The intensity level of a single tissue class can vary over the extent of the image, and internal materials (for instance surgical clips) may cause distortion in the imaged organ (Rani et al, 2011; Withey & Koles, 2007). Some of these effects are depicted in Figure 1.

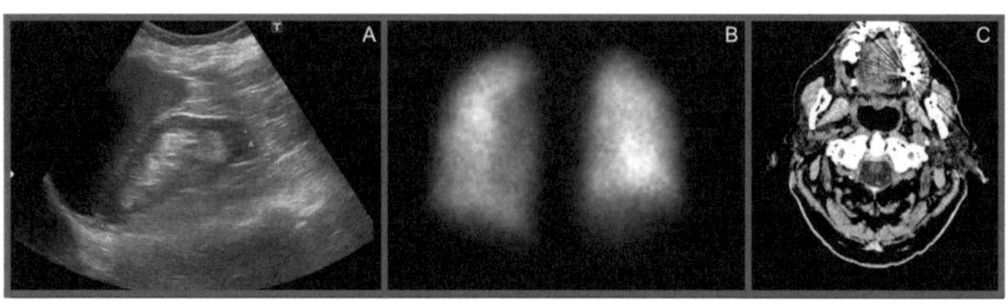


Fig. 1. Examples of effects that can affect structure identification can be seen in the three images: (A) kidney in Ultrasound (US), (B) lung in Nuclear Medicine (NM) and (C) brain in Computed Tomography (CT). The noise associated with each image modality has to be dealt with in different ways. In image (C) the presence of dental metal pieces degraded the reconstructed slice of the brain (images acquired at the Imaging Department - Heart Institute – HCFMUSP- with patient anonymization).

All these factors may affect the identification of organs due to poorly defined boundaries, blur or weak edges homogeneity. Moreover, the identification of organs in medical imaging presents some unique challenges as the creation of efficient models for representation of biological structures that are not easily described by mathematical models. All these factors, added to the variability in tissue distribution among individuals in the human population, means that some degree of uncertainty must be attached to all segmentation results. Figure 2 exemplifies the difficulty in identifying brain structures in Computerized Tomography (CT) and Magnetic Resonance (MR) images.

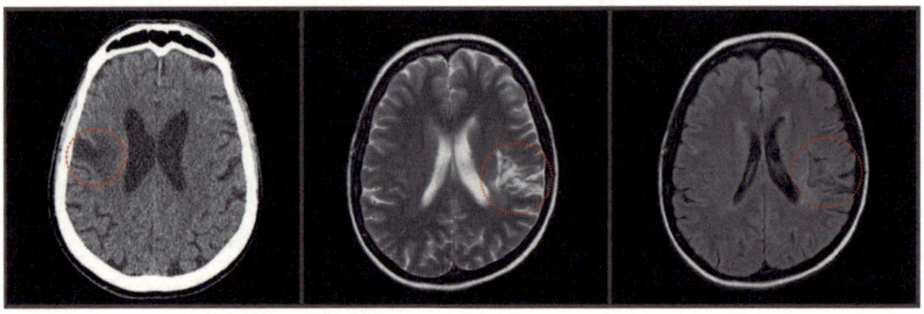

Fig. 2. Example challenging identification tasks in brain images. The areas inside the red circles are the areas to be identified. Due to the aforementioned problems, the identification of some tissues in medical images can be difficult even in modalities with high resolution as CT (left image) and MR (middle and right) (images acquired at the Imaging Department - Heart Institute - HCFMUSP- with patient anonymization).

### 3.1 Use of a priori information for identification in medical images

In the context of medical images, the concept of identification, as defined above, involves the discrimination against a particular organ or the discrimination between normality and abnormality for a particular organ, based on the attributes of the image. Although trained clinicians are able to find and classify body structures precisely, there is not a technique that can reproduce precisely their ability in computational environments. The use of simple methods that rely only on information contained in the image data, in general, does not produce satisfactory results. In other words, the intrinsic information of the image is not enough to characterize the structures present in real objects (Suetens et al, 1992). Effective procedures for identifying structures should incorporate knowledge of the model or the context.

There are several studies in the literature aiming the characterization of the knowledge about a particular organ in a medical image modality to aid the automatic processing of the image. Typically, the methods use information about shape, size, texture and position of a given structure. A major difficulty in using *a priori* information about the forms of the organs is to characterize them geometrically. Unlike the rigid objects from other applications of computer vision, most human organs have few calculable and stable invariants. Apart from that, the features to be detected in images may be small and subtle, sometimes characterized only by tiny changes in gray level. In many medical applications there is a significant amount of known information about the human anatomy. However, there is a major difficulty involving the creation of models to represent biological structures, comprising very complex forms that are not described easily. Furthermore, for a given population these structures usually show variations both in form and size.

### 3.2 A review of applications in medical imaging

Techniques specifically designed for computerized detection of abnormalities in chest radiographs were among the first works in the area of identification of structures in medical images (Duncan & Ayache, 2000). The field has evolved continuously since then and the amount of knowledge has grown constantly with a huge number of methods described in the literature, as pointed out in many survey papers (Bandyopadhyay, 2011; Duncan & Ayache, 2000; Kirbas & Quek, 2002; Lesage et al, 2009; Ma et al, 2008; Oliver et al, 2010; PetitJean & Dacher, 2011; Witney & Koles,2007).

The assumptions and requirements taken by identification methods vary substantially for different body organs and imaging modalities. Therefore, the choice of the method will be dependent on the particular application, regarding the organ or system under study, as well as the imaging modality (Bandyopadhyay, 2011). There have been described general methods that intended to be more comprehensive, and therefore can be applied to a number of applications. However, their performance is worse than that of methods designed for specific applications, as the latter generally use *a priori* information available about the problem under study (Bandyopadhyay, 2011).

In the next paragraphs we will present some methods proposed in recent years. A general overview of the methods described for medical image identification in the last decades is presented in the first section. The next sections are dedicated to clinical applications with emphasis on the organ under study, presenting the well-known specific challenges for identifying the particular organ and exploring some recently published methods. This text avoids performance comparisons due to fact that existing applications are so different in their purposes and practical applications, that direct comparisons do not make sense.

#### 3.2.1 Evolution of the methods along the last decades

There is a number of papers discussing the evolution of the algorithms for extraction or identification of medical structures. It is out of the scope of this chapter to present and compare all studies and methodologies for classifying the existing methods. Instead, we present a description of the field evolution based on two surveys, presented by Ma et al (2008) and Witney & Koles (2007), which we believe presents the evolution of the field in a simple and informative way. For the other reviews, readers are referred to the literature (Duncan & Ayache, 2002; Petitjean et al, 2011). Withey and Koles (2007) classified the medical image identification approaches in literature into three generations, while Ma et al (2008) classified the methods in three categories that can be fitted to the three generations model of Witney and Koles.

The first generation techniques are those almost based on intrinsic image information, without any *a priori* information. They include:

- Threshold: algorithms belonging to this type assume that the searched structures are related to clearly quantifiable features as image intensity and gradient.
- Region growing: from an initial seed located in the image, adjacent pixels are checked against a set of predefined homogeneity criteria. Pixels that meet the criteria are included in the region.
- Edge tracing: after the application of an edge detection algorithm, the edge pixels with adjacent neighbor connectivity are followed sequentially and collected into a list to represent an object boundary.

The second generation is composed of algorithms using image models, optimization methods, and uncertainty models, and includes:

- Pattern recognition and clustering: as certain structures in medical images can be treated as patterns, segmentation algorithms that combine pattern recognition techniques have been proposed to extract the searched structures.
- Deformable models: deformable models use curve evolution to perform segmentation. A moving equation should be defined to drive the initial curves to the right structure boundaries.
- Graph search: image pixels are used to form nodes in a graph and the nodes are interconnected to neighbors, mapping the corresponding pixel associations in the image. Costs are assigned for each interconnection. Algorithms from combinatorial optimization are used to obtain minimum-cost solutions.
- Multiresolution methods: multiresolution or multiscale analysis refers to the use of scale reduction to group pixels into image objects. A stack of images is formed by recursively reducing the scale of the original image by blurring followed by down sampling. The central idea in this category is that there may be scales that are more suited for processing some image features.

The third generation is characterized by algorithms that are capable of incorporating knowledge, such as:

- Shape and appearance models: the active shape model (ASM) was inspired by deformable models with the added intention of limiting the extent of the model deformation. A statistical representation of an object is formed by identifying a set of landmark points on an object boundary and analyzing the variation of each across a set of training images.
- Atlas-based: it is a generic technique for automatic delineation of structures in volumetric images, which starts by registering an anatomical image from an atlas with a target image to be segmented. A critical underlying assumption is that it is possible to find a deformation that aligns the atlas with the target image in such a way that label propagation lines up the objects of interest.
- Rule-based: image primitives are usually derived from first-generation and second-generation algorithms and then interpreted using anatomical and image knowledge applied as a set of rules.

### 3.2.2 Brain applications

Environmental factors, age and disease can affect neuroanatomical structures during the process of ageing. These structures are also affected by genetic factors in patients with degenerative diseases (Ashburner et al, 2003). Besides providing anatomical information, medical imaging procedures are able to provide extremely relevant information about brain physiology, which can be used to understand physical and psychological clinical conditions.

In order to capture the extraordinary morphological variability of the human brain, a number of automatic methods for identification and analysis of structures have been developed for different imaging modalities (Ashburner et al, 2003; Bandyopadhyay, 2011; Bresser et al, 2011; Ishii et al, 2009; Lopes et al, 2008; Ribbens et al, 2010; Rousset et al, 2007; Shiee et al, 2010; Tu & Bai, 2010; Yi et al, 2009; Zhang et al, 2011).

Most automatic systems for analysis of brain images have three processing steps: (i) brain tissue identification; (ii) registration: the voxels of interest are matched to a template or to an earlier scan from the same individual; (iii) statistical comparison of different groups of patients or same patient in different times.

In their review of the methods to assess brain structures, Ashburner et al (2003) discuss the strengths and limitations of algorithms for identification and registration of brain images, together with evidence of their usefulness at the clinical and research level. A more recent review of current methods used for computer automated identification in brain anatomical images is presented by Bandyopadhyay (2011). Most methods for extraction of brain structures and tissue segmentation use some kind of *a priori* information. Some authors, however, try to minimize the need of *a priori* knowledge. As an example, Scherrer et al (2009) extracted tissue and sub-cortical structures in MR images by considering a local approach to cope with intensity non-uniformity and a multi-agent based implementation.

### 3.2.3 Cardiovascular applications

Cardiovascular diseases are the leading cause of death in developed countries (Allender et al, 2008). Imaging techniques are nowadays among the most valuable tools in helping diagnosis, treatment and follow-up of cardiovascular pathologies, as they provide qualitative and quantitative information of the heart, which would be impossible to obtain otherwise (Cordero-Grande et al, 2011). Diagnosis and treatment follow-up of these pathologies can rely on numerous cardiac imaging modalities, which include echography, CT (computerized tomography), digital subtractive angiography, coronary angiography and cardiac MRI.

**Heart.** Quantitative analysis of the heart structure and function can be performed by the extraction of cardiac descriptors from medical images. These descriptors can provide information about global and local function. This includes estimating left ventricle volume, ejection fraction, cardiac output, myocardial mass, myocardial morphology, myocardial uptake rates, tissue viability, blood flow, local motion and deformation (wall thickening). The determination of most of these descriptors involves an appropriate 3D identification of cardiac structures - being the cardiac chambers, cardiac muscle or cardiac valves - as a prerequisite (Alattar et al, 2010; Cordero-Grande et al, 2011). The imaging modality of choice will depend on the problem under study and the complexity of the identification of the cardiac structures will depend on the modality chosen.

Automatic isolation of the heart structures in MR images is a challenging task because of the inherent noise associated with cine MRI, caused by factors such as patient movement, cardiac dynamics, and complex intensity characteristics (Lynch, 2008). Even in noiseless cases, MR images may present blurred edges due to the partial volume effect and can be affected by motion artifacts. In addition, low contrast between the myocardium and surrounding tissues complicates the identification of the cardiac structures. As an example, the papillary muscles, the trabeculae, or the liver have pixel intensity values which are virtually indistinguishable from those of the myocardium (Cordero-Grande et al, 2011). In the literature there is a huge number of recent works on heart identification in MR images (Alattar et al, 2010; Cordero-Grande et al, 2011; Lekadir et al, 2011; O'Brien et al, 2011; O'Donnell et al, 2006; Rouchdy et al, 2007; Schaerer et al, 2010; Zhao et al, 2009). A comprehensive survey focusing on extracting the heart cavities in short axis view from cardiac MR images has been published recently by Petitjean & Dacher (2011).

The analysis of cardiac conditions using CT images needs a highly consistent identification of the involved surfaces. To measure blood volume, segmentation should consistently follow the cavity border. Wall thickness measurements should be based on a convex hull around the cavity that excludes papillary muscles from the myocardium. For the epicardium, it is important to avoid local confusions with the nearby pericardium or lung transition (Peters et al, 2010). A number of authors have described methods to isolate the cardiac walls and chambers in CT images (Ecabert et al, 2008; O'Donnell et al, 2006; Peters et al, 2010; Zheng et al, 2010).

Ultrasound imaging is arguably the hardest medical imaging modality upon which to perform organ identification (Noble, 2010). The main problem in detecting, for example, heart boundaries in ultrasound images is related to the high level of multiplicative noise (mainly speckle noise), low contrast among structures, artifacts such as shadowing from the lungs and, attenuation. All these factors can hinder the automatic analysis of the images (Antunes et al, 2010). A recent work by Mora et al (2009) combined supervised neural networks with different image processing techniques to identify heart cavities. Antunes et al (2010) applied a geometric deformable model to identify the four heart chambers of newborns.

**Vascular system.** Vascular identification is a particular challenging problem. The network trees of vessels are complex structures, with high variability in size and curvature. The general tubular organ geometry can be perturbed by stents, calcifications, aneurysms, and stenosis, besides being embedded in complex anatomical scenes, surrounded by other organs. Lesage et al (2009) published a review on vessel lumen segmentation techniques focused on 3D contrast-enhanced imaging modalities (Magnetic Resonance Angiography - MRA and Computed Tomography Angiography - CTA). A former survey on vessel extraction techniques was presented by Kirbas and Kerk (2002). Destrempes et al (2009) describe a method for extracting carotid artery in ultrasound images. A segmentation and visualization of the left coronary heart arteries in CT images was presented by Rahman et al (2010). The arteries extraction methods tend to use a strong cylinder assumption. Qian et al (2009) presented a method in which they try to avoid this common strong prior knowledge. The analysis of temporal change in vessel images was addressed by Zhao et al (2009) who described a method to identify subjects with connective tissue disorder in 4D cardiovascular MRI.

### 3.2.4 Liver applications

Precise measurement of shape and composition of liver is the basis for diagnosis, surgery planning and therapy control of liver pathologies such as cirrhosis, liver cancer, and fulminant hepatic failure (Campadelli et al, 2009). CT images are preferred by the doctors for performing these tasks. Liver identification in CT scans poses problems due to the low contrast and blurred edges that characterize CT images. In their survey of liver extraction in CT scans, Campadelli et al (2009) identified the main applications of the technique as: (1) automatic detection of liver cancer from other liver diseases; (ii) measurement of liver volume - an important index in cases of living donor liver transplantation; (iii) 3D volume rendering of abdominal organs for surgical planning and radiation treatment programs. Another review of the methods for liver identification in CT images was published by Heimann et al (2009). Recent works in this area have also been described by Ruskó et al

(2009), Masuda et al (2010) and Pu et al (2009). Linguraru et al (2009) proposed a method to isolate both the spleen and liver in contrast-enhanced CT images by first aligning the images with models from an atlas and then improving the results by an active contour technique.

### 3.2.5 Lung applications

Pulmonary nodules are potential manifestations of lung cancer, and their detection and inspection are essential for screening and diagnosis of the disease (Kubota et al, 2011). Once the nodule has been detected, monitoring of its size, density, edge-smoothness and growth rate provide information about what treatment, if any, is appropriate (Murphy et al, 2009). An extensive review of computer aided diagnosis in chest radiography was published by van Ginneken et al (2001). Automated detection of nodules has been described by Murphy et al (2009) and Kubota et al (2011). Bouma et al (2009) proposed a system for the automatic detection of pulmonary embolism in contrast-enhanced CT images and Pu et al (2011) proposed an automated scheme to extract the airway tree depicted on CT images.

### 3.2.6 Other applications

**Mammography**. In mammography, the use of computer-aided diagnosis (CAD) systems is intended to assist radiologists in the automatic detection and classification of mammographic abnormalities. There is a large number of different types of mammographic abnormalities. In the majority of cases the abnormalities are either micro-calcifications or masses (Oliver et al, 2010). Mammography CAD systems usually start by a preprocessing step to extract the breast tissue, background tissue and pectoral muscle (Cheng et al, 2003; Samulski & Karssemeijer, 2010; Timp et al, 2007). Oliver et al (2011) published an extensive review on the theme in which they divide the automatic methods for detection of abnormalities in three groups: (i) Region-based methods: region growing and related methods, watershed methods, split and merge methods; (ii) Contour-based methods; (iii) Clustering methods.

**Thyroid**. Diseases of the thyroid gland are among the most frequent endocrine disorders. Ultrasound has become the most important technique for thyroid gland imaging and computerized systems have been described to aid doctors in the task of thyroid image analysis. Hegedüs (2004) and Kollorz et al (2008) presented methods to automatically isolate the thyroid gland in US images, using geodesic active contour level set based approach.

**Kidney**. In renal applications Oguro et al (2011) described a system to aid CT-guided percutaneous cryoablation of renal tumors. Xie et al (2005) used *a priori* information about texture and size to segment kidney in ultrasound images. The described method provides the ability to deal with objects with incomplete boundaries by taking into account their texture.

**Meniscal tears**. The meniscus is an important part of the knee supporting mechanism. The knee joint can be severely damaged by a variety of causes, such as arthritis or knee injury. This can cause pain and inability to walk. In some cases, replacing parts of the joint is the appropriate course of action (Andra et al, 2008). Meniscal tears are a knee injury that is common in both young athletes and the aging population. It requires accurate diagnosis and, if necessary, surgical intervention. Ramakrishna et al (2009) described a novel CAD diagnostic system for automatic detection of meniscal tears in the knee in MR images. Andra et al (2008) described a system for pre-operative surgical planning based on structural simulation of the bone-prosthesis system. The model of the bone was constructed based on information from CT datasets.

**Radiotherapy planning.** In the process of radiotherapy planning the most critical issue is the identification of the gross tumor volume and its relationship with surrounding tissues in order to decide the appropriate irradiation angles to minimize non-tumor tissue damage. Zaidi & El Naqa (2010) published a survey on methods for tumor identification in PET images.

### 3.2.7 General methods

Kohlberger et al (2009) described a method for general organ segmentation with level sets that incorporates local intensity statistics and local curvature by means of a point-based tracking mechanism. Campadelli et al (2010) described a method for extracting abdominal organs in CT images, using a gray-level based segmentation framework and an *a priori* anatomical knowledge that can be adapted to segment different abdominal organs. Noble (2010) made a review on segmentation techniques in ultrasound images as well as ultrasound tissue characterization for general applications. Crum et al (2004) reviewed non-rigid image registration, with emphasis in cardiac and brain applications. Van Rixoort et al (2010) described a framework for multi-atlas segmentation, in which the most appropriate atlases for a target image are automatically selected. The framework was applied to segment heart from non ECG gated volumetric chest CT scans and caudate nucleus from MR brain images.

## 4. Multiscale methods for identification, some research and examples

The fact that real objects appear different depending on the scale of observation has important consequences to their description. The concept of scale is very important when analyzing image data by means of automatic methods (Koenderink, 1984). An object in a scene can be described in several forms, such as: its edges, its geometrical properties, its density or color, or its surface area. Ideally, each object has a set of features that set it aside from the other structures in the scene. Any method for the interpretation of image content must involve a phase for the detection of those features. Such detection is performed by the application of some operator to the image data. The application raises some questions about the type and size of the operators: the result of the operation is strongly dependent on these choices. The use of multiple scales is a way to overcome the problem of determining the size of the operator (Yuille & Poggio, 1986; Witkin, 1983). For optimal detection in a single scale, the size of the structure to be found should be known *a priori*. Several multiscale methods have been described in the literature for detection and classification of tissues and organs (Amira et al, 2008; Bernard & Friboulet, 2009; Gooya et al, 2008; Ugarriza et al, 2009; Yoon et al, 2008; Yu et al, 2008). In the following section we present an example of a representation for identification of organ structures that uses prior information in a multiscale technique.

### 4.1 Example application

In this example we propose a representation for the identification of medical structures by using a multiresolution approach, the scale-space. We evaluate the use of a data representation that allows the inclusion of *a priori* knowledge about the structures in several scales and we also develop the idea of an optimal scale to perform the processing.

#### 4.1.1 Methodology

**Linear scale-space**. The linear scale-space concept was introduced in the Western literature by Witkin (1983) and Koenderink (1984). Weickert (1997) showed that the concept had already been introduced in Japan approximately 20 years before. One of the main requirements of the scale-space formalism is that structures at coarser scales in the multiscale representation should constitute simplifications of corresponding structures at finer scales. This requirement has been stated in different forms by several authors (Babaud et al 1986; Koenderink, 1984; Lindeberg, 1994; Yuille & Poggio, 1987). Adding the requisites of linearity and invariance to spatial displacement, those authors have shown that the Gaussian ( $g(\vec{x};\sigma)$ ) is the only filter that leads to monotonic destruction of detail under consecutive blurring. A blurred version of the original image $E(\vec{x})$ is obtained by its convolution with the Gaussian filter, for a specific σ (Equation 1). In Equation 1, $H(\vec{x};\sigma)$ is the intensity of element after convolution. The width σ determines the scale of the output image in each image dimension. In an isotropic condition, σ assumes the same value for all image dimensions. The stack of images, as a function of increasing scale parameter σ, is known as linear scale-space.

$$\begin{cases} H(\vec{x},\sigma)=E(\vec{x})*g(\vec{x},\sigma) \\ g(\vec{x};\sigma)=\dfrac{1}{\sqrt{2\pi\sigma^2}}\,e^{-\left(\frac{|\vec{x}|^2}{(2\sigma^2)}\right)} \end{cases} \tag{1}$$

In order to keep the property of scale invariance, the sampling of the scale parameter, σ, must be logarithmic (Keonderink, 1984). In the implementation of the Gaussian filter bank, a new parameter τ is usually introduced and it varies linearly throughout scales and relates to σ as: $\sigma_n = e^{n.\tau}$, where n is a natural number ($N$) consisting of zero and all positive integers, that represents the level in the scale space; σ is the parameter related to the resolution, or inner scale, of each level and τ determines the degree of spacing between the levels of the scale space. Linear scale space can be seen as a generic representation of image data that is common to different types of processing tasks. The main issues at this point are: how to describe properly the hierarchy throughout scales and how to extract important structures in each level of scale space and create a new data representation that can be suitable for high level processing routines.

**Multiscale representation - scale space primal sketch**. Primal sketch is an image structure first described by Marr (2010) based on the concept of gray level blobs (GLBlob), which are regions of the image that are lighter or darker than the surrounding background. Relating these regions to image structures results from the fact they have an intensity, or range of intensities, that may single them out among the other structures. Qualitatively, the concept of gray level blob for bi-dimensional images can be explained using the watershed operation from Mathematical Morphology (Lindeberg, 1994): the image function is seen as a flooded geographic area. As the water level decreases maxima points appear. At a certain point - or water level - two different peaks become connected. This point is called saddle. The difference between the image intensity at the maximum and at the saddle defines the contrast of each blob. The gray level of the saddle point is called blob base level. The support region of the blob is defined as the region containing the points with intensity values higher than the blob base level and can be reached from a local maximum without crossing points with intensity values lower than the blob base level. For 2D images, the gray level blob is defined as the tridimensional volume defined by the surface of the gray level and the base level.

A more formal definition of the blob concept is: the elliptical region associated to an extreme that is delimited by the above mentioned extreme and a saddle point. Differential geometry theory states that any image characteristic that has a geometrical meaning can be represented by a suitable differential operator. Florack et al (1992) presented an operator for the detection of elliptic regions - or blobs - in the images, the umbilicity operator. In 3D, it is given by Equation 2:

$$U = \frac{\partial^2}{\partial x^2} \cdot \frac{\partial^2}{\partial y^2} + \frac{\partial^2}{\partial x^2} \cdot \frac{\partial^2}{\partial z^2} + \frac{\partial^2}{\partial y^2} \cdot \frac{\partial^2}{\partial z^2} - \left( \frac{\partial^2}{\partial x \partial y} \right)^2 - \left( \frac{\partial^2}{\partial x \partial z} \right)^2 - \left( \frac{\partial^2}{\partial y \partial z} \right)^2 \tag{2}$$

Regions with positive values of the umbilicity define the gray level blob regions. To discriminate light from dark blobs the laplacian operator is used (Equation 3):

$$L = \frac{\partial^2}{\partial x^2} + \frac{\partial^2}{\partial y^2} + \frac{\partial^2}{\partial z^2}, \qquad \begin{cases} U > 0 \;\; and \;\; L > 0 & \Rightarrow \; dark\, blob \\ U > 0 \;\; and \;\; L < 0 & \Rightarrow \; light\, blob \end{cases} \tag{3}$$

Dark and light blobs are not only prominent in the original image, but also tend to maintain this prominence throughout the scales (Koenderink, 1984). That characteristic makes them a suitable choice for the elements of an image representation containing scale information. The Scale Space Primal Sketch (SSPS), first described by Lindeberg (1994), is an extension of the Primal Sketch and describes the characteristics of the blobs and their relations across scale space. Blobs in different scales are linked and form a new structure, the scale space blobs (SSBlob).

Figure 3 presents an example of a tree structure that maps blob relations in scale space. Figure 3.c depicts 5 levels of a scale space built for that image and their corresponding GLBlobs. Figure 3b presents the tree mapping of the relevant events occurring when following the blobs up in the scale space: creation, destruction and merging of blobs. These events are called bifurcations. A SSBlob is the object produced by the union of all GLBlobs that exist in the range between two bifurcations and is represented as a node in the tree. Each SSBlob is associated with a maximum scale (appearing scale) and a minimum scale (disappearing scale). The difference, given as number of scales, between the appearance and disappearance scales is called the life time. The information content of the tree nodes comprises the number of scales a structure survives, its appearance and disappearance scales, contrast with background, position at each survival scale, structure volume at each scale and total volume throughout scales. The linking between nodes reflects the behavior of the blobs during the smoothing process: creation, destruction and merging. This tree model is called Scale Space Primal Sketch.

Stable blobs in the SSPS must represent significant structures in the image (Koenderink, 1984, Lindeberg, 1994). Based on the stability of the SSBlobs significance measurement rates can be defined, allowing the classification of structures. The first significance measure proposed by Lindeberg (1994) was solely based on intrinsic characteristics of the image: blob volume and blob life time. The assumptions for this measurement were general and assumed there was not any *a priori* knowledge about the structures present in the image.

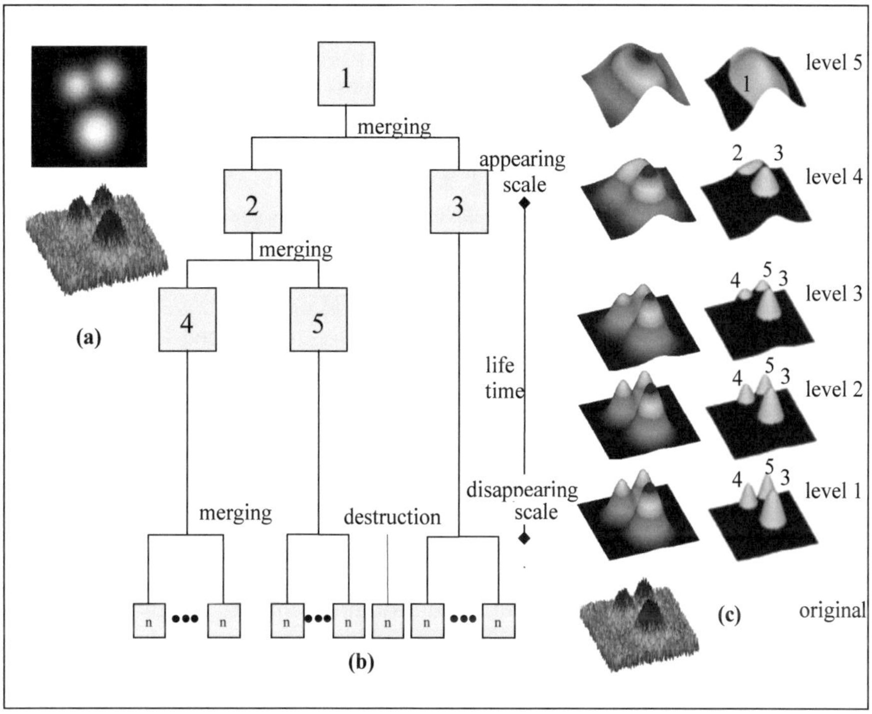


Fig. 3. (a) an image that comprises three regions with higher counts than their background. The lower image of (a) shows the image represented as isosurface; (b) SSPS built for the scale space shown in (c); (c) Six levels of the scale space of image (a) and their corresponding GLBlobs.

As an example, the general significance measure can be applied to extract significant structures in thoracic magnetic resonance images, such as cardiac cavities, arteries and veins, shown in Figure 4 left.

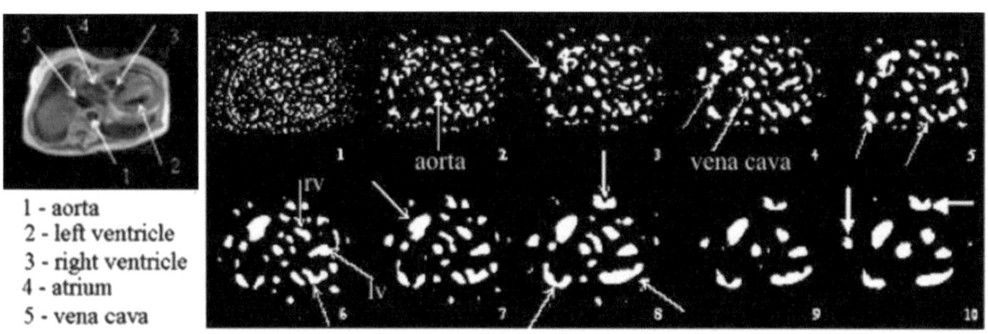


Fig. 4. (left): slice of a T1 spin echo MRI thoracic sequence, the arrows point to the five target structures. (right) Dark blobs from 9 levels of the scale space of the image shown in (a). Values of $\sigma$ are: $\sigma_1 = 1.0$ (original image), $\sigma_2 = 1.19$; $\sigma_3 = 1.41$; $\sigma_4 = 1.68$; $\sigma_5 = 2.00$; $\sigma_6 = 2.37$; $\sigma_7 = 2.82$; $\sigma_8 = 3.35$; $\sigma_9 = 3.97$; $\sigma_{10} = 5.61$. (Original image acquired at the Imaging Department - Heart Institute - HCFMUSP- with patient anonymization).

The thin arrows in Figure 4 right point to the 15 most significant dark blobs extracted using the general significance rate and the scale where the blob is more distinguished. Figure 4 right shows that almost all target structures are present amongst the set of significant blobs (exception is the atrium). Other anatomic structures are also present in the set, like the lungs (two lower arrows in scale 8). The general approach is not able, therefore, to set aside a particular structure from others present in the image. Furthermore, there are some structures that do not have any anatomic meaning, such as disconnected parts of organs in lower scales (lower arrows at scales 5 and 6) and some spurious structures originated from noise in upper scales, identified by the thicker arrows (Rebelo, 2000). In order to overcome the problems found with the application of the general approach, an important feature of medical images can be embedded in the image representation: the knowledge about the general characteristics and expected location of the target structure.

**Including *a priori* information on SSPS**. The SSPS is used as an image structure that serves as a guide to subsequent high level processing step where *a priori* knowledge about the desired feature is modeled and included in the representation. The image structure is first used to build patterns of known objects present in the image. A particular object can then be identified in new images by matching with symbolic features described in the pattern. Any kind of information can be embedded in the SSPS structure. The question that arises immediately regards defining the kind of information that is useful to include in the representation. The answer to this question is highly dependent on the problem domain, including the modality of the image under analysis, the kind of structure to be identified and the representation chosen for the biological structures. To validate the proposed method we have built a prototype application, which is described in detail in the next section.

### 4.1.2 Prototype application

In a previous work we proposed a prototype, in which geometrical information of the target structure and its relation with other structures present on the scene were included in SSPS (Rebelo, 2007). The set of parameters chosen for building the pattern was: (i) SSBlob volume, or the sum of the support regions of all GLBlobs; (ii) support region of the GLBlob; (iii) contextual information in the form of relative position of the target structure and the others present in the image, specifically distances and angles. For an image containing N GLBlobs at a given scale level the calculation of the set of parameters has a complexity of $O(N^3)$. In addition, the calculation has to be performed for the images in all levels of the scale space. A score is determined for each structure present in the image based on the closeness of its feature values to the pattern.

The matching procedure presents, therefore, a problem related to the huge amount of GLBlobs at the lower levels of scale. This can lead to an explosion in the number of parameters to be processed, especially the number of angles, greatly increasing processing time to detect the node with the highest score. In order to decrease the possible combinations for matching, we have developed the following strategy: (1) decrease the number of nodes for the contextual matching phase by performing a selection of the possible nodes, using a global parameter. The prototype uses SSBlob volume, since the previous experiments with thoracic images showed its potential for recognition of relevant structures in medical images. A set of candidate nodes is created by eliminating the nodes with SSBlob volume too distant from the pattern; (2) choosing a suitable scale in the scale space for the contextual matching.

The concept of suitable scale for processing is based on the idea that the smoothness degree for which an object vanishes in the scale space is related to the object size. This issue links directly to the subject of scale selection, a task that is not trivial and that has been studied by some authors (Lindeberg, 1994; Majer, 2000; Pauly et al, 2003). These authors articles considered the case when image analysis is performed without any *a priori* knowledge about the structures present in the scene. In the present work the suitable scale is determined by constructing the SSPS representation for the pattern images. The analysis of the survival scales for the structure under study and all other structures representing real entities in the image allows the determination of the best scale for the geometrical matching. The following steps are performed: (1) inspect all scales at which the target structure can be detected as a single blob; (2) the levels of the scale space where all blobs representing real structures in the image are present are considered informative and (3) the upper informative scale is considered the most suitable for the contextual matching.

The reasons behind that choice are: (1) the occurrence of spurious structures in lower scales is higher. This fact would highly increase the number of useless calculation of distances and angles; (2) although structures are smoother in higher scales, the determination of angles and distances is based on the geometrical centers of each structure. These points should not change their position under the smoothness process. There is a problem with this strategy when there is not a single level in which all blobs representing real structures exist as a unique structure. This is the case when a small and low contrast structure is present and its corresponding blobs appear only in low scale levels, when bigger objects do not constitute a single blob anymore due to noise. In such cases, the suitable scale is chosen as the higher scale where the blob representing the target structure appears.

### 4.1.3 Schema of the prototype application

The identification of structures modeled in the prototype comprises the following steps: (1) creation of the scale space by using the linear Gaussian filter; (2) detection of GLBlobs through the application of the umbilicity operator; (3) creation of the Scale Space Primal Sketch; (4) comparison of the SSBlob volumes from all nodes with the pattern. Elimination of nodes with values outside a defined range; (5) determination of the distance and angles for the remaining SSBlob in the suitable scale; (6) contextual matching between each candidate node and the features' pattern: support region, angles and distances and (7) the node with the best matching is identified as the target structure.

**Similarity criteria.** In the simplification of the SSBlob tree processing phase, the candidate nodes are defined as those having SSBlob volume values lying in a range defined as a function of the pattern. That range was initially set to 20% around the pattern. The suitability of this choice are analyzed in the experiments. The similarity criterion for contextual matching consists in minimizing the Euclidean distance between each of the feature values obtained for each node of the test image and the pattern.

**Pattern creation**. The pattern is obtained by applying the proposed method to a set of data. The following parameters of the blob representing the target structure are stored in the pattern: SSBlob volume, the suitable scale, the support region of the GLBlob in this scale, all distances and angles between the target structure and the others present in this scale, the spatial resolution of the original image, the value of $\tau$ used for the construction of the scale space.

### 4.1.4 Experiments

The Mathematical Cardiac Torso (MCAT) phantom is an anthropomorphic phantom, developed at the University of North Carolina that models size, shape and configurations of the major thoracic structures and organs by using of mathematical formulae (Tsui, 1993). A set of experiments was performed with two-dimensional images obtained from manipulations - adding and mirroring - of MCAT images. The manipulation aimed at creating frames with more organs, to make the matching step more complex. The goal was to analyze the ability of the method to identify organs at different levels of noise and contrast. The results for each case are described in the following sections.

**Behavior for different noise levels**. Five images were generated from the MCAT frames without noise. Three different levels of additive Gaussian noise with zero mean were then added to each image. For computing the noise level, we used the signal-to-noise ratio (SNR) described by Rangayan (2005).

$$SNR = 20 * \log_{10}\left(\frac{\sigma_{signal}}{\sigma_{noise}}\right) dB \tag{4}$$

In equation 4, $\sigma_{signal}$ is the standard deviation of the intensity values of the original image (not corrupted with noise); $\sigma_{noise}$ is the standard deviation of the intensity values of the noise image added to the original to generate the final corrupted image. The signal-to-noise ratio of the three different levels were 8dB (high noise level), 19 dB (medium level) and 33 dB (low level).

The five groups of images were classified into two distinct sets, according to their geometry. Figure 5 shows two images representatives of these sets: an image from Set 1 in first line and Set 2 in second line. In each set, one structure was chosen to be identified: structure 4 in Set1 and structure 5 in Set 2. The pattern was built based on the original images without noise. In Figure 5 the original images (not corrupted by noise) are shown in column A. The noisy images are presented in column B (low level of noise), C (medium level of noise) and D (high level of noise).

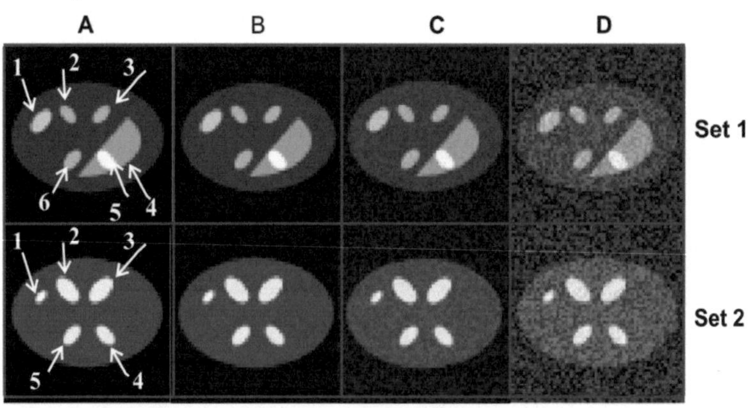


Fig. 5. Two images representative of the two Sets (image 3 from Set 1 and image 4 from Set 2). Column (A) shows the original images (without noise), column (B) the low noise images, column (C) medium noise images and column (D) high noise images.

After the construction of the scale space, using $\sigma$ = 0.19, the GLBlobs were detected in 12 levels of scale. Figure 6 depicts the GLBlobs detected for the images of Set 1 and Set 2, presented in Figure 5. In Figure 6 it is possible to observe that the number of blobs in lower scales increases for higher noise images. This effect tends to disapear for upper scale levels.

The application of the proposed method led to the successful identification of the chosen structures in most experiments, exception made to two with the highest noise level.

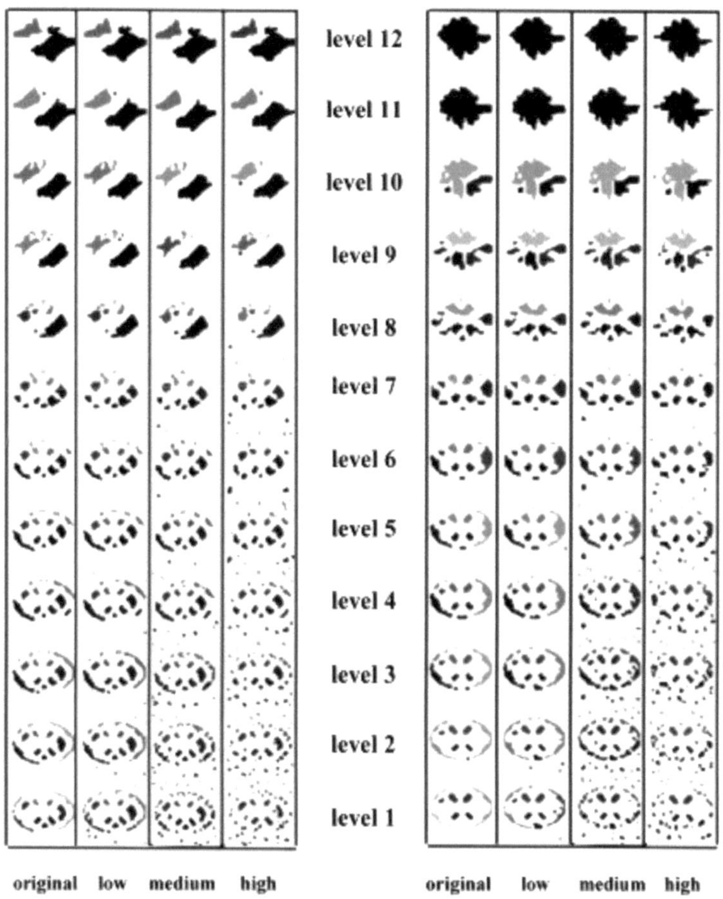


Fig. 6. Set of GLBlobs determined in 12 levels of scale for two groups of images shown in Figure 5. The set from Set 1 (original without noise, low level noise, mid level noise and high level noise) is shown on the left and the set from Set 2 is shown on the right.

**Behavior for different contrast levels.** The contrast between a structure and its background is one of the factors affecting the survival of the structure in the scale space, or, in other words, it affects the shape of the SSPS. In order to test the application of the method at several levels of contrast a simpler version of image 3 from Set 1, shown in Figure 5 (first line), was used. From the original image, two sets of images were created to assess how contrast influences SSPS shape. The first set was created by changing the counts of the thoracic region. The second set was created by changing both the counts of the thoracic region and the counts of the background, in such a way that the contrast between thorax and background remained constant. The contrast C(s,b) between a target structure S and its local background B, was calculated by Equation 5:

$$C = \frac{\mu_S - \mu_B}{\mu_B} . \tag{5}$$

$\mu_S$ is the mean value of intensity inside the structure; $\mu_B$ is the mean value of intensity in its background B. For each contrast manipulated image a set of noisy images with three different noise levels was created. For this experiment, noise was quantified by the contrast to noise ratio, defined in relation to the target structure S by Equation 6 (Rangayan, 2005):

$$CNR = \frac{|\mu_S - \mu_B|}{\sigma_B} \tag{6}$$

where $\sigma_B$ is the standard deviation of intensity in the background.

The structure number 2 (Figure 5 upper A) was chosen as the target. An interesting observation was that when the contrast between thorax and background remained at the same value, the blobs of the images with low contrast between the internal structures and the thorax had a behavior not very different from the one observed in the images with high contrast. However, all internal structures survived in a lower number of levels as the contrast decreased.

The results of identification were satisfactory. In 87% of the experiments the target structure was identified correctly. The pattern was built based on the original image with the lowest contrast between the internal structures and the thorax.

## 5. Conclusion

In this chapter we discussed the challenges, methods and clinical examples of medical image identification. We pointed out the importance of this task as a previous step for medical image applications such as visualization and the quantitative analysis of organs and systems. A classification for the methods described in the literature and a brief review of their clinical applications were presented.

It was shown that identification of structures in medical images is a very difficult task due to the complexity of the anatomical structures and their changing with different physiological states. A simplification of the task can be achieved by dividing it in two phases: first, identification of the desired structures that includes a rough segmentation; then a post-processing phase for segmentation refinement.

In this text we presented a method for the first phase that uses an image representation based on a scale space approach that embeds *a priori* knowledge in it. One of the main goals of this proposal was to develop a powerful representation for images that would be suitable for application of high level processing routines, such as the matching used in the prototype implemented. A study with MCAT phantom images was performed in order to assess the method under controlled conditions reproducing anatomical structures. The results we have obtained were quite encouraging. However, further intensive investigation with real patient data should be carried out in order to assess the full clinical usefulness of the method. The presented method is general and can be classified as a third generation method, according to the classification presented in the review, as it is a second generation multiresolution representation capable of incorporating knowledge to be used in a specific application. Although the representation is generic, the information chosen for definition of the pattern will depend on particular applications, and can be easily inserted in the data structure.

The review presented in this chapter was intended to give the reader a general scenario of medical applications. We focused on clinical applications and the issues for identification of particular organs and not on detailed application and modality-dependent aspects. Methods and applications that have appeared in the recent literature were briefly described. The main goal was to to give the readers a glimpse of this broad and extremely active research field.

In spite of the huge number of existing methods, the problem of identification in medical images is still challenging, with no general and unique solution and remains an open and promising area in the field of image processing. The growing research in the clinical areas makes the number of objects of interest in medical images to grow constantly, which generates a continuous demand for automatic solutions to aid clinicians. On the other side, fast advances in radiological imaging systems result in increasingly higher volume (3D) images to be processed. Processing of these images in radiological diagnostic systems requires accurate and fast algorithms. Intense use of apparel techniques must be studied, and the use of new computing platforms, such as computational grids, must be explored.

The goal of automated systems is not to replace the experts, whose experience and knowledge are essential in any automatic systems for identification or analysis. Instead, the development of automated systems to assist the clinicians is intended to reduce their workload in the step of analyzing patient data, saving them time to other valuable tasks as strategies and decision making.

## 6. Acknowledments

This work is supported by National Council for Scientific and Technological Development, The National Institute for Science and Technology - Medicine Assisted by Scientific Computing (INCT-MAAC) and Zerbini Foundation.

## 7. References

Alattar, M. A., Osman, N.F. & Fahmy, A. S. (2010). Myocardial Segmentation Using Constrained Multi-Seeded Region Growing. *Lecture Notes in Computer Science - Image Analysis and Recognition*, vol. 6112/2010, pp. 89-98.

Allender, S., Scarborough, P., Peto, V., Rayner, M., Leal, J., Luengo-Fernandez, R. & Gray, A. (2008). *European cardiovascular disease statistics: 2008 edition,* British Heart Foundation, London.

Amira, A., Chandrasekarana, S., Montgomery, D.W. & Uzunb, I.S. (2008) A segmentation concept for positron emission tomography imaging using multiresolution analysis. *Neurocomputing* , vol.71 (2008), pp. 1954- 1965.

Andra, H., Battiato, S., Bilotta, G., Farinella, G.M., Impoco, G., Orlik, J., Russo, G. & Zemitis, A. (2008). Structural Simulation of a Bone-Prosthesis System of the Knee Joint. *Sensors*, vol 8 (2008), pp. 5897-5926.

Antunes, S.G., Silva, J.S. & Santos, J.B. (2010) A Level Set Segmentation Method of the Four Heart Cavities in Pediatric Ultrasound Images. *Lecture Notes in Computer Science*, vol. 6112/2010 (2010), pp.99-107.

Ashburner, J., Csernansky, J.G., Davatzikos, C., Fox, N.C., Frisoni, G.B. and Thompson, P.M. (2003). Computer-assisted imaging to assess brain structure in healthy and diseased brains. *Lancet Neurology*, vol. 2 2003, pp. 79–88.

Babaud, J., Witkin, A.P., Baudin, M. & Duda, R.O. (1986). Uniqueness of the Gaussian kernel for scale space filtering, *IEEE PAMI 8*, (1986), pp. 26-33.

Ballard, D.H., Brown, C.M. (1982). *Computer Vision*. Prentice-Hall, Inc. Englewood Cliffs

Bandyopadhyay, S.K. (2011). A Survey on Brain Image Segmentation Methods. *Journal of Global Research in Computer Science*, vol 2, no 2 (2011), pp. 4-7.

Bernard, O. & Friboulet, D. (2009) Fast medical image segmentation through an approximation of narrow-band B-spline level-set and multiresolution. *IEEE International Symposium on Biomedical Imaging: From Nano to Macro*, pp. 45 - 48.

Bouma, H., Sonnemans, J.J., Vilanova, A., Gerritsen, F.A. (2009) Automatic Detection of Pulmonary Embolism in CTA Images. *IEEE Trans on Med Imag*, vol. 28, no 8 (2009), pp. 1223 - 1230.

Bresser, J., Portegies, M.P., Leemans, A., Biessels, G.J., Kappelle, L.J. & Viergever, M.A. (2011). A comparison of MR based segmentation methods for measuring brain atrophy progression. *NeuroImage*, vol 54 (2011), pp. 760–768.

Campadelli, P., Casiraghi, E. & Esposito, A. (2009) Liver segmentation from computed tomography scans: A survey and a new algorithm. *Artificial Intelligence in Medicine*, vol. 45 (2009), pp.185—196.

Campadelli, P., Casiraghi, E. & Pratissoli, S. (2010) A segmentation framework for abdominal organs from CT scans. *Artificial Intelligence in Medicine*, vol. 50 (2010), pp. 3–11.

Cheng, H.D., Cai, X. , Chen, X., Hu, L. & Lou, X. (2003). Computer-aided detection and classification of microcalcifications in mammograms: a survey, *Pattern Recognition*, vol. 36 (2003), pp. 2967-2991.

Cordero-Grande, L., Vegas-Sánchez-Ferrero. G., Casaseca-de-la-Higuera, P., San-Román-Calvar. J.A., Revilla-Orodea, A., Martín-Fernández, M. & Alberola-López, C. (2011) Unsupervised 4D myocardium segmentation with a Markov Random Field based deformable model. *Medical Image Analysis*, vol. 15 (2011), pp. 283–301.

Crum, W.R., Phil, D., Hartkens, T. & Hill, D.L.G. (2004) Non-rigid image registration: theory and practice. *The British Journal of Radiology*, vol. 77 (2004),pp. 140–153.

Destrempes, F., Meunier, J., Giroux, M.F., Soulez, G., Cloutier, G. (2009) Segmentation in Ultrasonic B-Mode Images of Healthy Carotid Arteries Using Mixtures of Nakagami Distributions and Stochastic Optimization. *IEEE Trans on Med Imag*, vol 28, no 2 (2009), pp. 215-229.

Duncan, J.S., Ayache, N (2000). Medical Image Analysis: Progress over Two Decades and the Challenges Ahead, *IEEE Trans on Pat Anal and Mach Intell*, vol 22, no 1 (2000), pp. 85-106.

Ecabert, O., Peters, J., Schramm, H., Lorenz, C., von Berg, J., Walker, M.J., Vembar, M., Olszewski, M.E., Subramanyan, K., Lavi, G. & Weese, J. (2008) Automatic Model-Based Segmentation of the Heart in CT Images. *IEEE Trans on Med Imag*, vol. 27, no 9 (2008), pp. 1189-1201.

Florack, L.M.J., Romeny, B.M.T.H., Koenderink, J.J. & Viergever, M.A.. (1992). Scale and the differential structure of images, *Image and Vision Computing*, vol 10 (1992), pp. 376-388.

Gonzales, R., Woods, R.E. (2000). *Digital Image Processing*. Editora Edgard Blücher Ltda. São Paulo

Gooya, A., Liao, H., Matsumiya, K., Masamune, K., Masutani, Y. & Dohi, T. (2008). A Variational Method for Geometric Regularization of Vascular Segmentation in Medical Images. *IEEE Trans on Imag Proc,* vol. 17, no 8 (2008), pp. 1295-1312.

Hegedüs, L. (2004) Thyroid ultrasound as a screening tool for thyroid disease. *Thyroid,* vol. 14, no 11 (2004), pp. 879–880.

Heimann, T., van Ginneken, B., Styner, M.A. et al (2009). Comparison and Evaluation of Methods for Liver Segmentation from CT Datasets, *IEEE Trans on Med Imag,* vol 28, no 8 (2009), pp. 1251-1265.

Ishii, K., Kanda, T., Uemura, T., Miyamoto, N., Yoshikawa, T., Shimada, K., Ohkawa, S. & Minoshima, S. (2009) Computer-assisted diagnostic system for neurodegenerative dementia using brain SPECT and 3D-SSP. *European Journal of Nuclear Medicine and Molecular Imaging,* vol 36 (2009), pp. 831–840.

Jain, A.K. (1989). *Fundamentals of Digital Image Processing,* Prentice Hall Englewood Cliffs.

Kirbas, C. & Quek, K. (2002). A Review of Vessel Extraction Techniques and Algorithms, *ACM Computing Surveys,* vol-36 (2002), pp. 81-121.

Koenderink, J.J. (1984). The structure of images. *Biological Cybernetics,* vol. 50 (1984), pp. 363-370.

Kohlberger, T., Uzunba, M.G, Alvino, C. & Kadir, T. (2009) Organ Segmentation with Level Sets Using Local Shape and Appearance Priors. *MICCAI 2009, Part II, LNCS,* vol. 5762, pp. 34–42.

Kollorz, E.N.K., Hahn, D.A., Linke, R., Goecke, T.W., Hornegger, J. & Kuwert, T. (2008) Quantification of Thyroid Volume Using 3-D Ultrasound Imaging. *IEEE Trans on Med Imag,* vol 27, no 4 (2008), pp. 457-466.

Kubota, T., Jerebko, A.K., Dewan, M., Salganicoff, M. & Krishnan, A. (2011) Segmentation of pulmonary nodules of various densities with morphological approaches and convexity models. *Medical Image Analysis,* vol. 15 (2011), pp. 133–154.

Lekadir, K., Keenan, N.G., Pennell, D.J. & Yang, G-Z. (2011) An Inter-Landmark Approach to 4-D Shape Extraction and Interpretation: Application to Myocardial Motion Assessment in MRI. *IEEE Trans on Med Imag,* vol 30, no 1 (2011), pp. 52-68.

Lesage, D., Angelini, E.D., Bloch, I. & Funka-Lea, G. (2009) A review of 3D vessel lumen segmentation techniques: Models, features and extraction schemes. *Medical Image Analysis,* vol. 13 (2009), pp. 819–845.

Lindeberg, T. (1994). Scale-space theory: a basic tool for analyzing structures at different scales, *Journal of Applied Statistics,* vol 21, (1994), p. 225-270.

Linguraru, M.G., Sandberg, J.K., Li, Z., Pura, J.A. & Summers, R.M. (2009) Atlas-Based Automated Segmentation of Spleen and Liver Using Adaptive Enhancement Estimation. *MICCAI 2009, Part II, LNCS,* vol. 5762/2009, pp. 1001–1008.

Lopes, R., Dubois, P., Makni, N., Szurhaj, W., Maouche, S. & Betrouni, N. (2008) Classification of brain SPECT imaging using 3D local multifractal spectrum for epilepsy detection. *International Journal of CARS 2008,* vol 3, pp. 341–346.

Lynch, M., Ghita, O. & Whelan, P.F. (2008) Segmentation of the Left Ventricle of the Heart in 3-D+t MRI Data Using an Optimized Nonrigid Temporal Model. *IEEE Trans on Med Imag,* vol. 27, no 2, pp. 195-203.

Ma, Z., Tavares, J.M.R.S. & Jorge, R.N. (2008) Segmentation of Structures in Medical Images: Review and a New Computational Framework. *Proceedings of International Symposium on Computer Methods in Biomechanics and Biomedical Engineering,* Porto, Portugal, Feb-March 2008.

Majer, P.A. (2000) *Statistical Approach to Feature Detection and Scale Selection in Images,* PhD Thesis, University of Göttingen, Germany, 122p.

Marr, D. (2010). *Vision: A Computational Investigation into the Human Representation and Processing of Visual Information*. The 2010 Edition. ISBN-13: 978-0-262-51462-0 The MIT Press. Cambridge, MA.

Masuda, Y., Foruzan, A.H., Tateyama, T. & Chen, Y.W. (2010) Automatic liver tumor detection using EM/MPM algorithm and shape information. *2nd International Conference on Software Engineering and Data Mining (SEDM)* 2010, pp. 692–695.

Mora, M., Leiva, J. & Olivares, M. (2009) Heart Cavity Segmentation in Ultrasound Images Based on Supervised Neural Networks. *Lecture Notes in Computer Science*, vol. 5496/2009, pp. 58-68.

Murphy, K., van Ginneken, B., Schilham , A.M.R., de Hoop, B.J., Gietema, H.A. & Prokop, M. (2009) A large-scale evaluation of automatic pulmonary nodule detection in chest CT using local image features and k-nearest-neighbour classification. *Medical Image Analysis*, vol. 13 (2009), pp. 757–770.

Niessen, W. (1997) *Medical Image Analysis*. PhD Thesis. Utrecht University, The Netherlands.

Noble, J.A. (2010) Ultrasound image segmentation and tissue characterization. *Proceedings of the Institution of Mechanical Engineers, Part H: Journal of Engineering in Medicine* 2010, pp. 224-307.

O'Brien, S.P., Ghita, O. & Whelan, P.F. (2011). A Novel Model-Based 3D Time Left Ventricular Segmentation Technique. *IEEE Trans on Med Imag*, vol 30, no 2 (2011), pp. 461-474.

O'Donnell, T., Funka-Lea, G., Tek, H., Jolly, M.-P. & Rasch, M. (2006). Comprehensive cardiovascular image analysis using MR and CT at Siemens Corporate Research. *International Journal of Computer Vision*, vol. 70, no 2 (2006), pp. 165–178.

Oguro, S., Tuncali, K., Elhawary, H., Morrison, P.R., Hata, N. & Silverman, S.G. (2011). Image registration of pre-procedural MRI and intra-procedural CT images to aid CT-guided percutaneous cryoablation of renal tumors. *International Journal CARS*, vol. 6 (2011), pp. 111–117.

Oliver, A., Freixenet, J., Martí, J., Pérez, E., Pont, J., Denton, E.R.E. & Zwiggelaar, R. (2010). A review of automatic mass detection and segmentation in mammographic images. *Medical Image Analysis*, vol.14 (2010), pp. 87–110.

Pauly, M., Keiser, R. & Gross, M. (2003) Multi-scale Feature Extraction on Point-sampled Surfaces, *EUROGRAPHICS 2003*, pp. 22.

Peters, J., Lessick, J., Kneser, R., Wächter, I., Vembar, M., Ecabert, O. & Weese, J. (2010). Accurate Segmentation of the Left Ventricle in Computed Tomography Images for Local Wall Thickness Assessment. *MICCAI 2010, Part I, LNCS*, vol. 6361, pp. 400–408.

Petitjean, C. & Dacher, J-N. (2011). A review of segmentation methods in short axis cardiac MR images. *Medical Image Analysis*, vol. 15, no 2, pp. 169-184.

Pu, J., Fuhrman, C., Good, W.F., Sciurba, F.C. & Gur, D. (2011). A Differential Geometric Approach to Automated Segmentation of Human Airway Tree. *IEEE Trans on Med Imag*, vol. 30, no 2 (2011), pp. 266-278.

Pu, J., Leader, J.K., Zheng, B., Knollmann, F., Fuhrman, C., Sciurba, F.C. & Gur, D. (2009). A Computational Geometry Approach to Automated Pulmonary Fissure Segmentation in CT Examinations. *IEEE Trans on Med Imag*, vol 28, no 5 (2009), pp. 710-719.

Qian, X., Brennan, M.P., Dione, D.P., Dobrucki, W.L., Jackowski, M.P., Breuer, C.K., Sinusas, A.J. & Papademetris, X. (2009). A non-parametric vessel detection method for complex vascular structures. *Medical Image Analysis*, vol. 13 (2009), pp. 49–61.

Rahman, M., Uddin, S. & Hasan, M. (2010). 3D Segmentation and Visualization of Left Coronary Arteries of Heart Using CT Images. *IJCA Special Issue on "Computer Aided Soft Computing Techniques for Imaging and Biomedical Applications"*, 2010, pp. 88-92.

Ramakrishna, B., Liu, W., Saiprasad, G., Safdar, N., Chang, C.-I., Siddiqui, K., Kim, W., Siegel, E., Chai,I.W., Chen, C., Lee, S-K. (2009). An Automatic Computer-Aided Detection System for Meniscal Tears on Magnetic Resonance Images. *IEEE Trans on Med Imag*, vol. 28, no 8 (2009), pp. 1308 - 1316. (verificar autores)

Rangayan, R.M. (2005). *Biomedical Image Analysis*, 1st edition Boca Raton Florida © CRC Press, 1272p.

Rani. U.N., Subbaiah, P.V. & Rao, D.V. (2011). Segmentation of Brain Tumors from Medical Scan Images Using DRLSE Variational Levelsets. *International Journal of Computer Science and Security (IJCSS)*, vol. 1, no 3, 7p.

Rebelo, M.S., Furuie, S.S., Gutierrez, M.A., Costa, E.T., Moura, L.A. (2007). Multiscale representation for automatic identification of structures in medical images. *Computers in Biology and Medicine*, vol. 37, no 8, pp. 1183-1193

Rebelo, M.S., Gutierrez, M.A., Furuie, S.S. & Moura, L.. (2000). Extraction of cardiac structures through the incorporation of *a priori* knowledge in a multi-scale approach, *Proc. Computers in Cardiology*, vol 27 (2000), pp. 611-614.

Ribbens, A., Hermans, J., Maes, F., Vandermeulen, D. & Suetens, P., (2010). SPARC: Unified Framework for Automatic Segmentation, Probabilistic Atlas Construction, Registration and Clustering of Brain MR Images. *IEEE International Symposium on Biomedical Imaging: From Nano to Macro (2010)*, pp. 856 - 859.

Rouchdy, Y., Pousin, J., Schaerer, J. & Clarysse, P. (2007). A nonlinear elastic deformable template for soft structure segmentation: application to the heart segmentation in MRI. *Inverse Problems*, vol. 23 (2007), pp. 1017–1035. (checar autores)

Rousset, O., Rahmim, A., Alavi, A. & Zaidi, H. (2007). Partial Volume Correction Strategies in PET. *PET Clinics*, vol. 2 (2007), pp. 235–249.

Ruskó, L., Bekes, G. & Fidrich, M. (2009). Automatic segmentation of the liver from multi- and single-phase contrast-enhanced CT images. *Medical Image Analysis*, vol. 13 (2009), pp. 871–882.

Samulski, M. & Karssemeijer, N. ( 2011). Optimizing case-based detection performance in a multi-view CAD system for mammography. *IEEE Trans on Med Imag*, vol. 30, no 4 (2011), pp. 1001–1009.

Schaerer, J., Casta, C., Pousin, J. & Clarysse, P. (2010). A dynamic elastic model for segmentation and tracking of the heart in MR image sequences. *Medical Image Analysis*, vol. 14 (2010), pp. 738–749.

Scherrer, B., Forbes, F., Garbay, C. & Dojat, M. (2009). Distributed Local MRF Models for Tno and Structure Brain Segmentation. *IEEE Trans on Med Imag*, vol. 28, no 8 (2009), pp. 1278–1295.

Shiee, N., Bazin, P-R., Ozturk, A., Reich, D.S., Calabresi, P.A. & Pham, D.L. (2010). A topology-preserving approach to the segmentation of brain images with multiple sclerosis lesions. *NeuroImage*, vol 49 (2010), pp. 1524–1535.

Sonka, M., Hlavac, V., Boyle, R. (1998). *Image processing, analysis, and machine vision*. Brooks/Cole Publishing Company, Pacific Grove.

Suetens, P., Fua, P. & Hanson, A.J. (1992). Computational strategies for object recognition. *ACM Computing Surveys*, vol. 24, no 1 (1992), pp. 5-55.

Timp, S., Varela, C. & Karssemeijer, N. (2007). Temporal Change Analysis for Characterization of Mass Lesions in Mammography. *IEEE Trans on Med Imag*, vol. 26, no 7 (2007), pp. 945-953.

Tsui, B.M.W., Terry, J.A. & Gullberg, G.T. (1993). Evaluation of cardiac cone-beam SPECT using observer performance experiments and ROC analysis, *Investigative Radiology*. vol. 28, no 12 (1993), pp. 1101-12.

Tu, Z. & Bai, X. (2010). Auto-Context and Its Application to High-Level Vision Tasks and 3D Brain Image Segmentation. *IEEE Trans on Pat Anal and Mach Intel*, vol. 3, no 10 (2010), pp. 1744-1757.

Ugarriza, L.G., Saber, E., Vantaram, S.R., Amuso, V., Shaw, M. & Bhaskar, R. (2009). Automatic Image Segmentation by Dynamic Region Growth and Multiresolution Merging. *IEEE Trans on Imag Proc*, vol. 18, no 10 (2009), pp. 2275-2288.

van Ginneken, B., Romeny, B.M.T.H. & Viergever, M.A. (2001). Computer aided diagnosis in chest radiography: a survey. *IEEE Trans on Med Imag*, vol. 20, no 12 (2005), pp. 1228-1241.

van Rikxoort, E.M., Isgum, I., Arzhaeva, Y., Staring, M., Klein, S., Viergever, M.A., Pluim, J. P.W. & van Ginneken, B. (2010). Adaptive local multi-atlas segmentation: Application to the heart and the caudate nucleus. *Medical Image Analysis*, vol. 14 (2010), pp. 39–49.

Weickert, J. (1997). Recursive separable schemes for nonlinear diffusion filters, In: *Scale-space theory in computer vision 1252.* Romeny, B.T.H., Florack, L., Koenderink, J., Viergever, M. pp. 260-271, Springer-Verlag, Berlin Heidelberg.

Withey, D.J. & Koles, Z.J. (2007). Medical Image Segmentation: Methods and Software. Proceeding of Noninvasive Functional Source Imaging of the Brain and Heart. *International Conference on Functional Biomedical Imaging* (2007), pp. 140-143.

Witkin, A.P. (1983). Scale space filtering. *Proc. Int "l Joint Conference Artificial Intelligence*, pp. 1019-1022, Karslruhe, Germany, Aug. 1983.

Xie, J.; Jiang, Y. & Tsui, Y. (2005). Segmentation of Kidney From Ultrasound Images Based on Texture and Shape Priors. *IEEE Trans on Med Imag*, vol. 24, no 1 (2005), pp. 45-57.

Yi, Z.; Criminisi, A.; Shotton, J. & Blake, A. (2009). Discriminative, Semantic Segmentation of Brain Tno in MR Images. *Lecture Notes in Computer Science*, Volume 5762 (2009), pp. 558-565.

Yoon, S.W.; Lee, C.; Kim, J.K. & Lee, M. (2008). Wavelet-based Multi-resolution Deformation for Medical Endoscopic Image Segmentation. *Journal of Medical Systems*, vol. 32 (2008), pp. 207–214.

Yu, G.; Lin, P.; Cai, S. (2008). Robust Vessel Segmentation Based on Multi-resolution Fuzzy Clustering. *Lecture Notes in Computer Science*, vol. 5326/2008, pp. 338-345.

Yuille, A.L. , Poggio, T.A. (1986). Scaling theorems for zero-crossings, *IEEE PAMI*, vol. 8 (1986), pp. 15–25.

Zaidi, H. & El Naqa, I. (2010). PET-guided delineation of radiation therapy treatment volumes: a survey of image segmentation techniques. *European Journal of Nuclear Medicine and Molecular Imaging*, vol. 37 (2010), pp. 2165–2187.

Zhang, N., Ruan, S., Lebonvallet, S., Liao, Q. & Zhu, Y. (2011). Kernel feature selection to fuse multi-spectral MRI images for brain tumor segmentation. *Computer Vision and Image Understanding*, vol. 115 (2011), pp. 256–269.

Zhao, Z., Zhang, H., Wahle, A., Thomas, M.T., Stolpen, A.H., Scholz, T.D. & Sonka, M. (2009). Congenital aortic disease: 4D magnetic resonance segmentation and quantitative analysis. *Medical Image Analysis*, vol. 13 (2009), pp. 483–493.

Zheng,Y., Vega-Higuera,F.V., Zhou,S.K. & Comaniciu, D. (2010). Fast and Automatic Heart Isolation in 3D CT Volumes: Optimal Shape Initialization. *Lecture Notes in Computer Science*, vol. 6357/2010, pp. 84-91

# 2

# Detection of Abnormalities in a Biological Tissue by Diffuse Optical Tomography: A Computational Study

H. Trabelsi, M. Gantri and E. Sediki
*University of Tunis El Manar, Faculté des Sciences de Tunis*
*Unité de Rayonnement, Département de Physique, Tunis*
*Tunisia*

## 1. Introduction

Diffuse optical tomography (DOT) has a real potential as a new medical diagnostic tool. This fact has stimulated considerable research interest in the last years. When it is possible, this technique has some advantages not available in classical medical imaging methods. Among the benefits of this technique, nonionizing radiation, low-cost instrumentation, mobility and possible functional imaging are the most important. Also, DOT could be used in combination with other imaging methods to provide high-resolution structural information. The transparency of tissues is related to absorption and scattering of light and it reaches its maximum in the near-infrared. Interaction of radiation from this range with biological tissues is widely studied [1-5]. In particular, some works was interested to detection of tumor-like inclusions within a biological tissue [6-8].

Most of models of light interaction with biological matter are based on radiative transfer theory [9-13]. The most used parameters in modelling Laser radiation interaction with biological tissue is absorption and scattering. However some other studies evoked a significant variation of refractive index of abnormal biological tissues especially in the near infrared range. More precisely, experimental results [14-17] showed that the tissue of malignant tumors could manifest an increase of the refractive index which could attain until 10 % of that of a normal tissue which encircles them. So, medical imaging by diffuse optical tomography should take advantage from the emergence of a third contrast parameter which is the refractive index. This drove to the appearance of a big number of numerical and fundamental works in the field of radiative transfer in a varying refractive index medium. Among them some papers are interested to varying refractive index biological tissues [18-22].

In this chapter, infrared laser radiation interaction with a biological tissue including a spatially variation of refractive index is studied through a time-dependent radiative transfer model. Our general concern is to contribute at the usability of the radiative transfer theory in a potential optical tomography setting in medical imaging. At this level, studying the effect of refractive index on the transmitted light through a biological rectangular layer is crucial. This should be a contribution to obtaining information about abnormal tissue in a typical DOT scheme. However, it is important to note that in a varying refractive index medium, the rays are not straight lines but curves. So even in a rectangular geometry, the varying refractive index radiative transfer equation displays angular derivative terms [23-25]. In this paper, these terms are treated with finite differencing scheme. More precisely, we present a computational model that could be suitable for basic optical tomography forward problem with spatially varying refractive index. We investigate cases concerning optical tomography applications. We consider a biological tissue-like domain submitted to a near infrared light source. Transmitted intensity detected on the boundary is computed. The effect of the embedded non-homogenous objects on the transmitted signal is studied. Particularly, a possible detection of these objects is discussed. Also, the model is used to study infrared radiation in a multilayered heterogeneous medium. The effect of optical parameters on the transmitted signal is presented. In particular, the effect of refractive index variation is pointed out.

## 2. Physical model and numerical implementation

In this work, the radiative transfer in a human biological tissue is described by using a varying refractive index RTE [26, 27]

$$\begin{aligned}&\frac{n(\vec{r})}{c}\frac{\partial I(\vec{r},\Omega,t)}{\partial t}+\vec{\Omega}.\nabla I(\vec{r},\vec{\Omega},t)+(\mu_a(\vec{r})+\mu_s(\vec{r}))I(\vec{r},\Omega,t)+\frac{1}{n(\vec{r})}\nabla n.\nabla_{\vec{\Omega}}I(\vec{r},\vec{\Omega},t)\\&-\frac{2}{n(\vec{r})}(\vec{\Omega}.\nabla n)I(\vec{r},\vec{\Omega},t)=S(\vec{r},\vec{\Omega},t)+\mu_s(r)\int_0^{2\pi}p(\vec{\Omega},\vec{\Omega}')I(\vec{r},\vec{\Omega}',t)d\vec{\Omega}'\end{aligned} \tag{1}$$

where $I(\vec{r},\vec{\Omega},t)$ is the directional energetic radiance at the spatial position $\vec{r}$ and $n(\vec{r})$ is the refractive index distribution. Equation (1) takes into account the fact that the rays are not straight lines but curves. It involves terms that illustrate the expansion or the contraction of the cross section of the tube of light rays in the medium. On the boundary, the radiance is the sum of the external source contribution and the partly-reflected radiance due to the refractive index mismatch at the boundary

$$I(\vec{r},\vec{\Omega},t)=S(\vec{r}_b,\vec{\Omega},t)+RI(\vec{r},\vec{\Omega}_{ref},t),\ \vec{n}_b.\vec{\Omega}<0\ and\ \vec{n}_b.\vec{\Omega}_{ref}=-\vec{n}_b.\vec{\Omega}\ ,$$

where $\vec{r}_b$ is a position on the boundary and $\vec{n}_b$ is an outer normal unit vector. The reflectivity $R$ can be calculated for each direction using Fresnel's relations. For a two-dimensional problem and in Cartesian coordinate system of the x-y plane, the terms due to the refractive index variation can be expressed as

$$\frac{1}{n}\nabla n.\nabla_{\vec{\Omega}}I-\frac{2}{n}(\vec{\Omega}.\nabla n)I=-\frac{1}{n}\frac{\partial n}{\partial x}(\sin\varphi\frac{\partial I}{\partial\varphi}+2\cos\varphi I)+\frac{1}{n}\frac{\partial n}{\partial y}(\cos\varphi\frac{\partial I}{\partial\varphi}-2\sin\varphi I)\ , \tag{2}$$

where cosφ and sinφ are the Cartesian coordinates of the unit direction vector in the x-y plane. In fact we assume that the radiance of out of plane directions is negligible. By using notations $\xi=\cos\varphi$ and $\eta=\sin\varphi$, equation (2) displays the classical form of the angular redistribution term commonly appearing when dealing with spherical and cylindrical geometries with uniform refractive index [28, 29]

$$\frac{1}{n}\nabla n.\nabla_{\vec{\Omega}} I-\frac{2}{n}(\vec{\Omega}.\nabla n)I=\frac{1}{2n^2}\left\{\frac{\partial n^2}{\partial x}\frac{\partial}{\partial \xi}[(1-\xi^2)I]+\frac{\partial n^2}{\partial y}\frac{\partial}{\partial \eta}[(1-\eta^2)I]\right\} \tag{3}$$

The angular redistribution terms will be noted

$$D_x=\frac{\partial}{\partial \xi}[(1-\xi^2)I] and D_y=\frac{\partial}{\partial \eta}[(1-\eta^2)I],$$

so equation (3) becomes

$$\frac{1}{n}\nabla n.\nabla_{\vec{\Omega}} I-\frac{2}{n}(\vec{\Omega}.\nabla n)I=\frac{1}{2n^2}\left\{\frac{\partial n^2}{\partial x}D_x+\frac{\partial n^2}{\partial y}D_y\right\}$$

In our numerical implementation, we use a rectangular domain which is divided into a set of I x J elementary uniform volumes ΔV with a uniform unitary depth. The angular discretization is obtained through a discrete ordinate technique. This yields a set of M discrete directions, $\{\varphi_m, m=1..M\}$ giving a set of angular discrete direction cosines $\{(\xi_m,\eta_m), m=1,...M\}$. An orientation depending on the incident ray direction is adopted for each cell [12]. Calculations are done by using integration of equation (1) over an elementary volume ΔV for each discrete direction. This gives

$$\begin{aligned}&\frac{n}{c}\frac{\partial I_{m,P}}{\partial t}+\Delta y\xi_m(I_{m,E}-I_{m,W})+\Delta x\eta_m(I_{m,N}-I_{m,S})+\Delta x\Delta y(\mu_a+\mu_s)I_{m,p}\\&+\frac{1}{n}\frac{\partial n}{\partial x}D_{x,m}+\frac{1}{n}\frac{\partial n}{\partial y}D_{y,m}=\Delta x\Delta y(S_{m,P}+\mu_s w_m p_{mm} I_{m,p}\\&+\mu_s\sum_{m'=1,m'\neq m}^{M} w_{m'}p_{mm'}I_{m',p})\end{aligned} \tag{4}$$

where $D_{x,m}$ and $D_{y,m}$ are the discrete angular derivative terms at the angular ordinate $\xi_m$ and $\eta_m$ respectively and $w_m$ is a weighting factor. The discrete term of Henyey-Greenstein phase function is written as

$$p_{mm'}=\frac{1-g^2}{4\pi(1+g^2-2g(\xi_m\xi_{m'}+\eta_m\eta_{m'}))^{3/2}}$$

If the direction cosines are positive, the directional radiances are known on the faces W and S and they are unknown on the faces E and N of the (i,j)-cell and also in the centre P. Therefore, we need two complementary relations to eliminate $\Psi_{m,N}$ and $\Psi_{m,E}$, this can be obtained by using interpolation formula

$$\begin{cases}I_{m,P}=\alpha I_{m,E}+(1-\alpha)I_{m,W}\\I_{m,P}=\alpha I_{m,N}+(1-\alpha)I_{m,S}\end{cases},$$

where α is an interpolation parameter. Using these relations, equation (3) becomes

$$\frac{n}{c}\frac{\partial I_{m,P}}{\partial t}+\frac{\Delta y \xi_m}{\alpha}(I_{m,P}-I_{m,W})+\frac{\Delta x \eta_m}{\alpha}(I_{m,P}-I_{m,S})+\Delta x \Delta y(\mu_a+\mu_s)I_{m,p}$$
$$+\frac{1}{2n^2}\left\{\frac{\partial n^2}{\partial x}D_x+\frac{\partial n^2}{\partial y}D_y\right\}=\Delta x \Delta y(S_{m,P}+\mu_s w_m p_{mm} I_{m,p} \tag{5}$$
$$+\mu_s \sum_{m'=1,m'\neq m}^{M} w_{m'} p_{mm'} I_{m',p})$$

For time discretization, an implicit three level second order time differencing scheme is used:

$$\frac{\partial I_{m,P}}{\partial t}=\frac{3I_{m,P}^{n+1}-4I_{m,P}^{n}+I_{m,P}^{n-1}}{2\Delta t}; \qquad n=1,\ldots n_{\max}$$

where $\Delta t$ being the discrete time step.

Theoretically, if we know the solution in the (i,j)-cell, we can do calculus over the cells (i+1,j) and (i,j+1) using the boundary conditions and the following relations

$$\begin{cases} I_{m,w}(i+1,j)=I_{m,E}(i,j); i=1,\ldots I-1 \\ I_{m,S}(i,j+1)=I_{m,N}(i,j); i=1,\ldots J-1 \end{cases}$$

If the direction cosines are both positive, we get the following equation

$$\frac{n}{c}\frac{3I_{m,i,j}^{n+1}-4I_{m,i,j}^{n}+I_{m,i,j}^{n-1}}{2\Delta t}+\frac{\Delta y \xi_m}{\alpha}(I_{m,i,j}^{n}-I_{m,i-1,j}^{n})+\frac{\Delta x \eta_m}{\alpha}(I_{m,i,j}^{n}-I_{m,i,j-1}^{n})+$$
$$\Delta x \Delta y(\mu_a+\mu_s)I_{m,i,j}^{n}+\frac{1}{2n^2}\left\{\frac{\partial n^2}{\partial x}D_x+\frac{\partial n^2}{\partial y}D_y\right\}$$
$$=\Delta x \Delta y(S_{m,i,j}+\mu_s w_m p_{mm} I_{m,i,j}^{n}+\mu_s \sum_{m'=1,m'\neq m}^{M} w_{m'} p_{mm'} I_{m',i,j}^{n})$$

## 3. Numerical treatment of angular derivative terms

The numerical treatment of the angular redistribution terms can be done by using the classical angular differencing scheme [23, 28].

$$D_{x,m,i,j}=\frac{A_{m+1/2}I_{m+1/2,i,j}-A_{m-1/2}I_{m-1/2,i,j}}{w_m}.$$

$$D_{y,m,i,j}=\frac{B_{m+1/2}I_{m+1/2,i,j}-B_{m-1/2}I_{m-1/2,i,j}}{w_m}$$

where

$$I_{m+1/2,i,j}=\frac{1}{2}(I_{m+1,i,j}+I_{m,i,j}) \text{ and}$$

$$I^{k}_{m-1/2,i,j}=\frac{1}{2}(I^{k}_{m-1,i,j}+I^{k}_{m,i,j}) \text{ with } I_{M+1,i,j}=I_{1,i,j}, I_{0,i,j}=I_{M,i,j}.$$

The coefficients A and B are given through the recurrent relations

$$A_{m+1/2}-A_{m+1/2}=-2w_m\xi_m,$$

$$B_{m+1/2}-B_{m+1/2}=-2w_m\eta_m \text{ with } A_{1/2}=B_{1/2}=0,$$

and $w_m$ being a quadrature weight factor. In this paper, we use a constant weight quadrature and an equally spaced distribution of angular ordinates $(\xi,\eta)$. To solve the above equation we use successive iterations in order to actualise the implicit internal source term in the right member. So, this gives

$$\left(I^{n+1}_{m,i,j}\right)^{k+1}=\left[\frac{3n_{i,j}}{2c\Delta t}+\frac{\Delta y\xi_m}{\alpha}+\frac{\Delta x\eta_m}{\alpha}+\Delta x\Delta y\left(\mu_{a,i,j}+\mu_{s,i,j}\right)\right]^{-1}\times$$

$$\left[\begin{array}{l}\frac{2n_{i,j}}{c\Delta t}\overline{I^{n}_{m,i,j}}-\frac{n_{i,j}}{2c\Delta t}\overline{I^{n-1}_{m,i,j}}+\frac{\Delta y\xi_m}{\alpha}\left(I^{n+1}_{m,i-1,j}\right)^{k+1}+\frac{\Delta x\eta_m}{\alpha}\left(I^{n+1}_{m,i,j-1}\right)^{k+1}\\ +\frac{1}{2n^2_{i,j}}\left(\Delta y\left(n^2_{i,j}-n^2_{i-1,j}\right)D^k_{x,m,i,j}+\Delta x\left(n^2_{i,j}-n^2_{i,j-1}\right)D^k_{y,m,i,j}\right)\\ +\Delta x\Delta y\left(S_{m,i,j}+\mu_s w_m p_{mm}\left(I^{n+1}_{m,i,j-1}\right)^k+\mu_{s,i,j}\sum_{m'=1,m'\neq m}^{M}w_{m'}p_{mm'}\left(I^{n+1}_{m',i,j-1}\right)^k\right)\end{array}\right]$$

The iteration process is repeated until a convergence criterion is attempted. To improve convergence speed, we use a successive over relaxation method. So the updated value $\left(I^{n}_{m,i,j}\right)^{k+1}$ is a linear combination of the iterated value $\left(I^{n}_{m,i,j}\right)^{k}$ and the previously computed value:

$$\left(I^{n}_{m,i,j}\right)^{k+1}_{updated}=\rho\left(I^{n}_{m,i,j}\right)^{k}+(1-\rho)\left(I^{n}_{m,i,j}\right)^{k+1}$$

where ρ is a relaxation parameter whose value is usually between 1 and 2. The solution is obtained when the relative discrepancy value:

$$\varepsilon=\left|\frac{\left(I^{n}_{m,i,j}\right)^{k+1}-\left(I^{n}_{m,i,j}\right)^{k}}{\left(I^{n}_{m,i,j}\right)^{k}}\right|$$

is smaller than a tolerance value. In that case the result is noted $\overline{I}_{m,i,j}$. In all our calculus, we have taken $10^{-8}$ as a tolerance value. As initial condition, we take a field of null radiances. Also, all our calculations are done in the case of interpolation diamond scheme (α=0.5).

If the direction cosines are not both positive, the precedent equations are valid provided that the orientation WESN of cells is done according to the direction of propagation. In all our investigations, the injected power source is assumed to be equivalent to a forward collimated monochromatic intensity placed at a source point on the middle of the bottom side of the boundary. Results shown below are obtained by using a near infrared collimated source with a uniform equivalent intensity value of 50 mW.cm$^{-1}$. To present our results, we use the detected fluence rate which is given in a ($i_d$,$j_d$)-detector point on the boundary as

$$\Phi_d = \sum_{m=1}^{M}(1-R_{m,i_d,j_d})w_m \bar{I}_{m,i_d,j_d}, \text{ with}$$

$$R_{m,i_d,j_d}=\begin{cases} 1 \, if \, \varphi_m \succ \arcsin\left(\dfrac{n_{air}}{n_{i_d,j_d}}\right) \\ \dfrac{1}{2}[(\dfrac{n_{i_d,j_d}\cos\varphi_m - n_{air}\cos\varphi_t}{n_{i_d,j_d}\cos\varphi_m + n_{air}\cos\varphi_t})^2 + (\dfrac{n_{i_d,j_d}\cos\varphi_t - n_{air}\cos\varphi_m}{n_{i_d,j_d}\cos\varphi_t + n_{air}\cos\varphi_m})^2], else. \end{cases}$$

where

$$\varphi_t = \arcsin\left(\frac{n_{air}\sin\varphi_m}{n_{i_d,j_d}}\right) \text{ and } n_{air} \approx 1 .$$

Also, we make use of a normalized detected fluence rate defined as

$$\Phi_N = \frac{\Phi_d}{1/D\sum_{d=1}^{D} w'_d \Phi_d},$$

where $D$ is the number of the detector points on one side of the boundary and $w'_d$ is a weighting factor from the generalized trapezoidal integration rule. In all calculations, we have used 28 detector points on each side. Also, all calculus is carried out by using 16 uniformly distributed discrete directions and a space grid of 121x121cells.

## 4. Results and discussion

### 4.1 First test: A continuous varying refractive index medium

As a first investigation, we study near infrared radiation transport in a rectangular medium exposed to a continuous collimated source which is placed on the bottom side of the boundary. Figure 1 shows the considered medium, it is assumed to be 3cmx3cm sized with varying refractive index. Within the medium, we consider a y-axis linear varying refractive index between the extreme values 1.33 and 1.58. It is an increasing- decreasing variation of refractive index RI. To show the effect of the refractive index on detected fluence rate, we have used a weakly absorbing and forward scattering background medium whose optical parameters are shown in figure1. Figure 2 shows the medium response detected on the right side of the boundary in the case of linear and parabolic variation respectively. The detected fluence rate curve presents distinguish increasing and decreasing regions with a peak of transmission when refractive index is close to the minimum value 1.33. Transmission on the boundary is relatively augmented when the refractive index is the closest to the air index.

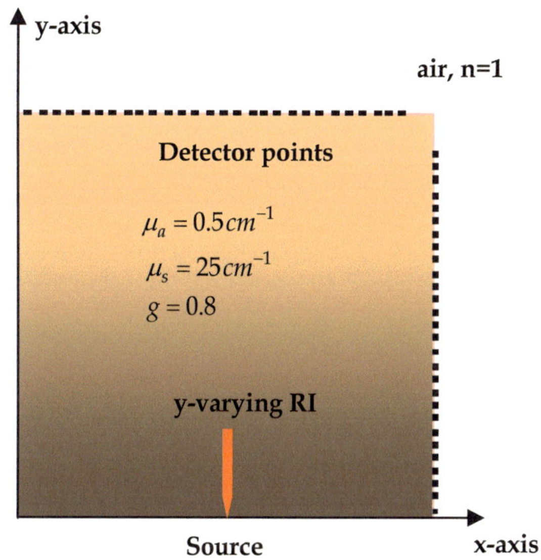


Fig. 1. A test-medium with background properties and detector points

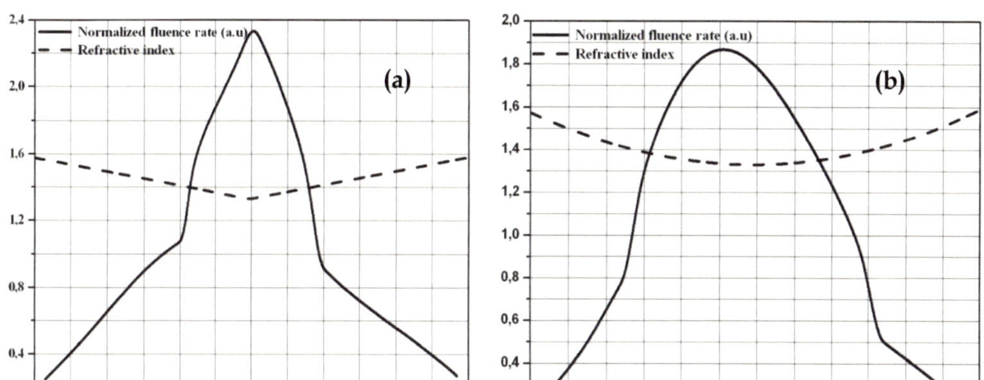


Fig. 2. Response of a continuous varying refractive index medium (a) in the case of a linear variation and (b) in the case of a parabolic variation.

### 4.2 Second investigation: Detection of heterogeneous object

In this investigation, we consider a 3cmx3cm sized background medium containing a circular heterogeneous object. The area of the object is 0.5 $cm^2$. We limit the analysis to the effect of heterogeneity by increase of the refractive index only. The background refractive index is taken 1.33. The other optical properties are the same as in the precedent investigation for the background and the object. The geometry of the medium and the position of the heterogeneous object are shown in figure 3. The detected signal on different sides of the medium is shown for an increase of refractive index by 5% and 10% respectively. There is no significant effect of the object presence on the detected signal on the left side because it is far from the detectors on that side. However there is a visible effect of the object on the right side and on the top side where the detectors are relatively near by the object. In such cases, there is an obvious effect of the heterogeneity on the detected signal especially when the refractive index is increased by 10%. The response shows a distinct distortion of the fluence rate curve. It is occurring on the targets where the object centre is laying exactly. This distortion allows a principled decision on the existence of such object in the medium. These findings highlight the potential of refractive index as a possible detection parameter of a tumour in a surrounding safe tissue.

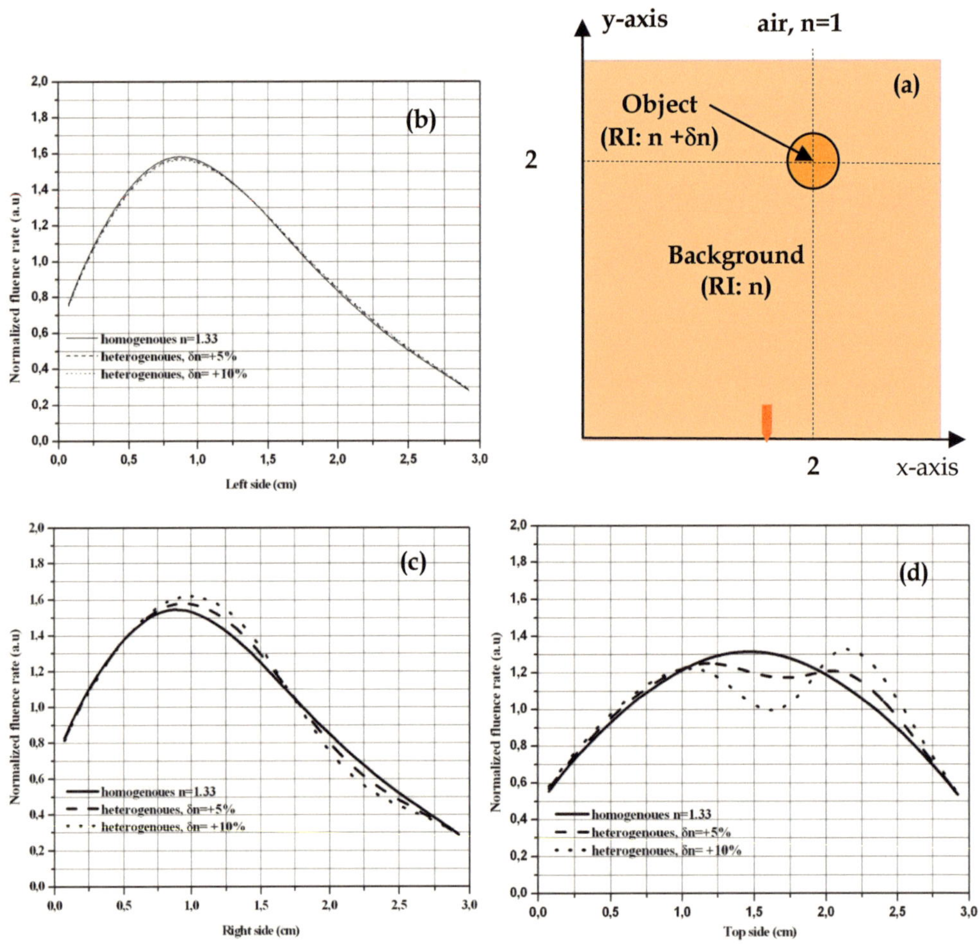


Fig. 3. Detection of heterogeneous objects by the effect of refractive index variation. (a) Geometry of the considered medium and object, (b) Detected fluence rate on the left side,(c) Detected fluence rate on the right side (d) Detected fluence rate on the top side.

### 4.3 Third investigation: Detection of inclusions in a biological tissue

In the course of this investigation, we simulate a post-mortem human prostate tissue-like medium containing two inclusions. The geometry of the medium and the targets of the inclusions are shown in figure 3. Each inclusion is a circle of area 0.5cm$^2$. The background medium properties at 850nm wavelength are taken from [30, 31]. Inclusion 1 is double scattering only and inclusion 2 is double absorbing only. The refractive index of the two inclusions is taken the same and it is noted $n_2$. Detected fluence rate on the top and on the lateral sides of the medium is computed and presented in figure 5 and figure 6. In particular, we confront results from refractive matching case ($n_1$=$n_2$) and from refractive mismatching case ($n_2$>$n_1$) on each side. According to figure 5, the introduction of refractive index with scattering and absorbing parameters gives a distinguish effect on top side detected signal. However this effect is more attenuated in lateral sides because of the strong forward scattering within the medium. This is shown in figure 6.

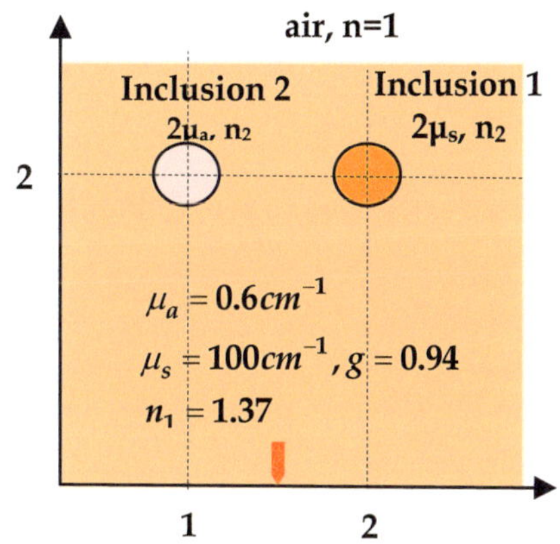


Fig. 4. Heterogeneous inclusions in human prostate-like tissue: geometry of the medium and inclusions.

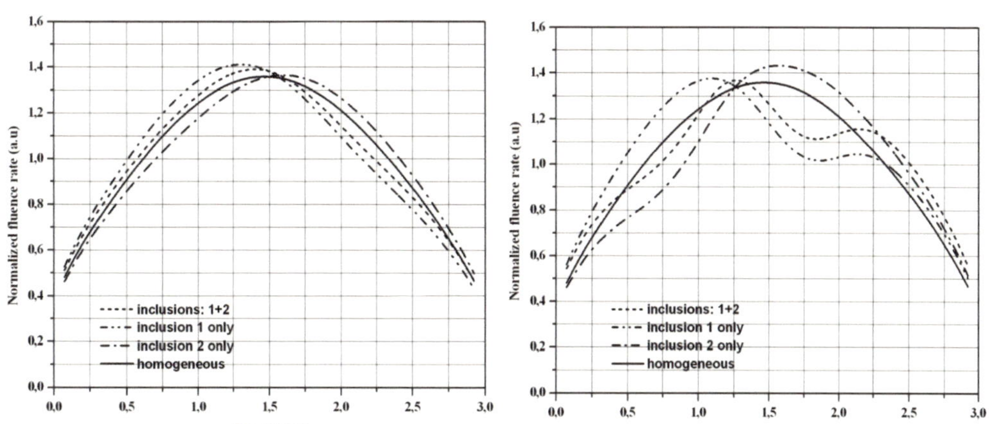


Fig. 5. Effect of heterogeneous inclusions on detected fluence rate on the top side (a) in the case of refractive matching ($n_1$=$n_2$=1.37) and (b) in the case of refractive mismatching ($n_1$=1.37 and $n_2$=1.51).

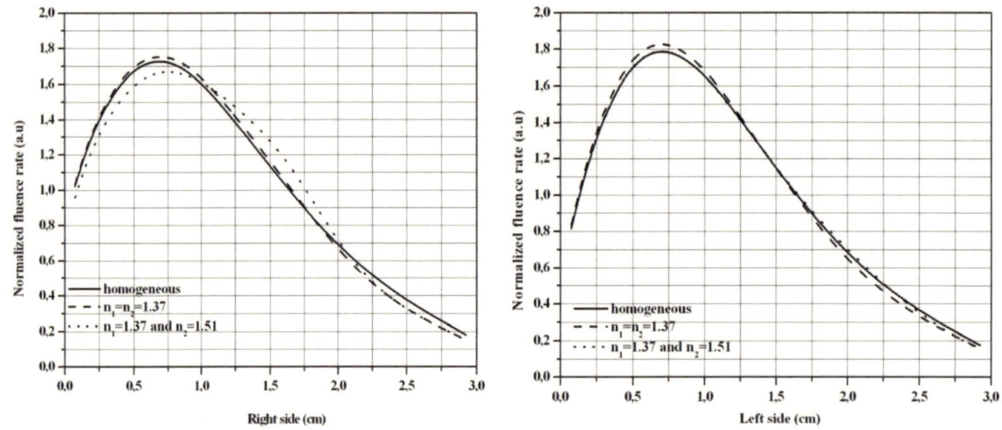


Fig. 6. Detected fluence rate on lateral sides in both cases refractive matching and mismatching cases: (a) Response on the right side (effect of inclusion 1) and (b) Response on the left side ( effect of inclusion 2)

### 4.4 Fourth investigation: Effect of refractive mismatching in multilayered tissue

As a fourth investigation, we consider a multilayered biological tissue-like medium. It contains three superposed layers of skin, fat and muscle. Figure 7 shows the considered medium. It is 3cmx3cm-sized medium with a fixed layer of skin (2mm) and with a varying fat-layer thickness of 3mm, 6mm and 9mm respectively. Optical properties of different tissues at 850nm-wavelength and refractive indices of the layers are taken from [30, 31]. Calculus is carried out as in the just previous section.

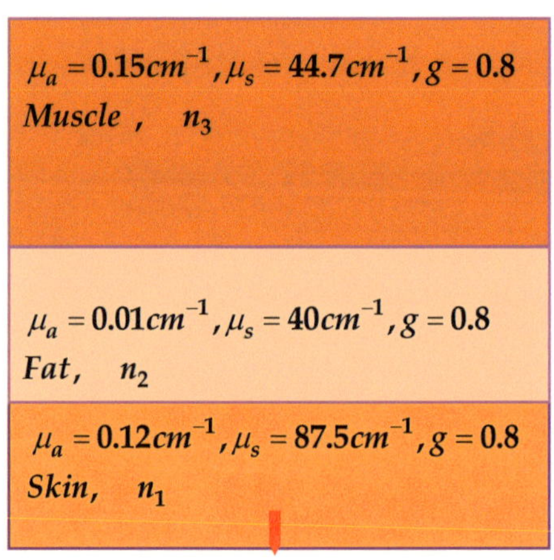


Fig. 7. A three-layered biological tissue-like medium with optical properties of skin, fat and muscle at 850 nm-wavelength.

Figure 8 shows results concerning transmitted fluence rate on the right side of the boundary in the case of a continuous wave source. We can see that in most detector points and for the three fat-layer thicknesses transmitted fluence rate profiles are almost superposed in the case of refractive matching with evidence of detected intensity increase when the fat thickness increases. When taking different refractive indices, a distinct distortion in the curves at every interface is observed especially at the fat-muscle interface. In all cases much more intensity is transmitted from the muscle layer.

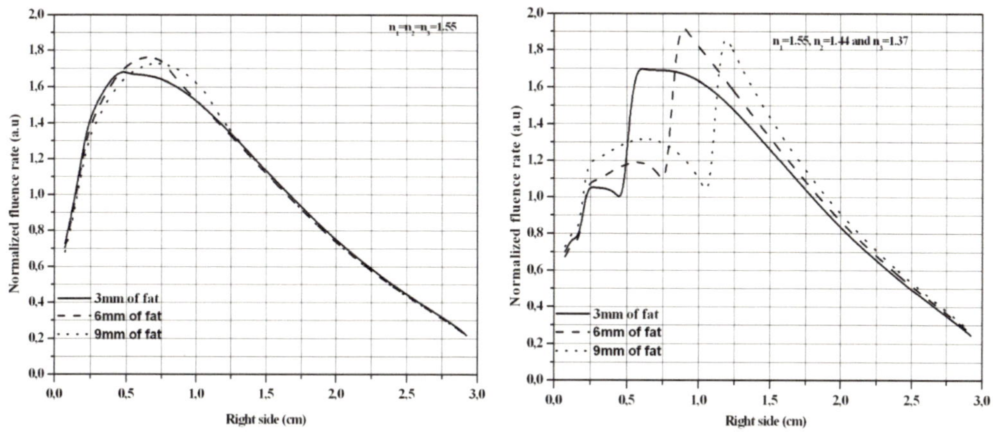


Fig. 8. Response of the three layered medium: (a) for uniform refractive index and (b) for different refractive indices.

### 4.5 Fifth investigation: Detection with a short pulse

In this investigation, we study the effect of abnormalities laying in a homogenous background medium as in the just precedent paragraph but we use a short-pulsed source. It is a 100fs-laser pulse injected in the medium through a point source on the middle of the bottom side of the boundary. Figure 9 shows the considered medium and the geometry and the properties of the

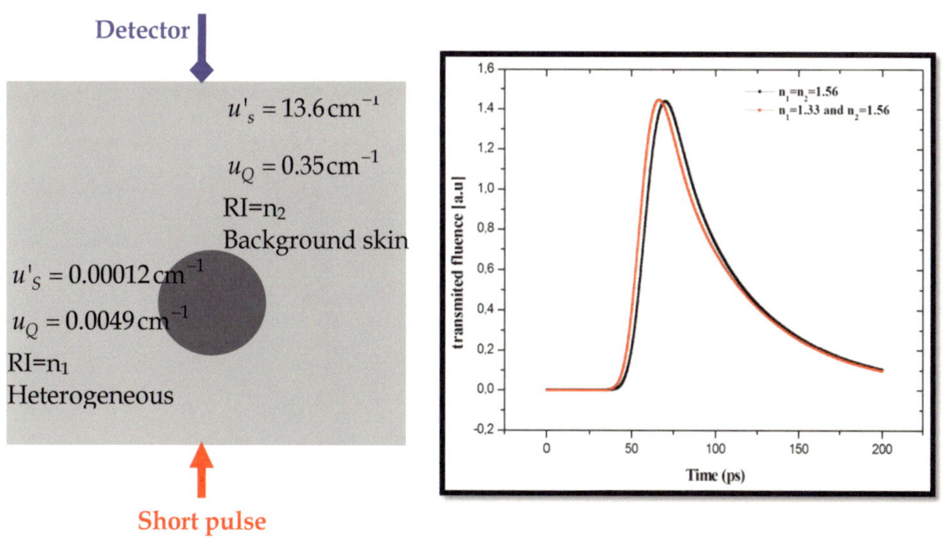


Fig. 9. A skin-like tissue containing a heterogeneous cyst-like inclusion submitted to short pulse and the detected signal.

a circular cyst-like object laying just forward the source. The detected signal on the opposite side of the source is shown in same figure. There is a distinct phase shift due to refractive mismatching showing the presence of the cyst within the background tissue.

### 4.6 Sixth investigation: Spectroscopy on a rat-liver

In this investigation, we consider a rat liver tissue-like medium as it is shown in figure 10. Optical properties of the tissue are taken from reference [30] from a set of several wavelengths. The response illustrate transmission through the considered medium on the top side. Only near infrared light displays a relative appreciable transmission. A maximum of detected fluence rate is noted at 800nm-light. A little delay of the maximum detection of radiation is observed when wavelength increases. Figure 11 shows fluence rate distribution into the medium at different moments after the pulse. In all moments, symmetric propagation of light is observed into the medium. Also, it can be observed that scattering prevails in 488nm while more and more absorption is observed in 2100 nm. At 488nm, the phenomenon of multiple scattering is dominant into the medium. The dispersion of the pulse is accentuated in all sides. Light disappears after 250ps. At 2100nm, more light is absorbed into the medium so a fraction of energy persists into the medium for more time.

Figure 12 shows typical movement of different photons in the medium at three different wavelengths. Calculations in our studied medium are carried out by using Monte Carlo simulations as it is described in reference. It can be observed that a typical 800nm-photon is almost snake. For 488nm-photon, the mean scattering free path is very small. Multiple scattering is dominant. The typical trajectory in this case is not ballistic and the photons are almost diffusive. For 2100nm, the mean scattering free path is longer than the 488nm-photon but the absorption mean free path is narrower. A typical photon in this wavelength is almost absorbed into the medium.

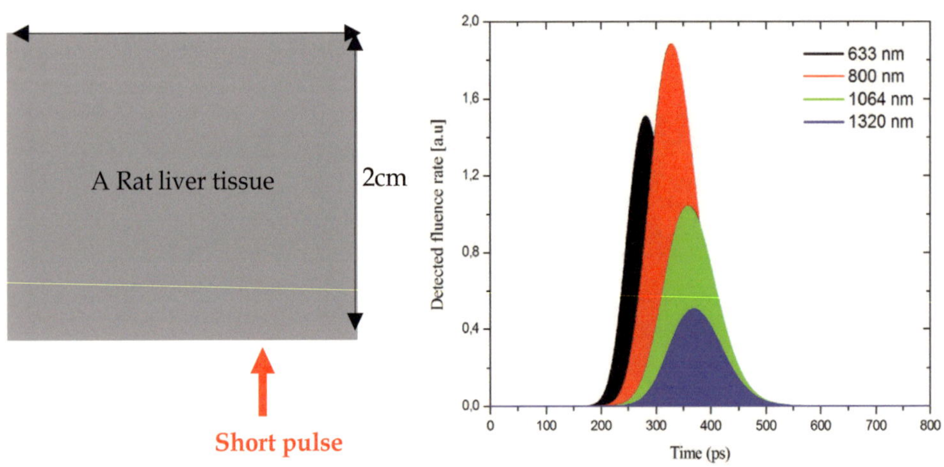


Fig. 10. Geometry of rat-liver tissue and detected signal for different wavelengths.

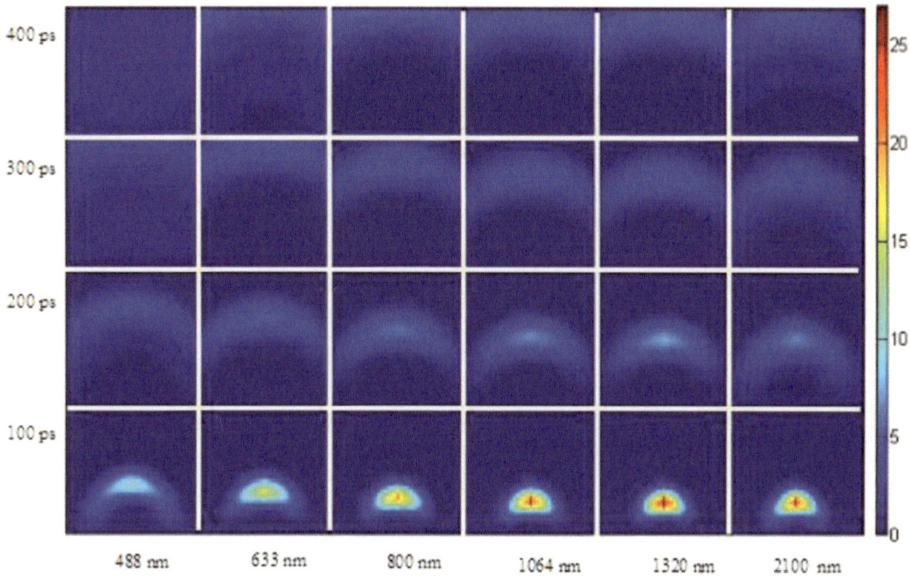


Fig. 11. Internal light distribution in the rat-liver tissue-like medium for different instants after the pulse.

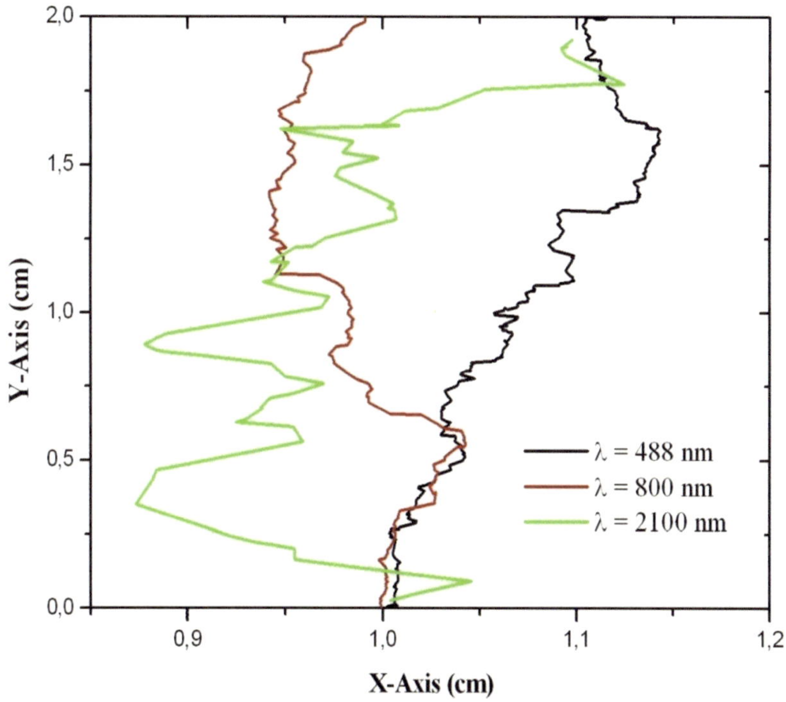


Fig. 12. Typical trajectory of photons for different values of the wavelength-source as obtained through Monte Carlo simulations.

## 5. Conclusion

In this chapter, we attempted to develop a computational way helping in detection of abnormalities in a biological tissue. This should enable predictions of eventual tumor existence when using a diffuse optical tomography scheme. The used model is based on radiative transfer theory including a possible variation of refractive index. The model is implemented to investigate some practical situations in DOT setting and near infrared spectroscopy. Obtained results showed that variation of refractive index can yield useful predictions about the target and the location of abnormal inclusions within the tissue.

## 6. Nomenclature

| | |
|---|---|
| c | Speed of light, (in vacuum), [cm/s] |
| DOT | Diffuse Optical Tomography |
| $D_{x,y}$ | Angular derivative terms |
| g | anisotropy factor |
| I | intensity, [$W.cm^{-2}sr^{-1}$] |
| n | refractive index |
| $p(\Omega,\Omega')$ | phase function |
| r | position vector, [cm] |
| R | reflectivity coefficient, |
| $r_b$ | position vector in the boundary |
| R I | Refractive Index |
| S | source term, [$W.cm^{-3}sr^{-1}$] |
| $w'_d$ | weighting factor from trapezoidal integration, |
| $w_m$ | weight associated with discrete direction |
| x,y | cartesian coordinates, [cm] |

**Greek symbols**

| | |
|---|---|
| $\alpha$ | interpolation parameter |
| $\Phi$ | fluence rate, [$W.cm^{-2}$] |
| $\Phi_d$ | Detected fluence rate, [$W.cm^{-2}$] |
| $\lambda$ | wavelength, [nm] |
| $\Omega$ | direction solid angle, [sr] |
| $\mu_a$ | absorption coefficient, [$cm^{-1}$] |
| $\mu_s$ | scattering coefficient, [$cm^{-1}$] |
| $\mu'_s$ | reduced scattering coefficient, [$cm^{-1}$] |
| $\rho$ | relaxation parameter, [-] |
| $\theta$ | scattering angle , [rad] |
| $\xi$, $\eta$ | direction cosines, [-] |

## 7. References

[1] Selser J C, Yeh Y, Baskin R J. A light scattering characterization of membrane vesicles. Biophysical Journal; 16 (4): 337-356, (1976)

[2] Jacques S L, Prahl S A. Modeling optical and thermal distributions in tissue during laser irradiation. Lasers in Surgery and Medicine; 6: 494-503, (1987)

[3] Arridge S R, Hebden J C. Optical imaging in medicine: II. Modeling and reconstruction. Phys Med Biol; 42: 841-853, (1997)

[4] Arridge S R, Schweiger M. A gradient-based optimisation scheme for optical tomography. Opt Express; 2 (6): 213-226, (1998)

[5] Hielscher A H, Bluestone AY, Abdoulaev AY, Klose A D, Lasker M, Stewart M, Netz U, Beuthan J. Near-infrared diffuse optical tomography. Disease Markers; 18: 313-337, (2002)

[6] Mourant J R, Hielscher A H, Eick A A, Johnson T M, Freyer J P. Evidence of intrinsic differences in the light scattering properties of tumoregenic and nontumorigenic cells. Cancer (Cancer Cytopathology); 84 (6): 366-384, (1998)

[7] Ntziachristos V, Hielscher A H, Yodh A G, Chance B. Diffuse Optical Tomography of Highly Heterogeneous Media. IEEE transactions on medical imaging; 20(6) :470-478, (2001)

[8] Pu Y, Wang W.B , Das BB, Alfano RR.Time-resolved spectral wing emission kinetics and optical imaging of human cancerous and normal prostate tissues. Optics communications; 282:4308-4314, (2009)

[9] Klose, A, D, Netz,U, Beuthan,J and Hielscher, A, H, Optical tomography using the time-independent equation of radiative transfer. Part I: Forward model, *JQSRT*, 72: 715-736, (2002)

[10] Cai W, Xiaohui Ni, Gayen S K, and Alfano R R. Analytical cumulant solution of the vector radiative transfer equation investigates backscattering of circularly polarized light from turbid media. Phys. Rev. E (74) 056605, (2006)

[11] Gantri M, Trabelsi H, Bensalah R and Sediki E. Solution of a radiative transfer problem in a biological tissue. An optical tomography model. AIP Conf. Proc; 935: 237-243, (2007)

[12] Trabelsi H, Gantri M and Sediki E. Visible and Near Infrared Laser Radiation in a Biological Tissue. A Forward Model for Medical Imaging by Optical Tomography. Lasers in Med Sci; 25:41-53, (2010)

[13] Gantri M, Trabelsi H, Sediki E, Ben Salah R. Computational Laser Spectroscopy in a Biological tissue. Journal of Biophysics, article ID 253763, 9pages, (2010)

[14] Li H, Xie S. Measurement method of the refractive index of biotissue by total internal reflection. Applied Optics; 35(10):1793-1795, (1996)

[15] Das B B, Liu F , Alfano R R. Time-resolved fluorescence and photon migration studies in biomedical and model random media. Rep. Prog. Phys; 60: 227-292, (1997)

[16] Ohmi M, Ohnishi Y, Yoden K, Haruan H. In vitro simultaneous measurement of refractive index and thickness of biological tissue by the low coherence interferometry. IEEE Transactions on Biomedical Engineering; 47(9):1266-1270, (2000)

[17] Lai J, Li Z, Wang C, He A. Experimental measurement of the refractive index of biological tissues by total internal reflection. Applied Optics; 44(10):1845-1849, (2005)

[18] Beuthan J, Minet O, Helfmann J, Herrig M, Muller G. The spatial variation of the refractive index of biological cells. Phys Med Biol; 41:369-82 (1996)

[19] Dehghani H, Brooksby B, Vishwanath, K, Pogue B W, Paulsen K D. The effects of internal refractive index variation in near-infrared optical tomography: a finite element modelling approach, Physics in Medicine and Biology; 48 (16):2713-2727, (2003)

[20] Khan T, Jiang H. A new diffusion approximation to the radiative transfer equation for scattering media with spatially varying refractive indices. J. Opt. A: Pure App. Opt; 5:137-141 (2003)
[21] Shendeleva M L, Molly, J, A, Scaling property of the diffusion equation for light in a turbid medium with varying refractive index, Journal of the Optical Society of America A; 24 (9): 2902–2910, (2007)
[22] Trabelsi H, Gantri M, Sediki E, Ben Salah R. A Time-dependent Computational Model for Radiation in a Spatially Varying Refractive Index Biological Medium. Proceedings of Eurotherm 83, Computational Thermal Radiation in Participating Media III; Lisbon, Portugal, (2009)
[23] Lemonnier D, LeDez V. Discrete ordinate solution of radiative transfer across a slab with variable refractive index. *JQSRT*; 72(2/5): 195–204, (2005)
[24] Liu, L, H, Benchmark numerical solutions for radiative heat transfer in two-dimensional medium with graded index distribution, *JQSRT*; 102: 293 – 303, (2006)
[25] Bal G. Radiative transfer equations with varying refractive index: a mathematical perspective, Journal of the Optical Society of America A; 23: 1639–1644 (2006)
[26] Ferwerda, H, A, Radiative transfer equation for scattering media with a spatially varying refractive index, Journal of Optics A: Pure and Applied Optics; 1(3): L1–L2, (1999)
[27] Tualle J M, Tinet E. Derivation of the radiative transfer equation for scattering media with a spatially varying refractive index, Optics communications; 228:33-38, (2003)
[28] Modest M, F. Radiative heat transfer; ISBN 0-12-503-163-7, Academic Press, (2003)
[29] Trabelsi H , Sghaier T et Sifaoui M S. Theoretical Study of Radiation between two Concentric Spheres Using a Modified Discrete Ordinates Method associated with Legendre Transform, JQRST; 93:415-428, (2005)
[30] Cheong W F, Prahl S A, Welch A J. A Review of the Optical Properties of Biological Tissues. IEEE J. Quantum Electronics; 26:2166-2185, (1990)
[31] Mobley J and Vo-Dinh T. optical properties of tissues, biomedical photonics handbook; ISBN 0-8493-1116-0, CRC Press LLC (2003)

# 3

# 3D Ultrasound Image Segmentation: Interactive Texture-Based Approaches

Julien Olivier[2,1] and Ludovic Paulhac[1]
[1]*Université François Rabelais Tours, Laboratoire Informatique (EA2101)*
[2]*École Nationale d'Ingénieurs du Val de Loire*
*France*

## 1. Introduction

The recent breakthroughs in 3D medical imaging technologies open new promising perspectives in the health domain. Significant efforts have being carried out and the precision of acquisition systems keeps on being improved. These devices are becoming widespread in the hospitals and the constantly increasing queues for this kind of exams prove the interest in these technologies. On the contrary, it seems that the evolution of 3D image analysis tools does not generate the same interest. It may be because, for a long time, people believed that considering 3D images as a succession of 2D frames was a sufficient and efficient way to make precise analysis. In our opinion, it is not the case and huge advancements can be obtained by considering 3D images with their entire complexity. This approach needs the development of specific models which can deal with multiple knowledge and are able to process huge information quantities. As a consequence, this chapter will present two original and efficient approaches of computer science for 3D image analysis and more particularly 3D ultrasound images.

Ultrasound techniques present a certain number of advantages when compared to other acquisition techniques like magnetic resonance imaging (MRI), X-ray computed tomography (CT), etc. Ultrasounds are not ionizing, which means they are not invasive for the patients. Moreover this technique is inexpensive and allows real time acquisitions. Nevertheless, the interpretation of ultrasound images is very complex and specialists are usually needed throughout the examination. In the same way, the segmentation (extraction of specific regions in the image) of ultrasound images is a very difficult task as these medical images present characteristic artifacts like shadows, speckle, attenuations, missing boundaries etc.

(Noble & Boukerroui (2006)) proposed a complete survey about native B-mode ultrasound image segmentation in which they tried to point out what makes a good ultrasound segmentation method. Among efficient techniques, the authors have identified methods dealing with image features such as gray level distribution, intensity gradient, phase, similarity measures and texture measures. As described in (Noble & Boukerroui (2006)), texture analysis is very efficient for ultrasound classification and segmentation. The classical method of Haralick's co-occurrence matrices (Haralick et al. (1973)) has often been used and has obtained good performances in several applications (Basset et al. (1993); Valckx &

Thijssen (1997)). Despite the great number of methods, results are still imprecise and the proposed solutions often focus on a given problematic, dedicated to one type of application. Nevertheless, it could be interesting to develop generic tools, automatic or semi-automatic, which would allow a more important usability and interactivity.

In this chapter, two original interactive systems for 3D skin ultrasound image segmentation are presented. Section 2 describes the interests of using 3D ultrasound images for contents analysis and presents classical methods to acquire this images. In section 3, we quickly explain the different families of texture analysis and we provide a discussion about the interest of using an interactive system in a man-aided application. In section 4, the first approach focuses on the development and the combination of efficient perceptual volumetric texture attributes easily understandable by humans. In section 5, the second one is based on a supervised segmentation model, interactively allowing the user to give useful information to the algorithm before the segmentation. To conclude, we discuss about our work and introduce the main prospects.

## 2. 3D ultrasound images

This section presents how to construct an acquisition of a 3D ultrasound image. We quickly explain the interest of the three-dimensions and what it is possible to analyze in ultrasound images of the skin.

### 2.1 Ultrasound image acquisition using a 3D probe

A 3D ultrasound image is acquired using a 3D probe that allows the user to obtain a volume of echo ($16 \times 16 \times 8\ mm^3$) using the scanning of an acoustic beam. For the acquisition of 2D ultrasound images, three main methods have been used (Grégoire et al. (2006)):

- The linear scanning: gives rectangular images well adapted to superficial exploration but the acquisition is slow.
- The sectorial scanning: faster method but the obtained image is not rectangular and presents an angulation.
- The circular scanning: very simple method but the image shape is a disk.

By combining two 2D scanning modes, following two different axis, it is possible to obtain a 3D scanning. To construct a 3D acquisition, it is also possible to move manually a 2D probe according to its perpendicular axis. In this case, the quality of the acquisition depends on the operator dexterity. Then, it is preferable to use a real 3D probe, with small size and weight, to obtain the best acquisition quality. This kind of probes has been used to acquire the 3D ultrasound images in this paper.

### 2.2 Ultrasound images of the skin

Today, manufacturers propose echographic systems with a resolution ranging from 100 $\mu m$ down to 30 $\mu m$. This requires ultrasonic frequencies ranging from 20 $MHz$ to 60 $MHz$. The increase of ultrasonic frequencies allows a resolution improvement but the wave in the media is attenuated, which limits the applications to superficial exploration. Resolution

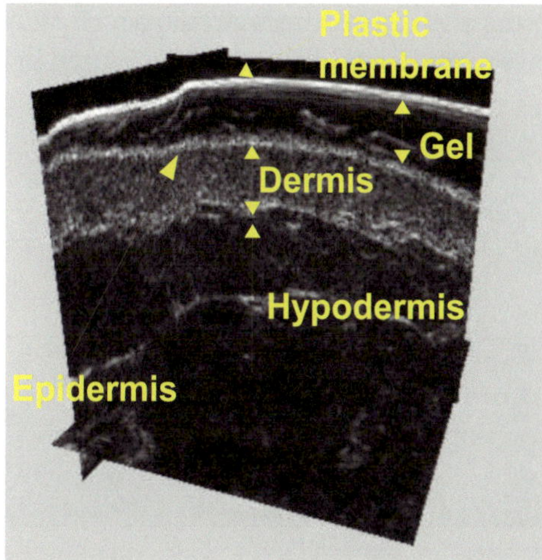


Fig. 1. Example of a three-dimensional image of the skin obtained with 20 $MHz$ ultrasound scanner (Atys Medical France)

provided with high frequencies ultrasound allows to observe the skin perfectly and especially the dermis that has an average thickness ranging from 1 to 2 $mm$. It is also possible to explore a part of the hypodermis. On the other hand, the resolution is insufficient to explore the epidermis (Figure 1). Indeed, its thickness vary between 0.05 to 0.3 $mm$ which need ultrasound frequencies higher than 80 $MHz$. Sonography of the skin allows tumor visualizations (cyst, nevus, melanoma, basal cell carcinoma (BCC) etc.), inflammatory pathologies, scars. The discrimination between the different lesions is not always obvious but cutaneous sonography is an important help for detection and diagnosis. The possibility to segment and characterize a lesion in three dimensions is very useful to establish therapeutic strategies. The three-dimensional sonography of the skin is rarely used because of the lack of three-dimensional image analysis tools but the recent evolution of three-dimensional probes should allow the emergence of new techniques. With a three-dimensional acquisition, it is possible to obtain features that are inaccessible with two dimensions. Moreover three-dimensional sonography is well adapted to supervise the evolution of a structure or a lesion notably using volume measures.

As it has been briefly presented in section 1, Noble & Boukerroui (2006) established that texture analysis was a very efficient way to process ultrasound images. Thus, the next section present the principle of this kind of analysis.

## 3. Texture analysis

### 3.1 Definition

When dealing with complex images (such as medical images), relying only on first order statistics such as gray level intensity means, standard deviations or histograms is not sufficient to carry out a precise analysis. Indeed, two objects with close intensity statistics and different visual aspects can generally be found in this kind of images (see figure 2). Such objects require to use analysis of higher order such as texture analysis, which allow us to study not only the intensity statistics of the pixels but also their spatial distribution in the image.

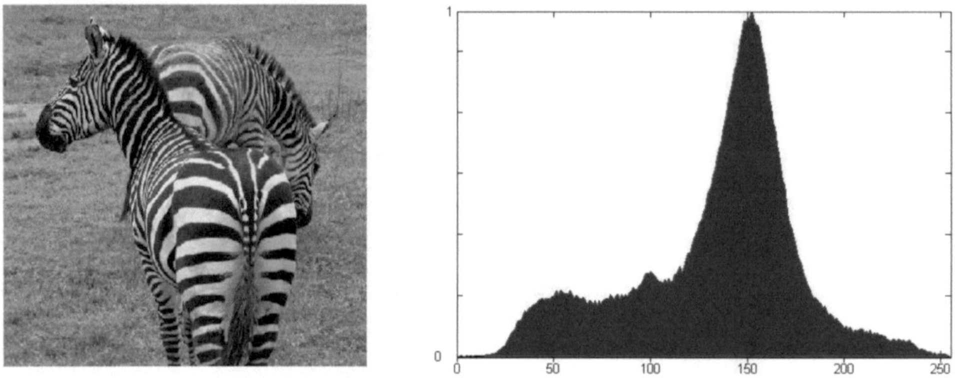


(a) Grey level intensity mean : 133.9 ; Standard deviation : 42.7

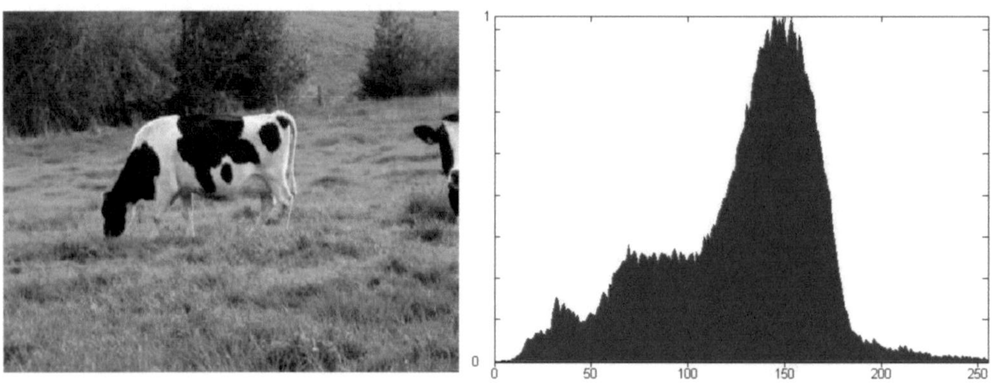


(b) Grey level intensity mean : 126.5 ; Standard deviation : 40.7

Fig. 2. First order analysis limitations: images a) and b) possess the same first order statistics (mean, standard deviation and gray level histogram) but their visual aspects are clearly different. Thus a high order analysis becomes necessary

Before presenting the main texture features, let us try to present a definition for the notion of texture.

Even if several definitions appear in the literature (see Tuceryan & Jain (1993)), if we stay in a general point of view we can define a textured zone in an image as a gray level distribution respecting an ordered scheme and for which the determination of unique features is possible.

However, three main texture types are identified in the literature (Richards & Polit (1974)).

- Deterministic textures: they are composed of one unique element, called a texton (see Julesz (1975)), which is regularly repeated in the space according to specific orientation and period. Even if this kind of textures can easily be characterized, it remains very rare in natural images. That is why, most of the time, deterministic textures are artificial ones.

- Stochastic textures: they are composed of non-regular pattern. These textures can be considered as bi-dimensional random fields.
- Quasi-deterministic textures: they are composed of several patterns that are very close to each other, but rarely identical. For this reason it remains difficult to isolate one unique pattern. The natural textures often belong to this type of textures.

These three texture types are illustrated in figure (3).

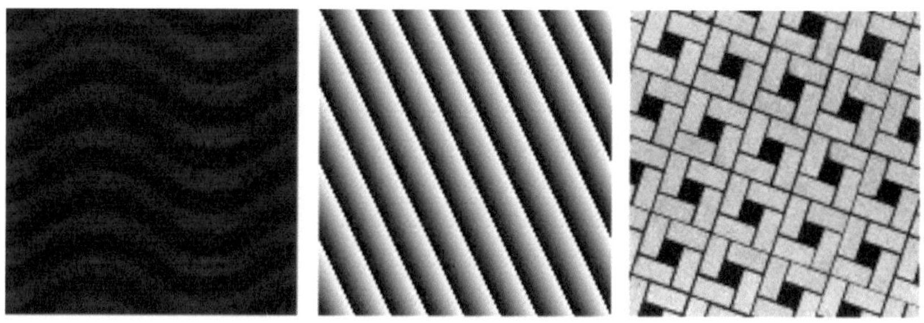

(a) Deterministic textures

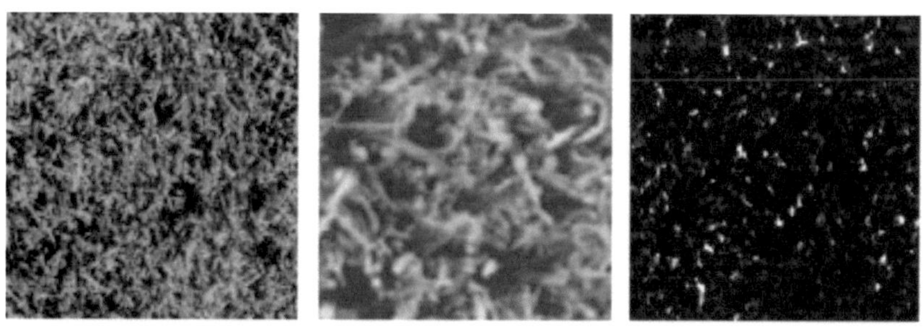

(b) Stochastic textures

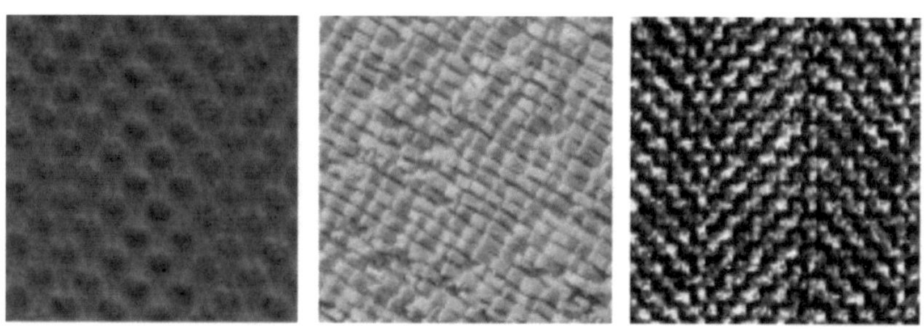

(c) Quasi-deterministic textures

Fig. 3. The three main texture types

The next part of this chapter presents the most used texture features.

### 3.2 Texture features

The purpose of a texture feature is to describe a textured zone with, at least, one numerical value. In an ideal scheme, two different textures will have two different values for one given feature. Unfortunately, this rarely happens because, usually, the discriminating power of each texture feature is strongly dependent to the kind of treated textures. In Richards & Polit (1974), four principal texture feature families are identified: statistical methods, geometric methods, model-based methods and, finally, frequency-based methods. Here, we will voluntary not give details about the feature calculations but will only present their principles. If interested, the reader will find further details by following the reference of each approach.

The statistical methods represent the oldest approaches in the texture analysis field. Their principle is to study the pixel's gray level spatial distribution in the image. They usually use statistics of at least second order (*i.e.* the pixels are studied by pair instead of independently). The features from this family represent the best choice for non-expert users because of their implementation easiness. Among the statistical features, the following ones can be considered as the most used: the Haralick coefficients of the coocurrence matrix (Haralick et al. (1973)), the autocorrelation measure (Otsu & Kurita (1988)) and the Local Binary Pattern (LBP) (Ojala et al. (1996)).

The approaches from the geometric method family are based on the principle of repetitiveness present in most of the textures. Indeed, they try to identify and characterize the texture primitive of a texture zone (the texton). As a consequence, this methods are very efficient on deterministic textures but encounter more difficulties when dealing with natural textures such as stochastic or quasi-deterministic ones. The Voronoï tessellation (Shamos & Hoey (1975)) and the structural methods (Voorhees & Poggio (1987); Zucker (1976)) can be considered as the two principal approaches of this family.

The principle of the model-based methods is to build an artificial texture model which must be as similar to the studied texture as possible. The evolution of this artificial model characteristics is observed during its construction and once the model is close enough to the studied texture, these characteristics are kept as the texture features. The Markov random fields (Li (1995)) and the fractal approaches (Mandelbrot (1977)) represent the two principal model-based methods.

The frequency-based methods consider that a texture can be characterized by analyzing the repetition of one or several pattern according to various spatial frequencies. Thus, several methods, initialy developed for 1D signals (like sound), have been adjusted to 2D signals such as images. The most popular frequency-based methods are the Fourier analysis (Azencott et al. (1997)), the Gabor filters (Turner (1986)) and the wavelet transform (Mallat (1989)).

### 3.3 Choosing the right texture feature

As it has been presented in the previous section, several texture features have been developed over the past thirty years. Unfortunately, most of these methods do not have a general applicability and cannot identify some classes of texture. For example, some of these approaches are not able to describe the directionality properties. In comparison, the human visual system can adapt to all types of textures even in the case of an unfavorable context. As a consequence, when developing an texture-based image analysis application, it would seems natural to think of including the maximum of texture features in order to obtain the best accuracy. Unfortunately, this strategy does not represent a good choice as some of the included features will alter the segmentation if they are not discriminating enough.

When dealing with ultrasound images, the various number of applications, each using different texture features, confirm this observation. As shown in (Noble & Boukerroui (2006)), the classical method of Haralick's co-occurrence matrices (Haralick et al. (1973)) has been widely used and has obtained great performances in several applications (Basset et al. (1993); Valckx & Thijssen (1997)). However, the increasing use of three-dimensional acquisition technologies in clinical practices requires three-dimensional segmentation or analysis methods. Boukerroui et al. (2001) propose a multi-resolution segmentation of three-dimensional ultrasound data (2D+T, 3D) using gray scale intensity, three-dimensional Haralick texture features and three-dimensional tissue characterizing information obtained from the local frequency spectra of the radio-frequency signals. The authors conclude that the use of complementary and/or redundant texture features allows a more robust segmentation. Sahiner et al. (2004) characterize breast masses on three-dimensional ultrasound images. They developed 2D and 3D active contour models for an automated segmentation. Then, they extracted three-dimensional texture and morphological features from the segmented mass. In their study, classification results of malignant and benign breast masses are similar to those experienced by breast radiologists. Zhan & Shen (2003; 2006) present a deformable model to segment three-dimensional ultrasound images. They compute texture features using two banks of two-dimensional Gabor filters located in the two orthogonal planes. Indeed, the use of a three-dimensional Gabor filter bank should have increased the number of filters and computation time. Nevertheless with two banks of two-dimensional Gabor filters, information is lost in comparison with a bank of three-dimensional Gabor filters.

Thus, as no unique efficient texture feature can be identified, it remains very important to choose the right texture features but this task is very difficult for a non-expert user because no single mathematical model describing all the features exists. Moreover, the names of the texture features rarely refer to something easily understandable.

This aspect of the texture analysis motivated us to develop interactive approaches which allow a non expert user to carry out texture-based segmentations without having to choose some precise texture features. This two approaches are presented in the following two sections.

## 4. Human Understandable Features (HUF)

In this first approach, a set of 3D texture features, inspired by the human way to describe a texture, is proposed. By using human understandable texture features, it is easier and possible for an operator (specialist or not in image analysis) to select the relevant features to process an image. Moreover in a given application it allows a better contents interpretation.

The set of characteristics has been chosen using analysis results from some previous works (Amadasun & King (1989); Tamura et al. (1978)). The chosen characteristics are the following: Granularity, which can be represented by the number of three-dimensional patterns constituting the texture, shape information about these patterns (volume, compacity, regularity), contrast and, finally, roughness of the image.

In sub-section 4.1, we present a multiresolution scheme for segmentation and we detail the HUF computation. Sub-section 4.2 presents psychological experiments proving the correspondence between our texture features and a human description of textures. Finally,

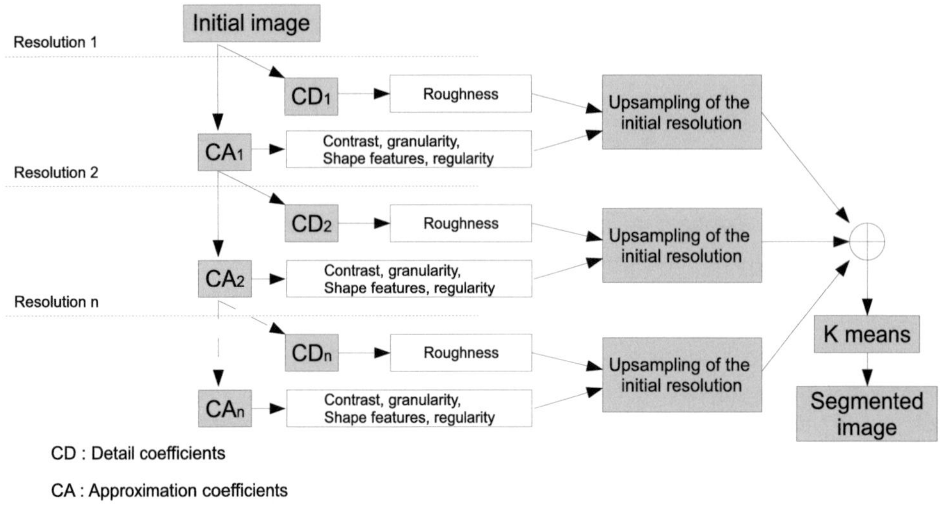


Fig. 4. Multiresolution segmentation

sub-section 4.3, shows segmentation results of 3D ultrasound images of the skin. More details about this work are available in Paulhac, Makris, Gregoire & Ramel (2009).

#### 4.1 A multiresolution scheme for texture segmentation

The proposed approach allows us to give an image description using texture features for several resolutions by using the 3D discrete wavelet transform (Figure 4). Mallat (1989) proposes a decomposition scheme using filters: a highpass filter, which allows to obtain detail coefficients and a lowpass filter which gives approximation coefficients. Roughness is computed using detail coefficients whereas the other proposed features are computed using approximation coefficients. Before the segmentation process, the proposed features are computed for each voxel and for several resolutions. In order to obtain a segmentation of the start image, a step of feature upsampling is necessary for each resolution. Thus, a voxel of the initial image is described by a vector containing $6n$ different features with $n$ the number of resolutions and 6 the number of proposed features. The user is then asked to choose the features that seem the most relevant from his point of view. And it is because they are human understandable that this choice will be easy. Finally, the K-means algorithm (Coleman & Andrews (1979)) allows to generate a segmentation using the set of computed vectors.

##### 4.1.1 A geometric approach for 3D texture analysis

We have chosen to describe the geometric structure of the textures with the help of the three-dimensional connected components which can be viewed as the patch patterns in the texture. To compute connected components, we propose a similar method to the one presented in (Shoshany (2008)): a gray-level textured image is decomposed into a progressive sequence of binary textures in order to study patterns and their evolution. In our approach, a clustering algorithm applied on the voxels of the initial 3D image allows us to identify a set of thresholds used to compute the sequence of binary versions of the image. Then, connected

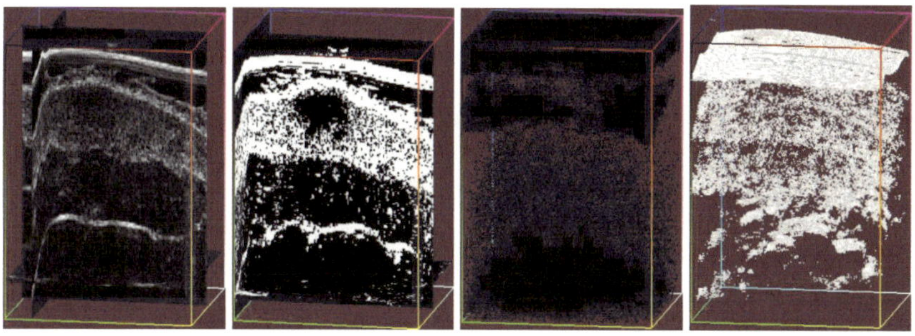


Fig. 5. a) One ultrasound image, b) The same ultrasound image after a binarization, [c-d] Connected components extracted from different binary images

components are computed for each binary textures of the produced sequence. Figure 5 presents a binarized image with examples of connected components.

Connected components represent the basic objects inside binary textures. Their analysis can provide important geometrical and volume information and it allows computation of features like granularity which corresponds to the number of patterns per volume unit, the volume and compacity of each connected components providing information about the shape of texture patches. The regularity can also be estimated using the variance of these patterns. In our case, the number of patterns corresponds to the number of connected components ($nbCC$) per volume unit. For a given texture, if the number of connected component is important for the resolution $\beta$ then, there is an important number of patterns and the granularity ($f_{gran_\beta}$) of the texture is significant.

Besides the number of connected components, we compute shape characteristics with the average volume and the average compacity of connected components. Like the number of connected components, the volume is an additional information to identify the fineness of a texture. The average volume of connected components is computed as follows:

$$f_{vol_\beta}(x,y,z) = \left(\sum_{i=1}^{nbCC_\beta} V_{i,\beta}\right)/nbCC_\beta \quad (1)$$

where $V_{i,\beta}$ is the volume of the $i^{th}$ connected component for the resolution $\beta$. The considered connected components are located in a cube of size $N^3$ centered at the coordinates $(x,y,z)$.

Compacity of connected components gives information about pattern shape. A texture with an important compacity is a texture with compact patterns. Otherwise this is a texture with elongate shapes. This characteristic is invariant by translation, rotation but also to scale changes (Zhang & Tan (2002)). It has been used to texture characterization in (Goyal et al. (1995)). The compacity of a connected component can be computed as follows:

$$C_{i,\beta} = \frac{S_{i,\beta}^{\frac{3}{2}}}{V_{i,\beta}} \quad (2)$$

where $S_{i,\beta}$ is the surface and $V_{i,\beta}$ is the volume of the $i^{th}$ connected component for the resolution $\beta$.

It is then possible to compute the average compacity $f_{comp_\beta}$ :

$$f_{comp_\beta}(x,y,z) = \frac{1}{nbCC_\beta} \sum_{i=1}^{nbCC_\beta} C_{i,\beta} \tag{3}$$

We can also obtain information about the regularity of a texture from the study of the connected components. Therefore, we decided to use the compacity variance. We have seen that this characteristic is invariant by any transformation (Zhang & Tan (2002)). The shape of patterns is the only element that affects the variance feature. A low variance of the compacity indicates an important regularity of the connected components whatever their spatial organization is.

$$f_{reg_\beta}(x,y,z) = E(C_\beta^2) - (E(C_\beta))^2 \tag{4}$$

where $E$ is the expected value.

#### 4.1.2 Statistical and frequency based method for contrast and roughness measure

The surface of a rough texture presents a high number of asperities. In an image, roughness can be described as a set of quick spatial transitions with varying amplitude. From a frequential point of view, the image asperities in the spatial domain correspond to the presence of high frequencies. Detail coefficients from the wavelet transform give a description of high frequencies in an image among several directions. It is then possible to have an estimation of the texture roughness for a specific resolution.

Finally, we propose to compute the roughness attribute as follows:

$$f_{rgh_\beta}(x,y,z) = \sum_{\alpha=1}^{M}(\sum_{i=1}^{N}\sum_{j=1}^{N}\sum_{k=1}^{N}\left|w_{\alpha,\beta}(i,j,k)\right|)/M \tag{5}$$

where $f_{rgh_\beta}$ is the roughness at the resolution $\beta$. $w_{\alpha,\beta}(i,j,k)$ corresponds to the set of detail coefficients in a cube of size $N^3$ centered at a voxel of a sub-band $\alpha$ at the coordinates $(x,y,z)$ and $M$ represents the number of detail coefficient sub-bands for a resolution.

Haralick et al. (1973) propose a measure to estimate contrast by computing the moment of inertia from the main diagonal of the co-occurrence matrix. Nevertheless, the construction of a co-occurrence matrix, only to obtain an estimation of the contrast, can be expensive in computing time. Tamura et al. (1978) claim that four factors are supposed to influence the contrast difference between two textures. They are the dynamic range of gray-levels, the polarization of the distribution of black and white on the gray-level histogram or ratio of black and white areas, the sharpness of edges, and the period of repeating patterns. They propose to approximate the contrast with a measure incorporating the two first factors. We use this approximation in our work. To obtain a measure of polarization the kurtosis $\alpha_4$ is used. It allows a measurement of the disposition of probability mass around their center.

$$\alpha_{4,\beta} = \frac{\mu_{4,\beta}}{\sigma_\beta^4} \tag{6}$$

where $\mu_4$ is the mean fourth moment and $\sigma^2$ the variance of gray-levels for the resolution $\beta$. In order to take into account the dynamic range of gray-levels, they combine the kurtosis with the standard deviation as follows:

$$f_{cont_\beta}(x,y,z) = \frac{\sigma_\beta}{\alpha_{4,\beta}^n} \tag{7}$$

where $n$ is a positive value. In their paper, Tamura et al make comparisons between psychological experiments and their operators before concluding that the value $n = 1/4$ gives the best approximation. At last, the values of $\sigma_\beta$ and $\alpha_{4,\beta}^n$ are computed in a cube of size $N^3$ centered at the coordinates $(x,y,z)$.

### 4.2 Psychological experiments

These experiments have been carried out to prove that a strong correspondence exists between the proposed features and the human vision. Thus, we propose to construct psychometric prototypes and to compare them to our texture measures.

The set of textures presented in Figure 6 has been used in our experiments. These textures have been constructed using methods presented in (Kopf et al. (2007); Paulhac, Makris & Ramel (2009)) except for textures (j) and (l) that are subsets of ultrasound images. Each of them is a volumetric texture (texture in the 3D domain) of size $128^3$ with 256 gray-levels. They have been printed using a printer HP Color LaserJet 3700 and presented to human subjects.

The group of human subjects was composed of 15 men and 11 women, and the majority of them had no knowledge in image and texture analysis. We distributed to each one of them a questionnaire containing the set of textures (Figure 6) and an explanation of the texture features used in our model. For each feature, textures had to be classified in descending order, *i.e.* from the most rough to the most smooth, from the most regular to the most irregular, etc. Using these questionnaires, we constructed a ranking of these textures for each texture attribute. For a given characteristic, a score has been assigned to a texture according to its ranking. For example, The most rough takes the value +12 (for the roughness feature), the second one +11, the last one +1, and this for all the questionnaires. The addition of the questionnaire scores for each texture allowed us to obtain a final ranking for a given texture feature.

Using the proposed texture attributes, we also generate a feature ranking. A vector of 6 features has been computed for each texture in the questionnaire. Here only the first resolution has been considered ($\beta = 1$), because this is the one which corresponds the best to the observation of textures by human subjects through questionnaires.

#### 4.2.1 Comparison between human and computational ranking

To compare human and feature ranking, the degree of correspondences between them has been determined. In this respect, we chose to use the well-known Spearman's coefficient of

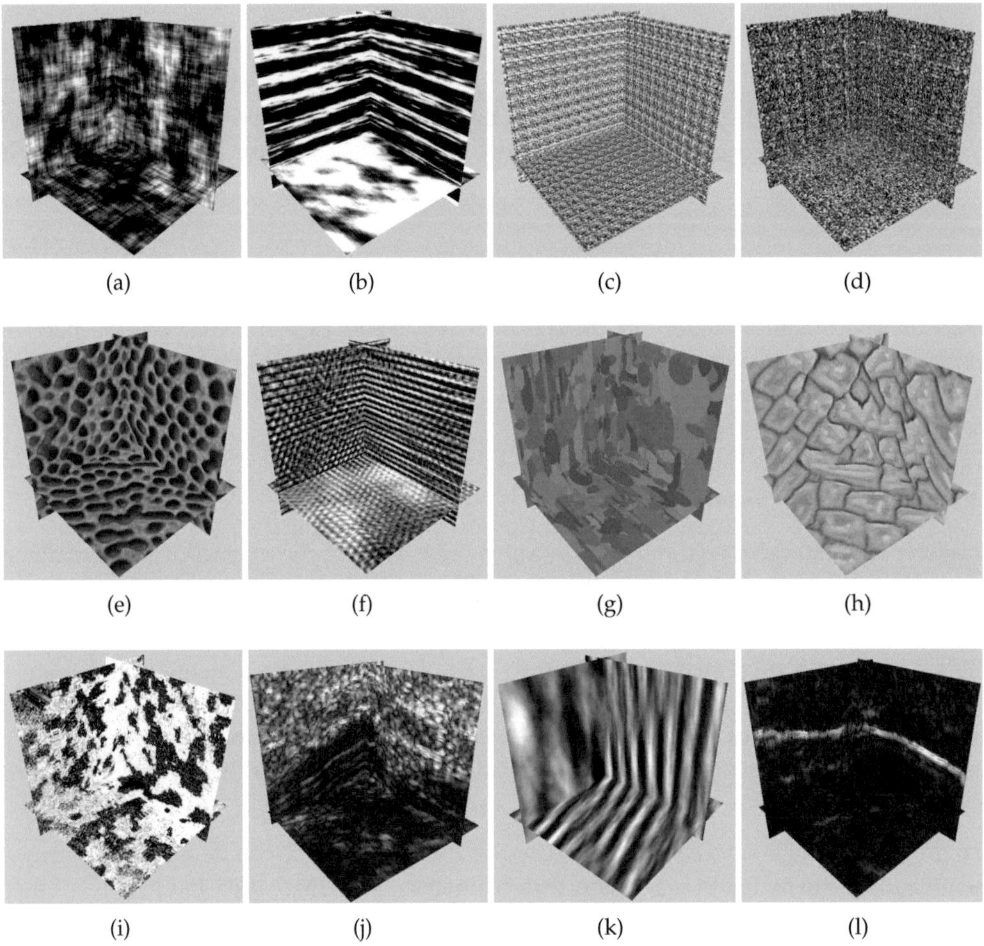


Fig. 6. Set of Solid textures used for psychological experiments

rank correlation:

$$r_s = 1 - \frac{6}{n^3 - n} \sum_{i=1}^{n} d_i^2 \tag{8}$$

where $n$ is the number of individuals, and $d_i$ is the difference between the ranks assigned to the $i^{th}$ object in the two measurements. The value of this coefficient varies between $-1$ and 1. Value 1 corresponds to the complete agreement of the two rankings whereas value $-1$ indicates complete disagreement. Table 1 presents coefficients of rank correlations between human and feature ranking.

| $f_{gran}$ | $f_{comp}$ | $f_{vol}$ | $f_{reg}$ | $f_{rgh}$ | $f_{cont}$ |
|---|---|---|---|---|---|
| 0.83 | 0.9 | 0.61 | 0.82 | 0.75 | 0.65 |

Table 1. Coefficients of rank correlations between human and feature ranking

| Region | Description | Texture attributes scoring |
|---|---|---|
| Nevus, Histiocytofibroma, Cyst, Melanoma, BCC | These lesions are present in the dermis and have an average or low echogenicity. | granularity:+, compacity:+++, contrast:+, roughness:+, regularity:++ |
| Normal Dermis | In this zone, there is a regular echogenicity. | granularity:+++, compacity:+, contrast:++, roughness:++, regularity:+ |
| Hypodermis | This region of the skin can contain more or less echogenicity according to zones. | granularity:++, compacity:++, contrast:++, roughness:++, regularity:+ |
| Epidermis | Resolution is to low to analyze epidermis. Moreover it is similar to the plastic membrane in ultrasound images with a high echogenicity. | granularity:+, compacity:+, contrast:++, roughness:+, regularity:++ |

Table 2. 3D interesting textures in skin images

These results show a huge correlation between human and feature ranking. For the volume, the Spearman's coefficient indicates that there is a link between the two measurements with a confidence rate included between 95 and 98 percent. The compacity feature gives the best result with a confidence rate which tends toward 100 percent. The volume feature has the smallest correlation results. It can be supposed that it is sometimes difficult for our human subjects to visualize the volume of patterns because of the 3D.

### 4.3 Segmentation of 3D ultrasound images with the HUF system

As explained in Noble & Boukerroui (2006), the scatterer distribution and their relative volumes to the wavelength of the incident ultrasound pulse produces different three-dimensional texture patterns. During an ultrasound examination, echogenicity represents the ability of a cellular tissue to create an echo. In an ultrasound image, echogenic zones contain a large number of white three-dimensional patterns and this is an important characteristic used by specialists to identify pathologies. From a texture analysis point of view, echogenicity of a zone can be described mainly by granularity measures carried out on these three-dimensional patterns. The interest of each of the proposed HUF features has been validated by specialists in dermatology. Table 2 presents a synthesis of the correspondence between the HUF features and the characteristics according to the regions in the skin. It was not possible to predict the exact value of the HUF features and a score (low:+, medium:++, high:+++) has been proposed for each texture attribute according to the regions in the skin.

#### 4.3.1 Presentation of the segmentation software

The architecture of the proposed system is composed of three main modules. The first one computes texture features according to user-defined parameters. Then, HUF features are used in the second module of segmentation. Finally, the segmented image can be exploited by the 3D visualization and manipulation module. This module allows to visualize the initial segmentation and to improve, in an interactive way, this first result. It is also possible to represent regions using a mesh or to compute volume information to help specialists in their diagnostic.

Before running the segmentation, the user needs to select the features that seem the most relevant to process a 3D image. A graphic interface allows the user to define his choice (Figure 7). The selected textural features, the parameters and the processed volumetric image are then exploited by the module of feature computation. For each voxel, the selected textural features are computed. Then, the segmentation module uses the set of computed feature vectors to generate a first segmentation with the K-means algorithm (Coleman & Andrews (1979)). Finally, using the graphical interface, the user can improve the segmentation using merging and splitting operations. Then, it becomes possible to merge two regions or to focus on a particular region by running, once more, a segmentation (a Kmeans clustering) of this region.

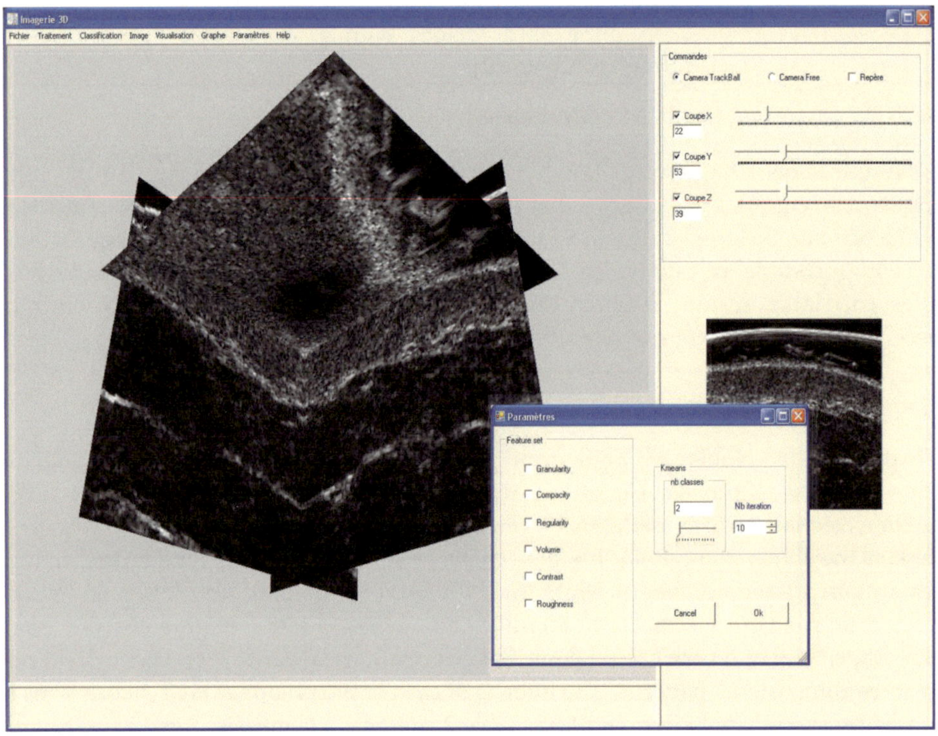


Fig. 7. Interface of the proposed software for segmentation of 3D ultrasound images.

### 4.3.2 Segmentation results

Our software has been provided to several dermatologists in order to help them to collect 3D information about pathologies. Figure 8 presents segmentation results for different skin ultrasound images. Using a segmentation, many extractions are possible: lesions, tendons, skin layers etc. Figure 8[a-b] shows two naevi, figure 8[c-d] shows two Histiocytofibroma, figures 8[a-d] contain at the left the original three-dimensional ultrasound image, at the center an image of classified voxels and on the right a mesh of the lesion built using the segmented image. With these results, it becomes possible to perform measures like volume and depth,

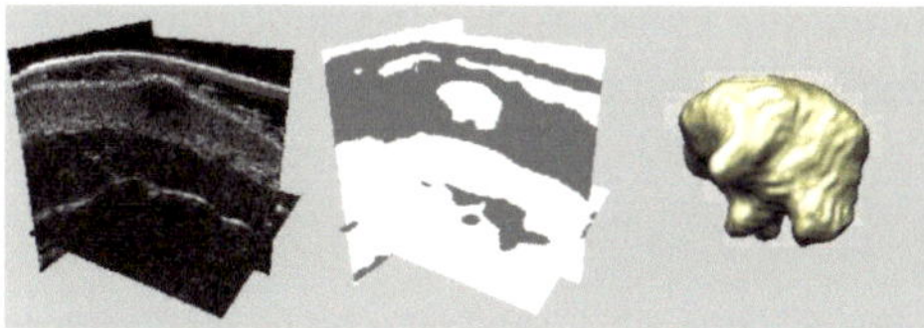

(a) Nevus, K=2

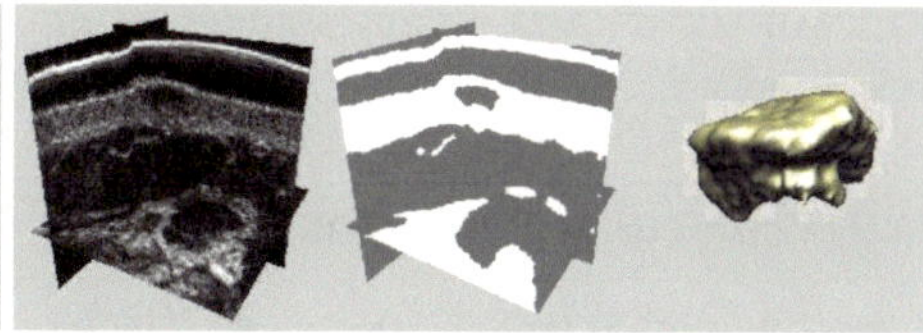

(b) Nevus, K=2

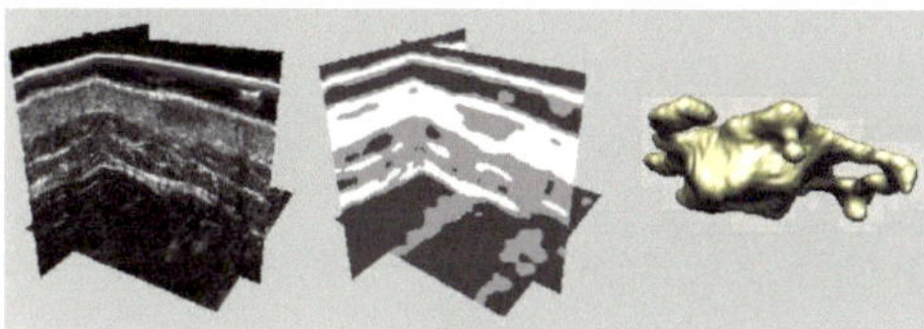

(c) Histiocytofibroma, K=3

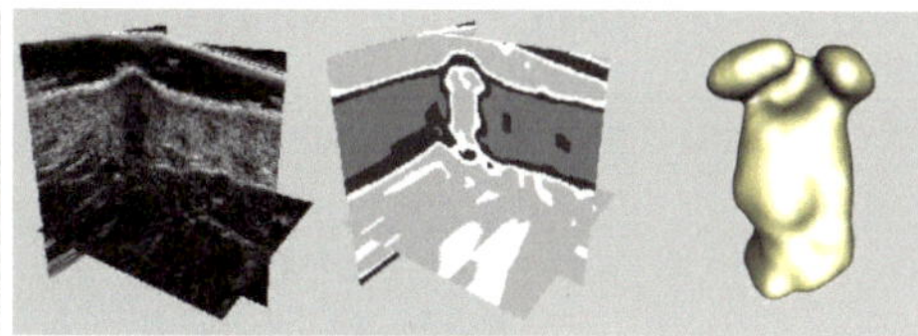

(d) Histiocytofibroma, K=4

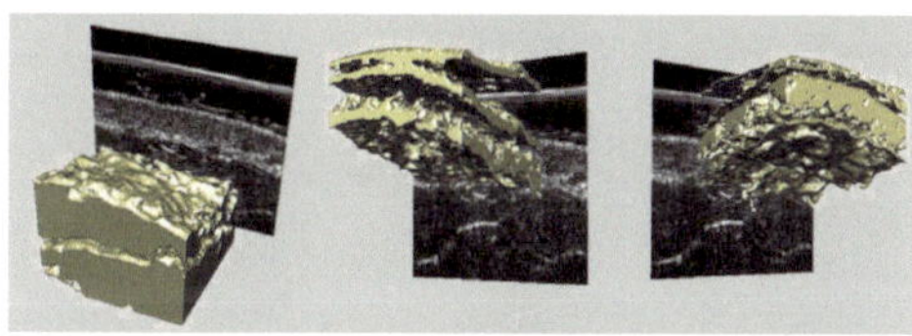

(e) Layers of the skin

Fig. 8. Segmentation of three-dimensional ultrasound images of the skin

in order to help specialists in their diagnostic, to track pathologies evolution or to carry out more precise extractions etc. With a clustering, all the voxels of an image are classified and it is possible to make a visualization of the different skin layers(figure 8(e)). For a specialist, this visualization is interesting because skin layers evolve according to the patient age and it is interesting to supervise the healing of a burned skin. This visualization is also of high interest for the evaluation of cosmetic product effects. To evaluate our results, the segmented images and their corresponding meshes have been presented to specialists in ultrasound images. The evaluation is only a qualitative one for the moment because producing ground truth for 3D images is a very hard task. Indeed, it is necessary to produce an expert segmentation for each two-dimensional cut (for example in z-axis direction) of a three-dimensional ultrasound image. With these set of two-dimensional ground truths it could be possible to construct a three-dimensional one but the gathering of the two-dimensional images could generate holes as well as precision problems. Thus, it stays difficult or even impossible to obtain a fine resolution for the evaluation.

## 5. Texture-based supervised active contours driven by a classifier for 3D ultrasound image segmentation

In this section, we present our second interactive texture-based model. The heart of the system is a 3D active contour, but for the user to easily deal with texture features, it has been chosen to guide the active contour segmentation with a supervised binary classifier. First, the principle of active contour segmentation will be presented. In a second part, we will describe the principle of supervised binary segmentation. Then, the complete segmentation process will be presented and finally, the segmentation software will be described.

### 5.1 Active contour segmentation

Initially developed by Kass et al. (1988), active contours are powerful segmentation approaches widely used in the segmentation field. An active contour is defined as a parametrized curve $\mathbf{C}$ mapping a parameter $s$ to a pixel $\mathbf{x}(s)$ in the image $\Omega$. The curve is initialized in $\Omega$ and evolves, under some constraints, according to its normal and tangential directions until it stops on the boundary of the object to be segmented. (see figure 9)

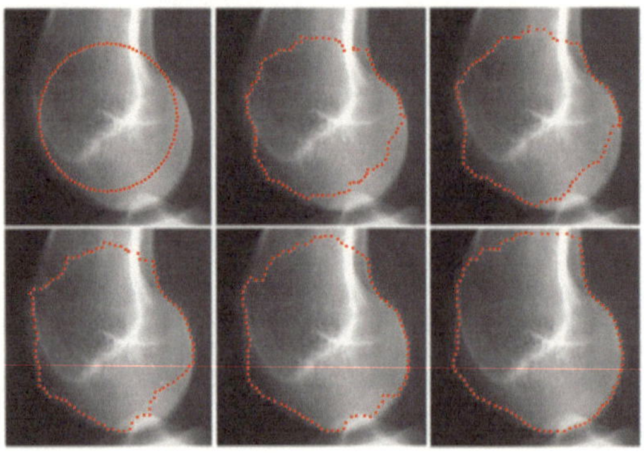

Fig. 9. Example of active contour segmentation

As the curve evolves in time, $\mathbf{C}(s,t)$ represents the family of curves obtained during the evolution. An energy is attached to the model and defined to control its evolution as:

$$E(\mathbf{C}(s,t)) = \int f(s,t)ds\,, \tag{9}$$

$f$ being a force composed of geometric criteria and external terms computed from the image (data terms). By minimizing (9), the model evolves until the final curve is placed on a position corresponding to a local minimum of $E$. Initially, the energy attached to the model was obtained by integrating $f$ only along the curve (Caselles et al. (1997); Xu & Prince (1998)). These models are called boundary-based but their application is restricted to objects whose boundaries can be defined by gradients and are not very efficient on complex images like textures. Later, region-based models emerged by integrating $f$ inside the curve or over the entire domain of $\Omega$ (Paragios & Deriche (2002); Zhu & Yuille (1996)).

Originally, Kass *et al* chose to represent the curve explicitly (the curve is sampled and its evolution is guided by several control points) but this prevents the model from handling topology changes without additional implementation. Yet, an implicit representation called the level set implementation emerged from the work of Osher and Sethian (Osher & Sethian (1988)). The main advantage of level sets is to allow the curve to handle topology changes automatically, as it can actually split or merge with others naturally. In order to implicitly represent a curve $\mathbf{C}$, it is necessary to define its evolution with a partial differential equation

(PDE or motion equation) such as:

$$\frac{\partial \mathbf{C}(s,t)}{\partial t} = F\mathbf{N}\,, \tag{10}$$

with $F$ the speed function of the model and $\mathbf{N}$ its inward normal vector.

PDE of models implicitly represented with level sets are usually deduced from the energy of the curve using Euler-Lagrange equations (Caselles et al. (1997); Zhu & Yuille (1996)), even though the first models were geometric ones, directly defined by their PDE (Caselles et al. (1993); Malladi et al. (1995)).

As the goal of the presented application was to ensure the most precise segmentation on 3D ultrasound images, the developed model is implicitly represented and uses Haralick texture features (Haralick et al. (1973)). Moreover, in order to let our model choose the best texture features, we introduce a supervised binary classifier in the motion equation of the active contour. The next section presents the principle of supervised binary classification. Details about the introduction of the classifier in the motion equation can be found in (Olivier et al. (2008)).

### 5.2 Supervised binary classification

The principle of supervised binary classification is to observe a learning dataset $\mathbf{X}$ composed of several samples such as $\mathbf{X} = \{\mathbf{x_1}, ..., \mathbf{x_n}\}$. For each sample $\mathbf{x_i} \in \mathbb{R}^m$, $i \in \{1, ..., n\}$, its $m$ features as well as the class to which its belongs are known and used to define a classification rule $\widehat{l} = f(\mathbf{x})$ allowing the classifier to automatically determine the class $\widehat{l}$ of each sample $\mathbf{x} \notin \mathbb{R}^m$.

In other words, given a set of already classified samples, a supervised classifier is able to determine the class of every unknown sample according to its features, automatically.

In the presented model, it has been chosen to give the classification task to a artificial neuron network (Rosenblatt (1958)).

The next section present the complete segmentation process.

### 5.3 Interactive segmentation process

As it as been presented in the previous section, using a supervised classifier requires the definition of a learning dataset composed of classified samples. As a consequence, our model evolves in two step. First, during an interactive step, an expert segmentation is carried out on one single slice of the 3D ultrasound image. The local Haralick texture features of some pixels from this segmentation are used to create the samples of a learning dataset, allowing the classifier to achieve its learning task. In a second step, a 3D active contour driven by this classifier is launched on the 3D image to carry out the desired segmentation. Figure 10 depicts the complete segmentation process. The extraction of the learning dataset is detailed in the following section.

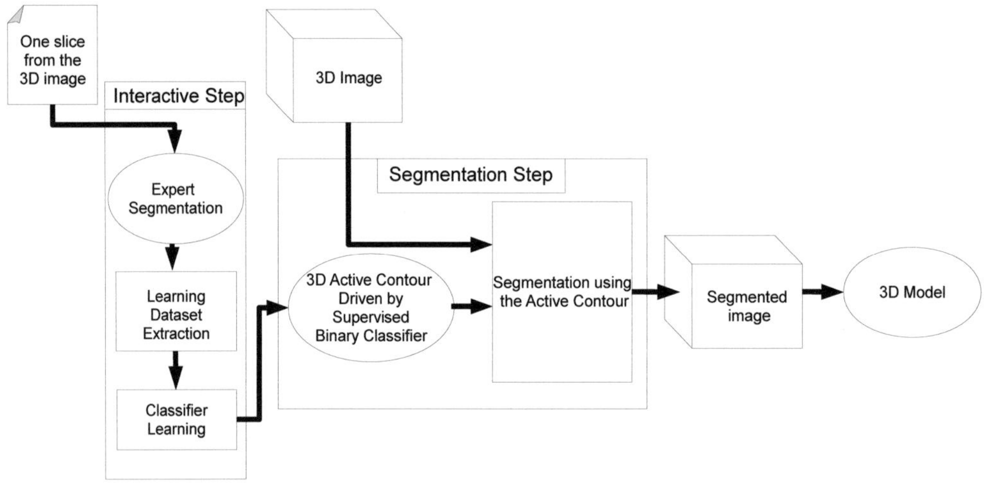


Fig. 10. The complete segmentation process: the expert segmentation is used to determine the learning dataset and to carry out the classifier's learning task. The segmentation is then launched on the 3D image.

### 5.3.1 Extraction of the learning dataset

During this step, one single slice $\Omega^*$ is extracted from the complete 3D utrasound image. Then, the user is asked to carry out an expert segmentation $C^*$. This segmentation must be composed of two ideal regions $C^{in}$ and $C^{out}$. $C^{in}$ will contain pixels from the object to be segmented while $C^{out}$ will be composed of pixels belonging to a narrow band surrounding $C^{in}$. Intuitively, $C^{in}$ should be taken as the interior of $C^*$ and $C^{out}$ as all the remaining image, giving $\Omega^* = C^{in} \cup C^{out}$. But in real images the region outside the segmented object is rarely homogeneous and sometimes even contains regions with textures very close to those of the inside region. Moreover, even if this phenomenon does not appear in $\Omega^*$, it can be present in other slices of the 3D image. This may involve a high variability in the textures from $C^{out}$ in the 3D image, making it hard for the classifier to correctly carry out its task. Thus, in order to maximize the distance between textures from $C^{in}$ and $C^{out}$ (giving a higher discriminant power to the Haralick texture features and to keep texture properties as constant as possible, we chose to define $C^{in}$ and $C^{out}$ as respectively the interior of $C^*$ and a narrow band giving homogeneous information about the boundary region of $C^*$.

Once the two regions determined, $m$ Haralick features are computed for each of their pixels. Thus, a learning dataset $\mathbf{X}$ composed of $n = n_1 + n_2$ samples, $n_1$ belonging to $C^{in}$ and $n_2$ belonging to $C^{out}$, is determined. $\forall i \in [1, n]$, a sample $s(i)$ will be described as:

$$s(i) = \{\ k_1(i), k_2(i) ... k_m(i), l(i)\},$$
$$l(i) = \begin{cases} -1 \text{ if } s(i) \text{ belongs to } C^{in} \\ 1 \text{ if } s(i) \text{ belongs to } C^{out}, \end{cases} \tag{11}$$

with $k_1(i), ..., k_m(i)$ the $m$ Haralick coefficients of the $i^{th}$ extracted pixel and $l(i)$ a label representing the region to which it belongs. Figure 11 shows an example of a manual segmentation carried out during the interactive step.

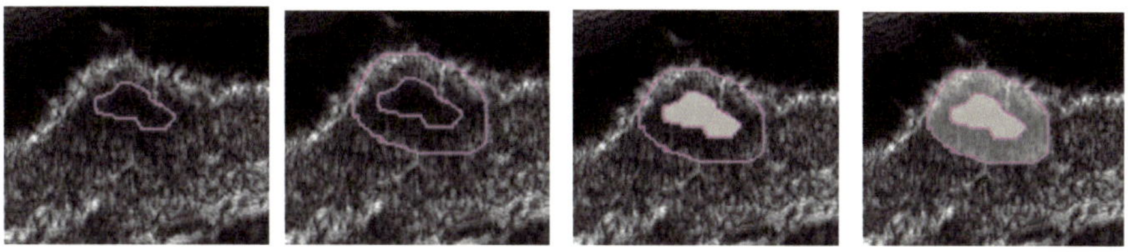

(a) (b) (c) (d)

Fig. 11. Example of expert segmentation. a): definition of $C^*$, b) definition of the narrow band, c) definition of $C^{in}$, d) definition of $C^{out}$.

#### 5.3.2 3D segmentation

Once the learning dataset is extracted, the automatic segmentation of the image is carried out. The learned classifier is used to guide the 3D active contour in the 3D image. The segmentation is stopped as the model reaches the boundaries of the object to be segmented. Once the segmentation is carried out, the final result is obtained by transforming the segmentation into a 3D mesh. Such a representation allows the user to easily understand the geometry of the object.

### 5.4 Segmentation software

#### 5.4.1 Interface

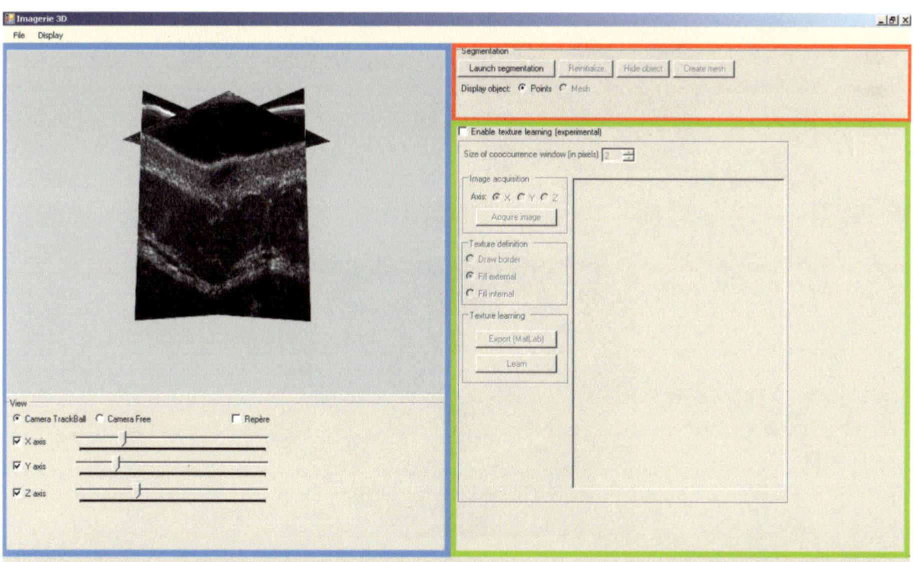


Fig. 12. The segmentation software interface.

The figure 12 presents the complete segmentation interface. The left part (blue square) is the visualization area. It allows the user to see the complete 3D ultrasound image. The red square in the right shows the segmentation command buttons while the green square surrounds the interactive part dealing with the manual segmentation and the supervised classification.

### 5.4.2 Interactive step

Once the 3D image is open, the user select one slice from it and carry out the manual segmentation (see fig 13.a). Then, the learning step of the artificial neural network is launched by pressing the "Learn" button. This step will allow the software to extract Haralick texture features and to determine the best ones.

### 5.4.3 Segmentation step

Now that the texture features have been determined, the 3D segmentation can be launched. When pressing the "Launch segmentation" button, the user will see the 3D active contour grow in the image until it stops on the boundaries of the object to be segmented (see figure 13.b). It can be noticed that the average segmentation duration is about half a minute on a common computer. The final step of the segmentation is the 3D reconstruction of the model.

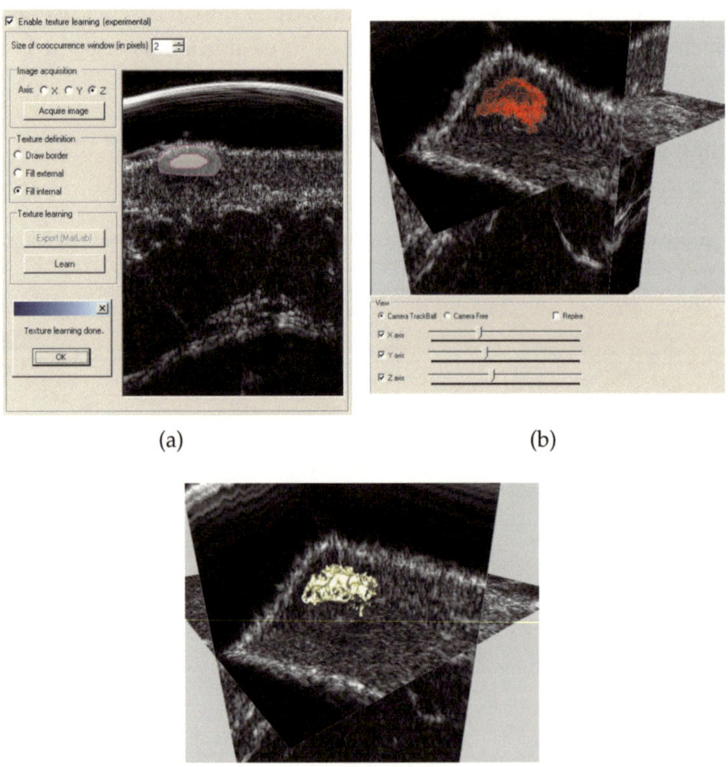


(a) (b)

(c)

Fig. 13. a) Interactive part of the software. b) 3D segmentation. c) 3D mesh

The segmentation can be turned into a 3D mesh by pressing the "Create mesh" button (see figure 13.c). Figures 14.a and 14.b shows other segmentation results. As it has been presented in section 4.3.2, numerically validating a 3D segmentation method is not easy as 3D ground truths are hard to obtain. As a consequence, all segmentation results have been presented to dermatologists and visually validated.

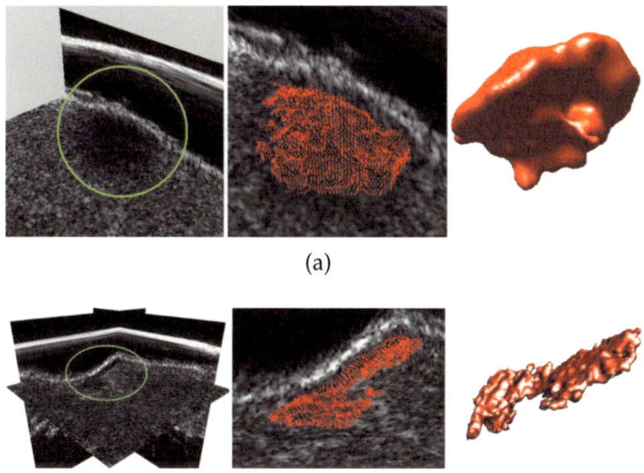

(a)

(b)

Fig. 14. Other segmentation results using the software.

## 6. Conclusion

In this chapter, two texture-based approaches for 3D ultrasound image segmentation have been presented. These methods have been developed for the user comfort and propose an important usability and interactivity.

In the first method a multiresolution scheme for volumetric texture segmentation have been defined. It includes perceptual features inspired by a human way to describe textures. The main interests of this approach are an easier way for an operator (specialist or not in image analysis) to select the relevant texture features to process an image and a better contents interpretation in a given application. We also presented psychological experiments that prove the strong correspondence between the proposed features and human perception of textures.

In the second approach, an interactive step is used where the user is asked to carry out a manual 2D segmentation on one single slice from the 3D image. Then, this segmentation is used to carry out the learning task of a supervised binary classifier. This last will determine the best texture features and will guide the segmentation of a 3D active contour among the 3D image, automatically. Thus, the major innovation of this work is to allow any non-expert user (in the image analysis domain) to achieve a texture-based segmentation. In some future work, this method will include more texture features in order to increase its adaptability.

Even if the applications presented in this chapter were focuses on ultrasound images, the two presented systems has also been successfully applied for the segmentation of MRI images as well as images obtained by confocal microscopy.

## 7. References


Amadasun, M. & King, R. (1989). Texture features corresponding to textural properties, *IEEE Transactions on Systems, Man, and Cybernetics* 19(5): 1264–1274.

Azencott, R., Wang, J.-P. & Younes, L. (1997). Texture classification using windowed Fourier filters, *IEEE Transactions on Pattern Analysis and Machine Intelligence* 19(2): 148–153.

Basset, O., Sun, Z., Mestas, J. & Gimenez, G. (1993). Texture analysis of ultrasonic images of the prostate by means of co-occurrence matrices, *Ultrasonic Imaging* 15: 218–237.

Boukerroui, D., Basset, O., Baskurt, A. & Gimenez, G. (2001). A multiparametric and multiresolution segmentation algorithm of 3-d ultrasonic data, *TUFFC '01: Proceedings of the IEEE transactions on ultrasonics, ferroelectrics, and frequency control*.

Caselles, V., Catte, F., Coll, T. & Dibos, F. (1993). A geometric model for active contours, *Numerishe Mathematik* 66: 1–31.

Caselles, V., Kimmel, R. & Sapiro, G. (1997). Geodesic active contours, *International Journal of Computer Vision* 22(1): 61–79.

Coleman, G. & Andrews, H. (1979). Image segmentation by clustering, *Proceedings of the IEEE*, pp. 773–785.

Goyal, R., Goh, W., Mital, D. & Chan, K. (1995). Scale and rotation invariant texture analysis based on structural property, *IECON '95: Proceedings of the International Conference on Industrial Electronics, Control, and Instrumentation*.

Grégoire, J.-M., Serrière, S., Georgesco, G., Jamet, F., Bleuzen, A., Ossant, F., Levassort, F., Tranquart, F. & Patat, F. (2006). Techniques et applications de l'échographie haute résolution non invasive, *Journal de Radiologie* 87: 1920–1936.

Haralick, R. M., Shanmugam, K. & Dinstein, I. (1973). Texture features for image classification, *IEEE Transactions on Systems, Man, and Cybernetics* 3(6): 610–621.

Julesz, B. (1975). *Experiments in the visual perception of texture*, Vol. 232, Scientific American.

Kass, M., Witkin, A. & Terzopoulos, D. (1988). Snakes: active contour models, *International Journal of Computer Vision* 1(4): 321–331.

Kopf, J., Fu, C.-W., Cohen-Or, D., Deussen, O., Lischinski, D. & Wong, T.-T. (2007). Solid texture synthesis from 2d exemplars, *SIGGRAPH '07: Proceedings of the 34th International Conference on Computer Graphics and Interactive Techniques*.

Li, S. Z. (1995). *Markov Random Field Modeling in Computer Vision*, Springer-Verlag New York, Inc.

Malladi, R., Sethian, J. A. & Vemuri, B. C. (1995). Shape modeling with front propagation: a level set approach, *IEEE Transactions on Pattern Analysis and Machine Intelligence* 17(2): 158–175.

Mallat, S. G. (1989). A theory for multiresolution signal decomposition: the wavelet representation, *IEEE Transactions on Pattern Analysis and Machine Intelligence* 11: 674–693.

Mandelbrot, B. B. (1977). *Fractals, Forms, Chance and Dimension*, Freeman, San Fransisco.

Noble, J. A. & Boukerroui, D. (2006). Ultrasound image segmentation: A survey, *IEEE Transactions on Medical Imaging* 25(8): 987–1010.

Ojala, T., Pietikäinen, M. & Harwood, D. (1996). A comparative study of texture measures with classification based on feature distributions, *Pattern Recognition* 29(1): 51–59.

Olivier, J., Rousselle, J.-J., Boné, R. & Cardot, H. (2008). Active contours driven by supervised binary classifiers for texture segmentation, *the 4th International Symposium on Visual Computing : ISVC 08*, Las Vegas, Nevada.

Osher, S. & Sethian, J. A. (1988). Fronts propagation with curvature-dependent speed: algorithms based on Hamilton-Jacobi formulations, *Journal of Computational Physics* 79: 12–49.

Otsu, N. & Kurita, T. (1988). A new scheme for practical flexible and intelligent vision systems, *IAPR Workshop on Computer Vision*, Tokyo, Japan, pp. 431–435.

Paragios, N. & Deriche, R. (2002). Geodesic active regions and level set methods for supervised texture segmentation, *International Journal of Computer Vision* 46(3): 223–247.

Paulhac, L., Makris, P., Gregoire, J.-M. & Ramel, J.-Y. (2009). Human understandable features for segmentation of solid texture, *ISVC '09: Proceedings of the 5th International Symposium on vision computing*, pp. 379–390.

Paulhac, L., Makris, P. & Ramel, J.-Y. (2009). A solid texture database for segmentation and classification experiments, *VISSAPP '09: Proceedings of the Fourth International Conference on Computer Vision Theory and Applications*.

Richards, W. & Polit, A. (1974). Texture matching, *Kibernetic* 16: 155–162.

Rosenblatt, F. (1958). The perceptron: A theory of statistical separability in cognitive systems, *Technical report VG-1196-G-1* M. A. Cornell Aeronautical Laboratory.

Sahiner, B., Chan, H.-P., Roubidoux, M. A., Helvie, M. A., Hadjiiski, L. M., Ramachandran, A., Paramagul, C., LeCarpentier, G. L., Nees, A. & Blane, C. (2004). Computerized characterization of breast masses on three-dimensional ultrasound volumes, *Medical Physics* 31: 744–754.

Shamos, M. I. & Hoey, D. (1975). Closest-point problems, *the* $16^{th}$ *Annual Symposium on Foundations of Computer Science* pp. 131–162.

Shoshany, M. (2008). An evolutionary patch pattern approach for texture discrimination, *Pattern Recognition* 41: 2327–2336.

Tamura, H., Mori, S. & Yamawaki, T. (1978). Texture features corresponding to visual perception, *IEEE Transactions on Systems, Man, and Cybernetics* 8(6): 460–473.

Tuceryan, M. & Jain, A. K. (1993). *Texture analysis*, World Scientific Publishing Co., Inc., River Edge, NJ, USA, pp. 235–276.

Turner, M. R. (1986). Texture discrimination by Gabor functions, *Biological Cybernetics* 55: 443–457.

Valckx, M. J. F. & Thijssen, J. M. (1997). Characterization of echographic image texture by cooccurrence matrix parameters, *Ultrasound in Medicine and Biology* 23(4): 559–571.

Voorhees, H. & Poggio, T. (1987). Detecting textons and texture boundaries in natural images, *proceedings of the International Conference on Computer Vision (ICCV87)*, London, England, pp. 250–258.

Xu, C. & Prince, J. (1998). Snakes, shapes, and gradient vector flow, *IEEE Transactions on Image Processing* 7(3): 359–369.

Zhan, Y. & Shen, D. (2003). Automated segmentation of 3d us prostate images using statistical texture-based matching method, *MICCAI '03: Proceedings of the International Conference on Medical Image Computing and Computer-Assisted Intervention*.

Zhan, Y. & Shen, D. (2006). Deformable segmentation of 3d ultrasound prostate image using statistical texture matching method, *IEEE Transactions on Medical Imaging* 25(3): 256–272.

Zhang, J. & Tan, T. (2002). Brief review of invariant texture analysis methods, *Pattern Recognition* 35: 735–747.

Zhu, S. & Yuille, A. (1996). Region competition: unifying snake/balloon, region growing, and Bayes/MDL/energy for multi-band image segmentation, *IEEE Transactions on Pattern Analysis and Machine Intelligence* 18(9): 884–900.

Zucker, S. W. (1976). Toward a model of texture, *Computer Graphics and Image Processing* 5: 190–202.

# 4

# Radiation Protection in Medical Imaging

Horațiu Colosi[1], Dan Colosi[2], Vlad Mureşan[3] and Marius Roman[3]
[1]*Iuliu Hațieganu University of Medicine and Pharmacy, Cluj-Napoca*
[2]*State University of New York, School of Dental Medicine, Stony Brook, New York*
[3]*Technical University, Cluj-Napoca*
[1,3]*Romania*
[2]*USA*

## 1. Introduction

Life on Earth has developed continuously in the presence of natural radiation. Radiation is a form of energy transfer through space and matter. The ability of radiation to transfer energy at the molecular level to living organisms is at the root of current efforts to understand and limit the effects of radiation on humans.

The radiation spectrum includes forms of radiation that carry various energy levels. Radiation forms, such as x-radiation, which carry sufficient energy to overcome binding energies of electrons and to eject them from their atomic orbits, can cause the formation of ions in the matter through which they travel, and are termed ionizing radiation. Ionizing radiation may also dissociate molecular bonds, leading to the formation of free radicals.

### 1.1 Biologic effects of ionizing radiation

A great proportion of the effects of ionizing radiation on living matter are a result of the interaction of these forms of radiation with water, a ubiquitous molecule that is present in most tissues and organs. This interaction leads to the generation of highly reactive radical species, mainly from the hydroxyl and hydroperoxyl categories, which, in turn, can interact with cellular DNA, leading to the formation of strand breaks and base damage (Hall & Giaccia 2005). To a lesser extent, radiation can also directly ionize or damage DNA and other biologic molecules: RNA, proteins, lipids. Many occurrences of damage limited to one DNA strand are rapidly detected by the surveillance mechanisms of the cell and the DNA integrity is restored using the intact complementary DNA strand as template. However, double-strand breaks, in which an intact DNA template is not available, are more difficult to repair accurately (Mladenov & Iliakis 2011). As a result, radiation-induced DNA double strand breaks may often lead to misrepaired DNA, resulting in point mutations, deletions or chromosomal translocations. Radiation-induced DNA damage that escapes detection by cell cycle checkpoints during cellular mitosis can result in an uncontrolled, accelerated rate of mitotic division of the affected cell (Hall & Giaccia 2005), a cellular hallmark of cancer. The association between exposure to radiation and cancer induction is well documented through epidemiological studies (Ron 2003).

### 1.2 Radiation doses

Various quantities are used to describe the radiation dose to organisms and the resulting risk. The absorbed dose refers to the radiation energy absorbed by tissues per unit of mass. It is measured in grays (Gy), with 1 gray equivalent to 1 joule of radiation energy absorbed per kilogram.

The effective dose accounts for the type of radiation and the biologic tissue that is exposed, by applying a radiation weighting factor and a tissue-weighting factor to the absorbed dose. The radiation-weighting factor of x-radiation is one. Tissue weighting factors have been assigned to various tissues and organs based on their estimated susceptibility to radiation damage. The effective dose, measured in Sieverts (Sv), is used to estimate risks from radiation exposure. For exposures to limited parts of the body, as is often the case in medical imaging, the calculated effective dose is equivalent to the whole body exposure that carries the same risk.

| | **Effective radiation dose (μSv)** | **Background Equivalent (days)** |
|---|---|---|
| Cosmic radiation | 390 | 59 |
| Radon and other radioactive gases | 1260 | 190 |
| Other terrestrial radiation | 770 | 116 |
| **Total natural** | **2.420** | 1 year |
| Medical exposure | **600** | 90 |
| **Total annual average dose** | **3020** | 455 |

Table 1. Sources of natural radiation and their average contribution to human exposure (adapted from United Nations Scientific Committee on the Effects of Atomic Radiation Report 2008)

Natural radiation contributes approximately 2.4 milliSieverts (mSv) annually to the average human radiation exposure of 3.0 mSv (United Nations Scientific Committee on the Effects of Atomic Radiation [UNSCEAR] Report 2008). Main natural sources of ionizing radiation are cosmic radiation, mainly from the sun and other stars, and terrestrial radiation, originating from naturally occurring radioactive elements (table 1).

Because the Earth's atmosphere acts as a radiation absorber and attenuator, exposure to cosmic radiation is greatly impacted by altitude. The exposure value to cosmic radiation at sea level approximately doubles with each 2000 m of elevation. While the yearly exposure to cosmic radiation at sea level is on average 0.24 mSv, at an altitude of 1600 m it is approximately 0.5 mSv. Similarly, airplane travel contributes to radiation exposure in the general population, with doses estimated to approximately 0.025 mSv for every 5 hours flown at 12,000 m (White & Pharoah, 2009).

Terrestrial radiation includes that originating from radionuclides in the soil, such as potassium 40, uranium 238 and thorium 232, some of which are taken up by ingestion. Together, these sources result in an annual dose of approximately 0.8 mSv. However, the main single source of natural radiation exposure is radon, a gas and uranium decay product, which contributes roughly 50% of the total natural radiation exposure to the general population (table 1). Radon may enter buildings through imperfectly sealed foundations and tends to accumulate in basements, from where it may leak into adjacent living spaces. Its radioactive decay products are inhaled, taking residence in the respiratory epithelium and contributing to the occurrence of lung cancer. Radiation exposure from radon varies widely with the geologic composition throughout the world.

Human activity has led to the development of new sources of radiation over the past decades. Medical radiation is the greatest peaceful contributor to radiation exposure in the general population, with an average annual effective dose of approximately 0.6 mSv (table 1).

## 2. Radiation exposure and current practices for radiation protection

### 2.1 Radiation exposure in diagnostic imaging

Medical use of radiation has increased continuously throughout the world, irrespective of the economic level of various regions. While therapeutic use of radiation in the treatment of cancer contributes a significant amount of radiation to a small number of individuals, the use of diagnostic radiation imparts a smaller amount of radiation to a large, and constantly growing, number of individuals.

The development of computed tomography (CT) over the past few decades has revolutionized diagnostic imaging. Its use has increased exponentially, and it is estimated that in the United States more than 62 million CT scans have been performed in 2006, compared to less than 20 million in 1995, and just 3 million in 1980 (Brenner & Hall, 2007). Due to the relatively higher radiation dose from a typical CT scan compared to that from conventional imaging modalities (table 2), and due to its widespread and increasing use, medical CT is currently estimated to contribute a significant amount of radiation exposure to the general population.

| | **Effective Dose (μSv)** | **Background Equivalent (days)** |
|---|---|---|
| Head plain radiograph | 27 - 100 | **4 - 15** |
| Dental radiographs (set of 19-20) * | 33 - 150 | **5 - 23** |
| Chest plain radiographs (PA + lateral) | 100 - 290 | **15 - 44** |
| Mammography | 230 - 400 | **35 - 123** |
| Abdomen plain radiograph | 370 - 810 | **56 - 123** |
| Head computed tomography | 900 - 2800 | **137 - 426** |
| Abdomen and pelvis computed tomography | 3100 - 15300 | **1.3 - 6.4 years** |

Table 2. Medical diagnostic imaging procedures and their contribution range to patients' radiation exposure (data: United Nations Scientific Committee on the Effects of Atomic Radiation Report 2008, * White and Pharoah, 2009)

Due to the large number of CT scans being administered in the present, and the trend of this number to increase in the future, radiation exposure from CT may gain significance as a public health concern (Brenner and Hall, 2007).

As a result, current radiation safety efforts carry a significant focus on monitoring and limiting medical radiation exposure from CT to the general population.

### 2.2 Radiation protection measures in diagnostic imaging

The main concern from medical imaging involving ionizing radiation is the risk of cancer induction. Radiation-induced cancer may occur at any time, including after decades, following the radiation exposure event, and, if it occurs, it is indistinguishable from spontaneously induced cancer.

The progressive understanding of biologic effects of radiation led to the development of guidelines for radiation protection by the international community. Evidence-based guidelines are outlined in the 2007 Recommendations of the International Commission for Radiological Protection (International Commission for Radiological Protection, 2007) and in the recommendations of the National Council on Radiation Protection and Measurements (NCRP) of the United States (Kase 2004).

The overarching goal of radiation protection in medical diagnostic imaging is to obtain a maximum of information relevant to the diagnostic task with the least amount of exposure to ionizing radiation (White & Pharoah, 2009). In practice, economic and individual factors, such as availability or access to imaging modalities of choice must also be taken into account.

The application in diagnostic imaging of this principle, also referred to "As Low As Reasonably Achievable" (ALARA), involves the implementation of general protective measures, including the following:

1. Imaging decision. Selection of the imaging examination to answer a specific diagnostic question should take into consideration all modalities that are likely to provide the sought information. When the diagnostic question can be answered through a study that involves no ionizing radiation - such as magnetic resonance or ultrasound imaging - the added radiation dose from the diagnostic procedure is reduced to zero. The selection of the imaging modality involving exposure to ionizing radiation should follow a justification process based on the patients' individual clinical circumstances and on scientific evidence. This process should suggest that the potential diagnostic benefit of the examination outweighs the estimated risk carried by the specific radiation exposure. Decision support software, which can assist the clinician in determining the appropriateness of a given imaging study to the clinical situation, has recently become available (Rosenthal et al., 2006). Preliminary studies have suggested that its utilization can contribute to the decreased prescription of examinations that are deemed of "low-utility" to the diagnostic task (Coakley et al., 2011).
2. Patient information: Providing easy-to-understand information to patients is an effective measure for bringing radiation exposure into context and for dispelling exaggerated fear of radiation in patients. Radiation doses from medical examinations can be compared with the amount of background radiation to which we are all exposed by living on Earth (see table 2). Risk comparison with common daily activities, such as driving or air travel, may also be effective (Coakley et al., 2011). For instance, travelling 64,000 km by car is associated with a risk of death from a motor vehicle accident of approximately 1:2000 in the United States (National Highway Traffic Safety Administration Fatality Analysis Reporting System, 2011). This risk is roughly equal to the risk of developing a fatal cancer from an effective radiation dose of 10 mSv, a dose five times higher than that from a typical CT scan of the head.

3. Shielding of the examination room, to limit or eliminate radiation exposure to neighbouring areas;
4. Shielding the patient's anatomic areas that are not in the region of interest of the examination, to reduce radiation exposure to sensitive organs, such as the thyroid, gonads, eye lens;
5. Filtration of the x-ray beam, which removes low energy photons that would otherwise be absorbed by the patient, and hence would not contribute to the radiographic image;
6. Optimal film-screen combinations that maximize photon-to-image conversion, while achieving the image quality required for the diagnostic task;
7. Appropriate x-ray source –to-skin distance, whenever this factor is adjustable;
8. Collimation of the exposed field strictly to the region of interest;
9. Optimal combination of exposure factors (kVp, mA, seconds) to achieve low radiation doses, while maintaining diagnostic image quality;
10. Quality assurance of the imaging and film processing equipment, to ensure consistent optimal quality of images with minimum exposure to patients and personnel.
11. Personal dose monitors and area dose monitors that assist in documenting individual exposure and area radiation levels. Personal dose monitors used in clinical practice include thermoluminescent dosimeters (TLD) and, more recently, optically stimulated dosimeters (OSLD). TLDs use lithium fluoride or calcium sulphate crystals laced with magnesium, titanium, copper or phosphorus impurities, which store the energy from radiation to which they are subjected. When the crystals are heated, the stored energy is released as luminescence proportional to the radiation exposure. While TLDs are small and they allow measurements of radiation doses ranging from microGy to kGy, accurate and reproducible readings are heavily technique-dependent (Kron 1994). OSLDs use aluminium oxide laced with carbon impurities to store radiation energy, which is released as luminescence proportional to the radiation exposure in response to stimulation light. OSLDs have a linear dose-response relationship in the 1-300 cGy range but can be calibrated for a significantly wider range of radiation exposures that are relevant in medical imaging (Jursinic 2007, Yukihara, 2008).

Due to the exponential growth in its utilization and its higher radiation effective dose compared to plain film radiographs, computed tomography (CT) is one of the most significant contributors to medical diagnostic radiation exposure today. While many of the general principles outlined above apply to CT as well, several measures specific to CT can be implemented to reduce patients' radiation risk:

1. Bismuth shields are used in the exposure path in front of sensitive organs, such as the breast. They partially absorb the direct radiation beam to underlying anatomic structures, without significantly impacting the image quality of adjacent structures. Bismuth shields can reduce radiation dose to the adult female breast by up to 40% (Yilmaz et al., 2007). However, when bismuth shields are used together with automatic exposure modulation, the latter may compensate for the radiation attenuation caused by the shield, offsetting the radiation savings benefits of the shield. To circumvent this situation, bismuth shields may be applied after exposure of the scout view, and before acquisition of the volumetric data (Coakley et al., 2011).
2. Optimization of CT imaging protocols involves tailoring imaging protocols to the patient and the diagnostic task. The radiation dose can be modified by adjusting one or several scan parameters:

i. The maximum tube electric potential (kVp): while the typical exposure setting used in routine CT scanning is between 100 and 140 kVp, a lower kVP can reduce radiation dose, albeit at the expense of increased image noise.
ii. Tube current (mA): a CT scan conducted with lower mA results in noisier images, but radiation exposure is diminished by an amount proportional to the decreased tube current.

Lower values can be selected for both parameters when scanning children or small adults, or in cases in which noisier images are unlikely to have a significant impact on the diagnostic task outcome (e.g. a study to evaluate renal calculi).

3. X-ray tube current modulation and automatic exposure control refer to systems in which the user (the radiologist, through the radiological technologist) indicates the desired level of image quality, based on which the CT software calculates the radiation output required to match that image quality in all regions of the scanned volume (McCollough et al., 2005). During acquisition of each sectional image, as the gantry rotates around the patient, angular tube current modulation works to modulate x-ray tube current to equalize the average photon flux reaching the detectors (x-, y-axis tube current modulation). As the patient progresses through the gantry, longitudinal (z-axis) tube current modulation acts to maintain constant image noise levels along the longitudinal axis of the patient as body regions with different attenuation properties are scanned (McCollough et al., 2005).
4. Enhanced CT reconstruction algorithms: most current CT scanners utilize reconstruction algorithms based on the filtered back-projection (FBP) method. When used in combination with low tube currents, this method tends to generate noisy images. The implicit radiation exposure threshold, below which the diagnostic image quality decreases to unacceptable levels, limits the potential for radiation savings with FBP reconstruction algorithms. Alternative solutions include iterative reconstruction algorithms, based on complex mathematical models that aim to correct the noise in images acquired with low tube currents. These algorithms are computation-intensive and lead to longer reconstruction times (Coakley et al., 2011). A recent, enhanced, iterative reconstruction method, known as adaptive statistical iterative reconstruction (ASIR), shows great promise for improved reconstruction speeds. Furthermore, by attempting to identify and correct for photon flux fluctuations that are unlikely to be caused by anatomic features, ASIR can reduce image noise, as well as certain types of image artefacts (Marin et al., 2010, Miéville et al., 2011, Renker et al., 2011). As a result, images reconstructed using ASIR from raw data acquired with low tube current may show similar or improved image quality compared to FBP reconstructions, while low current settings allow radiation savings in the range of 32-65% for a variety of clinical utilization scenarios (Cornfeld et al., 2011, Flicek et al., 2010, Hara et al., 2009). Together, these characteristics of ASIR protocols may lead to CT studies of overall similar or better diagnostic quality compared to FBP reconstruction methods, with a potential for significantly reduced patient radiation exposure.
5. Calculation and reporting of radiation dose: Most CT scanners have the integrated capability to calculate radiation exposure as a dose-length product (measured in mGy/cm), which can be recorded in the patient's clinical record. This facilitates tracking CT radiation exposure to patients.

## 3. Modelling and simulation for radiation control of imaging devices

### 3.1 Preliminaries

Automated control of radiation field intensity generated during medical imaging and radiation therapy, constitutes an efficient method to reduce unnecessary radiation exposure for both patients and device operators (Sajin et al., 2003, McCollough et al., 2006).

This heading presents an original method for automated control of radiation field intensity. Its implementation in medical imaging devices employing ionizing radiation can offer important exposure savings to both patients and medical personnel.

The goal of this study has been to develop an original and flexible model for radiation field control, in order to allow an exact administration of the minimum necessary radiation dose at any desired tissue depth, even through non-homogeneous tissue layers that intensify or attenuate the electromagnetic field generated by an imaging device. Therefore, we modelled and simulated the spread of radiation through non-homogeneous media, as is the case when using medical imaging devices to investigate human tissues.

A general model of radiation field spread using Cartesian coordinates (0p; 0q; 0r) can be represented as seen in figure 1. Patterns of spread have been considered, in relation to three spatial axes and in relation to time (t).

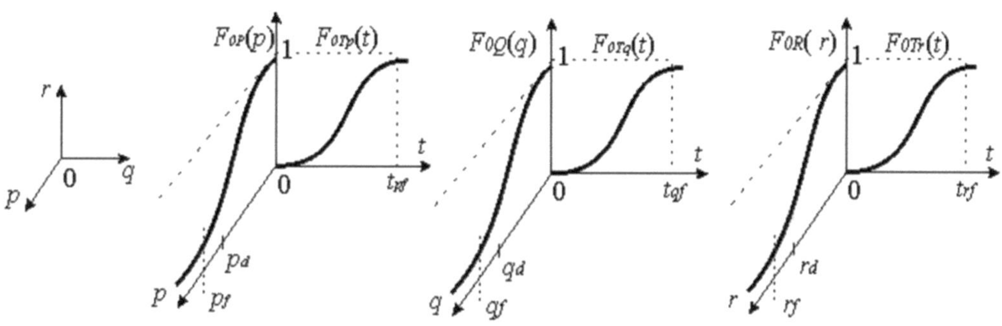


Fig. 1. General model of radiation field intensity, y(t, p, q, r) in Cartesian coordinates

Radiation field intensity y(t, p, q, r) shown in figures 1b, 1c, and 1d, can be expressed as:

$$y(t,p,q,r)=y_{00}[t,s,u(t)]=K_y \times F_{0T}(t) \times F_{0S}(s) \times u(t) \tag{1}$$

The output variable y=y[t, s, u(t)] is the intensity of the radiation field, u(t) is the input (command) signal applied for the radiation source, Ky is a weighting coefficient and (2) stands for the usual form of compression of the Cartesian space variable on the axes of coordinates (0p), (0q) and (0r), as illustrated in figure 2.

$$s=\pm\sqrt{p^2+q^2+r^2};\quad s_f=\pm\sqrt{p_f{}^2+q_f{}^2+r_f{}^2} \tag{2}$$

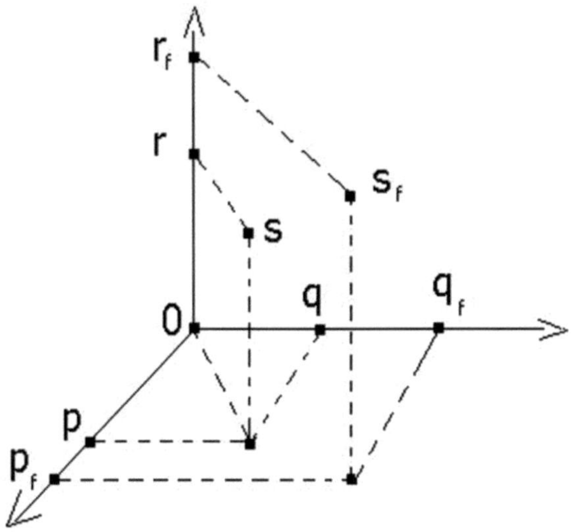


Fig. 2. Cartesian coordinates system and Cartesian space variable (s)

$$F_{0S}(s)=\pm\sqrt{F_{0P}^{\,2}(p)+F_{0Q}^{\,2}(q)+F_{0R}^{\,2}(r)} \tag{3}$$

where:

$$F_{0P}(p)=\frac{P_1}{P_1-P_2}\times\varepsilon^{-\frac{abs(p)}{P1}}+\frac{P_2}{P_2-P_1}\times\varepsilon^{-\frac{abs(p)}{P2}} \tag{4}$$

$$F_{0Q}(q)=\frac{Q_1}{Q_1-Q_2}\times\varepsilon^{-\frac{abs(q)}{Q1}}+\frac{Q_2}{Q_2-Q_1}\times\varepsilon^{-\frac{abs(q)}{Q2}} \tag{5}$$

$$F_{0R}(r)=\frac{R_1}{R_1-R_2}\times\varepsilon^{-\frac{abs(r)}{R1}}+\frac{R_2}{R_2-R_1}\times\varepsilon^{-\frac{abs(r)}{R2}} \tag{6}$$

The axes (0p) and (0q) define the horizontal plane, in which the electromagnetic field generator is located. Field intensity expressed in (1), and axis (0r) correspond to the depth of field propagation. The constants in (4), (5) and (6) can be approximated by expert procedures, namely:

$$P_1=\frac{p_f}{\mu_P(1+\lambda_P)}\ ;\ P_2=\lambda_P\times P_1,\ \text{where: } \mu_P=(4\div 6) \text{ and } \lambda_P>1 \tag{7}$$

$$Q_1=\frac{q_f}{\mu_Q(1+\lambda_Q)}\ ;\ Q_2=\lambda_Q\times Q_1,\ \text{where: } \mu_Q=(4\div 6) \text{ and } \lambda_Q>1 \tag{8}$$

$$R_1=\frac{r_f}{\mu_R(1+\lambda_R)}\ ;\ R_2=\lambda_R\times R_1,\ \text{where: } \mu_R=(4\div 6) \text{ and } \lambda_R>1 \tag{9}$$

in which the final abscises $(p_f)$, $(q_f)$, $(r_f)$ correspond to negligible values (for example ≤ 0.05). For $F_{0P}(p)$, $F_{0Q}(q)$, $F_{0R}(r)$, the abscises $(p_d)$, $(q_d)$, $(r_d)$ may show disturbances due to discontinuities in tissue structure, estimated by:

$$F_{0S}(s)=\frac{S_1}{S_1-S_2}\times\varepsilon^{-\frac{abs(s)}{S1}}+\frac{S_2}{S_2-S_1}\times\varepsilon^{-\frac{abs(s)}{S2}} \tag{10}$$

where

$$S_1=\frac{s_f}{\mu_S\times(1+\lambda_S)};\quad S_2=\lambda_S\times S_1 \tag{11}$$

$$\mu_S=\frac{p_f+q_f+r_f}{\frac{p_f}{\mu_P}+\frac{q_f}{\mu_Q}+\frac{r_f}{\mu_R}};\quad \lambda_S=\frac{P_2+Q_2+R_2}{P_1+Q_1+R_1} \tag{12}$$

Therefore, $F_{0S}(s)$ can also be written:

$$F_{0S}(s)=\frac{1}{1-\lambda_S}\times\left[\varepsilon^{-\frac{\mu S(1+\lambda S)}{sf}\times abs(s)}-\lambda_S\times\varepsilon^{-\frac{\mu S(1+\lambda S)}{sf}\times abs(s)}\right] \tag{13}$$

or

$$F_{0S}(s)=C_0\times\left(\varepsilon^{C1\times\sqrt{p^2+q^2+r^2}}+C_2\times\varepsilon^{C3\sqrt{p^2+q^2+r^2}}\right) \tag{14}$$

in which

$$C_0=\frac{1}{1-\lambda_S};\quad C_1=\frac{\mu_S(1+\lambda_S)}{s_f};\quad C_2=-\lambda_S;\quad C_3=\frac{1}{\lambda_S}\times C_1 \tag{15}$$

The results of $F_{0S}(s)$ in (4), (10), (13) and (14) also represent spatial curves deformed by multiple degrees of freedom, for example $(\mu_S)$, $(\lambda_S)$ and $(s_f)$, while the "length constants" (P...), (Q...) and (R...) may exhibit "inertia" or "attenuation" of radiation field propagation through different tissue layers.

Function components $F_{0P}(p)$, $F_{0Q}(q)$ or $F_{0R}(r)$ can be approximated by:

$$F_{0vd}(v)=A_{vd}\times\varepsilon^{-Kvd(vd-v)^2} \tag{16}$$

in which variable (v) becomes (p), (q) or (r), according to case.

The disturbance index (d) refers to the homogeneity disturbance due to tissue heterogeneity located on the abscissa $(v_d)$, while $(A_{vd})$ in (16) represents the amplitude of heterogeneity illustrated in figure 3.a.

A more or less steep, respectively a more or less symmetrical slope can result from the convenient choice of parameter $(K_{vd})$. The deformation effect of function $F_{0vd}(v)$ on the right abscissa $(v_d)$ over the component $F_{0v}(v)$ can be seen in figure 3.b.

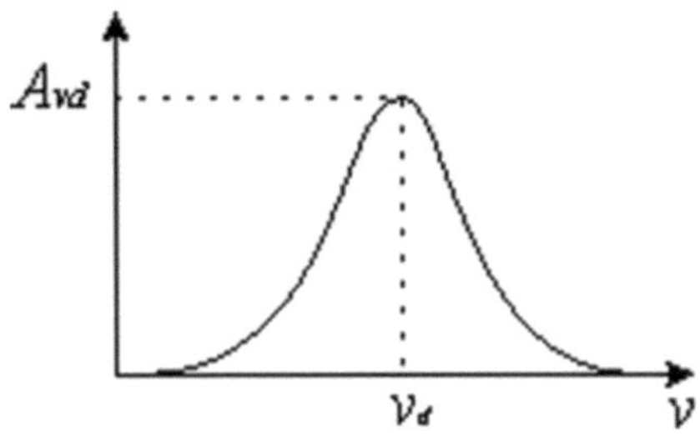


**a.** Amplitude

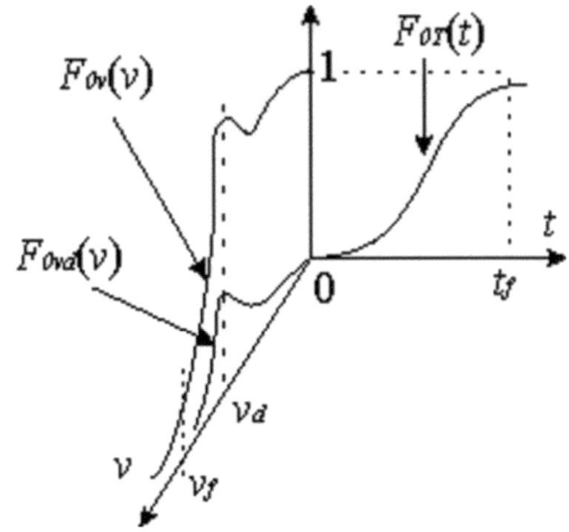


**b.** Trajectory in Cartesian space

Fig. 3. Tissue heterogeneity may lead to homogeneity disturbances of field intensity

If, with respect to time, the spread of radiation field intensity y(t,p,q,r) is identical on all three axes (0p), (0q) and (0r) depicted in figures 1a, 1b and 1c, then:

$$F_{0Tp}(t)=F_{0Tq}(t)=F_{0Tr}(t)=F_{0T}(t) \tag{17}$$

which may also be approximated as a customary form of step response, related to a control signal u(t) applied to the radiation source.

Thus:

$$F_{0T}(t)=1-\frac{T_1}{T_1-T_2}\times\varepsilon^{-\frac{t}{T1}}-\frac{T_2}{T_2-T_1}\times\varepsilon^{-\frac{t}{T2}} \tag{18}$$

The final values $(p_f,q_f,r_f,v_f)$ in figures 1a, 1b, 1c, 2 and 3 show the depth of radiation field penetration, which will depend on this control signal u(t) and on the more or less homogeneous structure of the tissue. The length $(t_f)$ of this transient phenomenon (figure 4) reflects a radiation propagation inertia, identical on axes (p, q, r, s) for which $t>t_f$ tends to a unitary asymptote.

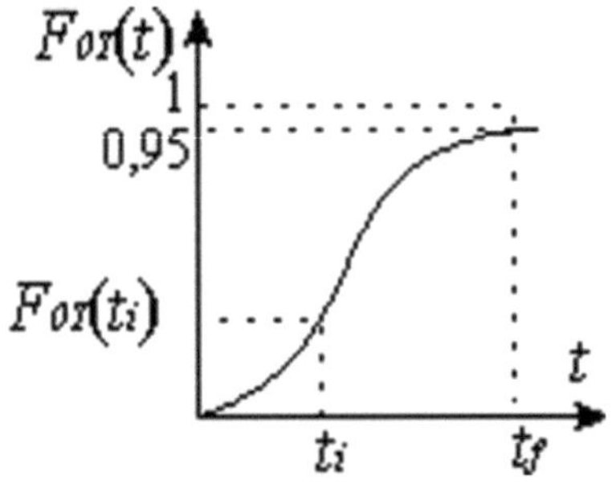


Fig. 4. Transient phenomenon

For a slow to fast ascending evolution we considered $\mu_T \cong 4 \div 6,\ \lambda_T > 1$, resulting in the following time constants:

$$T_1 = \frac{t_f}{\mu_T \times (1+\lambda_T)};\ T_2 = \lambda_T \times T_1;\ t_i = \frac{T_1 \times T_2}{T_2 - T_1} \times \ln\left(\frac{T_2}{T_1}\right) \tag{19}$$

where $(t_i)$ is the moment corresponding to the inflexion $F_{0\tau}(t_i)$.

If, with respect to time, the spread of radiation field intensity y(t,p,q,r) is not identical on all three axes (0p), (0q) and (0r) depicted in figures 1a, 1b and 1c, then condition (17) is no longer accomplished, resulting in:

$$F_{0Tp}(t) \neq F_{0Tq}(t) \neq F_{0Tr}(t) \tag{20}$$

In this case, formally identical to relation (19), each axis will exhibit:

$$T_{1p} = \frac{t_{pf}}{\mu_{Tq} \times (1+\lambda_{Tp})};\ T_{2p} = \lambda_{Tp} \times T_{1p} \tag{21}$$

$$T_{1q} = \frac{t_{qf}}{\mu_{Tq} \times (1+\lambda_{Tq})};\ T_{2q} = \lambda_{Tq} T_{1q} \tag{22}$$

$$T_{1r} = \frac{t_{rf}}{\mu_{Tr} \times (1+\lambda_{Tr})};\ T_{2r} = \lambda_{Tr} T_{1r} \tag{23}$$

where (t…f), ($\mu_T$…) and ($\lambda_T$…) are specifically established for each axis.

In order to transform into Cartesian coordinates it can be shown that:

$$\mu_\tau = \frac{t_{pf} + t_{qf} + t_{rf}}{T_{1p} + T_{2p} + T_{1q} + T_{2q} + T_{1r} + T_{2r}};\ \lambda_\tau = \frac{T_{2p} + T_{2q} + T_{2r}}{T_{1p} + T_{1q} + T_{1r}} \tag{24}$$

finally resulting in:

$$T_1 = \frac{t_f}{\mu_\tau \times (1+\lambda_\tau)};\ T_2 = \lambda_\tau \times T_1 \tag{25}$$

which are the equivalent time constants of the Cartesian space, assuming that inertial propagations are different along the three axes (p, q, r).

Following this method, $F_{0T}(t)$ in equation (1) becomes:

$$F_{0T}(t) = \frac{T_1}{T_1 - T_2} \times \varepsilon^{-\frac{t}{T1}} + \frac{T_2}{T_2 - T_1} \times \varepsilon^{-\frac{t}{T2}} \tag{26}$$

which together with $F_{0S}(s)$ from (10), allows the computation of the radiation field intensity defined by (1) and depicted in figure (1).

### 3.2 Analogical modelling

Figure 5 presents the proposed control block diagram for adjusting radiation fields. It's components have been modeled by algebraic and differential equation systems (27) and (28), as well as by partial differential equation (29).

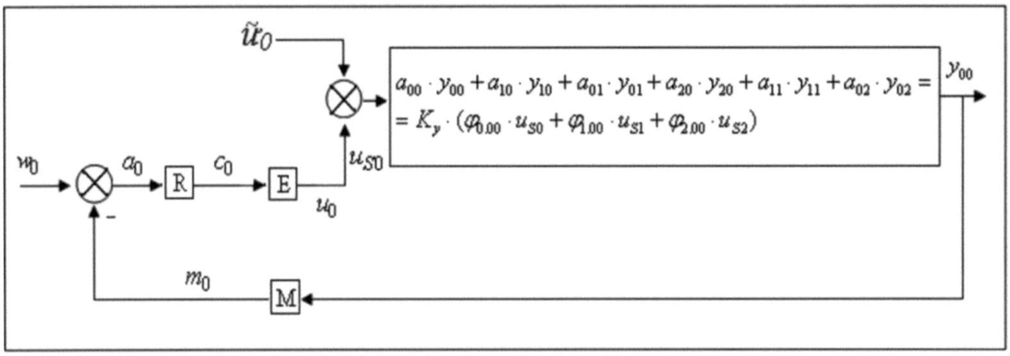


Fig. 5. Control block diagram of the proposed adjustment system

$$a_0=w_0-m_0\ ; \quad K_m \times y_{00}=m_0+T_m \times m_1 \tag{27}$$

$$K_{IR} \times a_0+K_{PR} \times a_1+K_{DR} \times a_2=c_1+T_R \times c_2 \sqrt{a^2+b^2}\ ; \quad K_E \times c_0=u_0+T_E \times u_1 \tag{28}$$

$$a_{00} \times y_{00}+a_{10} \times y_{10}+a_{01} \times y_{01}+a_{20} \times y_{20}+a_{11} \times y_{11}+a_{02} \times y_{02}=K_y \times (\varphi_{0.00} \times u_{S0}+\varphi_{1.00} \times u_{S1}+\varphi_{2.00} \times u_{S2}) \tag{29}$$

The indexes in relations (27), (28) and the first parameter in relation (29), correspond to the order of derivative with respect to time (t). The second parameter in (29) corresponds to the order of derivative with respect to variable (s), defined in relation (2).

The radiation field intensity $(y_{00})$ defined by (1) is converted by the measurement transducer M into electrical signal $(m_0)$ found in (27). The control error $(a_0)$ results from (27), in which $(w_0)$ is the reference signal.

In the above presented adjustment scheme, the R controller with proportional integrative derivative (PID) behaviour defined in (28) emits a control signal $(c_0)$ which adjusts the electromagnetic field generator E, as defined in relation (28).

The radiation emitting unit, E, generates the execution signal $(u_0)$ representing the incident radiation field applied to various environments (e.g. air, tissues), together with a resultant disturbance signal $(\tilde{u}_0)$, resulting in:

$$u_{S0}=u_0 \pm \tilde{u}_0 \tag{30}$$

In the above equation, $(u_{S0})$ is the resulted electromagnetic field and $(\tilde{u}_0)$ corresponds to the homogeneity disturbance $F_{ovd}(v)$ from (16), where $v=s_d$, which may be defined in Cartesian space as seen in figure 6 and expressed in (31).

$$t_f=\sqrt{t_{pf}^2+t_{qf}^2+t_{rf}^2}\ ;\ \ s_f=\sqrt{p_f^2+q_f^2+r_f^2}\ ;\ \ s_d=\sqrt{p_d^2+q_d^2+r_d^2} \tag{31}$$

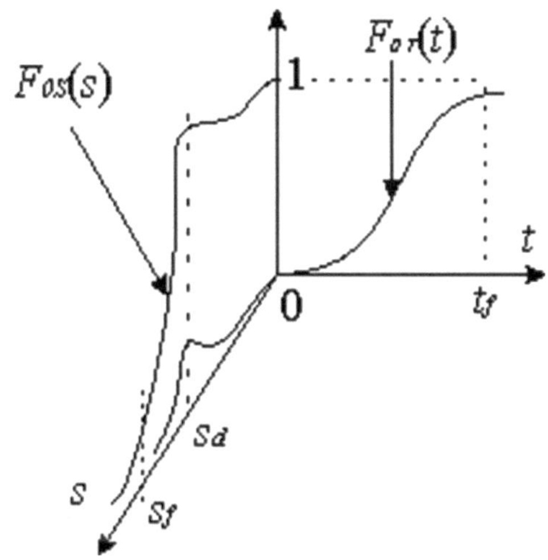


Fig. 6. $F_{OT}$ and $F_{OS}$ including homogeneity disturbance at $s_d$

Thus, the complex phenomenon of radiation spread can be estimated and adjusted by partial differential equation (29).

In the left side of this equation we introduced the approximated solution

$$y_{00}[t,s,u(t)]=K_y\times F_{00}(t,s)\times u_{S0}(t) \tag{32}$$

where $F_{00}(t,s)=F_{0T}(t)\times F_{0S}(s)$ and $(K_y)$ is a weighting coefficient.

This resulted for the right side of equation (29) in:

$$\varphi_{0.00}=a_{00}\times F_{00}+a_{10}\times F_{10}+a_{01}\times F_{01}+a_{20}\times F_{20}+a_{11}\times F_{11}+a_{02}\times F_{02} \tag{33}$$

$$\varphi_{01.00}=a_{10}\times F_{00}+2\times a_{20}\times F_{10}+a_{11}\times F_{01} \tag{34}$$

$$\varphi_{2.00}=a_{20}\times F_{00} \tag{35}$$

in which partial derivatives $(F_{0...})$, $(F_{11})$ and $(F_{...0})$ are obtained from (32). Only signal $(u_0)$ is included in the block diagram. The homogeneity disturbance $(\tilde{u}_0)$ is an independent external signal.

From the equation system (27)…(31), the matrix containing partial derivatives of the state vector ($M_{dpx}$) represented in (36) has been deduced for the entire adjustment system depicted in figure 5.

$$\boxed{\mathbf{M}_{dpx}} = \begin{array}{|c|c|}\hline x & x_S \\ \hline x_T & x_{TS} \\ \hline \end{array} = \begin{array}{|c|cccc|}\hline m_0 & & & 0 & \\ m_1 & & & 0 & \\ c_0 & & & 0 & \\ c_1 & & & 0 & \\ u_0 & & & 0 & \\ u_1 & & & 0 & \\ y_{00} & y_{01} & y_{02} & \cdots & y_{08} \\ y_{10} & y_{11} & y_{12} & \cdots & y_{18} \\ \hline m_2 & & & 0 & \\ c_2 & & & 0 & \\ u_2 & & & 0 & \\ y_{20} & y_{21} & y_{22} & \cdots & y_{28} \\ \hline m_3 & & & 0 & \\ c_3 & & & 0 & \\ u_3 & & & 0 & \\ y_{30} & y_{31} & y_{32} & \cdots & y_{38} \\ \hline & & \cdots & & \\ \hline m_6 & & & 0 & \\ c_6 & & & 0 & \\ u_6 & & & 0 & \\ y_{60} & y_{61} & y_{62} & \cdots & y_{68} \\ \hline \end{array} \qquad (36)$$

Because the signals m=m(t), c=c(t) and u=u(t) are functions only of time, all their partial derivatives with respect to (s) are equal to zero. Details concerning analogical modelling of systems through $\left(M_{dpx}\right)$ may be found in T. Colosi et al., 2009.

### 3.3 Numerical simulation

Numerical simulation has been performed using $\left(M_{dpx}\right)$ and Taylor series, which required knowledge of initial conditions CI($t_0$,s), for $x_{CI}=x(t_0,s)=x_{k-1}$. Hence, by partial derivative with respect to (s), $x_{S,CI}=x_s(t_0,s)=x_{S,k-1}$, in which sequence (k-1) corresponds to the moment $t_{k-1}=(k-1)\times\Delta t$, and sequence (k) corresponds to $t_k=k\times\Delta t$, where $(\Delta t)$ is a sufficiently small integration step.

By means of $(x_{CI})$ and $(x_{S,CI})$ we computed the composing elements of $(x_T)$ and $(x_{TS})$, using specific operations based on symbolic derivatives by indices: $x_{T,CI}=x_T(t_0,s)=x_{T,k-1}$ and $x_{TS,CI}=x_{TS}(t_0,s)=x_{TS,k-1}$.

After setting these initial conditions, we approximated through iterative calculus:

$$x_k=x_{k-1}+\sum_{T=1}^{6}\frac{\Delta t^T}{T!}\times x_{T,k-1}\ ; \qquad x_{S,k}=x_{S,k-1}+\sum_{T=1}^{6}\frac{\Delta t^T}{T!}\times x_{TS,k-1} \qquad (37)$$

For each integration step ( $\Delta t$ ) we operated with a number of 20 Taylor series, of which 6 for ( $m_{0k}, m_{1k}, c_{0k}, c_{1k}, u_{0k}, u_{1k}$ ) and 14 for ( $y_{00k}, y_{01k}, ..., y_{06k}$ ).

It can be observed that 8 elements (signals) included in Taylor series are from the state vector component $(x)$ while the other 12 are from the matrix component $(x_S)$, all of them included in $(M_{dpx})$.

The truncation error at each integration step ( $\Delta t$ ) is proportional to $(\Delta t^7 / 7!)$, for ( $m$, $c$, $u$, $y_{00}$ ), as well as to $(\Delta t^6 / 6!)$, for ( $y_{10}$ ).

### 3.4 Examples of simulated radiation control

In order to illustrate the radiation control that would result from an electronic implementation of the above adjustment system, we present the simulated results regarding field intensity and its automatic adjustment for three simulated tissue types:

1. homogenous tissue
2. **heterogeneous** tissue with an intensity-**increasing** homogeneity disturbance located between body surface and the tissue depth targeted for imaging
3. **heterogeneous** tissue with both an intensity-**decreasing** and an intensity-**increasing** homogeneity disturbance, located between body surface and the targeted tissue depth

For every case, the intensity and spread of electromagnetic radiation has been simulated in open loop (without radiation field control) and in closed loop (with radiation field control).

In all simulated cases the adjustment goal was to ensure a predefined, constant and uniform intensity level of 5 units (e.g. 5 mGy) at a tissue depth of 50 units (e.g. 50 mm), regardless of potential intensity disturbers (radiation absorbing or intensifying environments) localized between body surface and the targeted tissue depth of 50 units.

Numerical simulation was performed using Matlab 7.5.0.

Since our goal has been to develop a general model, we did not impose certain scales or units of measurement. The scales and units of measurement constitute flexible choices that may be conveniently defined for every imaging technique for which our method would be implemented. Given that initialization parameters need to be conveniently chosen and experimentally calibrated for every targeted imaging technique (CT, cone-beam CT, conventional radiography, etc.), we will not undergo a presentation regarding the initial parameters used for these simulated examples. Details regarding the choice of these initial parameters may be found in Roman et al., 2009, 2010 and Colosi et al., 2010.

Simulation results regarding field intensity have been plotted against time and tissue depth, as seen in figures 7-12. Colour coding has been employed in order to highlight different intensity levels of the electromagnetic radiation field.

For every simulated case (figures 7 and 8; figures 9 and 10; figures 11 and 12), significant changes regarding electromagnetic field intensity at different tissue depth can be observed between the unadjusted systems and the ones adjusted by the PID controller.

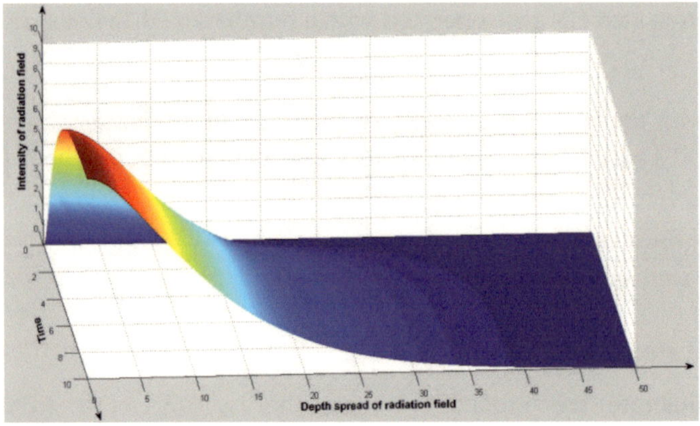


Fig. 7. Intensity of the electromagnetic radiation field, simulated in open loop (without radiation field adjustment), for a homogenous tissue.

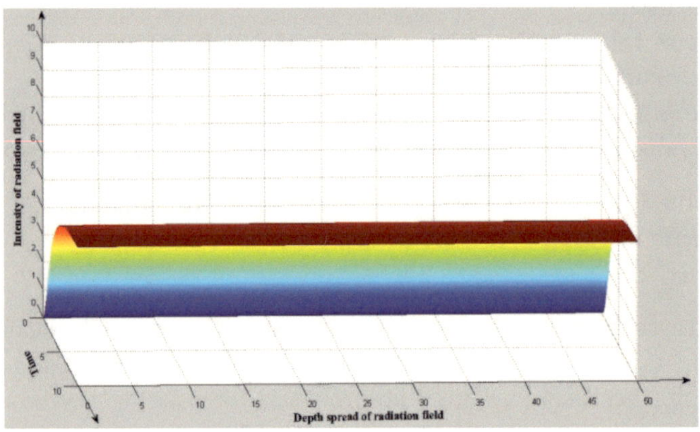


Fig. 8. Adjustment of the electromagnetic radiation field towards a constant intensity of 5 units at a tissue depth of 50 units, simulated in closed loop, for a homogenous tissue.

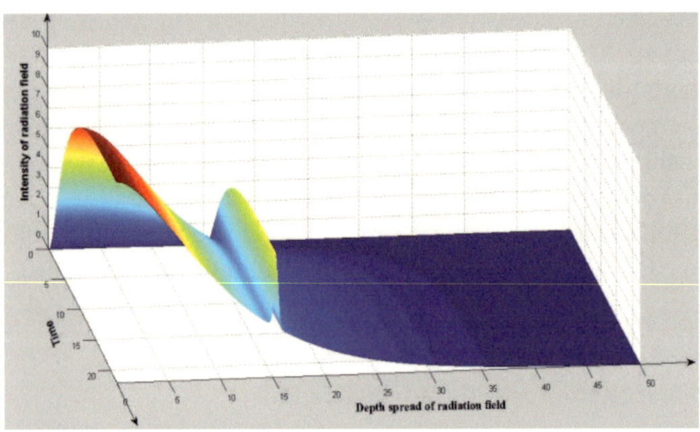


Fig. 9. Intensity of the electromagnetic radiation field, simulated in open loop (without radiation field adjustment), for a heterogeneous tissue with an intensity-increasing homogeneity disturbance at a depth of 15 units.

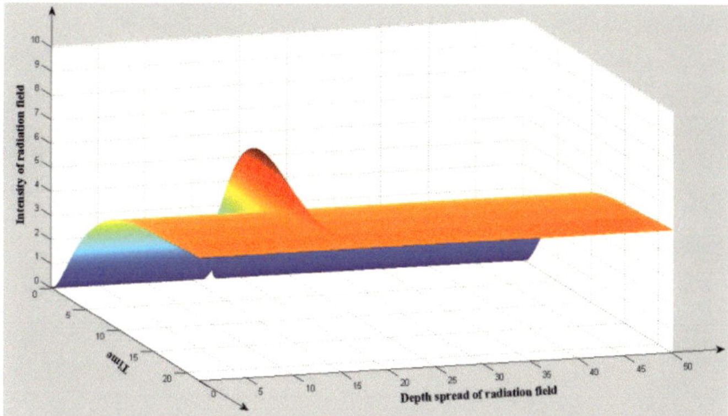


Fig. 10. Adjustment of the electromagnetic radiation field towards a constant intensity of 5 units at a tissue depth of 50 units, simulated in closed loop, for a heterogeneous tissue with an intensity-increasing homogeneity disturbance at a depth of 15 units.

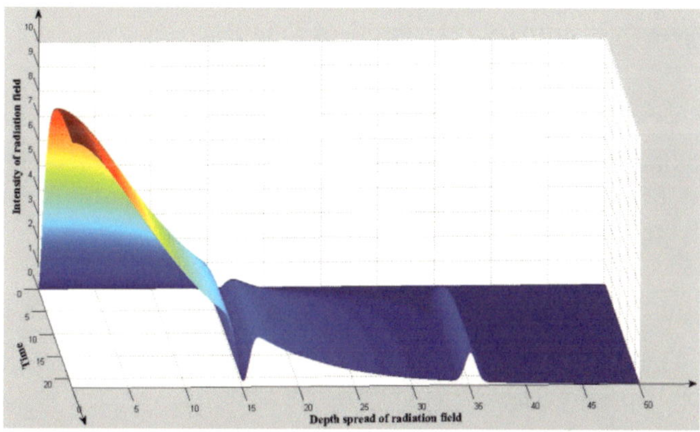


Fig. 11. Intensity of the electromagnetic radiation field, simulated in open loop (without radiation field adjustment), for a heterogeneous tissue with an intensity-decreasing homogeneity disturbance at a depth of 15 units and an intensity-increasing homogeneity disturbance at a depth of 35 units.

Figures 7, 9 and 11 illustrate the fact that, due to radiation absorption from a dense environment, an unadjusted systems can not achieve the targeted dose of 5 intensity units at the desired depth of 50 units, unless a significantly higher field intensity is administered to begin with.

On the other hand, when the systems are adjusted by the PID controller, the electromagnetic field intensity at a tissue depth of 50 units is stabilized at the targeted value of 5 units, in all simulated cases.

Thus, the controlled systems in figures 8, 10 and 12 ensure a minimization of the total administered radiation dose necessary to achieve 5 intensity units at 50 units of tissue depth.

As may be inferred from the examples above, this general and highly flexible model offers a foundation for very precise electromagnetic field adjustments. Experimental validation and calibration for concrete imaging techniques, as well as an electronic implementation of the model, remain to be performed in order to implement this model for practical use.

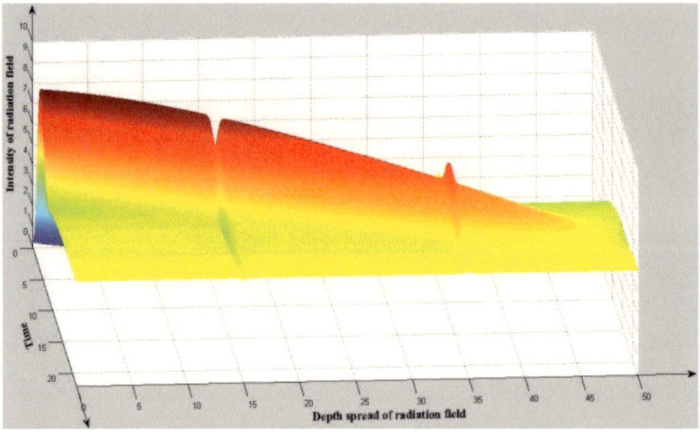


Fig. 12. Adjustment of the electromagnetic radiation field towards a constant intensity of 5 units at a tissue depth of 50 units, simulated in closed loop, for a heterogeneous tissue with an intensity-decreasing homogeneity disturbance at a depth of 15 units and an intensity-increasing homogeneity disturbance at a depth of 35 units.

## 4. Conclusion

The proposed radiation adjustment model offers a precise tool to assist in meeting the overarching goal of radiation protection: to obtain a maximum of relevant imaging information, with the least amount of exposure to ionizing radiation.

## 5. References

Brenner, D.J. & Hall, E.J. (2007). Computed Tomography – An Increasing Source of Radiation Exposure. *New England Journal of Medicine*, Vol. 357, No. 22, pp.2277-2284, ISSN 0028-4793.

Coakley, F.V. et al. (2011). CT radiation dose: what can you do right now in your practice? AJR. American *Journal of Roentgenology*, Vol. 196, No. 3, pp.619-625, ISSN 1546-3141.

Colosi, H. & Roman, N.M. (2010). Digital Simulation and Control of Electromagnetic Field Effects in Heterogeneous Organic Tissues, *Proceedings of 2010 IEEE International Conference on Automation, Quality and Testing, Robotics*, pp. 321-326, ISBN 978-1-4244-6722-8, Cluj-Napoca, Romania, May 28-30, 2010

Colosi, T.; Ungureşan, M.L.; Dulf, E.H. & Cordoş, R.C. (2009). *Introduction to Anlogical Modeling and Numerical Simulation, with (Mpdx) and Taylor Series for Distributed Parameters Processes*, Ed. Galaxia Gutenberg, ISBN 978-973-141-192-7, Târgu-Lăpuş, Romania

Cornfeld, D. et al. (2011). Impact of Adaptive Statistical Iterative Reconstruction (ASIR) on Radiation Dose and Image Quality in Aortic Dissection Studies: A Qualitative and Quantitative Analysis. *Am. J. Roentgenol.*, Vol. 196, No. 3, pp.W336-340.

Flicek, K.T. et al. (2010). Reducing the radiation dose for CT colonography using adaptive statistical iterative reconstruction: A pilot study. *American Journal of Roentgenology*, Vol. 195, No. 1, pp.126-131, ISSN 1546-3141.

Hall, E.J. & Giaccia, A.J. (2005). *Radiobiology for the Radiologist.* (6th ed.), ISBN 978-0781741514 Lippincott Williams & Wilkins Publishing, Philadelphia, PA.

Hara, A.K. et al. (2009). Iterative reconstruction technique for reducing body radiation dose at CT: feasibility study. AJR. American Journal of Roentgenology, Vol. 193, No. 3, pp.764-771, ISSN 1546-3141

International Commission on Radiological Protection, 2007. The 2007 Recommendations of the International Commission on Radiological Protection. ICRP publication 103. Annals of the ICRP, 37(2-4), pp.1-332.

Jursinic, P.A., 2007. Characterization of optically stimulated luminescent dosimeters, OSLDs, for clinical dosimetric measurements. Medical Physics, 34(12), pp.4594-4604.

Kase, K.R., 2004. Radiation protection principles of NCRP. Health Physics, 87(3), pp.251-257.

Kron, T., 1994. Thermoluminescence dosimetry and its applications in medicine--Part 1: Physics, materials and equipment. Australasian Physical & Engineering Sciences in Medicine / Supported by the Australasian College of Physical Scientists in Medicine and the Australasian Association of Physical Sciences in Medicine, 17(4), pp.175-199.

Marin, D. et al. (2010). Low-Tube-Voltage, High-Tube-Current Multidetector Abdominal CT: Improved Image Quality and Decreased Radiation Dose with Adaptive Statistical Iterative Reconstruction Algorithm—Initial Clinical Experience1. *Radiology*, Vol. 254, No. 1, pp.145 -153

McCollough, C.H., Bruesewitz, M.R. & Kofler, J.M., Jr, (2006). CT dose reduction and dose management tools: overview of available options. Radiographics: *A Review Publication of the Radiological Society of North America*, Inc, Vol. 26, No. 2, pp.503-512, ISSN 1527-1323

Miéville, F.A. et al. (2011). Paediatric cardiac CT examinations: impact of the iterative reconstruction method ASIR on image quality - preliminary findings. *Pediatric Radiology*. Available at: http://www.ncbi.nlm.nih.gov/pubmed/21717165 [Accessed July 1, 2011]. ISSN 1432-1998

Mladenov, E. & Iliakis, G. (2011). Induction and repair of DNA double strand breaks: The increasing spectrum of non-homologous end joining pathways. *Mutation Research*, Vol. 711 No. 1-2, pp.61-72, ISSN 0027-5107

National Highway Traffic Safety Administration Fatality Analysis Reporting System, Fatality Analysis and Reporting System Encyclopedia. *National Highway Traffic Safety Administration Fatality Analysis Reporting System*. Available at: http://www-fars.nhtsa.dot.gov/Main/index.aspx [Accessed July 1, 2011].

Renker, M. et al. (2011). Evaluation of Heavily Calcified Vessels with Coronary CT Angiography: Comparison of Iterative and Filtered Back Projection Image Reconstruction. *Radiology*. Available at: http://www.ncbi.nlm.nih.gov/pubmed/21693660 [Accessed July 1, 2011], ISSN 1527-1315

Roman, N.M.; Colosi, H. & Pusca, M. (2009). Digital Simulation for Computer Control of Radiological Devices: A Preliminary Model Using Partial Differential Equations, *Proceedings of MediTech 2009 International Conference on Advancements of Medicine and Health Care through Technology*, pp. 37-42, ISBN 978-3-642-04291-1, Cluj-Napoca, Romania, September 23-26, 2009

Roman, N.M.; Colosi, H. & Pusca, M. (2010). Numerical Simulation Using Partial Differential Equations for Modeling and Control of Medical Radiation Fields.

*Annals of the Academy of Romanian Scientists, Series on Science and Technology of Information*, Vol.3, No.1, (2010), pp. 59-74, ISSN 2066-2742

Ron, E. (2003). Cancer risks from medical radiation. *Health Physics*, 85(1), pp.47-59, ISSN 0017-9078

Rosenthal, D.I. et al. (2006). Radiology order entry with decision support: initial clinical experience. *Journal of the American College of Radiology*. Vol. 3, No. 10, pp.799-806, ISSN 1558-349X

Sajin, G.; Sajin, M. & Gavriloaia, G. (2003). *Aplicații biologice ale radiațiilor electro-magnetice*, Ed. Academiei Tehnice Militare, ISBN 973-640-010-7, Bucureşti, Romania

United Nations Scientific Committee on the Effects of Atomic Radiation (2010). *Sources and Effects of Ionizing Radiation. [UNSCEAR] 2008 Report to the General Assembly with Scientific Annexes (2010): Vol. 1 Annex A*. United Nations Publications, ISBN 978-92-1-142274-0 New York, NY

United Nations Scientific Committee on the Effects of Atomic Radiation (2010). *Sources and Effects of Ionizing Radiation. [UNSCEAR] 2008 Report to the General Assembly with Scientific Annexes (2010): Vol. 1 Annex B*. United Nations Publications, ISBN 978-92-1-142274-0 New York, NY

White, S.C. & Pharoah, M.J. (2009). *Oral Radiology - Principles and Interpretation* (6th ed.), Mosby Elsevier ISBN 978-0323049832 St. Louis, MO

Yilmaz, M.H. et al. (2007). Female breast radiation exposure during thorax multidetector computed tomography and the effectiveness of bismuth breast shield to reduce breast radiation dose. *Journal of Computer Assisted Tomography*, Vol. 31, No. 1, pp.138-142, ISSN 0363-8715

Yukihara, E.G. & McKeever, S.W.S., 2008. Optically stimulated luminescence (OSL) dosimetry in medicine. Physics in Medicine and Biology, 53(20), pp.R351-379.

# Part 2

## Image Processing Techniques

# Current Trends in Archiving and Transmission of Medical Images

Luís S. Ribeiro, Carlos Costa and José Luís Oliveira
*Universidade de Aveiro, IEETA*
*Portugal*

## 1. Introduction

The traditional Picture Archiving and Communication System (PACS) model consists of one PACS serving one healthcare institution (i.e. hospital-centered). Typically, a healthcare institution does not possess all the modalities or experts to evaluate a patient. Therefore, patients tend to move across several healthcare institutions to undergo all the required exams or diagnosis. These high levels of patient mobility produce huge amounts of medical data spread among different healthcare institutions without being shared conveniently, making the traditional PACS model obsolete. The current solutions for sharing non-anonymous medical images (i.e. HIPAA's Protected Health Information - PHI) rely mainly on point-to-point trust relationships (e.g. the radiologist trusts the physician sending image reports by e-mail) or ad-hoc solutions between few institutions (Jacq, 2007). The main problem of the ad-hoc solutions is interoperability, caused by the heterogeneity of methods to exchange information. To overcome this and other issues, the health industry, research and professionals around the world joined forces and started an initiative entitled Integrating the Health Enterprise [1] (IHE) with the main purpose of defining which standards (e.g. DICOM, HL7, ISO, OASIS, etc) may be used in a given situation of the healthcare workflow. IHE does not design standards, but defines integration profiles, i.e. blueprints that describe real-world scenarios or specific characteristics for building integration-ready systems (Størkson & Aslaksen, 2009). Among several integration profiles, one stands out: the Cross-Enterprise Document Sharing (XDS). XDS is gaining momentum and nowadays there are several implementations working in the field. XDS for imaging (XDS-I) is a content profile based on XDS that takes into consideration the particularities of the medical imaging field. However, XDS or XDS-I assume that their architectural components are located inside trustworthy domains, i.e. owned and maintained by Healthcare institutions. Planning and maintaining the IT infrastructure required to support the XDS-I architecture is not simple and demands a significant human and financial effort. Therefore, it would be desirable to delegate this task to a third-party entity and pay for it as a service. For instance, delegating the IT infrastructure to a Cloud Computing provider where the healthcare institutions would just pay to use the data-sharing service and not for the entire IT infrastructure required to support XDS.

Cloud is a computing paradigm that intends to deliver computation and data storage as a utility service (Faruqui, 2005; Michael Armbrust, 2009; Rajkumar Buyya, 2009). A utility

[1] http://www.ihe.org

service in the Cloud follows the same approach as a utility service in currently established utility facilities (e.g. electricity, gas, or telecommunications). Utility services are accessed so frequently that they need to be available anywhere and whenever the consumer requires them. This approach brings obvious advantages since consumers no longer need to plan, invest heavily at the outset or maintain a complex IT infrastructure.

However, combining the concepts of PACS/XDS-I and Cloud computing raises other problems, mainly regarding protection of the patient's private information from unauthorized entities. In this chapter we intend to: (i) - describe the XDS-I and Cloud computing; (ii) - highlight the challenges and opportunities of combining these two concepts; (iii) - present several complementary solutions allowing discussion of whether the benefits of outsourcing the XDS infrastructure on Cloud are worth the associated risk.

## 2. Background

Medical imaging is a non-invasive technique used to create internal images of the human body for clinical or medical science purposes (i.e. "virtual dissecting" of the human body). The genesis of medical imaging occurred in the final decade of the 19th century (1895), when Professor Wilhelm Roentgen noticed electromagnetic radiation while performing vacuum tube experiments. Not understanding the plenitude of that radiation he decided to call it x-rays (Roentgen, 1898). After these first steps, radiology evolved at a good rate until World War II. The intense use of x-rays during the Second World War, and the arrival of the digital computer and new modalities such as ultrasound and magnetic resonance have triggered a boom in diagnostic imaging techniques in the past years (Hendee & Ritenour, 2002). Digital imaging techniques have been in use since the 1970s after the clinical acceptance of Computer Tomography (CT scanner). Currently, digital medical imaging technology is globally acknowledged and an important part of the healthcare workflow.

### 2.1 Current medical imaging scenario

Nowadays, the importance of medical imaging in the healthcare system is irrefutable. To physicians it represents a key factor in supporting their clinical thesis and, as a result, delivering high quality healthcare decisions. Images and studies are stored in local repositories following a PACS concept (Huang, 2010). PACS embraces a set of technologies for the archiving, distribution, visualization and acquisition of medical images over a computer network. Compared with the traditional analogue film, the PACS concept brings significant benefits for the productivity, economy and management of a healthcare institution (De Backer et al., 2004; Huang, 2010; Langer, 2009). At the present time, PACS is a widespread concept in the majority of medical centers. This acceptance was encouraged by introduction of the DICOM, a standard for handling, storing, printing and transmitting medical images. It includes data format definition, storage organization and a network communication protocol (Costa et al., 2007; Mustra et al., 2008; Pianykh, 2008). In this way, PACS devices from different vendors are able to interact with each other in a transparent manner. The PACS architecture began mainly on an ad-hoc basis, serving small subsets, called modules, of the radiology department. Each module functioned as an independent island, unable to communicate with other modules (Huang, 2010). Later it evolved into a PACS infrastructure solution, integrating the hospital information system and the radiology information system, serving the entire hospital (figure 1). The core element of a PACS is one (or more) archive that holds all the DICOM images and studies. Although the various PACS archives that serve the institution are typically accessible within the institution, they tend to be independent from each other. This may be useful to create federations of clinical specialities within the institution, but if a workstation needs to access the full picture of one patient it has to query archive by archive. Furthermore, when the central PACS archive of the healthcare institution or department deteriorates (e.g. not capable of delivering an acceptable Quality of Service), the institution typically replaces it with a more powerful machine (scales up) or appends a new and independent PACS archive, bringing problems regarding data migration and lack of a unified view within the archive of the same department. If inside the healthcare institution such problems still persist, the magnitude and complexity of the problem amplifies when we reach the inter-institutional document-sharing level. Medical imaging exchange among different institutions and e-health in general poses a range of legal and ethical challenges, such as ownership, confidentiality, privacy and integrity of medical data or licensure, accreditation and liability of the health professional or institutions. Legal issues have been a major barrier to inter-institutional medical imaging exchange (Pattynama, 2010). The transmission of PHI across different institutions is not just transferring data from one spot to another. A major problem regarding inter-institutional cooperation is the trust establishment (Lovis et al., 2007; Ruotsalainen, 2009). Due to the rigid laws regarding data privacy and security protection, institutions are reluctant to exchange sensitive data such as non-anonymous medical images. Compromising sensitive data is a present risk when data leaves the institution walls because the institution that controls the data (data controller) may be accountable for any malpractice performed on it, even if the data is sent to other institutions and the malpractices were performed there (Mora et al., 2008). This scenario leads to institutional closure and prevents inter-institutional cooperation due to the lack of trust in third party institutions. Therefore, in order for a group of healthcare institutions to cooperate and share clinical data they must trust each other in the first place. Moreover, besides trusting each other, they must trust in the IT infrastructure that supports the medical imaging cross-transmission.

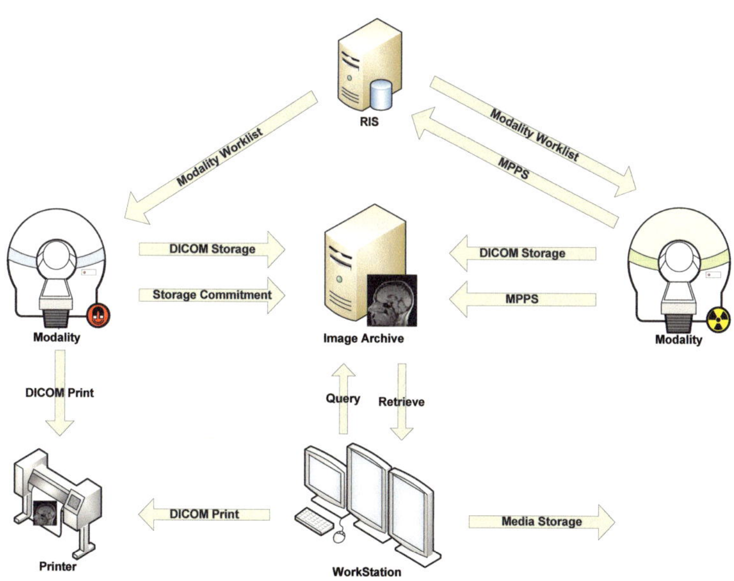


Fig. 1. PACS traditional workflow.

### 2.2 Integrating the healthcare enterprise

As mentioned before, DICOM supports interoperability inside the healthcare institution, but inter-site interoperability is a different situation. Ideally, an authorized entity would have access to the entire clinical history of the patient, relevant for one specific episode, whether or not the exams were performed by the institution. IHE aims to make this possible by improving system integration and eliminating barriers to achieving optimal patient care. IHE provides integration profiles, every one composed of several actors and transactions. The IHE actors and transactions are abstractions of the real-world healthcare information system environment. While some of the transactions are traditionally performed by specific product categories (e.g. HIS, Electronic Patient Record, RIS, PACS, Clinical Information Systems or imaging modalities), IHE intentionally avoids associating functions or actors with such product categories. For each actor, the IHE defines only those functions associated with integrating information systems. The IHE definition of an actor should therefore not be taken as the complete definition of any product that might implement it, nor should the framework itself be taken to comprehensively describe the architecture of a healthcare information system. The reason for defining actors and transactions is to provide a basis for defining the interactions among functional components of the healthcare information system environment (IHE, 2006a).

#### 2.2.1 Cross-Enterprise Document Sharing for imaging

Cross-Enterprise Document Sharing (XDS) is IHE's integration profile that provides core guidelines for sharing documents among any healthcare institution, more precisely it supports: querying, retrieving, publishing and registering Electronic Health Records (EHR) documents. However, XDS is content neutral this means that its architecture was designed to support any type of EHR document. This document independence allows XDS to be a generic framework and more resilient to the appearance of future document standards or formats. In the other hand, being so generic could raise challenges dealing with more specialized domains (e.g. radiology, cardiology). Therefore, it is possible to extend the XDS integration profile and create more specific profiles, entitled content profiles. XDS for Imaging (XDS-I) is a content profile scoped to the medical imaging domain, where systems like PACS, RIS or DICOM objects are taken into account on the XDS architecture.

XDS-I profile facilitates the registration, distribution and access of medical images and imaging related documents across multiple healthcare institutions. Its focus is to provide a standard-based specification for managing the sharing of documents between any healthcare provider, ranging from a small physician office to a metropolitan Hospital (IHE, 2006a; 2008). XDS-I may be seen as a content profile of the integration profile XDS specialized in the radiology domain. Like XDS, XDS-I is document type independent however XDS-I takes in consideration some radiology particularities such as the integration of PACS and RIS in the conceptual architecture.

XDS, and as a consequence XDS-I, assumes that the healthcare institutions belong to one, or more, XDS Affinity Domains (XAD). XAD is a community of healthcare providers that agreed to cooperate using a common set of policies, share a common infrastructure of repositories and a common document registry. Inside an Affinity Domain policies must be defined, such as patient identification (e.g. using IHE Patient Identifier Cross-Reference - PIX), control of access, security model, as well as the format, content, structure, organization and

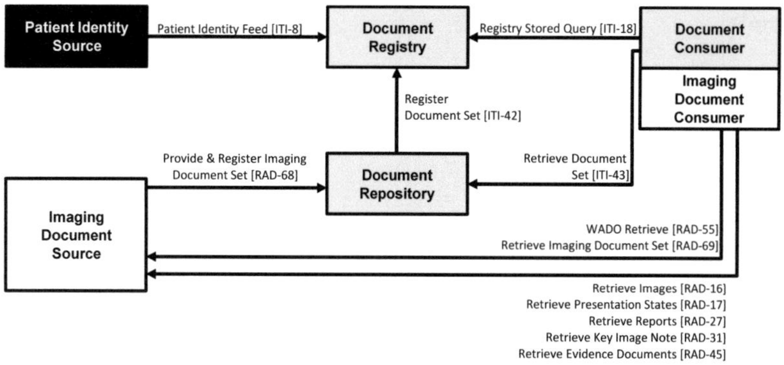


Fig. 2. Diagram of the XDS-I content profile with respective actors and main transactions.

representation of the clinical information (IHE, 2006b). Although XAD is a trust community and authorized participants may access the documents, the healthcare provider that produces the documents may select which documents are to be shared and which are just for internal use.

As mentioned before, the IHE actors communicate through well defined IHE Transactions. These Transactions are based on ebXML messages developed by the OASIS standards [2]. So, the exchanged XDS documents are wrapped in ebXML. The receiving actor by analyzing the message will know what type of information the message contains and who the sender entity was. Figure 2 shows the actors taking part in the XDS-I profile and the transactions between the actors. The Imaging Document Source is the actor that provides or holds the clinical documents (e.g. PACS) typically within the healthcare institutions. It is responsible for pushing the documents and its metadata to the respective Document Repository. If the document is a DICOM object the Repository will only hold the DICOM Key Object Selection (KOS). The KOS objects are small DICOM objects containing a list of UID references (instead of the image data itself) in order to the Document consumer retrieve the images from the Imaging Document Sources. Besides being responsible for the persistent storing of the documents, the Document Repository actor is also responsible for registering the document's metadata in the appropriate Document Registry. The Document Registry actor is the central player of the entire XDS Affinity Domain. It maintains the metadata of each registered document and its mapping to the respective Document Repository, where the actual document is stored. Furthermore, the Document Registry responds to queries from the Document Consumer actor with the locations of the matching documents. Moreover, the Document Consumer actor queries the Document Registry to find the location and the identifier of the document. With this information, it contacts the respective Imaging Document Source (or Sources) requesting the access to the respective image (or images). If the Imaging Document Source authorizes the access, the set of images are typically retrieved through the WADO retrieve protocol - a sub-protocol of the DICOM standard. Finally, Patient Identity Source from the PIX integration profile, and not from XDS, is the actor that provides a unique patient identifier within the Affinity Domain.

[2] http://www.oasis-open.org

### Usage example

Figure 3 illustrates a real world application of the XDS-I approach on the inter-institutional cooperation within an Affinity Domain. At this example, the XAD is composed by a shared document registry and each institution owns a document repository and an imaging document source within its walls. This example highlights possible interactions between professionals, institutions and patients in an inter-institutional clinical episode enabled by the XDS-I content profile:

- **Physician Office:** A referring physician, working in a private office, orders one examination and the patient goes to the Imaging Acquisition Center to perform the exam.
- **Imaging Acquisition Center:** An imagiology institution with modality equipment and a RIS/PACS to manage report and imaging information. The healthcare professional queries the Document Registry for previous studies relevant to this clinical episode. Then, the images studies (acquisition and report) are preformed and, finally, the new documents are registered on the Document Registry.
- **Diagnostic Center:** Eventually, the private physician determines that a consult with a specialized physician is required after analyzing the new exams. At the healthcare institution with specialized physicians (e.g. oncologist) the physician queries the document registry and fetches, from the distributed document repositories, all the needed documents. It performs the evaluation reports of the clinical episode and, finally, registries the documents on the Document registry of the Affinity Domain.
- **XDS Document Registry:** The Document Registry it is the heart of the affinity domain. It is this entity that enables the lookup of documents by indexing the documents' metadata.

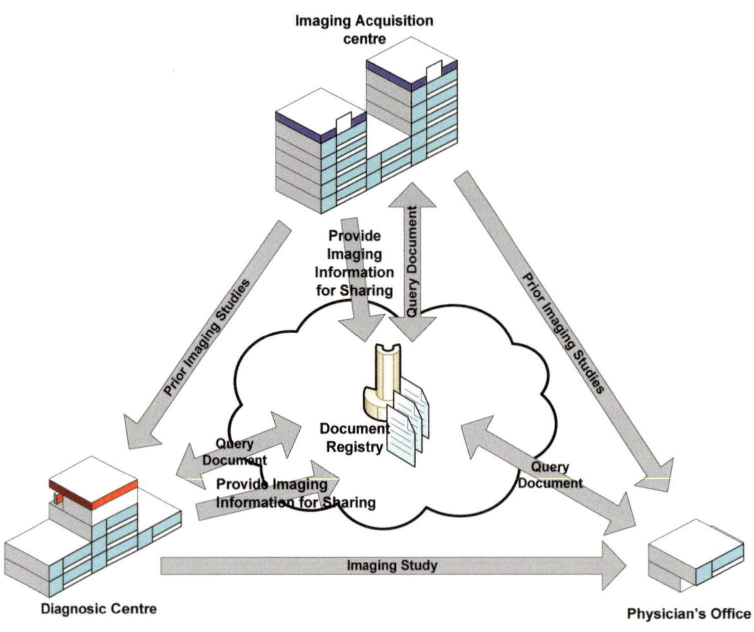


Fig. 3. Data flow within an XDS-I Affinity Domain for a clinical consult.

### 2.2.2 Cross-community access for imaging

In the last section, the reader learned how XDS enables the creation of trust communities for document sharing. However, the scenario of a unified cluster of healthcare institutions sharing documents is not always possible. As mentioned before, the participants of a XAD have to agree a priori to several matters that might slow down the creation of XAD or even make it impossible. For instance, XDS assumes that the patient identifiers are globally unique inside the XAD. However, each institution has their own patient identifiers and the effort of merging, or mapping, the identifiers into a master patient identifier can be great and, as a consequence, jeopardize the project. Whether for technical or conjectural reasons it is certain that patients will flow across several XADs or independent care communities. Therefore, having a way to access documents from outside the community is a desirable feature. Foreseeing this scenario, IHE proposed the Cross Community Access (XCA) integration profile that enables independent communities to exchange documents.

The Cross-Community Access (XCA) integration profile was designed to complement XDS. If XDS creates islands of institutions and XCA creates bridges between those islands. In other words, XDS provides the blueprints for building concise domains of document sharing. While on the other hand, XCA defines a way for extra-domain entities to access the documents shared within the community.

Although XCA does not specify that communities must be XDS Affinity Domains, the reality is that its design makes it the natural choice to connect XDS Affinity Domains. However, the actions allowed to an entity using XCA are not the same as if the entity belonged to the XAD. XCA only allows search and retrieval of documents among communities and does not support pushing or registering of documents inside those communities.

## 2.3 Cloud computing

Cloud computing is a new buzz word for an old dream of computing as a utility, more precisely the 5th utility after water, electricity, gas and telecommunications. Cloud computing does not stand for a completely new concept, as several computing paradigms have promised to deliver this utility computing vision such as Cluster computing, Grid computing, and more recently Cloud computing. A utility service in the Cloud follows the same approach as a utility service in the current established utility facilities (e.g. electricity). Cloud's business model is based on Economies of Scale where efficiency of the provided service increases as the number of services being delivered increases. Hence, the average unitary cost of the service decreases, because the fixed costs of the service are shared over the increased number of provided services. For instance, state of the art magnetic resonance (MR) modalities have high purchase costs; if every healthcare institution (independently of its dimension) had a MR modality, the unitary price of each exam would be higher because there would not be enough patients to fill the modality's schedule. Therefore, the usage efficiency of the provided service would be low and, as a consequence, the service would have to be more costly. As result, typically there are imaging centers that own several modalities and sell the service to the patients of nearby healthcare institutions. This scenario brings several advantages: (i) - healthcare institutions do not need to invest heavily up-front in modalities to conduct their healthcare core business; (ii) - the institutions do not need to maintain the modalities; (iii) - there is more efficient use of the modality and therefore the costs of patients' exams may become lower.

In addition to economic advantages, the quality of service is a major incentive to use Cloud services: high availability, high reliability and high scalability (Binnig et al., 2009). Technologically, Cloud may be seen as a Grid with a different business model, managed by a single entity and with a virtualization strategy (Foster et al., 2008; Rajkumar Buyya, 2009). Its economic approach could make Cloud computing more sustainable than the Grid in the long term, because it is driven by economic goals and does not rely on uncertain and ephemeral project founding. As a consequence, Cloud computing could be seen as the next step of the Grid's technology to deliver computing as the 5th utility (Rajkumar Buyya, 2009; Rimal et al., 2009).

Cloud computing relies on virtualization. Virtualization fits the extremely dynamic Cloud environment very well. With it, computing environments may be dynamically created, expanded, shrunk, replicated or moved according to demand (Rimal et al., 2009). With virtualization, it is possible to easily build scalable and fault-tolerant systems according to the quality of service purchased by the cloud consumer. Virtualization is boosted by the increasing ability of hardware to run applications within Virtual Machines efficiently (Rajkumar Buyya, 2009), more precisely the recent advance in the field of multi-core microprocessor. Cloud Computing stands for the applications, the hardware resources and everything in between is delivered as a service.

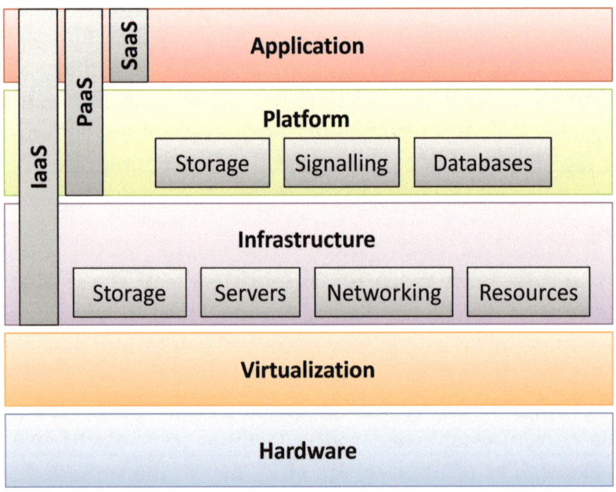


Fig. 4. Cloud Computing layers.

Figure 4 illustrates Cloud's abstract layers (Fu & Chen, 2010):

- **Hardware layer:** refers to the actual physical machines that compose the data center.
- **Virtualization layer:** the hardware resources of the below layer are shared among all the virtual machines supported (i.e. the hardware capabilities are sliced into virtual machines). Each virtual machine has a self-contained operating system and may be seen as an individual and independent machine.
- **Infrastructure layer:** Known as Infrastructure as a Service (IaaS) extends the services provided by the virtualization layer. It provides the mechanisms to manage, monitor, and configure all the supported virtual machines into a utility computing manner. IaaS is the

abstraction allowing access to infrastructure resources (e.g. storage, computation, server, data center) on-demand and paid according to the required quality-of-service (QoS).

- **Platform layer:** Known as Platform as a Service (PaaS) extends the IaaS layer by hiding the IaaS complexity. PaaS is accessed as one big system and not by accessing individual virtual machines. Therefore, it provides an abstraction where the virtual machines are automatically managed by the cloud service provider. Offering reliable services by default such as storage, databases and signalization.
- **Application layer:** Layer usually entitled as Software as a Service (SaaS) where the applications hosted on the Cloud are deployed on local computers typically through web-browser. On this layer, the payment is associated with the application itself and not with the platform or infrastructure below it. Typically, this layer is where developers build their applications.

The services themselves have long been referred to as Software as a Service (SaaS) and Cloud does not change that (Michael Armbrust, 2009). Nevertheless, Cloud Computing allows the application providers the choice of deploying their product as SaaS without providing a data center.

## 3. Challenges

Cloud promises to deliver financial benefits to enterprises by reducing the costs of the IT department. The IT infrastructure supporting the storage of medical images is a heavy burden for healthcare institutions. Besides storing the clinical data in a reliable manner, it is also required to make that data available 24/7 and provide appropriate access performance - a true management nightmare (Huang, 2010). When the scope of the IT infrastructure ranges from an intranet to a cross-enterprise solution, the associated costs, complexity and effort of deployment also increase. Regarding the financial dimension, Cloud's business model is attractive to build cross-enterprise solutions, such as XDS-I, due to the fact that the costs associated with components shared by the community (e.g. XDS Document Registry, XDS Document Repository) would be paid as a service and according to each institution's use. In this way, the significant costs of developing and maintaining such infrastructure would be eliminated. Unfortunately, the outsourcing of clinical data to the Cloud faces many challenges that must be considered before moving the clinical data or components of the IT infrastructure to the Cloud.

### 3.1 Privacy and confidentiality

The privacy and confidentiality of the data placed on the Cloud are the main barriers that delay Cloud's general acceptance. The World Privacy Forum (WPF) released a report spelling out the risks to privacy and confidentiality posed by Cloud computing. The report unveils concerns regarding Cloud's current state: what happens to the data after the consumer uploads it to the Cloud and how its confidentiality will be protected. The answer to this question is somehow disappointing. In the current state of Cloud computing it does not ensure privacy or confidentiality of the stored data. The simple fact of uploading data to the Cloud makes that data more suitable for disclosure or unauthorized usage. The WPF published several privacy advices in order to aware the cloud consumers:

- Read the Terms of Service before placing any information in the cloud. If the Terms of Service are not understandable, a different cloud provider must be considered.

- Information in the cloud is legally easier to access through the Cloud than by seizing a private computer. Therefore, sensitive information should not be uploaded to the Cloud.
- In the Term of Services one must notice if the Cloud provider reserves rights to use, disclose, or make the uploaded information public.
- Read the Privacy Policy before placing any information in the cloud. If the Privacy Policy is not understandable, a different cloud provider must be considered.
- Beware if the Cloud provider retains rights over removed data by the consumer.
- Beware if the cloud provider notifies their consumers when the Terms of Service or Privacy Policy change.

Furthermore, WPF extends its advices to companies or governments that are considering the upload of data or the migration of the IT infrastructure to the Cloud:

- Caution on ad-hoc Cloud computing is advised. Organizations should have standardized rules for employees to know which data they may (or not) upload to the cloud.
- Sensitive information that is of the interest of the organization to keep away from the government, other competitive organizations or other governments should not be uploaded.
- Information disclosure of cloud's data should be considered before uploading the actual data.
- Hire professional support for understanding the Terms of Service or Privacy Policies of the Cloud provider.

After analyzing these advices, answering the question: Is the current state of Cloud computing suitable for storing any PHI? The answer is pretty straightforward: No! Any cloud consumer should consider that any uploaded data could be used by others e.g. statistics, publicity or even be sold to competitors. For instance, health insurance companies may buy information regarding the health history of a patient in order to assert fees or deny the health insurance to the patient. At this case, the patient privacy right was jeopardized and there was a confidentiality breach. Even if the uploaded medical data is anonymous for safeguarding the patient's privacy, it is still possible to infer statistical analysis to the data identifying geographical regions propitious to certain pathologies and sell that information to health insurance companies. Terms of Service and rigid Privacy Policy agreements may raise the protection of the stored data by adding liability to the Cloud provider. However, is extremely difficult to prove that the stored data was violated, or not, by the Cloud provider. Therefore, Cloud computing, without any privacy and confidentiality protection system built over the Cloud, is not suitable to store any data undesirable to be disclosed.

### 3.2 Interoperability and standardization

Although some efforts towards reaching standardization among for Cloud Computing, such as the Cloud Computing Interoperability Forum (CCIF) or the European Telecommunications Standards Institute (ETSI), the reality is that cloud standardization is far from being achieved and at some levels maybe it never will, as a consequence, the lack of interoperability inter-cloud provider is a resilient issue. If it is possible and relatively easy to guarantee cloud interoperability at the IaaS level even without standardization (e.g. DeltaCloud [3]),

[3] http://incubator.apache.org/deltacloud/

accomplishing interoperability between the several PaaS is a more demanding task. Not only due to possible economical interests of the Cloud providers, but as well at the technical level. PaaS APIs abstract the complexity of the IaaS and provides the developers with embedded functionalities (e.g. automatic scaling) that at the IaaS level have to be implemented from scratch . This facilitated API of PaaS is more convenient for the developer but less flexible at the same time (Michael Armbrust, 2009). PaaS automatic features turn the standardization or interoperability efforts more complex. Each Cloud provider follows its unique IT architecture - especially above the IaaS level (PaaS or SaaS). If some features are easy to accomplish in some cloud architectures, the same features could be extremely difficult to achieve at other architectures. This heterogeneity of features and architectures may push back standardization, and turn full interoperability above the IaaS level extremely difficult.

### 3.3 Geographical distribution

The Cloud providers are private companies adjudicated to a country obligated to follow the countries laws. However, they compete with each other on a global market, ignoring countries borders. Enabled by the Internet, a Cloud provider from the USA may easily offer its Cloud services to a consumer from Singapore or Australia. At the same level, a Cloud provider may have several data centers around the world. For instance, one of the major expenses of a data center is the energy consumed for refrigerating the machines and, if the data center is placed in a cold natural geographical location (e.g. Alaska) the cooling costs will be much lower and the Economics of Scale enhanced. However, this cross-border logistics of the Cloud business model may aggravate liability and jurisdiction risks, due to the fact that cross-border litigation is typically more complex and high-staked than litigations within borders, and is not clear which court have jurisdiction over the Cloud where the illegality occurred: would it be treated in the jurisdiction of the consumer, the provider or the vendor?

### 3.4 Consumer lock-in and bankruptcy

Consumer lock-in and bankruptcy of the Cloud provider are two serious risks and both have a similar consequence, which is losing control of the data trusted by the cloud consumer to the cloud provider. Consumer Lock-in may be performed at two different levels: data lock-in and vendor lock-in. Trusting valuable data to a single provider may lead to opportunistic reprising, where the provider uses the held data at its data centers to blackmail the costumer and rise prices while renegotiating contracts. Vendor lock-in is more subtle type of consumer lock-in. Due to the fact that each Cloud provider offers, to its customers, a unique development API which turns the applications specific to the Cloud provider. Therefore, the consumer is locked-in with the Cloud provider since migrating the applications to other Clouds means recoding the applications following the new cloud API. As a result, the cost of migration does not compensate the eventual competitive prices of other Clouds. As it was mentioned before, other risk that could lead to losing control of the consumer's data is the bankruptcy of the Cloud Provider. Cloud Providers are companies and companies may go bankrupt. The obvious question that arises is what happens to the consumer's data and applications if such scenario becomes a reality? Migrating data (e.g. images or documents) probably would be less demanding than migrating applications developed with specific PaaS API. As a result, the lack of interoperability at the PaaS may turn the migration process extremely difficult, requiring the refractor of the majority of the source code.

## 4. Available solutions and new opportunities

As we mentioned at the Challenges section, the architecture of Cloud Computing is not suitable by itself to sustain PHI. There were identified several issues that turn the outsourcing of PHI on the Cloud inappropriate or even illegal. However, when the challenges are identified, opportunities also may emerge to mitigate them. At this following section we will present some design approaches, built over the Cloud, in order to enable XDS-I IT infrastructure to be outsourced to the Cloud taking into consideration the previous identified challenges.

### 4.1 Encryption and decryption client-side

The public Cloud design permutes the previous trust patterns of older computing paradigms such as Client-Server. For instance, at the Client-Server paradigm the Server is considered the most trustworthy entity of the architecture. This trust assumption fades away when the data to be dealt on the Cloud is PHI. At this scenario of storing PHI on the Cloud the trustworthy entities are the clients and it must be assumed that the Cloud's data center is untrustworthy. Therefore, besides the transmission channels between nodes, the information must be hidden from the central node where the information is stored or relayed, more precisely the Cloud's data center. To do so, the encryption must be performed on the client machine and stored ciphered at the Cloud data center. Consequently, a reverse procedure must be performed while retrieving the information from the Cloud: download the ciphered data and decrypt it at the client machine. The described workflow may seem trivial but is the core essence of several systems that use the Cloud to connect trustworthy nodes. With this strategy two approaches may emerge: Cloud as a Relay or Cloud as a Repository.

#### 4.1.1 Cloud as a eelay

In the Cloud as a Relay approach the Cloud is used to create a virtual bridges between the intranets of different healthcare institutions enabling the exchange, search and store of medical images within a wide domain (Ribeiro, Costa & Oliveira, 2010; Ribeiro, Silva, Costa & Oliveira, 2010). They add at each trust node (i.e. intranet of the healthcare institutions) one device that acts as a proxy for the income data and as a gateway for the outcome data. The proxy/gateway device installed within the healthcare institution speaks DICOM (i.e. the device is DICOM compliant and implement several DICOM services) and with the outside it communicates through Internet standards such as IMAP and HTTPS (figure 5). The mentioned solutions are interoperable within the institution due to the fact that they implement the DICOM services. However, at the cross-enterprise scale the communication is ad-hoc. Nevertheless, they were managed to enable the exchange of medical images through a Cloud bridge without jeopardizing the confidentiality and privacy of the clinical data. Furthermore, because the Cloud is just used as a relay and the PHI is stored temporally it mitigates identified issues, namely consumer's lock-in, bankruptcy of the Cloud provider, and the geo-distributed nature of the Cloud is irrelevant. However, the major drawbacks of such solutions are: (i) - the Cloud is just used as a relay and the IT infrastructure remains at within the institution. Therefore, the Cloud's benefit, of outsourcing at lower prices, is not ideal. Furthermore, a VPN connection would have the same effect (although in several countries opening a VPN connection in a public healthcare institution is a bureaucratically and procedure and such solutions may diminish the initial inertia of inter-site cooperation). (ii) - The performance of the relay strategy decreases while comparing with storing the data at the Cloud in a repository approach, since the data must be uploaded to the cloud and downloaded from the cloud for all inter-site interactions. (iii) - Such solutions may not be considered pure cross-enterprise because, for instance, they do not deal with cross identification of patients so that task is managed manually.

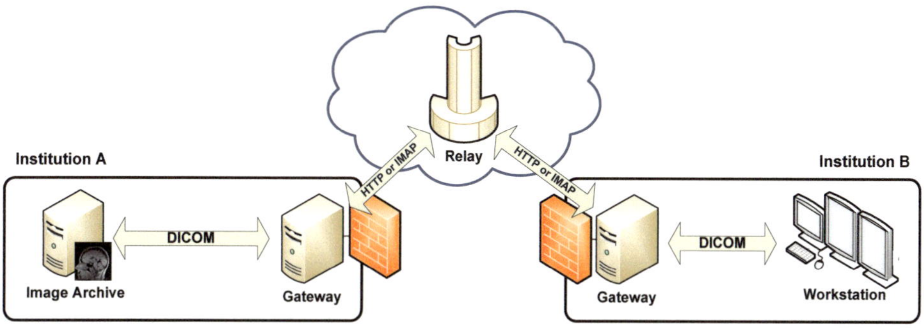


Fig. 5. Example of using Cloud as a Relay inter-connecting two different healthcare institutions.

### 4.1.2 Cloud as a repository

In the Cloud as a Repository approach the Cloud is used as repository of medical images (i.e. Image Document Source) (Silva et al., 2011). The architecture is similar to the Cloud as a Relay: there is a device (e.g. gateway) that encrypts/decrypts the clinical data client-side. However, the ciphered data is stored in a persistent manner at the cloud (figure 6). Furthermore, the trivial approach does not enable rich search queries (e.g. by patient demographics) only queries by unique identifier of the document. To overcome this problem Silva et al. (2011) decoupled the searchable text based data of the images (metadata) from the image data pixel itself. The pixel component data is encrypted and stored at the Cloud while the searchable metadata is stored is a server that is owned (therefore trustworthy) by the healthcare institution. This approach diminishes the IT infrastructure more than the Cloud as a Relay approach, since the metadata represents a small portion of the data required to be stored. Furthermore, the privacy and confidentiality of the clinical data is guaranteed and the geo-distribution nature of the Cloud is diminished. However, this approach may be affected from Cloud bankruptcy or data lock-in due to the fact that the actual pixel data is at the Cloud-side. These risks are minimized since the gateway of Silva et al. (2011) enables Cloud provider redundancy, by following a similar approach of DeltaCloud. This way, healthcare institutions are able to store the ciphered pixel data at more than one cloud provider in a transparent manner for the institutions' DICOM devices, increasing the reliability of the system. The Silva et al. (2011) PACS solution is ideal for a multi-site healthcare institution enabling the institution's distributed nodes to share the same PACS archive. However, the trust community created does not follow the communication standards recommended by the XDS-I content profile and vendor lock-in is still possible at the cross-enterprise scale. Nevertheless, XDS-I does not predicts the outsourcing of the IT infrastructure and Silva et al. (2011) was capable of developing a cross-site solution enabling it without jeopardizing the privacy and confidentiality of the clinical data, and with an acceptable performance degradation while comparing with local PACS archive.

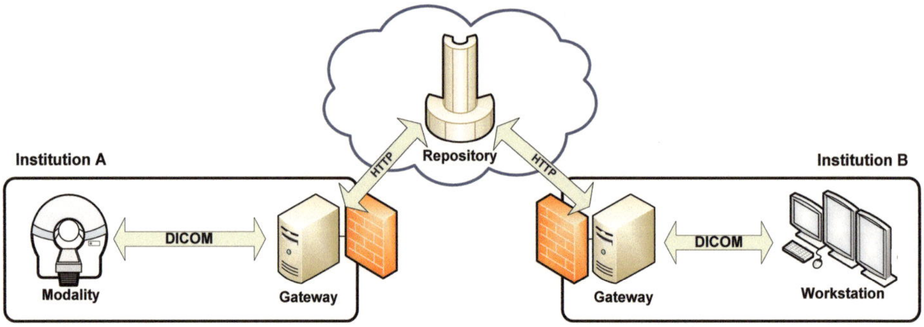


Fig. 6. Example of using Cloud as a Repository of clinical information.

### 4.2 XDS-I infrastructure on the cloud

The current state of Cloud Computing does not guarantee privacy or confidentiality of the stored data. Even if the Service Terms and the Privacy Policy of the Cloud provider claim privacy and confidentiality of the trusted data, it is extremely difficult (if not impossible) to prove that there was not any leak of information or if there was some data mining processes to extract patterns of the clinical data. Therefore, the system's design running above the Cloud must take this issue in consideration. As we mentioned previously, XDS-I assumes that the nodes where its actors are instantiated are trustworthy. Therefore, the clinical data may be stored in a readable manner - assumption possible to have in private Clouds owned by trustworthy entities (e.g. hospital, National Healthcare System) but inappropriate to have in public Clouds. In order to combine these two concepts (public Cloud and XDS-I) one must ensure privacy and confidentiality of the PHI without removing the interoperability of the XDS-I content profile. Analyzing the XDS-I actors (figure 2) we have three candidates to be migrated to the Cloud: Document Registry, Document Repository and Imaging Document Source. The only central and unique component of the Affinity Domain is the Document Registry, which searches the registry to locate documents that meet the criteria specified in the query request by the Document Consumer IHE (2006b). The queries supported by the Document Registry are well defined by the transaction Registry Stored Query (IHI-18). This transaction reduces directly or indirectly the scope of the search to the global patient ID of the respective affinity domain. For instance, to find documents' metadata the patient ID must always be supplied and within that patient scope the search query may filter according other attributes (e.g. document's type, author's ID). Therefore, queries only based on patient demographics are not supported. Patient demographics are an optional field only intended as an audit/confirmation mechanism for the Document Consumers (IHE, 2010). Ribeiro et al. (2011) was able to launch XDS Document Registries on the public Cloud in a secure manner and keeping the privacy and confidentiality of the metadata. Any fields of the metadata on the XDS Registry possible to extract meaning (e.g. patient demographics, institution's name) are protected. The level of protection is defined by the administrator of the Affinity Domain that may vary from storing the meaningful fields encrypted to not allowing those fields to be stored at all. This is possible due to the fact that the readable metadata with meaning is optional. Nevertheless, from the three above mentioned candidate actors the XDS Document Registry is the one that offers less consequences if disclosure of the meaningful fields occurs. In the other hand, the other two candidate actors, Document Repository and Imaging Document Source, hold valuable clinical information and must be protected accordantly from disclosure.

The approaches to ensure privacy and confidentiality, and at the same time interoperability while migrating these two actors to the Cloud may pass by:

1. **Encrypted Storing and on-the-fly Decryption:** The PHI is cloud-side encrypted with one symmetric key generated by the XDS-I actor (unknown to any other entities). The encrypted PHI is stored on the cloud. Whenever transaction triggers the access to the encrypted data, the data is decrypted on-the-fly and the transaction is answered with readable data. This approach guarantees interoperability and adds some level of data privacy/confidentiality protection. However, it is possible that when the data is being decrypted on-the-fly the Cloud provider sniff it leaking the PHI.
2. **Middleware encryption/decryption:** One middleware device is added between the communication of the Document Consumer and the Document Repository or Image Document Source placed on the cloud. The middleware device is owned by the healthcare institution and is responsible for translating (encrypting/decrypting) the flow of data between the two end actors. The middleware device implements the XDS-I transactions and therefore it is interoperable. Furthermore, privacy and confidentiality of PHI is ensured due to the fact that PHI is stored ciphered and encrypted in a trustworthy node. However, this approach may bring performance degradation compared with the previous approach since the message flow required is always bigger. Finally, the middleware machine owned by the healthcare institution would be a bottleneck and scalability and availability issues could rise.
3. **XDS for private imaging:** The XDS integration profile was designed to be document format independent, i.e. it supports any document type. When the Document Consumer retrieves data from the Document Repository like, for instance, a report in the Portable Document Format (PDF) the document requires a PDF reader in order to be accessed by the healthcare professional. The same occurs at XDS-I when a DICOM object is retrieved from the Imaging Document Source. XDS-I is a content profile based on the XDS integration profile for dealing with medical imaging. Following the same thread of thought and taking in account that XDS is format independent it is possible to design a new content profile XDS for private images (XDS-$\pi$). At XDS-$\pi$ the three candidate actors could be migrated to the public cloud, storing the documents and the medical images encrypted, and the encryption/decryption would be performed client-side. This approach ensures the PHI privacy and confidentiality and interoperable at the architecture level since the transactions and the actors of the XDS-I would be the same. However, the drawback of this approach would be the lack of interoperability at the document level since it is not yet predicted by IHE.

Furthermore, the three above approaches may follow a Searchable Symmetrical Encryption (SSE) to discover wanted documents among the encrypted resources stored on the cloud. Single private-key encryption inhibits the search document among encrypted blobs of data. SSE enables the search of keywords over the encrypted data without the need to decrypt the data or disclosure the keyword (Curtmola et al., 2006). Therefore, SSE ensures privacy and confidentiality of the data and at the same time the ability of retrieve selectively documents from the Cloud is maintained. Finally, comparing the risk associated with each approach the $1^{st}$ approach is the one that offers less privacy and confidentiality protection. In the other hand, the $2^{nd}$ and $3^{rd}$ approaches offer higher levels of protection from disclosure which, in our opinion, are adequate for storing PHI on the Cloud.

## 5. Conclusion

It is expected that the production of medical imaging will continue to increase in the following decades. For instance, the PET-CT modality requires space for storing the PET images, the CT images and the outcome fusion images and, the same situation happens with the new modality PET-MRI. Furthermore, there is a new research trend of content-based image retrieval, where it is possible to discover and retrieve images based on the pixel data of the image. This content-based retrieval is enabled by models describe the image and these models also require store space. As result, the storing requirements of the medical imaging fields are demanding and will be even more demanding in the future. Therefore, new storage solutions with flexible business models are needed more than ever. The Cloud computing paradigm offers an elastic framework to allocate or release computational resources on-the-fly and enabling a more efficient usage and, as a consequence, reducing costs. Current PACS architectures, hospital oriented, with their own short-term and long-term archives with no or little interaction with other institutions or PACS are difficult to extrapolate to the cross-institutional environment. XDS-I allied with XCA integration profile set the roadmap to enable the cross-enterprise medical imaging sharing. The conjugation of both integration profiles offers to the healthcare institutions flexible levels of inter-institutional coupling: through XDS-I the institutions create a common trust community (XAD) aggregating their federations into one single federation of medical imaging inter-site sharing or through XCA allowing access to the documents of other XADs without the need of federation fusion. Ribeiro, Costa & Oliveira (2010); Ribeiro, Silva, Costa & Oliveira (2010); Silva et al. (2011) proved that storing and/or distribute medical images and related exams using public Cloud providers is possible. Although, these solutions are interoperable within institution (since are DICOM compliant) at the cross-enterprise level they do not follow the transactions defined by the IHE. Nevertheless, based on their experience and on the hypothesis analysis performed at the new opportunities section we conclude that the public Cloud Computing utility has potential to host several actors of the XDS-I content profile safeguarding the privacy and confidentiality of the PHI.

## 6. Acknowledgment

The research leading to these results has received funding from Fundação para a Ciência e Tecnologia (FCT) under grant agreement PTDC/EIA-EIA/104428/2008.

## 7. References

Binnig, C., Kossmann, D., Kraska, T. & Loesing, S. (2009). How is the weather tomorrow?: towards a benchmark for the cloud, *DBTest '09: Proceedings of the Second International Workshop on Testing Database Systems*, ACM, pp. 1–6.

Costa, C., Silva, A. & Oliveira, J. (2007). Current Perspectives on PACS and a Cardiology Case Study, *Computational Intelligence (SCI)* 65: 79–108.

Curtmola, R., Garay, J., Kamara, S. & Ostrovsky, R. (2006). Searchable symmetric encryption: improved definitions and efficient constructions, *Proceedings of the 13th ACM conference on Computer and communications security*, CCS '06, ACM, pp. 79–88.

De Backer, A., Mortele, K. & De Keulenaer, B. (2004). Picture archiving and communication system–part 2 cost-benefit considerations for picture archiving and communication system., *JBR-BTR: organe de la Société royale belge de radiologie (SRBR)= orgaan van de Koninklijke Belgische Vereniging voor Radiologie (KBVR)* 87(6): 296.

Faruqui, S. A. (2005). *Utility computing: certification model, costing model, and related architecture development*, California State University.
URL: *http://books.google.pt/books?id=wMdENwAACAAJ*

Foster, I., Zhao, Y., Raicu, I. & Lu, S. (2008). Cloud computing and grid computing 360-degree compared, *IEEE Grid Computing Environments* .

Fu, L. & Chen, T. (2010). Building enterprise application based on cloud computing, *E-Health Networking, Digital Ecosystems and Technologies (EDT), 2010 International Conference on*, Vol. 2, pp. 534 –537.

Hendee, W. R. & Ritenour, R. (2002). *Medical Imaging Physics; 4th ed*, Wiley, New York, NY.

Huang, H. (2010). *PACS and Imaging Informatics: Basic Principles and Applications*, John Wiley & Sons.

IHE (2006a). It infrastructure (iti) technical framework integration profiles, revision 6.0 - final text, *Technical report*, Integrating the Healthcare Enterprise.

IHE (2006b). Iti technical framework supplement: Cross-enterprise document sharing for imaging, *Technical report*, Integrating the Healthcare Enterprise.

IHE (2008). It radiology technical framework integration profiles, revision 9.0 - final text, *Technical report*, Integrating the Healthcare Enterprise.

IHE (2010). It infrastructure technical framework: Cross-transaction specifications and content specifications, *Technical report*, Integrating the Healthcare Enterprise.

Jacq, N. (2007). *From genes to personalized healthcare: grid solutions for the life sciences : proceedings of HealthGrid 2007*, Studies in health technology and informatics, IOS Press.

Langer, S. (2009). Issues Surrounding PACS Archiving to External, Third-Party DICOM Archives, *Journal of Digital Imaging* 22(1): 48–52.

Lovis, C., Spahni, S., Cassoni, N. & Geissbuhler, A. (2007). Comprehensive management of the access to the electronic patient record: Towards trans-institutional networks, *International Journal of Medical Informatics* 76(5-6): 466–470.

Michael Armbrust, e. a. (2009). Above the clouds: A berkeley view of cloud computing, *Technical Report UCB/EECS-2009-28*, EECS Department, University of California, Berkeley.

Mora, L., Nevid, J. & Chaplin, W. (2008). Psychologist treatment recommendations for internet-based therapeutic interventions, *Comput. Hum. Behav.* 24(6): 3052–3062.

Mustra, M., Delac, K. & Grgic, M. (2008). Overview of the DICOM standard, *ELMAR, 2008. 50th International Symposium*, Vol. 1.

Pattynama, P. M. T. (2010). Legal aspects of cross-border teleradiology, *Eur J Radiol* 73(1): 26–30.

Pianykh, O. S. (2008). *Digital Imaging and Communications in Medicine: A Practical Introduction and Survival Guide*, Springer Publishing Company, Incorporated.

Rajkumar Buyya, e. a. (2009). Cloud computing and emerging it platforms: Vision, hype, and reality for delivering computing as the 5th utility, *Future Generation Computer Systems* 25(6): 599–616.

Ribeiro, L. S., Blanquer, I., Costa, C. & Oliveira, J. L. (2011). On demand ihe xds document registries on the cloud, *international Journal of Computer Assisted Radiology and Surgery*, Springer, pp. 297–298.

Ribeiro, L. S., Costa, C. & Oliveira, J. L. (2010). A proxy of dicom services, *Advanced PACS-based Imaging Informatics and Therapeutic Applications*, SPIE Medical Imaging.

Ribeiro, L. S., Silva, L., Costa, C. & Oliveira, J. L. (2010). Email-p2p gateway to distributed medical imaging repositories, *3th International Conference on Health Informatics*, pp. 310–316.

Rimal, B. P., Choi, E. & Lumb, I. (2009). A taxonomy and survey of cloud computing systems, *Networked Computing and Advanced Information Management, International Conference on* 0: 44–51.

Roentgen, W. (1898). Ueber eine neue art von strahlen, *Annalen der Physik* 300: 12–17.

Ruotsalainen, P. (2009). Privacy and security in teleradiology, *European Journal of Radiology* .

Silva, L., Costa, C. & Oliveira, J. (2011). A pacs archive architecture supported on cloud services, *International Journal of Computer Assisted Radiology and Surgery* pp. 1–10. 10.1007/s11548-011-0625-x.
URL: *http://dx.doi.org/10.1007/s11548-011-0625-x*

Størkson, S. A. & Aslaksen, A. (2009). Pacs: Beyond radiology, *International Journal of Computer Assisted Radiology and Surgery* 4: 168–170. 10.1007/s11548-009-0321-2.

# 6

# Large-Scale User Facility Imaging and Scattering Techniques to Facilitate Basic Medical Research

Stephen D. Miller[1], Jean-Christophe Bilheux[1], Shaun S. Gleason[2], Trent L. Nichols[2], Philip R. Bingham[2] and Mark L. Green[3]
*[1]Neutron Scattering Science Division, Oak Ridge National Laboratory*
*[2]Measurement Science & Systems Engineering Division*
*Oak Ridge National Laboratory*
*[3]Tech-X Corporation*
*USA*

## 1. Introduction

Conceptually, modern medical imaging can be traced back to the late 1960's and into the early 1970's with the advent of computed tomography[1]. This pioneering work was done by 1979 Nobel Prize winners Godfrey Hounsfield and Allan McLeod Cormack which evolved into the first prototype Computed Tomography (CT) scanner in 1971 and became commercially available in 1972. Unique to the CT scanner was the ability to utilize X-ray projections taken at regular angular increments from which reconstructed three-dimensional (3D) images could be produced. It is interesting to note that the mathematics to realize tomographic images were developed in 1917 by the Austrian mathematician Johann Radon who produced the mathematical relationships to derive 3D images from projections - known today as the Radon Transform[2]. The confluence of newly advancing technologies, particularly in the areas of detectors, X-ray tubes, and computers combined with the earlier derived mathematical concepts ushered in a new era in diagnostic medicine via medical imaging (Beckmann, 2006).

Occurring separately but at a similar time as the development of the CT scanner were efforts at the national level within the United States to produce user facilities to support scientific discovery based upon experimentation. Basic Energy Sciences[3] within the United States Department of Energy[4] currently supports 9 major user facilities along with 5 nanoscale science research centers dedicated to measurement sciences and experimental techniques supporting a very broad range of scientific disciplines. Tracing back the active user facilities,

---

[1] Computed Tomography and History: http://en.wikipedia.org/wiki/Computed_tomography
[2] Radon Transform: http://en.wikipedia.org/wiki/Radon_Transform
[3] US DOE Basic Energy Sciences User Facilities:
http://science.energy.gov/user-facilities/basic-energy-sciences/
[4] US DOE: http://science.energy.gov/

the Stanford Synchrotron Radiation Lightsource[5] (SSRL) a SLAC National Accelerator Laboratory was built in 1974 and it was realized that its intense x-ray beam could be used to study protein molecular structure. The National Synchrotron Light Source[6] (NSLS) at Brookhaven National Laboratory was commissioned in 1982 and currently has 60 x-ray beamlines optimized for a number of different measurement techniques including imaging and tomography. The next generation NSLS-II facility is now under construction. The Advanced Light Source[7] (ALS) commissioned in 1993 has one of the world's brightest sources of coherent long wavelength x-rays suitable for probing biological samples in 3D. The Advanced Photon Source[8] at Argonne National Laboratory also has a number of x-ray beamlines dedicated to imaging and tomography suitable for biological and medical imaging research. The Spallation Neutron Source[9] (SNS) at Oak Ridge National Laboratory (ORNL) also has a number of beamlines suitable for studying the structure and dynamics of proteins and other biological systems. A neutron imaging and tomography beamline is currently being planned for SNS. Similarly, the High Flux Isotope Reactor[10] (HFIR) also at ORNL has beamlines suitable for examining biological matter and has an operational imaging beamline. In addition, the production of medical isotopes is another important HFIR function.

These user facilities have been intended to facilitate basic and applied research and were not explicitly designed with the intention to scan patients the same way commercial medical imaging scanners do. Oftentimes the instrument beam power is significantly more powerful than that produced by medical scanners. Thus the ionizing radiation effects of these beams must be considered when contemplating how these facilities can contribute to medical research. Suitable research areas involving user facilities include the study of proteins, human and animal tissue sample scanning, and in some cases, the study of non-human vertebrate animals such as various rodent species. The process for scanning biological and animal specimens must be approved by the facility biosafety review board.

However there is still a significant amount of bio and medical related research being performed at these national laboratory user facilities and below is a sampling of some of the published research which utilized imaging and scattering resources available via the above mentioned national laboratories:

- At NSLS: The study of thrombosis in rats utilizing Micro- and Nano-CT (Stolz et al., 2011), density quantification of Vasa Vasorum in tomographic coronary angiograms (Moritz et al., 2010), Micro-CT imaging of the human lung acinus (Litzlbauer et al., 2010), rat bone imaging (Rao et al., 2009), bone density using iliac crest biopsies (Jorgensen et al., 2008).
- At APS: sparse data reconstruction of biomedical samples using micro-tomography (Xiao et al., 2010), trabecular bone sample imaging (Xiao et al., 2008), high-energy x-ray scattering of a cortical bone specimen (Stock et al., 2008), visualization of trace metals in biological tissue (D de Jonge & Vogt, 2010).

---

[5] SSRL: http://www-ssrl.slac.stanford.edu/
[6] NSLS: http://www.nsls.bnl.gov/
[7] ALS: http://www-als.lbl.gov/
[8] APS: http://www.aps.anl.gov/
[9] SNS: http://neutrons.ornl.gov/facilities/SNS/
[10] HFIR: http://neutrons.ornl.gov/facilities/HFIR/

- At ALS: irradiation effects on human cortical bone fracture behavior (Barth et al., 2010), x-ray diffraction microscopy of whole biological cells (Nelson et al., 2010), and soft x-ray tomography to image antifungal drug molecules in action (Uchida et al., 2009).
- At SSRL: cell-cell and cell-matrix adhesion molecules (Choi & Weis, 2011), crystallographic analysis (Gupta & Kielkopf, 2011), X-ray absorption spectroscopy for DNA repair (Giri et al., 2011).
- At SNS & HFIR: protein-protein interactions in DNA replication and repair (Hinerman, 2008), lysosome diffusion dynamics of hydration water (Zhang et al., 2009), and enzymatic studies in aqueous ionic liquids (Baker & Heller, 2009).

Each of these facilities utilizes a similar process for how to get beam time at the instruments. There are periodic calls for proposals to which competing proposal teams will respond with descriptions of the experiments they seek to perform while also citing their experiment goals and objectives. Once the proposal call is closed, the proposals are reviewed by a committee comprised of technical experts from a variety of different research and academic institutions. The first pass is a feasibility review to determine if the proposed experiment can be done at the beamline for which time has been requested. This feasibility review will consider things such as the sample environment required, the nature of the material should it be hazardous in some way, and the experiment needs versus the resolution and capabilities of the instrument. The proposals that pass the feasibility review are then peer reviewed by an external scientific review committee which rates and rank the proposals. Subsequently, a beam time allocation committee will make determinations on the amount of time each experiment will then get according to the scientific review committee findings. The outcome will be a list of accepted and alternate proposals and the facility User Office will then initiate making contact with the corresponding experiment Principal Investigators informing them that their proposals have been accepted. As part of the scheduling process, the instrument team will interact with the approved experiment teams to determine experiment dates. As part of scheduling, a local contact will be assigned to each experiment team. This local contact is a valuable asset to the experiment team as this person will assist as necessary to help with making the experiment a success.

Each of these user facilities is a part of the national laboratory in which it resides. As such, there are a number of potential resources available to the research teams which may vary according to the capabilities, personnel, and support facilities available within a particular national laboratory. Across the national laboratory system, five Nanoscale Science Research Centers have been built, and one function of these centers is to help facilitate scientific research at the experimental user facilities. These centers include:

- Center for Nanophase Materials Sciences[11] (CNMS) at ORNL which provides clean rooms, wet and dry labs, sample fabrication, and analysis. CNMS is co-located with SNS to help provide unique capabilities for neutron scattering.
- Molecular Foundary at Lawerence[12] Berkeley National Laboratory which provides laboratories for material science, chemistry, biology, and molecular biology utilizing clean rooms, controlled environment rooms, DNA synthesizer and sequencer, NMR spectrometer, mass spectrometers, along with scanning tunnelling, transmission electron, fluorescence microscopes.

---

[11] CNMS: http://www.cnms.ornl.gov/

[12] Molecular Foundary: http://foundry.lbl.gov/

- Center for Integrated Nanotechnologies[13] (CINT) jointly administered by Los Alamos National Laboratory[14] (LANL) and Sandia National Laboratory[15] (SNL). CINT focus areas are nanophotonics and nanoelectronics, complex functional nonomaterials, nonomechanics, and the nonoscale/bio/microscale interfaces.
- Center for Functional Nanomaterials[16] (CFN) is located at Brookhaven National Laboratory[17] (BNL). CFN develops understandings of the chemical and physical nature of nanomaterials in order to make functional materials such as sensors, activators, and energy conversion devices.
- Center for Nanoscale Materials[18] (CNM) is located at Argonne National Laboratory[19] (ANL) and focuses on research pertaining to advanced magnetic materials, complex oxides, nanophotonics, and bio-inorganic hybrid materials.

In addition to these centers, the national laboratories have unique capabilities to interpret the data that is generated by these facilities. For example, the Imaging, Signals, and Machine Learning (ISML) group[20] within ORNL has expertise in imaging, image/data understanding, and machine learning methods to turn large experimental data sets into useful information for the scientist. A few of the relevant active research capabilities include high-resolution neutron image capture (new scintillators, coded apertures, etc.), tomographic reconstruction, and post reconstruction image analysis and data understanding. Application areas include biomedical imaging[21], telemedicine for retinal diagnostics, CAD for mammography, small animal high-resolution micro-tomographic medical imaging, image analysis for organ segmentation, neuron image analysis and phenotype screening. Such capabilities to analyze and interpret data are an important component of such user facilities to ensure that the ultimate goal of extraction of information from the collected data can be realized.

The remainder of this chapter will now examine the imaging and scattering capabilities of these instruments with special considerations for neutron imaging.

## 2. Imaging and scattering techniques

The measurement techniques at these user facilities vary more widely than those currently employed routinely within the field of medical imaging. In addition to traditional planar and tomographic imaging, additional scattering techniques such as spectroscopy, diffraction and small angle scattering are employed. In these cases, the scattered neutrons or x-rays are fit to physical models in order to determine structure or dynamics (Pynn, 1990). Structures can be at the atomic, molecular, or macro-molecular size scale depending upon the wavelength of the probing beam. An important distinction between x-ray and neutron scattering is that x-rays interact with the electron cloud while neutrons scatter off of the atomic nucleus. Thus in conceptual thinking, x-ray attenuation is approximately linear

[13] CINT: http://cint.lanl.gov/
[14] LANL: http://www.lanl.gov
[15] SANDIA: http://www.sandia.gov
[16] CFN: http://www.bnl.gov/cfn
[17] BNL: http://www.bnl.gov/
[18] CNM: http://nano.anl.gov/index.html
[19] ANL: http://www.anl.gov
[20] ISML: http://www.ornl.gov/sci/ees/mssed/isml/index.shtml
[21] ISML Biomedical Imaging: http://www.ornl.gov/sci/ees/mssed/isml/research-bio.shtml

according to the material density. However this is not the case with neutrons as the scattering cross section[22] is not linear with element density and neutrons scatter quite well off of hydrogen atoms where, in contrast, these atoms are difficult to image with x-rays, but aluminum and other metals are relatively transparent to neutrons. Thus these potentially complementary attenuation properties are useful to exploit for what they can provide.

## 2.1 Imaging

Contrasting imaging instruments and commercial medical imaging scanners reveals a drastically different scale required for hosting the devices. Typically the largest portion of the user facility is required to produce the interrogating beam. These beams have high power and can typically be shaped to produce a beam bandwidth of interest. Thus the instruments must be located at the facilities and people must come to them unlike the situation where many of the medical imaging modalities can be small enough to be mobile. Another important factor to consider is that imaging biological specimens, laboratory animals, and in rare cases, human tissue is the exceptions and not the rule for these facilities. To start with, one must make a convincing case via their proposal that it is worthwhile to scan the subject of interest. Then one must be prepared for additional scrutiny and review by the appropriate facility biological and bio-hazard review committees. Upon acceptance, one must then be prepared to follow proper specimen handling procedures. Note that science areas such as protein crystallography and soft matter are much more routine than described above. The instruments at the user facilities have powerful capabilities and one must carefully prepare in order to utilize them.

Despite these obstacles, there are active communities of researchers which utilize imaging instruments to help with their research. The context here for the definition of imaging refers to the various X-ray and neutron imaging instruments. Conceptually these instruments produce images in similar format as those produced by medical imaging scanners, however these instruments typically incorporate more flexibility for their capabilities and are less specialized and optimized as compared to the medical scanners. To illustrate imaging capabilities, some examples showing the differences in image contrast between neutron and x-ray imaging are shown in figures 1 through 3.

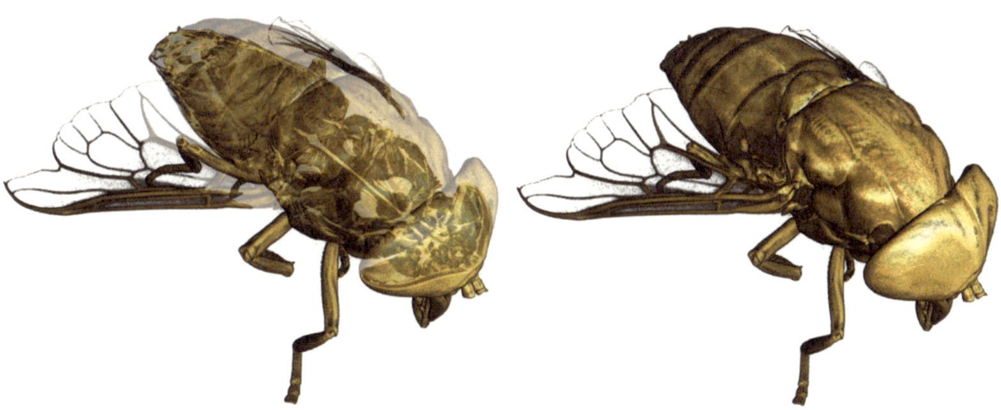

[22] Neutron scattering cross sections: http://www.ncnr.nist.gov/resources/n-lengths/list.html

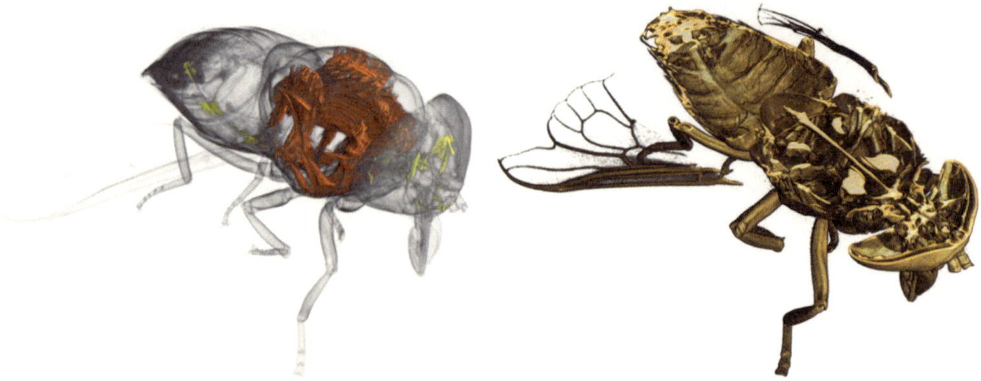

Fig. 1. Neutron tomography of a dried horsefly. Top right: outer surface, top left: upper portion sliced away, bottom right: mid-level slice, bottom left: contour of wing muscles. Note that the insect is approximately 1cm in length head to tail. Images courtesy of Dr. Eberhard Lehmann using the ICON beamline, SINQ, Paul Scherrer Institut, Switzerland[23].

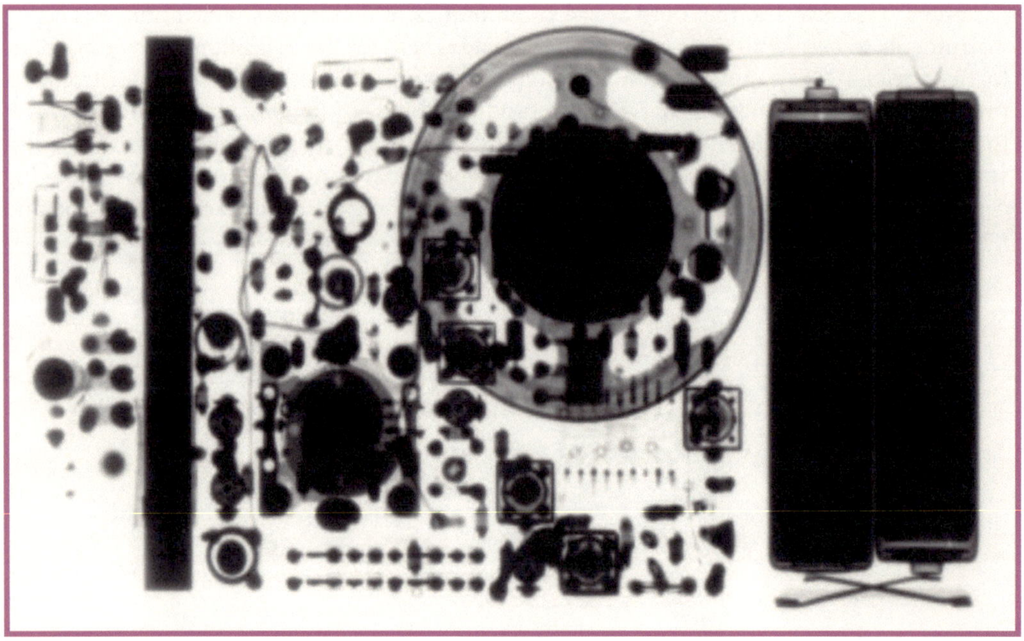

[23] ICON Instrument: http://neutra.web.psi.ch/facility/icon_index.html

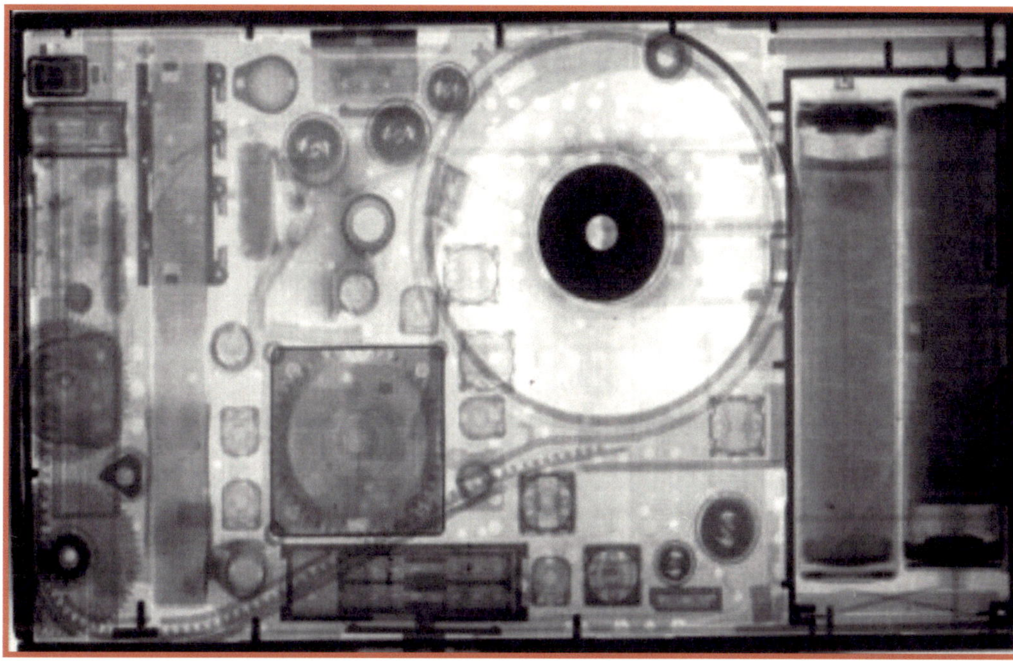

Fig. 2. X-ray (top) and neutron (bottom) images of a miniature transistor radio. Images courtesy of Dr. Eberhard Lehmann taken using the ICON beamline, SINQ, Paul Scherrer Institut, Switzerland.

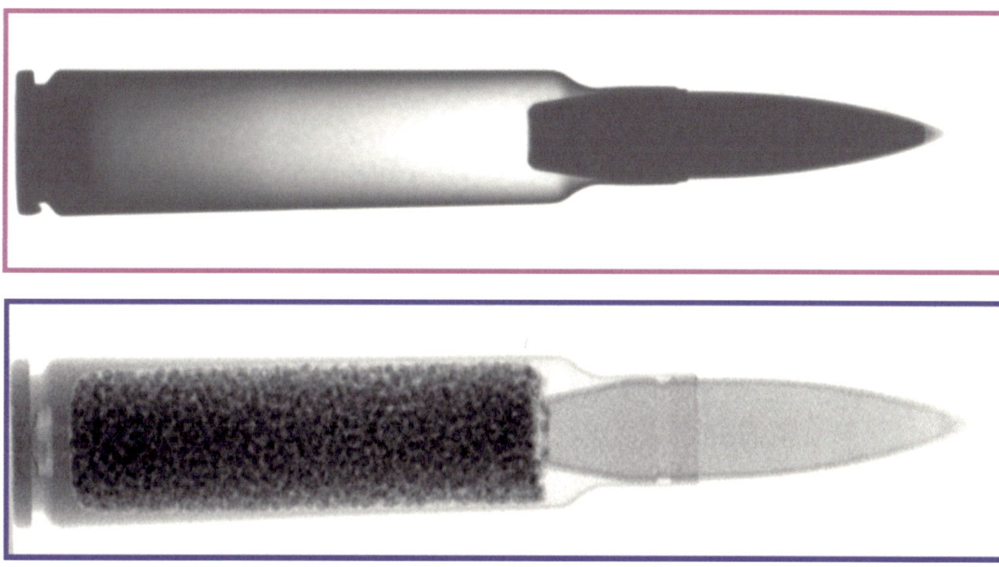

Fig. 3. X-ray (Top) and neutron (Bottom) image of a bullet. Note the difference in contrast where x-rays image illustrate metal density while neutrons are capable of imaging through metals to image materials containing hydrogen atoms. Images courtesy of Dr. Eberhard Lehmann taken using the ICON beamline, SINQ, Paul Scherrer Institut, Switzerland.

### 2.2 Scattering

From a medical imaging perspective, the usual case is to observe the attenuation pattern based upon the beam which transmits through the object being imaged. For tomography, a set of views are taken at angular increments around the object.

However a portion of the beam can scatter off of the object and can be detected outside the boundaries of the transmission image, and scattering techniques exist for both neutron and x-rays. For neutron scattering, a strong scattering object will scatter ~10% or less of the total transmission flux. The scattering angle can be vary across $4\pi$ Steradians (sr) depending upon a number of factors including beam properties such as wavelength and material properties such as structure. A conceptual illustration of transmission and small angle scattering is shown in figure 4. In contrast with transmission imaging, scattering detection systems may

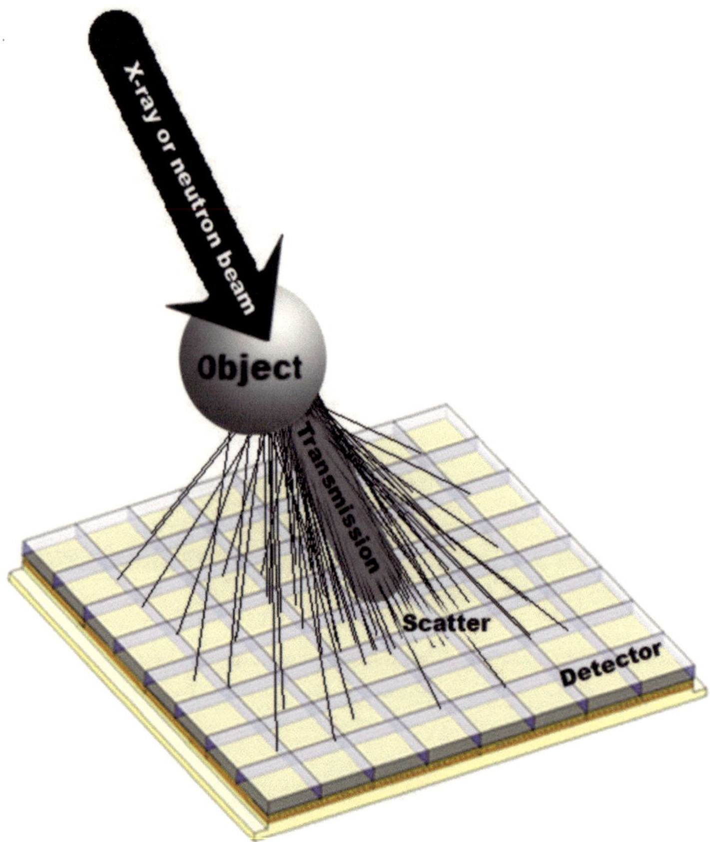


Fig. 4. Cartoon illustrating transmission and scatter detection locations for an object in an X-ray or neutron beam. Typically only one technique will be employed at a time but shown here together to illustrate differences between the detection techniques. The transmission image results from rays which strike the detector having passed directly through the object. The scatter pattern results from the rays being deflected at some angle here shown as small angle scattering though the scattering angles can be arbitrary in solid angle depending upon the sample and imaging beam characteristics.

utilize very small samples in comparison to the detector sizes. For example, a 1 $cm^3$ size sample or smaller is typical while the detection system sizes may range to 10+ meters tall in order to obtain the desired solid angle detection range. Other scattering systems fix detectors about the sample covering as much of the $4\pi$ space as possible. The necessary distance between the sample and the detectors must be considered when spacing the detectors so as to take into consideration adequate resolution, and this distance may be several meters for some instruments.

There are a number of elastic scattering techniques including small angle scattering shown in figure 5, reflectometry, powder and single crystal diffraction. There also exist inelastic scattering techniques such as direct and indirect geometry spectrometry. Typically the scatter patterns are not as visually intuitive as the transmission images as one must deduce the structure via model fitting in the case for scattering science. As previously mentioned, a good primer for neutron scattering has been written by Pynn (Pynn, 1990). For examining the statistical nature of structure, scattering techniques can be used to measure a wide range of length scales ranging from atomic to molecular, to macromolecular and thus has its advantages over other measurement techniques.

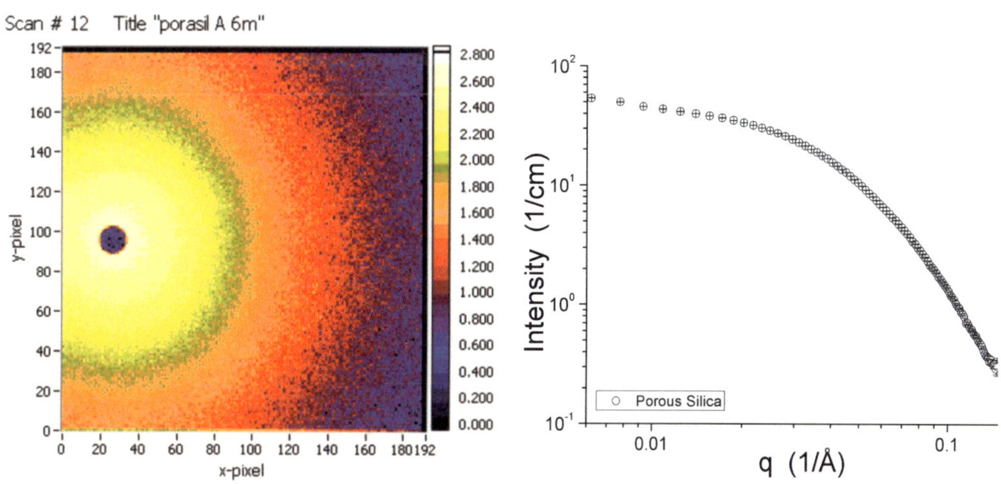


Fig. 5. Neutron scattering image of porous silica from a Small Angle Neutron Scattering instrument. Left: The raw detector data image - note that the center of scattering is offset to the left center of the image in this case to extend visibility of the data "tails" at the edge of the scattering pattern. Right: the corresponding reduced data illustrating intensity versus inverse Angstroms. Models can be fit to the reduced data to determine structure. Images courtesy of Dr. William T. Heller of the Spallation Neutron Source at Oak Ridge National Laboratory.

## 3. Neutron imaging beamline overview

The following section illustrates from acquisition to visualization working with neutron imaging data. The detection systems are explored as well as the processes for normalizing data and reconstructing images. A section discussing data management pertinent to the national laboratories is also included which illustrates some significant differences in data handling between the research and commercial medical imaging communities.

### 3.1 Data acquisition

Neutron radiography systems follow the same basic geometric design as x-ray system, so those familiar with resolution and magnification in x-ray systems will quickly feel comfortable working with neutrons. There are very few neutron imaging instruments, and they are built to accommodate a variety of types of materials research, so these instruments are designed to be flexible in their geometry in order to satisfy imaging requirements over a broad spectrum of applications from industrial to medical to archeological applications. This flexibility requires the user to have a basic understanding of neutron imaging instrument components and geometries to plan successful experiments. While the x-ray and neutron system geometries are similar, the commonly used designs are different due to differences in the available sources and detectors. Since x-ray and neutron imaging are so similar and x-ray is a well accepted and understood imaging modality, the following discussion of neutron radiography system will draw parallels and point out differences between the systems through the description of the sources, detectors, and geometric designs.

#### 3.1.1 Neutron sources

Neutron sources for radiography are large user facilities that are either reactor sources producing a continuous beam of neutrons or spallation sources producing neutron pulses (Arai & Crawford, 2009). Since the neutrons from both types of source are initially higher in energy than would be useful for most scattering and imaging experiments, the neutrons are passed through a moderator that scatters the neutrons to lower their energy. As a result of creating a large initial source to emit as many neutrons as possible and use of a moderator, neutron sources are quite large with ports to instruments having sizes in the tens of centimeters. In contrast, x-ray sources with similar flux are available having spot sizes down to 5μm in diameter. The large source size for neutrons is a key issue when designing the imaging geometry as discussed later.

Pulsed sources for both x-rays and neutrons can be used like a flash bulb to stop motion of the object being imaged; however, the reason for building pulsed neutron sources such as the SNS is to provide energy resolution. The speed that a neutron travels is directly proportional to the energy of the neutron; therefore, a neutron pulse spreads out over distance traveled. By placing a detector with timing resolution a sufficient distance from the source, images can be obtained over a range of neutron energies (wavelengths). In medical imaging, we see dual energy x-ray systems used to enhance the contrast between materials in the body and also achieve some level of elemental analysis. This is possible because a material's x-ray attenuation coefficient is a function of the x-ray energy, and this function varies between materials. For example, a dual energy X-ray image can determine if a kidney stone is composed of uric acid or if it contains calcium. Another common use of dual energy x-ray is to calculate bone mineral density for diagnosis of osteoporosis or osteopenia. Finally, dual (or more) energy x-rays are commonly used to enhance images of lung parenchyma because the bones can be removed from the final image. In this same sense, imaging over a range of neutron energies can provide contrast for different materials and even identify materials based on the transmission spectrum. One area of interest for imaging at multiple wavelengths is with respect to crystal structures and may have applications in imaging of interfaces between tissue and prosthetic joint devices. The polycrystalline materials of these metal joints has a unique transmission spectrum with large swings in attenuation at particular energies known as Bragg edges.

Imaging on both sides of a Bragg edge will provide two very different contrast images to help identify the interface between tissue, bone, and prosthetic device.

### 3.1.2 Neutron imaging devices

Two types of direct digital imaging devices are employed at neutron imaging instruments: scintillator based and micro channel plate (MCP) based. MCP based detectors provide the higher resolution than scintillators for neutron radiography, but they are much more expensive and degrade with use.

Scintillator based imaging devices use a $^{6}$Li based scintillator plate to convert neutrons to visible light which is imaged by a CCD or CMOS based camera as shown in figure 6. In these systems, a mirror is used to move the camera out of the direct neutron beam for protection of the electronics and to remove components that may become activated by the neutron beam and as a result produce noise in the images due to gamma ray emissions striking the CCD or CMOS electronics. The right side of this figure is a photograph of a scintillator based camera in use at HFIR.

The highest resolution of scintillator based neutron imagers is approximately 50μm and is a function of the scintillator, the lens, and the CCD or CMOS detector. Currently the resolution is limited by the scintillator resolution. $^{6}$Li Scintillator screens are available in varying thicknesses. Thinner screens provide the highest resolution but interact with fewer neutrons which leads to longer exposure times.

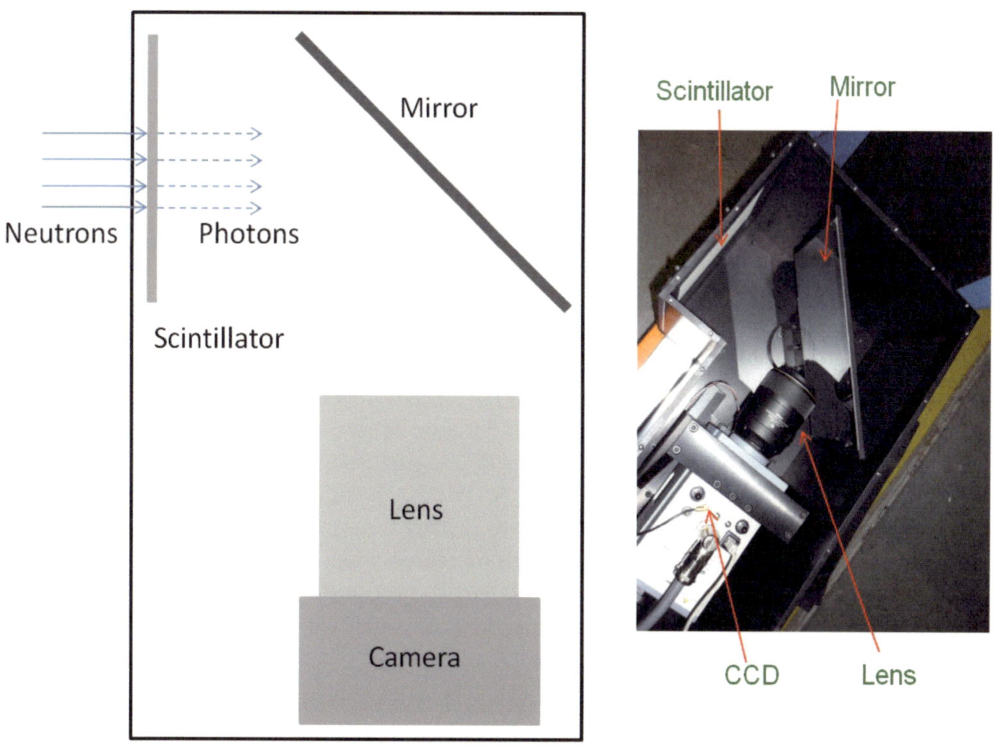


Fig. 6. Scintillator based neutron imaging device.

MCPs are thin slabs of material with an array of holes through the slab. Each hole or microchannel is an electron multiplier, so once a single electron is produced the signal is amplified by a 1000 times or more to enable detection of the single event. MCPs are glass based and have been developed for neutron imaging through the incorporation of $^{10}B$ in the glass. Interactions of the neutron with $^{10}B$ in the glass produces ions that can escape the glass into neighboring microchannels. These ions free electrons in the microchannel which then get multiplied and detected at the output. The latest microchannels are being produced with diameters <10μm leading to resolutions approaching 10μm. MCPs doped with $^{10}B$ are efficient for neutron detection due to the high cross section of $^{10}B$. Efforts to improve these devices further are attempts to further reduce the channel diameters for higher resolution and doping with Gd to further improve efficiency (Tremsin, 2011).

### 3.1.3 System design

Due to the difference in available source spot sizes, radiography system geometries in particular used for CT differ between x-ray and neutron systems in the position of the object between the source and detector. Neutron systems place the object as close as possible to the detector while x-ray CT systems place the object half way between source and detector. One reason x-ray systems will place object in the center is to allow rotation of source and detector around the object for CT. This isn't possible with the permanent neutron sources, so the object must be rotated and doesn't need to be centered. Another advantage of placing the object in the center is a magnification factor of two for the object projection on to the detector. Magnification eases resolution requirements for the detector, but restricts size of the source spot to maintain resolution.

Resolution of radiography systems (both x-ray and neutron) is determined by source size, system geometry, and detector resolution. Detectors for both x-ray and neutron imaging systems consist of a conversion material, optics, and a pixelated detector. Resolution of the detector is a function of the point spread of the conversion material, the modulation transfer function of the optics, and the pixel size of the pixelated detector. Resolution of an imaging system up to the detector plane is a result of the source and system geometry as shown in figure 7. In this figure, an edge is imaged by a source of finite size, D, at a distance, L, from the source. From parts a and b of the figure, the blur of the edge which is called penumbra, p, is obviously smaller with the reduced source size. The comparison between a and c shows an inverse relationship between the source to detector distance and the penumbra. As a result, instrument developers at neutron sources often specify the quality of their neutron beams with L/D. This value has a direct relationship to resolution of the beam for imaging. L/D values from 300-500 are typical at neutron imaging instruments. Most instruments will offer setups at several different L/D values. The L/D values are selected by placing an aperture in the beam line close to the source to restrict the size of the source. As the diameter of the aperture gets smaller, L/D (resolution) increases linearly and exposure time increases as a square of the diameter. Since one could easily produce a very high L/D value with a small aperture an instrument specifications must also include a neutron flux value for fair comparison between imaging instruments.

The example in figure 7 kept the object at the same distance from the imager. To understand why the object is placed close to the imager for neutron imaging with a relatively large spot size, consider the effect of pulling the object away from the imager. If an object is placed in contact with the imager, penumbra is reduced to zero. As the object moves away, the object is magnified onto the detector, but so is the penumbra or blur of the edges. For flexibility, neutron imaging instruments have stages to move the object position setup to accommodate various size objects and still keep them as close to the imager as possible.

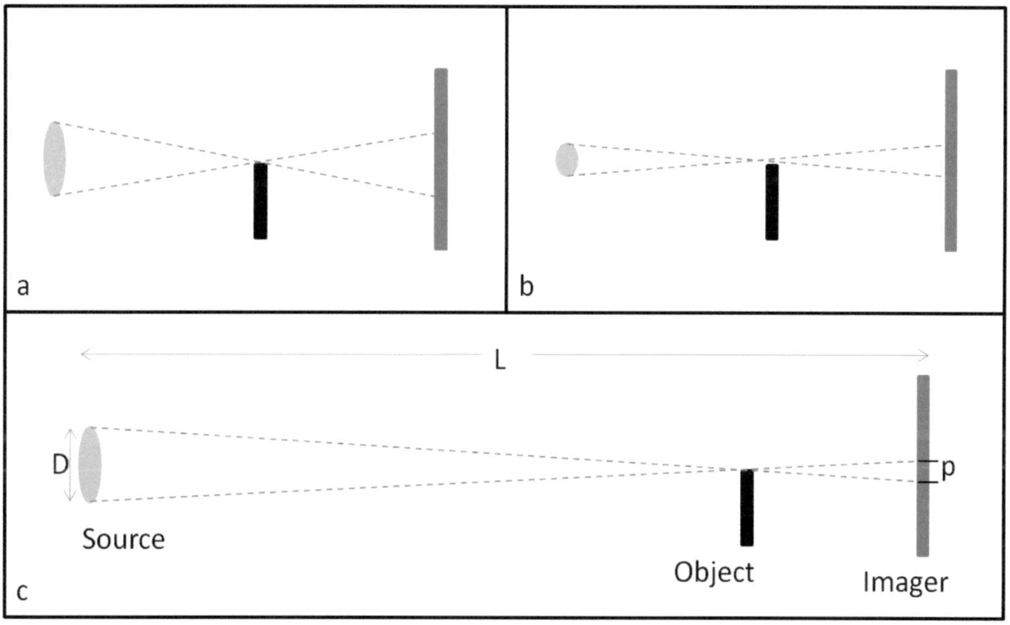


Fig. 7. Resolution of system depends on source size and geometry. Decrease in source size between a and b; Increase in source to detector distance between a and c.

Before a user submits a proposal to use a neutron imaging instrument, he/she should understand the capabilities of the beam line to determine whether the instrument provides the required field of view and resolution for their application. User facilities have specifications for their beam lines and will provide best resolution and field of view specifications, but it is difficult to include all potential imaging setups in descriptions of a neutron imaging instruments due to the flexibility. User facilities have beam line scientists assigned to each instrument. Consulting with the beam line scientist on a particular application is a recommended method to determine whether the instrument is capable of meeting the needs for the proposed research.

### 3.2 Data management

Data management at large-scale research facilities can be drastically different than commercially available smaller scale systems. In general commercially available system are static as well as propriety and perform in a highly regulated environment whereas research facilities are quite dynamic and utilize open source packages on unregulated open data files. Many research facilities do indeed have data policies and/or best practices that they follow but for the most part they follow an open research policy. These large-scale research facility data policies support an innovative and collaborative environment while still enabling a fair and competitive atmosphere.

In recent years we have seen a dramatic increase in data file sizes that are generated from research instruments. This size increase has afforded researchers the ability to produce high fidelity images with extremely fine-grained resolutions. As a result, scientific discovery has been enabled and it is now commonplace to process and transfer data files on the order of hundreds of gigabytes. These data files are part of collections that in some cases approach a terabytes of raw and reduced data. The ability to transfer these data sets over high-bandwidth modern networks is now not trivial especially when remote users require these data collections to be transferred to their home institutions. In most cases it is necessary to use multi-threaded streaming data file transfer applications in order to efficiently migrate these data collections. For instance, Orbiter Commander is currently used at the Spallation Neutron Source for transferring data collections utilizing streaming compressed mutli-threaded algorithms as seen in figure 8.

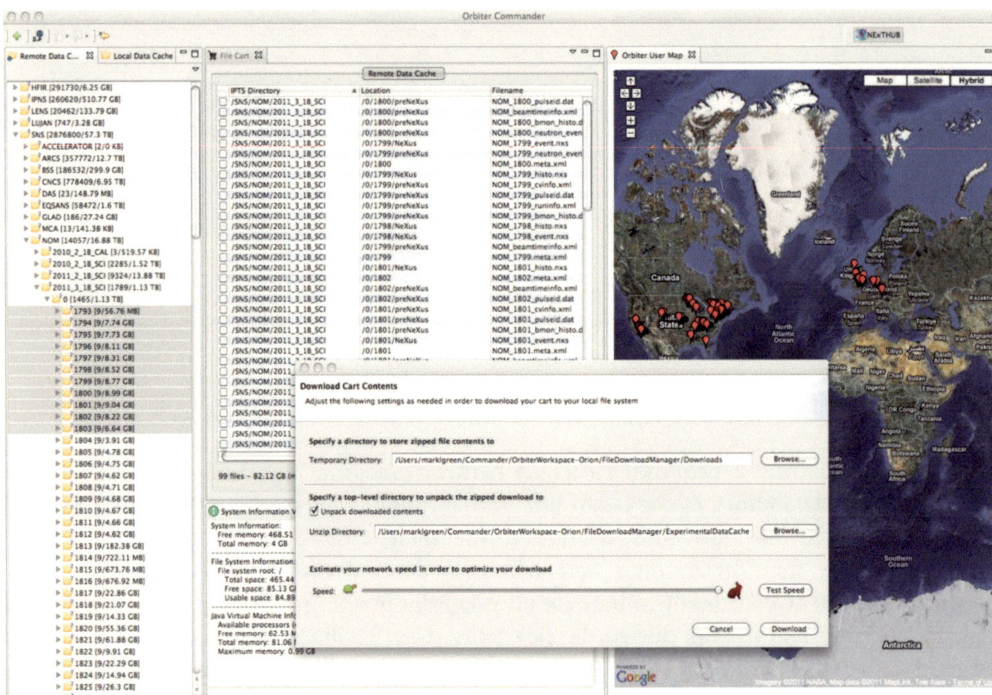


Fig. 8. The Commander file download manager application – https://orbiter.txcorp.com

### 3.3 Data reduction and normalization

Data from scintillation based detectors results in projections stored in common image storage formats. MCP imagers detect individual neutron interactions resulting in a list that includes the time and position of each acquired interaction instead of an image. Images are produced out of this list mode data through binning of the individual interactions based on the imaging setup (i.e. binning on time for pulsed sources provides energy resolution). X-ray CT systems encountered in medical imaging applications are well developed such that projection data is captured along with normalization shots and then normalized and passed to a reconstruction engine without requiring input from the user along the way. The flexibility of neutron imaging instruments makes full automation of this process difficult, since the user can select the number of projections, range of angles, number of normalization images, and rotational stage position. Acquisition will provide the user with a projection data set and normalization images (light and dark) based on the setup. Beam lines will have normalization and reconstruction capabilities for the users to analyze their data.

After acquisition, the sample data files produced need to be normalized. The normalization is a simple mathematical process that cleans up the data by removing imperfection of the incident beam, signal detected that are not related to the sample measured and noise due to the surrounding. To perform the normalization, two more data files called open beam and dark field are required.

The open beam measures the shape and intensity of the incident beam. The open beam is acquired using exactly the same set up and time duration as the sample data file but without the sample in the beam. Due to the way they are acquired, background signals of the open beam and sample data have to match. Because the intensity of the incident beam can vary over time, it is important to bring the intensity of the data file background to the same level as the open beam background. This is done by selecting several regions of interest, away from the sample, in the data file, and calculating their average intensities. The same process is repeated on the open beam. Average of the ratio of those intensities gives a corrector factor to apply to the sample data. The dark field measured the electronic noise (thermal noise and dark current) and background. It is acquired with incident beam turn off and shutter open.

Gamma rays detected also need to be removed from the various files. Gamma rays events have the particularity of being very concentrated (1 or 2 pixels for each event) and very intense. Because those events happen randomly, the files have to be treated individually. Different mathematical processes can be used to do so. In development of normalization routines at ORNL, we discovered that the Lee filtering works very well. After removing gamma strike spikes from all images include data, open beam and dark field, the data are normalized using the following mathematical formula:

$$ND = \frac{Data - DF}{OB - DF}$$

With ND: normalized data, Data: data sample, DF: Dark Field and OB: Open beam. Since the DF and OB images are used to normalize every projection, any noise in these images propagates into all normalized projections. To reduce the noise in the normalization images, multiple DF and OB images are collected and averaged together after removal of gamma spikes.

To facilitate this whole process, programs such as iMars, (iMAging Reduction Software), as shown in figure 9, can be used. This program, using the IDL[24] programming language, has been developed at the Spallation Neutron Source and works as follows. First, the user has to select the input files (data file, open beam and dark field) and select the regions of interest

---

[24] IDL: http://www.ittvis.com

using manual or graphical input. The program then automatically performs the normalization and produced various output file formats (fits, tiff or jpeg).

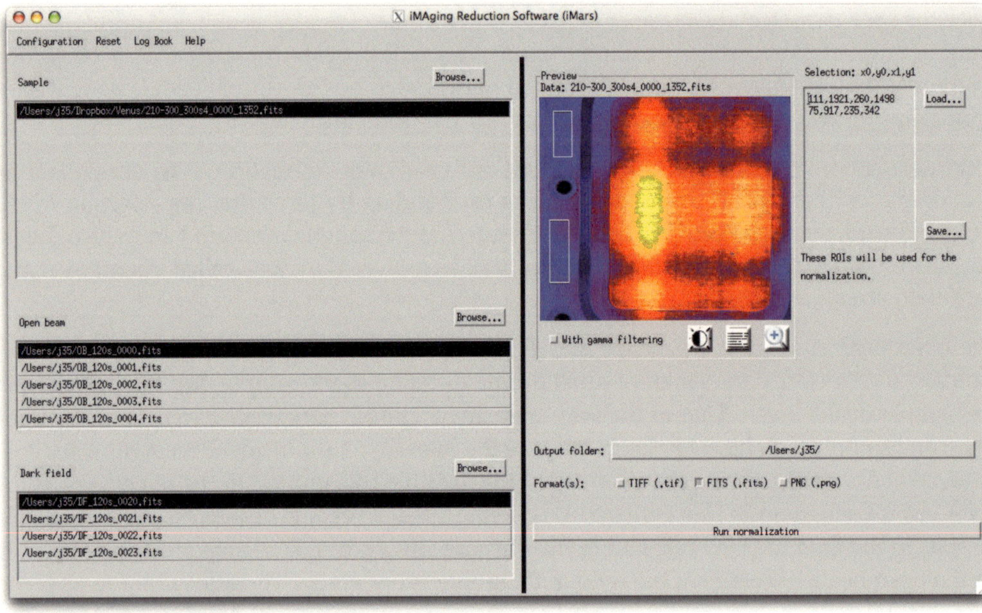


Fig. 9. iMars (iMAging Reduction Software) user interface in use with the HFIR imaging beamline.

### 3.4 Data reconstruction

Neutron radiography and computed tomography reconstruction can fully leverage techniques of medical imaging with x-rays and has benefited from the development of analysis and reconstruction algorithms developed by the medical imaging community. Two discrete classes of reconstruction algorithms are widely employed to generate tomographic images. Analytic algorithms calculate the image data directly using defined single-pass mathematical methods. These algorithms have the advantage of relative simplicity and speed, but tend to produce noisier reconstructed images. In contrast, iterative reconstruction algorithms employ complex models of the acquisition system and repeatedly estimate solutions and compare the estimate with a modeled "ideal" solution until pre-defined convergence criteria are met. Iterative algorithms typically produce superior images but can take much longer to execute. We will briefly introduce these two types in this chapter, and a more detailed treatment can be found in (Gleason et al., 2010).

As an example of an analytic type, Filtered Back Projection (FBP) algorithms are well developed for cone beam geometries seen in x-ray CT systems (Kak, 1988). Neutron radiography systems are cone beam systems as well and therefore use the exact same reconstruction algorithms with a change in system parameters for placement of the center of rotation closer to the detector. Again, flexibility of the neutron systems will challenge the user to set up the appropriate system parameters in any reconstruction code used so attention must be paid to the setup during data acquisition to ensure a proper reconstruction.

FBP basically spreads the attenuation measured by a single pixel within a projection equally across the 3D volume between the source and the pixel. With enough projections around the object, the attenuation on a true object piles up and the attenuation that is spread to incorrect positions in the volume becomes insignificant. This direct calculation method enables high speed reconstruction of 3D volumes, but places requirements on number and spacing of projections around the object. These requirements are easily met by x-ray systems due to the high flux from x-ray sources. Neutron sources have lower flux at the camera, so obtaining a data set with sufficient signal to noise ratio and number of projections may not be feasible due to time required to collect the projections.

Iterative reconstruction algorithms have seen considerable development for improvement of x-ray CT data, but do not see common use in medical imaging outside of research environments, because iterative reconstruction is computationally intense requiring much more time than FBP, and FBP reconstructions are suited for most medical applications. A CT projection data set represents a large set of linear equations to be solved for attenuation in each voxel of the volume. Using iterative methods for solving linear equations, reconstruction codes have been developed by many research groups with variation in the iterative methods focused on speeding up reconstruction through quicker convergence or parallel computation. Iterative reconstruction algorithms allow reconstruction with fewer and non-uniformly distributed projections and allow inclusion of more complex physics models. For these reasons, iterative algorithms should be considered as a reconstruction option for neutron radiography where the number and quality of projections are less than in medical x-ray CT. However, iterative reconstruction comes at a considerable cost in computation.

### 3.5 Image analysis and data visualization

In broad use across the national laboratories is a wide range of open-source and commercially licensed image analysis and data visualization applications. To illustrate, several are listed below:

**IDL[25]:** The Interactive Data Language (IDL) is a commercial array-processing language, which has been designed from its earliest inception for image processing applications development. IIDL implements an efficient array-processing engine combined with a large library of analysis routines, and is well suited for rapidly developing a wide variety of complex mathematical programs. This combination of array processing, image visualization, and data analysis functionality is why IDL is well suited for the tomography reconstruction. While a full version of IDL requires a license from ITT Visual Information Systems (ITTVIS), the IDL Virtual Machine is freely available and able to run compiled IDL programs. IDL is also capable of exporting compiled procedures as self-contained executables, making it an ideal platform for developing and sharing tomography algorithms.

**MATLAB[26]:** MATLAB is commercial a high-level array language with control flow statements, functions, data structures, file and data input/output, and object-oriented programming features with an integrated interactive development environment, and has pre-built extensive facilities for displaying vectors and matrices as graphs, as well as

---

[25] IDL: http://www.ittvis.com/
[26] MATLAB: http://www.mathworks.com/

capabilities for annotating and printing these graphs. It includes high-level functions for two-dimensional and three- dimensional data visualization and image processing. MATLAB is also a natural platform for rapidly prototyping and developing reconstruction algorithms.

**VisIt[27]:** Developed by Lawrence Livermore National Laboratory, VisIt is a free, open source, interactive parallel visualization and graphical analysis tool for viewing scientific data on Unix and PC platforms. Users can quickly generate visualizations from their data, animate them through time, manipulate them, and save the resulting images for presentations. VisIt contains a rich set of visualization features so that you can view your data in a variety of ways. It can be used to visualize scalar and vector fields defined on two- and three-dimensional (2D and 3D) structured and unstructured meshes. VisIt was designed to handle very large data set sizes in the terascale range and yet can also handle small data sets in the kilobyte range.

VisIt employs a distributed and parallel architecture in order to handle extremely large data sets interactively. VisIt's rendering and data processing capabilities are split into viewer and engine components that may be distributed across multiple machines:

VisIt-Viewer: Responsible for rendering and is typically run on a local desktop or visualization server so that it can leverage the extremely powerful graphics cards that have been developed in the last few years.

VisIt-Engine: Responsible for the bulk of the data processing and input/output (I/O) and is typically run on a remote compute server where the data is located. This eliminates the need move the data and makes high-end compute and I/O resources available to it. The engine can be run serially on a single processor or in parallel on thousands of processors.

VisIt also supports C++, Python and Java interfaces. The C++ and Java interfaces make it possible to provide alternate user interfaces for VisIt or allow existing C++ or Java applications to add visualization support. VisIt can be controlled by its Graphical User Interface (GUI), through the Python and Java programming languages, and can be integrated into custom user interfaces as well.

**VTK[28]/ITK[29]:** The VTK is an open source library, licensed under the GPL (section 1.1). It is entirely written in C++ and is available for many different platforms (Linux, Mac and Windows), and has support for writing platform independent applications. The library has a size of over 700 C++ classes and contains many algorithms for 2D and 3D image processing and visualization. It implements a data processing pipeline and numerous filters for reading, modifying and writing data. It also implements algorithms for volume and surface rendering. Although the library is written in C++, it was designed to be easily extensible and can be used within other programming languages. There are currently wrappers available for TCL/TK, Java and Python. For the surface rendering, VTK typically uses OpenGL to make use of the graphic card's hardware acceleration. In contrast to that, volume rendering will in most cases be performed "in software" by the computer's CPU.

[27] VisIt: https://wci.llnl.gov/codes/visit/
[28] VTK: http://www.vtk.org/
[29] ITK: http://www.itk.org/

ITK is an extension of the VTK, adding techniques for analyzing medical images, for example and registration/segmentation methods. Like the VTK, the ITK comes with an extensive class documentation that has the same features as the VTK documentation. ITK also includes several example applications that demonstrate the functionality of the library.

**ImageJ[30]:** ImageJ is a public domain Java image-processing program inspired by NIH Image for the Macintosh. It runs, either as an online applet or as a downloadable application, on any computer with a Java 1.4 or later virtual machine. Downloadable distributions are available for Windows, Mac OS, Mac OS X and Linux.

It can display, edit, analyze, process, save and print 8-bit, 16-bit and 32-bit images and read many image formats including TIFF, GIF, JPEG, BMP, DICOM, FITS and "raw". It supports "stacks", a series of images that share a single window. It is multithreaded, so time-consuming operations such as image file reading can be performed in parallel with other operations.

ImageJ does calculate area and pixel value statistics of user-defined selections and mea- sure distances and angles. It can create density histograms and line profile plots and it supports standard image processing functions such as contrast manipulation, sharpening, smoothing, edge detection and median filtering. It does geometric transformations such as scaling, rotation and flips. Image can be zoomed up to 32:1 and down to 1:32. All analysis and processing functions are available at any magnification factor. The program supports any number of windows (images) simultaneously, limited only by available memory. Spatial calibration is available to provide real world dimensional measurements in units such as millimeters. Density or gray scale calibration is also available.

ImageJ was designed with an open architecture that provides extensibility via Java plugins. Custom acquisition, analysis and processing plugins can be developed using ImageJ's built in editor and Java compiler. User-written plugins make it possible to solve almost any image processing or analysis problem.

**GPULib[31]:** Graphics hardware has been increasing in performance at a much faster rate than CPUs. Additionally, since they are designed for graphics applications, GPUs already include a great deal of parallelism and are optimized for vector- and matrix-based calculations. Until recently this power was used mostly for video games and computer-generated animations, and now the scientific community is taking advantage of GPU performance in visualization applications routinely. GPULib is a commercial product which provides a high-level, generalized interface that allows scientists and engineers to take advantage of the speed and performance of GPU hardware in their own applications. Using GPULib, vector calculations, matrix transforms, and array manipulations can be off-loaded from the CPU to NVIDIA graphics hardware, leveraging the optimizations and speed of the GPU to increase performance of their applications. Currently, language bindings for IDL, Matlab, Python, Java, and C exist. Generally GPULib can be integrated quickly and provide 30-100x speedup for reconstruction algorithms and 3D tomography visualizations.

---

[30] ImageJ: http://rsbweb.nih.gov/ij/

[31] GPULib: http://www.txcorp.com/products/GPULib/

GPULib can be used within all of these steps for increasing the processing speed substantially. To use GPULib from within an IDL script, you first need to call the gpuinit procedure. This will load the needed libraries and give you access to GPU-related functions. Once gpuinit is loaded, you will have access to over 135 GPULib functions.

## 4. Case study – Neutron imaging

Following is a case study examining the utility and issues for neutron based medical imaging. Currently there are no known neutron detection based commercial medical imaging scanners, though medical applications for neutron imaging are explored.

### 4.1 Medical applications of neutron imaging

Interest in neutron radiography dates back to shortly after Chadwick's discovery of the neutron (Chadwick 1932). In the 1950's and 1960's, neutron radiography came into use in non-destructive testing(Berger 1965) but it was the later when it interest in imaging biological samples emerged(Thewlis 1956; Berger and McGonnagle 1962; Barton 1964; Atkins 1965). Seminal articles on the subject outlined to problems of neutron detection, radiation dose, and multiple scattering events for in realistic thicknesses of tissue that degrade the images for everything but high energy neutrons (> 1 MeV)(Brown and Parks 1969; Parks and Brown 1969; Budinger, Bichsel et al. 1971; Budinger, Howerton et al. 1971). At that time, images were obtained by using a scintillator that exposed photographic film. Since that time, detectors have improved and cover much more of the energy spectrum than would be required to perform any imaging in humans. Despite advances, current detectors are specific for defined neutron energies, are not linear, and do not cover the entire energy spectrum (Vartsky, Mor et al. 2005; Marinelli, Milani et al. 2006; Marinelli, Milani et al. 2007; Mayer, Forkel-Wirth et al. 2007; Dangendorf, Bar et al. 2009; Mor, Vartsky et al. 2009; Ruddy, Flammang et al. 2009; Ruddy, Seidel et al. 2009; Vartsky, Mor et al. 2010).

The most significant problem for neutron imaging of tissues is multiple neutron scattering by the protons in hydrogen. The best transmission images, x-ray or neutron, occur when there is only a single scattering event in the sample before it reaches the detector. This goal is never practically achievable. A larger the percentage of multiple scattering events will result in greater the degradation of the image. Since tissue is composed of hydrocarbons, neutron radiography is currently confined to thin specimens or the neutron energies must be large. This is best understood by considering the scattering of neutrons from the protons in hydrogen atoms in the organic molecules that compose tissues.

From elementary kinematics, the energy transfer from the incident neutron to the proton (where the masses of the neutron and proton are taken to be equal) is given by:

$$E_p = \frac{1}{2} E_n \left(1 - \cos\phi\right)$$

where $E_p$ is the recoil proton energy, $E_n$ is the incident neutron energy, and $\phi$ is the center of mass scattering angle. Averaging over all scattering angles gives a result that on the average; the energy is divided evenly between the neutron and proton, i.e.

$$E_p = \frac{1}{2} E_n .$$

So even very energetic neutrons are converted to thermal neutrons (energy ~0.025 eV) within relatively few collisions. It can easily be shown that a 10 keV neutron requires ~19 collisions to reach a thermal energy while a 10 MeV neutron will only 28 collisions before becoming completely thermalized. After a very few collisions, the neutron distribution becomes isotropic and thus has lost all structural information. To understand how this applies to tissues, consider Table 1 which shows an approximate composition of human tissues (this will vary somewhat between organ systems but it is representative of the body as an average). The cross sections are for thermal neutrons only and Nσ represents the total elastic cross section as measured in the laboratory. This shows that the neutrons are scattered more by hydrogen than the next most significant element, carbon, by a factor of 20. Deuterium, which is hydrogen with a neutron or ${}^{2}_{1}H$, has a much smaller cross section for neutrons and therefore will not attenuate the beam as much. Thus, by using deuterated or heavy water, the number of multiple scattering events will decrease which will improve the image. The total cross section is important because it is related to the mean free path by:

$$\lambda = \left( \sum_i N_i \sigma_i \right)^{-1}$$

where the *i*'s refer to the different elements present. As noted above, most of the scattering is from the proton in hydrogen so the mean free path in tissues can be approximated by:

$$\lambda \approx 1 / (N_H \sigma_H) .$$

| Element | Tissue Abundance | Atomic Weight | Number Density ($cm^{-3}$) | σ (b) | Nσ($cm^{-1}$) |
|---|---|---|---|---|---|
| H | 0.11 | 1.008 | 6.51E+22 | 30.39 | 1.977084 |
| C | 0.51 | 12.010 | 2.53E+22 | 4.746 | 0.120158 |
| N | 0.02 | 14.010 | 8.51E+20 | 12.19 | 0.010372 |
| O | 0.36 | 16.000 | 1.34E+22 | 3.97 | 0.053320 |
| Na | 0.001 | 22.990 | 2.59E+19 | 3.92 | 0.000102 |
| P | 0.001 | 30.970 | 1.92E+19 | 4.37 | 0.000084 |
| S | 0.001 | 32.070 | 1.86E+19 | 1.52 | 0.000028 |
| Cl | 0.001 | 35.450 | 1.68E+19 | 65.32 | 0.001099 |

Table 1. A representative elemental composition of human tissues with number densities, thermal neutron ($E_{thermal}$ = 0.025 eV) cross sections, and total elastic scattering cross sections.

Table 2 shows the mean free path for neutron energies from 1 eV to 10 MeV for hydrogen scattering only. The table shows that to penetrate a human limb that the incident neutron spectrum will need to be between 1 and 10 MeV. As might be expected, increasing the neutron energy also increases the radiation dose (absorbed dose). The exact details of such radiation doses due to a neutron require a significant effort to calculate. Such calculations are typically performed by large Monte Carlo codes such as available from the Radiation Safety Information Computational Center at Oak Ridge National Laboratory[32]. Prior determinations of neutron doses would indicate that doses would be in an acceptable range but further work needs to be performed before human trials could be contemplated (Brown and Parks 1969; Budinger, Howerton et al. 1971; Kry, Howell et al. 2009).

| E(keV) | σ(b) | Nσ(cm-1) | λ(cm) |
|---|---|---|---|
| 0.001 | 20.470 | 1.33256 | 0.750 |
| 0.01 | 20.181 | 1.31380 | 0.761 |
| 0.1 | 20.153 | 1.31196 | 0.762 |
| 1 | 20.048 | 1.30510 | 0.766 |
| 10 | 19.196 | 1.24867 | 0.800 |
| 100 | 12.743 | 0.82957 | 1.205 |
| 1,000 | 4.246 | 0.27643 | 3.617 |
| 10,000 | 0.935 | 0.06088 | 16.427 |

Table 2. Neutron cross sections, total neutron cross sections, and mean free path lengths for hydrogen, as a function of energy.

One method to ameliorate the attenuation problem is to change the water composition from normal water to deuterated water (also referred to as heavy water)(Slatkin, Stoner et al. 1983; Nakagawa, Hatanaka et al. 1994; Kushner, Baker et al. 1999; Medina, Li et al. 2005). Studies have shown that approximately 20% of total body water (TBW) can be replaced with deuterated water without deleterious effects(Kushner, Baker et al. 1999). However, it is time consuming to replace 20% of the TBW, which would require several days of intravenous or oral deuterated water intake. Since deuterated water is also expensive, this is not currently a likely method to improve neutron transmission through tissue *in vivo*.

Even though there are problems with neutron attenuation and tissue dose for neutron imaging, there are real possibilities for the future. Images have been made of small amounts of tissue as can be seen in Figure 10. The images are of a rat lung in two views. The trachea, main stem bronchi and bronchial tree are well defined by the contrast afforded by air bronchograms. Several orders of bifurcation are clearly seen. Additionally, the cartilaginous rings in the trachea and main bronchi are clearly visible as well showing a difference in

[32] RSICC at ORNL: http://rsicc.ornl.gov

contrast between the two types of connective tissue. The cartilaginous bands are separated and covered by a fibrous connective tissue. The molecular composition and thickness is seen in the images. As detectors improve and imaging system geometries improve the resolution of such images will undoubtedly improve. Resolutions of 50-10 μm are readily available at most neutron imaging centers today. Resolutions of 1 μm appear to be routinely possible in the near future with sub-micron imaging a real possibility in the future.

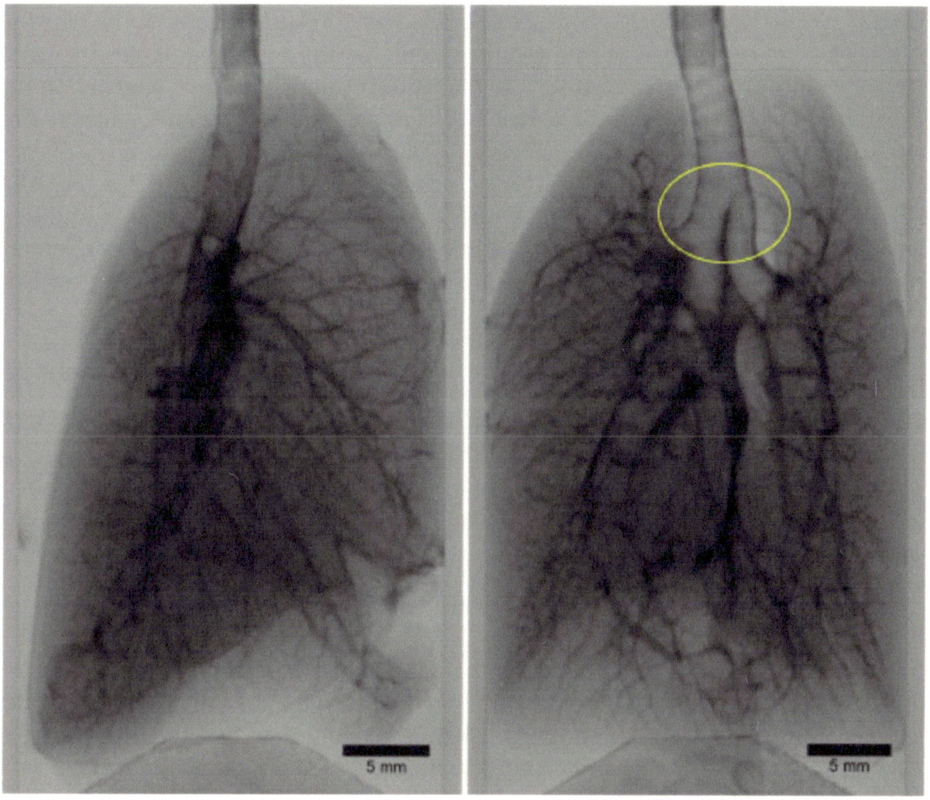


Fig. 10. Two neutron radiographs of the lungs of a rat from lateral (left) and anterolateral (right) views are shown. The air bronchograms are clearly visible as is the cartilaginous rings in the trachea and main bronchi. Courtesy: Dr. Burkhard Schillinger, Neutronentomographie ANTARES, Forschungsreaktor FRM-II, Technische Universität München, Germany.

### 4.2 Possible uses

Osteoarthritis (OA) is the most common of all joint diseases affecting 68% of persons over 68 years of age as based upon radiological criteria(Goldman and Ausiello 2008). Clinically, patients suffer from pain and functional limitations such as decreased range of motion and instability. Plain x-ray radiographs demonstrate osteophytes and joint space narrowing. Currently, there exist no treatment strategies that prevent or ameliorate the disease process so therapies are aimed at analgesia and improving the function of the joint. Not infrequently, the patient has a chronic course that eventually fails medical therapy which makes the patient a candidate for joint replacement surgery. When the joint has significant functional limitations and/or the pain becomes intractable, interfering with sleep or activity the patient may elect to have a total joint replacement. The bone prosthesis interface is very important to the success of the procedure. Even though not common, total knee replacement infection rates are 0.5 to 1.0 whereas total hip replacements have infection rates of 0.5 to 1.0 (1995; Berbari, Hanssen et al. 1998; Sperling, Kozak et al. 2001; Widmer 2001). It is important to make an accurate diagnosis because the treatment is the removal of the prosthesis followed by many weeks therapy with antibiotics. New prostheses are not always possible after infection. Therefore, it is very important to be certain that there an area of infection next to the metal. X-ray techniques such as CT suffer from significant degradation due to scattering from the metal prosthetic device. MRI scanning can still produce suitable images except in the case of cardiac pacemakers and defibrillators. The prevalence of cardiac pacemakers in all Medicare beneficiaries was increasing in time with 504.4 per 100,000 enrollees in 2000 as compared to 324.5 in 1990 and the prevalence increases significantly with age (Brown, Croft et al. 2005). So the patients with pacemakers or defibrillators and joint prostheses are increasing which leads to diagnostic dilemmas when the prosthesis is believed to be infected. Using a technique called Bragg edge imaging, the bone prosthesis interface should be amenable to relatively high resolution imaging which should demonstrate the fluid found in an infection in those patients with pacemakers.

Another case which is becoming far too common is that of a stroke patient who needs an MRI of the brain but cannot due to a pacemaker. Since both MRI and neutron radiography map the hydrogen atom distribution to create an image, neutron radiography should be able to provide images that would allow an accurate diagnosis to be made. Whether this is actually achievable will require more research.

Like positron emission tomography, magnetic resonance imaging, and x-ray computed tomography before it, neutron radiography will much research and engineering for it to become a clinically useful tool. Paul Lauterbur and Raymond Damadian doubtless had people shake their heads when told that their machines would image water in the body when that is the major constituent of the human body. They eventually developed the MRI which has revolutionized medical imaging of certain structures such as the brain. Originally, the MRI could not image the heart, lungs, or great vessels due to motion and slow acquisition rates. Those problems with time are being solved. So there is good reason to believe that neutron imaging could have a similar story. Since the mean free path of a positron is ~1 mm, it has been felt that PET cannot exceed a resolution of 1 mm. However, improved reconstruction algorithms are improving the resolution to the sub-millimeter range. Thus, it is reasonable to believe that the barriers for using neutron radiography for *in vivo* human imaging will be overcome. When that occurs, physicians will have new images that will improve their understanding of some disease processes and aid in the care of their patients.

## 5. Conclusion

The national laboratories provide a number of imaging and scattering instruments which can be used to facilitate basic medical research. These resources are available competitively via the scientific peer review process for proposals submitted through the user programs operated by each facility. Imaging human and animal tissue occurs but is not routine in most places, and strict procedures must be followed to do so. However research communities are burgeoning in a number of biomedical areas, and protein crystallography research is well established in the X-ray and neutron scattering communities. Novel here is the forward looking work on neutron imaging with potential medical and biomedical applications. Thus the national laboratories provide a research environment with capabilities and a culture conducive to researching new methods and techniques suitable for exploring new frontiers in medical and biomedical imaging.

## 6. Acknowledgement

The authors wish to thank the following for their contributions:

- The United Stated Department of Energy Basic Energy Sciences for the large scale user facilities which it designs, constructs, operates, and maintains. In FY 2010, these facilities cumulatively provided over 32,500 hours of service to over 12,700 unique users[33].
- Research at Oak Ridge National Laboratory's Spallation Neutron Source was sponsored by the Scientific User Facilities Division, Office of Basic Energy Sciences, U. S. Department of Energy.
- This manuscript has been authored by UT-Battelle, LLC, under Contract No. DE-AC05-00OR22725 with the U.S. Department of Energy. The United States Government retains and the publisher, by accepting the article for publication, acknowledges that the United States Government retains a non-exclusive, paid-up, irrevocable, world-wide license to publish or reproduce the published form of this manuscript, or allow others to do so, for United States Government purposes.
- DOE BES SBIR Grants DE-FG02-08ER85000
- DOE BES SBIR Grant DE-SC0004586
- Dr. Eberhard Lehmann for providing images from the ICON beamline, SINQ, Paul Scherrer Institut, Switzerland.
- Dr. Burkhard Schillinger for providing images from the FRM II reactor of Technische Universitat Munchen
- Dr. William T. Heller for providing SANS images from HFIR at Oak Ridge National Laboratory.

## 7. References

Arai, M. & Crawford, K. (2009). Neutron Sources and Facilities, In: *Neutron Imaging and Applications*, H. Z. Bilheux, R. L. McGreevy, & , I. S. Anderson, pp. 13-30. Springer, ISBN 978-1-4419-4619-5, New York.

Atkins, H. L. (1965). "Biological evaluation of neutron radiography." Materials Evaluation 23: 453-458.

Baker, G. A.; Heller, W. T. (April 2009), Small-angle neutron scattering studies of model protein denaturation in aqueous solutions of the ionic liquid 1-butyl-3-methylimidazolium chloride, *Chemical Engineering Journal*, Vol. 147, No. 1, pp. 6-12, Available from:
http://www.sciencedirect.com/science/article/pii/S1385894708007250

[33] BES Operations: http://science.energy.gov/~/media/budget/pdf/sc-budget-request-to-congress/fy-2012/Cong_Budget_2012_BES.pdf

Barth H. D., Launey, M. E. MacDowell, A. A. Ager III, J. W. Ritche, R. O. (2010), Irradiation Effects on Human Cortical Bone Fracture Behavior, *ALS Science Highlight #212.*

Barton, J. P. (1964). "Some Possibilities of Neutron Radiography." Physics in Medicine and Biology 278: 33-42.

Beckmann, E.C. (2006). CT scanning the early days, *The British Journal of Radiology*, Vol 79. (January 2006) pp 5-8, DOI: 10.1259/bjr/29444122

Berbari, E. F., A. D. Hanssen, et al. (1998). "Risk factors for prosthetic joint infection: case-control study." Clin Infect Dis 27(5): 1247-54.

Berger, H. (1965). Neutron Radiography. New York, Elsevier Press, Inc.

Berger, H. and W. J. McGonnagle (1962). Progress on neutron radiography, Argonne National Laboratory. USAEC Report ANL-6279.

Brown, D. W., J. B. Croft, et al. (2005). "Epidemiology of pacemaker procedures among Medicare enrollees in 1990, 1995, and 2000." Am J Cardiol 95(3): 409-11.

Brown, M. and P. B. Parks (1969). "Neutron radiography in biologic media. Techniques, observations, and implications." The American journal of roentgenology, radium therapy, and nuclear medicine 106(3): 472-85.

Budinger, T. F., H. Bichsel, et al. (1971). "Visual phenomena noted by human subjects on exposure to neutrons of energies less than 25 million electron volts." Science 172(985): 868-70.

Budinger, T. F., R. J. Howerton, et al. (1971). "Neutron radiography and dosimetry in human bengs: theoretical studies." Physics in Medicine and Biology 16(3): 439-50.

Chadwick, J. (1932). "Possible Existence of a Neutron." Nature 129(3252): 312.

Choi, H. J. & Weis, W. I. (2011), Crystal Structure of a Ridig Four-Spectrin-Repeat Fragment of the Human Desmoplakin Plakin Domain, *Mol. Biol.*, Vol 409, No. 800, DOI: 10.1016/j.jmb.2011.04.046.

Dangendorf, V., D. Bar, et al. (2009). "Multi-Frame Energy-Selective Imaging System for Fast-Neutron Radiography." Ieee Transactions on Nuclear Science 56(3): 1135-1140.

D de Jonge, M.; Vogt, S. (2010). Hard X-ra fluorescence tomography - an emerging tool for structural visualization. *Structural Biology*, Vol. 20, No. 5, pp. 606-614. DOI : 10.1016/j.sbi.2010.09.002.

Giri, N. C.; Sun, H., Chen, M., Costa, M., and Maroney, M. J., (2011), XAS Structural Investigation of Early Intermediates in the Mechanism of DNA Repair by Human ABH2, *Biochemistry*, DOI: 10.1021/bi101668x

Gleason, S.; Paulis, M., & Osborne, D. (2010). Molecular Imaging: Principles and Practice: Principles of Micro X-ray Computed Tomography, Weissleder, R., et al., eds., McGraw Hill, 2010, ISBN 9781607950059

Goldman, L. and D. Ausiello, Eds. (2008). Cecil Medicine. Philadelphia, Saunders, Elsevier.

Gupta, A. & Kielkopf, C. L. (2011). Purification, Crystallization and Preliminary X-ray Crystallographic Analysis of a Central Domain of Human Splicing Factor 1, *Acta Crystallogr.*, F 67, No. 486. DOI: 10.1107/S1744309111004623.

Hinerman, J. M. (2008). The Study of Protein-Protein Interactions Involved in Lagging Strand DNA Replication and Repair, Dissertation - University of Toledo, Available from:http://etd.ohiolink.edu/send-pdf.cgi/Hinerman%20Jennifer%20M.pdf?toledo1216824884

Jorgensen, S.; Eaker, D. Vercnocke, & A. Ritmin, E. (2008). Reproducibility of Global and Local Reconstruction of Three-Dimensional Micro-Computed Tomography of Iliac Crest Biopsies, *IEEE Transactions in Medical Imaging*, Vol. 27, No. 4, pp. 569-575.

Kak, A.C. and Slaney, M. (1988), *Principles of Computerized Tomographic Imaging*, IEEE Press.

Kushner, D. J., A. Baker, et al. (1999). "Pharmacological uses and perspectives of heavy water and deuterated compounds." Can J Physiol Pharmacol 77(2): 79-88.

Litzlbauer, H.; Korbel, K. Kline, T. Jorgensen, S. Eaker, D. Bohle, R. Riterman, E. & Langheinrich, A. (2010). Synchrotron-Based Micro-CT Imaging of the Human Lung Acinus, *Anatomical Record*, Vol. 293, No. 9. pp 1607-1614.

Marinelli, M., E. Milani, et al. (2006). "High performance (LiF)-Li-6-diamond thermal neutron detectors." Applied Physics Letters 89(14).

Marinelli, M., E. Milani, et al. (2007). "Synthetic single crystal diamond as a fission reactor neutron flux monitor." Applied Physics Letters 90(18).

Mayer, S., D. Forkel-Wirth, et al. (2007). "Response of neutron detectors to high-energy mixed radiation fields." Radiation protection dosimetry 125(1-4): 289-92.

Medina, D. C., X. Li, et al. (2005). "Pharmaco-thermodynamics of deuterium-induced oedema in living rat brain via 1H2O MRI: implications for boron neutron capture therapy of malignant brain tumours." Phys Med Biol 50(9): 2127-39.

Mor, I., D. Vartsky, et al. (2009). "High spatial resolution fast-neutron imaging detectors for Pulsed Fast-Neutron Transmission Spectroscopy." Journal of Instrumentation 4.

Moritz, R.; Eaker, D. Langheinric, A. Jorgensen, S. Bohle, R. & Ritman, (2010), E. Quantification of Vasa Vasorum Density in Multi-Slice Computed Tomographic Coronary Angiograms : Role of Computed Tomographic Image Voxel Size, Journal of Computer Assisted Tomography, Vol. 34, No. 2, pp 273-278.

Nakagawa, Y., H. Hatanaka, et al. (1994). "Partial deuteration and blood-brain barrier (BBB) permeability." Acta Neurochir Suppl (Wien) 60: 410-2.

Nelson J.; Huang, X. Steinbrener, J. Shapiro, D. Kirz, J. Marchesini, S. Neiman, A. M. Turner, J.J. Jacobson, C. (2010), High Resolution x-ray diffraction microscopy of specially labeled yeast cells, PNAS, Vol. 107, No. 16, DOI: 10.1073/pnas.0910874107.

Parks, P. B. and M. Brown (1969). "Antiscatter grids for low-energy neutron radiography." Radiology 92(1): 178-9.

Pynn, R. (1990). Neutron scattering A PRIMER, *Los Alamos Science*, Vol. 19, http://library.lanl.gov/cgi-bin/getfile?19-01.pdf

Rao, D.; Cesareo, R. Brunetti, A. Akatsuka, T. Yuasa, T. Takeda, T. Tromba, G. & Gigante, G. (2009). Micro-CT Imaging of Rat Bone and Lumber Vretebra using Synchrotron Radiation, *Application of Accelerators in Research and Industry : Twentieth International Conference*, Vol. 109, pp 896-899.

Ruddy, F. H., R. W. Flammang, et al. (2009). "Low-background detection of fission neutrons produced by pulsed neutron interrogation." Nuclear Instruments & Methods in Physics Research Section a-Accelerators Spectrometers Detectors and Associated Equipment 598(2): 518-525.

Ruddy, F. H., J. G. Seidel, et al. (2009). "Development of Radiation Detectors Based on Semi-Insulating Silicon Carbide." 2008 Ieee Nuclear Science Symposium and Medical Imaging Conference (2008 Nss/Mic), Vols 1-9: 5256-5262.

Slatkin, D. N., R. D. Stoner, et al. (1983). "Whole-body irradiation of deuterated mice by the 10B(n, alpha)7Li reaction." Proc Natl Acad Sci U S A 80(11): 3480-4.

Sperling, J. W., T. K. Kozak, et al. (2001). "Infection after shoulder arthroplasty." Clin Orthop Relat Res(382): 206-16.

Stock, S.; De Carlo, F. & Almer, J. (2008). High energy X-Ray scattering tomography applied to bone. Journal of Structural Biology, Vol. 161, No. 2, pp. 144-150. DOI: 10.1016/j.jsb.2007.10.001.

Stoltz E.; Yeniguen, M. Kreisel, M. Kampschulte, M. Doenges, S. Sedding, D. Ritman, E. Gerriets, T. & Langhinrich, (2011). Angioarchitectural Changes in Subacute Cerebral Venous Thrombosis, *NeuroImage*, Vol. 55, pp. 1881-1886.

Thewlis, J. (1956). "Neutron radiography." British Journal of Applied Physics 7: 345-350.

Tremsin, A.S., Phate, J.B., Vallerga, J.V., Siegmund, O.H.W., Feller, W.B., Lehmann, E., and Dawson, M.(2011), "Improved efficiency of high resolution thermal and cold neutron imaging," Nuclear Instruments and Methods in Physics Research Section A: Accelerators, Spectrometers, Detectors, and Associated Equipment, Vol. 628, No. 1, pp. 415-418.]

Uchida, M.; McDermott, G. Wetzler, M. Le Gros, M. A. Mylls, M. Knoechel, C. Baron, A. E. & Larabell, C. A., (2009), Soft x-ray tomography of phenotypic switching and the cellular response to antifungal peptoids in Candida albicans, Proc. Nat. Acad. Sci., Vol. 106, No. 46.

Vartsky, D., I. Mor, et al. (2010). "Novel detectors for fast-neutron resonance radiography." Nuclear Instruments & Methods in Physics Research Section a-Accelerators Spectrometers Detectors and Associated Equipment 623(1): 603-605.

Vartsky, D., I. Mor, et al. (2005). "Time-resolved fast neutron imaging: simulation of detector performance." Nuclear Instruments & Methods in Physics Research Section a-Accelerators Spectrometers Detectors and Associated Equipment 542(1-3): 206-212.

Widmer, A. F. (2001). "New developments in diagnosis and treatment of infection in orthopedic implants." Clin Infect Dis 33 Suppl 2: S94-106.

Xiao, X.; Xia, D. Bian, J. Han, X. Sidky, E.Y. De Carlo, F. & Pan, X. (2010). Image reconstruction from sparse data in synchrotron-based micro-tomography of biomedical samples, 1st International Conference on Image Formation in X-Ray Computed Tomography, UCAIR, pp 156-164.

Xiao, X.; De Carlo, F. & Stock, S. (2008). X-ray zoom-in tomography of calcified tissue, *Developments in X-Ray Tomography SPIE proceedings,* Vol. 7078. DOI: 10.1117/12.796638.

Zhang, Y.; Lagi, M., Liu, D. Z., Mallamace, F., Frantini, E., Baglioni, P., Mamontov, E., Hagen, M., Chen, S. H. (2009), Observation of high-temperature dynamic crossover in protein hydration water and its relation to reversible denaturation of lysozyme, *Journal of Chemical Physics*, Vol. 130, No. 13, Available from: http://jcp.aip.org/resource/1/jcpsa6/v130/i13/p135101_s1

# 7

# Tools to Improve the Patient's Processes at Imaging Centers

Liliana Neriz[1] and Francisco J. Ramis[2]
[1]*School of Economics and Business, Universidad de Chile, Santiago*
[2]*Department of Industrial Engineering, University of Bio-Bio, Concepcion*
*Chile*

## 1. Introduction

There is a worldwide concern for increased efficiency and cost effectiveness in healthcare delivery which in the USA represents about 16% of the Gross Domestic Product. The variability and complexity of the processes within healthcare systems demand the use of more sophisticated management tools, such as the recommended by a joint study by the National Academy of Engineering and the Institute of Medicine in the USA (NAE 2005), to improve the healthcare delivery system. In this chapter it is seen the integration of three management tools (Activity Based Costing, Lean Healthcare and Process Simulation) to facilitate the development of Medical Imaging Center (MIC) studies in order to improve the patient´s processes, which departs from traditional modeling because it uses a pull paradigm for the patients. Activity Based Costing (ABC Costing) is used to identify improvement opportunities from the managers' point of view, Lean Healthcare (Lean) to identify opportunities from the Customers´ point of view and Process Simulation (Simulation) to test the potential impact of any proposed alternative identified with ABC Costing or Lean, prior to its implementation. The center to be modeled might be as simple as having one x-ray machine, or, more complex having all kind of imaging machines (magnetic resonance, CT, x-ray, digestive radiology, ultrasound scan, angiography, mammography and others).

Medical Imaging Centers are important units in every hospital or medical center as they are a relevant link in generating a patient's diagnostic. Because of this, it is necessary that these centers be managed with high quality standards but also with efficiency. As an application, an integrated example is provided where ABC costing, Lean and Simulation are applied to an imaging center to improve the patient's waiting times and process costs.

Medical Imaging Centers have made an important investment in PACS systems, which provide data comprising from the reception of patients to the taking of the image. This kind of system gives relevant and detailed information, such as: number and kind of patient, frequency, type of exam, supplies and drugs utilized and personnel involved, all of these entry data are significantly useful to the proposed tools, and, furthermore complement and support the information for the management of MIC.

## 2. Patient flow

Traditionally, when studying a process, the first step is to build a flowchart of the process that the patient will undergo. A typical patient's process is presented in Figure 1. The process begins when a patient and his or her companions arrive to the reception desk at the MIC. The arrivals could be spontaneous, scheduled or sent from an emergency room. The receptionist asks the patient about the type of exams that he/she is requesting, proof of insurance or payment method and all the paper work required. Once this information is entered, the patient waits to be called by a technician/doctor to carry out a preliminary evaluation, preparation prior to the exam in case the patient may need anesthesia, contrast medium or other preparation, and the requested exams. The exams can be classified as: magnetic resonance, CT, X-Ray, digestive radiology, ultrasound scan, angiography, mammography and others. Once the exam is performed, the patient leaves the examination area and meets her/his companion, afterwards, back office activities are performed to digitalize/print the image or make a CD, finally, the results of the examination are communicated to the patient or reported to the physician.

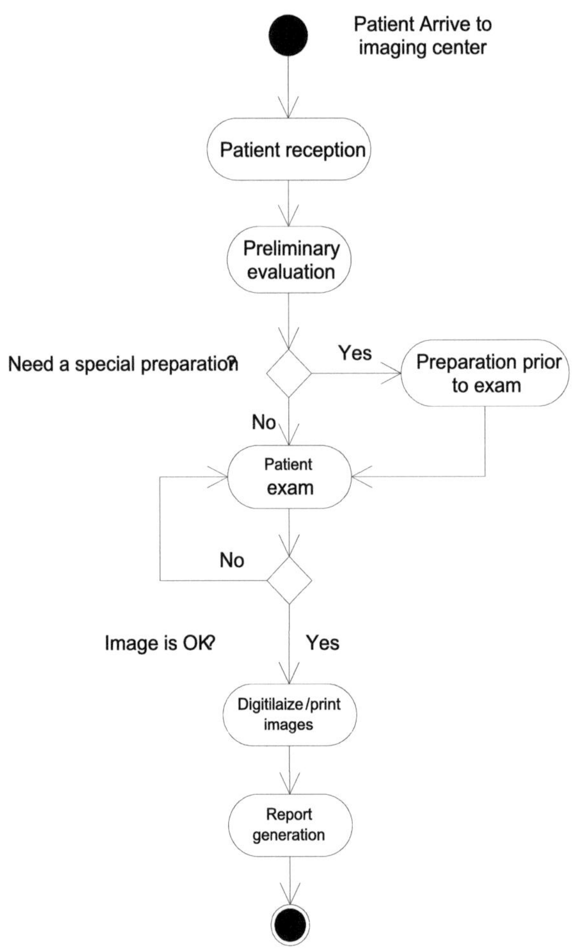


Fig. 1. Patient flow diagram at an Imaging Center

Building and understanding MIC workflow is usually conducted in a brute-force fashion; that is, by taking a stopwatch and physically timing each step of the clinical examination processes. This can be observed as taking a snapshot from the doctors'/technologists' daily activities focusing on a patient examination, including the room preparation prior to an examination, the examination itself, the report generation and the discharge of the patient from the MIC (Wideman and Gallet 2006).

The upper flow diagram is useful for representing the process and the activities involved, the sequence of such activities, and also, as a communication device for the persons working within the imaging center. However, it does not provide any guidelines to identify potential improvements. Because of this, a three steps approach is proposed in this chapter to identify opportunities for improvement: 1) ABC costing to identify important activities from a cost point of view, 2) Lean to identify one of the patients' concerns, the waiting times and process times and 3) Simulation to test the impact of proposed solutions before implementing them. These three tools are explained in the following section.

## 3. Description of management tools

There are several management tools that could be used to manage an imaging center. In particular, this chapter illustrates the use and integration of three of them, which are focused on the processes and generate synergies to support the decision making process more objectively. This way, the manager can get different points of view, take more effective decisions and promote the continuous improvement of the processes. The three tools to be used are described as Activity Based Costing, Lean Healthcare and Process Simulation.

### 3.1 Activity based costing

Activity Based Costing (ABC) was developed by Kaplan and Cooper (1997). The objective of ABC is to compute the cost of products or services (cost objects) in industries where indirect costs are significant and have more than one product. Traditional costing methods assign indirect costs directly to the products using an allocation criteria (units produced, patients, square feet, etc.), which do not reflect the current use of resources. This is the case of healthcare, where most of the costs are indirect, i.e., the resources utilized to produce the products are used by more than one product.

ABC relates the use of the resources to the products, through the allocation of costs of the resources to the processes, which are represented by activities. These activities consume resources, and then the costs of activities are allocated to the products generated (goods or services). For ABC, a process is a group of activities, i.e., a process is composed of at least two activities. A definition of the concept of activity is a "task that consumes resources."

The ABC basic elements are: direct and indirect resources, activities, drivers and products. Products are tangible goods or services. Drivers represent the way used to allocate resources to activities and then from the activities to the products. The methodology can be summarized as follows: (1) identify the processes in a company, (2) establish the activities associated to those processes, (3) choose drivers for each indirect resource and allocate the costs of the resources to the activities, and (4) calculate the costs of products by assigning activity costs through the predefined cost drivers.

The ABC costing process requires identifying the activities and their characteristics as well as recognizing the direct and indirect resources needed to operate the company. Once the indirect resources have been identified and valued, their costs should be allocated to the activities that use the resources by identifying the appropriate drivers (resource drivers). These drivers relate the activity level to the resources used. Once the activities have been valued, the next step is to allocate the costs of the activities to the products through other drivers (activity drivers), which link the activity with the products. Finally, direct costs are directly allocated to each product. See Figure 2.

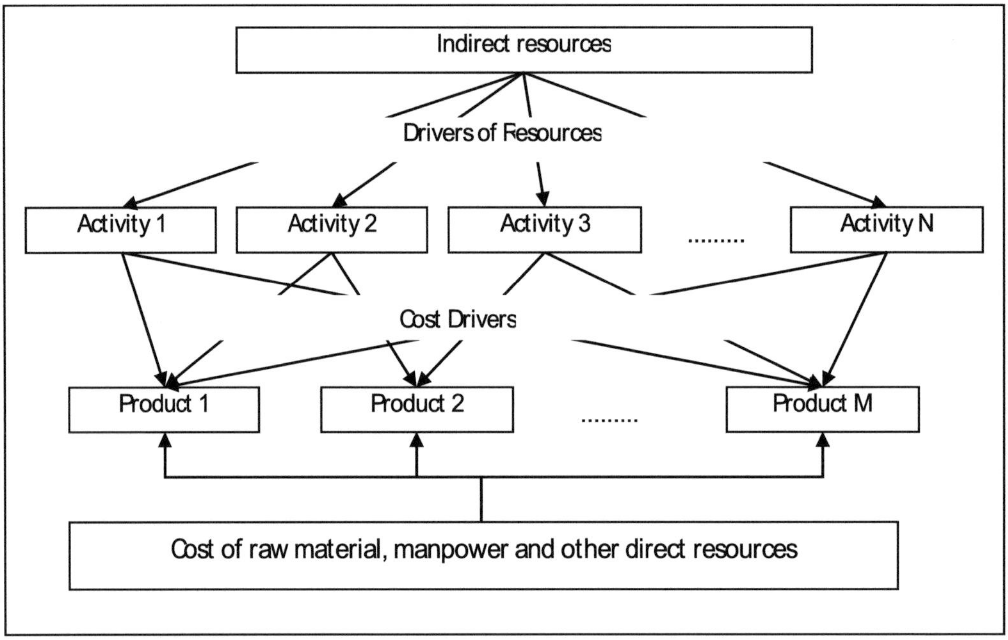


Fig. 2. Activity based costing method.

Figure 2 provides valuable information to the manager, as opposed to traditional costing methods that give the total cost and do not answer why or where the most expensive activities are going to be found or how the process might be improved. Managing the activities is called Activity Based Management (ABM), which is the basis for any initiative of process improvement. As managers know their real costs, therefore they could find original ways to improve their processes and reduce costs or add more value. ABM supports continuous improvement, cost reduction program, re-engineering and other process and quality initiatives (Kaplan and Cooper, 1997).

Imaging procedures are services with a high amount of indirect costs which require many activities; several authors have provided some evidence such as Canby (1995) who, using ABC principles and techniques, calculates costs associated with a x-ray process in a midsized outpatient clinic. Laurila et al. (2000) show an informative and detailed picture of resource utilization in a radiology department in order to support its pricing and management. Another research from Laurila et al. (2001), studied the efficacy of continuous quality improvement (CQI) compared to ordinary management from a radiology department. Cohen et al. (2000) applied ABC to test the hypothesis that academic radiology can be separated into three distinct businesses –clinical activity, teaching and research- in order to determine the effect of the current teaching paradigm on the clinical productivity. This analysis identifies opportunities to improve quality of service, productivity and cost within each business.

There are several ABC studies in different imaging areas such as Enzmann et al. (2001) in mammography services; Gray et al. (2003) in magnetic resonance imaging; Suthummanon et al. (2005) researched how applying ABC to the nuclear medicine unit at a teaching hospital for training interns; and Clevert et al. (2007) who analyzed methods to reduce cost in interventional radiology departments by reorganizing supplies.

### 3.2 Lean applied to healthcare

Lean healthcare tools are focused on those activities that an institution must develop to added value to their customers, represented by the patients of the clinical services. Lean is based in the Toyota Production System (TPS), which, by definition is how to produce more with less (Womack and Jones, 2005).

Lean has four principles: (i) Only perform activities that add value to the customer, (ii) Eliminate waste. (iii) Promote flows, and (iv) Continuously improve processes. Adding value to the customer means only perform those activities that the customer is willing to pay for, the activities are correctly executed at first, and the activity must change the product or service in some way. For example, waiting for an x-ray to be taken does not add value to the customer.

Waste can be eliminated by identifying the seven sources of waste: 1) Production of defects (wrong dose, wrong medication, rework, correction of defects), 2)overproduction(unnecessary tests, reading mails, production to inventory), 3) Unnecessary transportation (inappropriate layout, changing documents), 4) Waiting times(patients waiting for reviews, doctors/nurses waiting for results of exams), 5) Excess inventories (expired drugs), 6) Motion (travel to the laboratory, excessive file search) and 7) Extra-processes (data collection that are not used, defective samples).

The promotion of flows is reached by minimizing the time between activities that add value. For example, minimizing the waiting times of the patients between successive treatments, which is triggered by a pull discipline, where the patient requests successive services as he/she makes progress in the attention process.

The fourth principle states that by doing things a little better every day, this will lead to continuously improve the processes. Ideally, people should arrive to their workplace in the morning and ask themselves: what can I do better today?

This study uses a particular tool of lean called Value Stream Map (VSM), to illustrate the relationship customer - supplier, and also to show the waiting and process times for the entire imaging procedure; as a result, overcrowding and unbalanced flows can be identified. In order to build a value stream map, the following steps should be followed: 1) Identify the boundaries of interest, 2) Identify the activities performed within the unit, 3) Use a pencil and paper to collect field data, 4) Draw the flow based on demand, the customer requirements, and his employer, 5) It is important to consider the flow of material, information and production flow, 6) Check the value chain backwards in every step of the flow, 7) Add boxes to the data on each process, 8) The individual process steps must go from left to right in the flow of the value chain, sometimes many paths converge on several points, 9) Add the number of operators 10) Add the cycle time and processing time, 11) Calculate the total cycle time and total processing time, 12) Once traced the flow of the chain and when data has been entered in each step, it is necessary to add the information flow and 13) Finally, add the timeline at the bottom of the page.

For a comprehensive view of lean see Womack and Jones (2005) pioneers in the introduction of the concept of Lean. For the specific case of Healthcare, an excellent handbook is provided by Graban (2008), with specific examples and guidelines for implementing lean healthcare. A general overview about how lean has been applied in North American hospitals is provided by Poole et al. (2010).

### 3.3 Process simulation

Simulation is a tool that allows studying complex systems under dynamic conditions (Law, 2007). Healthcare simulation is different from the well known manufacturing simulation, where the entities go through a well defined and standardized process, requesting resources at different locations, waiting in a row if the resources are not available and both the processing and waiting discipline are according to a given priority. In healthcare, patients (the entities) request the resources at a fixed location, or in other words, are the resources (doctors, nurses, paramedics and others) that come to the patient and provide him with the required services. Also, patients cannot wait forever to get service or be stored as inventories in case they are not given service in a given day. Waits have dynamic priorities and physicians give preference to the patients with the highest severity.

In order to build a simulation model with any modern simulation software, for example with FlexsimHC that is the only object oriented simulation software for healthcare processes (www.flexsim.com), the typical steps are: 1) Import layout of the imaging center, 2) Drag & Drop objects into layout, 3) Adjust visual properties, names and areas of objects, 4) Create the Tracks, 5) Make connections according to tracks/patient flow, 6) Configure the experiment, scenarios and performance measures and 7) Run the model and view results.

Simulation has the flexibility to become a suitable tool for healthcare due to the complexity of these systems, which are integrated by different actors and a large number of parts interacting (Monsef, 1997). For a comprehensive healthcare simulation review see (Eldabi et al., 2007), (Young et al., 2009) and (Neriz et al., 2011). Specific examples of simulation of imaging centers can be found in (Ramis et al., 2008, 2009), where simulation focuses on providing an alternative to reduce the waiting time of the patients, improve the use of physical and human resources, evaluate different alternatives of plant layout, scheduling patients or simply, to study and better understand the inner working of the system.

## 4. Using ABC costing and lean to identify opportunities for improvement

To illustrate the integration of tools, it is presented the case of an Imaging Center at a research hospital, which is a high complexity center with different equipments such as Magnetic Resonance, CAT's, x-ray, Digestive Radiology, Mammography, Angiography, Echography among others. In this center, it was applied an activity-based costing model and as an example in Table 1 it is reported the X- ray section, which shows the annual breakdown of the costs of activities in this unit.

| Activity | Total annual costs (US$) | Activity | Total annual costs (US$) |
|---|---|---|---|
| Carry envelopes | 687.204 | Give the report to the patient | 7,805.274 |
| Record times | 834.288 | Give directions | 8,275.712 |
| Give indications to patients | 1,517.640 | Deliver reports to departments | 8,648.474 |
| Coordinate people's schedules | 1,999.228 | Call and receive the patient | 8,724.822 |
| Give contrast to patient | 1,531.640 | Check exams (images) | 9,303.936 |
| Assign envelopes | 1,999.228 | Finish the process | 10,217.488 |
| Carry reports (into the envelopes) | 2,227.104 | Proceed with the process | 11,315.038 |
| Label envelopes | 2,441.644 | Do anamnesis | 12,025.192 |
| Arrangements | 2,459.968 | Digitalize exams | 12,089.694 |
| Bring reports | 2,576.066 | Release exams | 12,089.694 |
| Carry cartridge | 3,511.320 | Admit patient | 15,208.386 |
| Building Maintenance | 3,732.934 | Receive payments | 23,444.442 |
| Obey safety measures | 4,789.020 | Print pictures | 23,654.790 |
| Remove safety measures | 4,789.020 | Check inventory stock | 27,519.104 |
| Print report | 5,749.998 | Check report | 36,406.510 |
| Dismiss the patient | 6,289.120 | Do report | 38,048.202 |
| Back to the imaging center | 7,397.258 | Manage academic duty | 84,917.472 |
| Settle the patient | 7,469.516 | Equipment Maintenance | 14,6236.436 |
| Check report | 7,501.822 | Manage the Center | 341,832.954 |
| Go to X-ray portable examination | 7,647.588 | Take exams | 795,188.264 |
| | | **Total Cost** | **1,721,125.714** |

Table 1. Activities in X-ray area

The information from table 1 is summarized in Figure 3. It can be observed that the costliest activity is of taking the exam, a situation that is explained because most of the resources employed in the X-ray section are fixed costs, and correspond to personnel, equipment and facility costs, as can be seen in Figure 4.

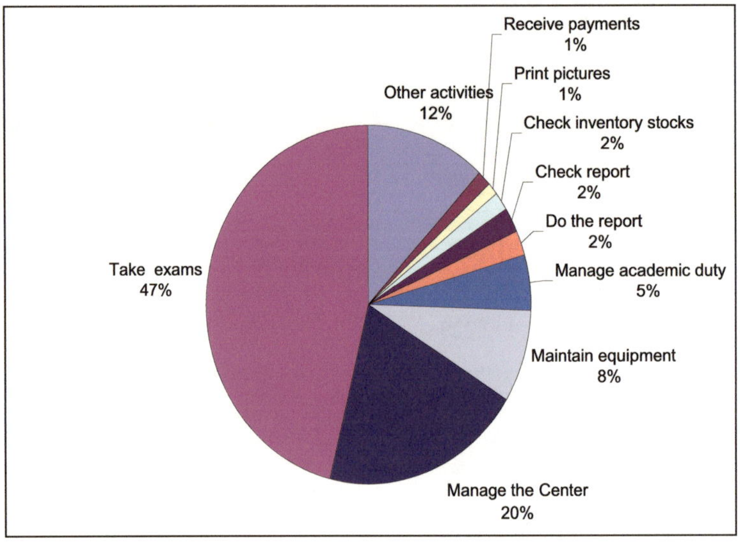


Fig. 3. Activities costs in X-Ray area

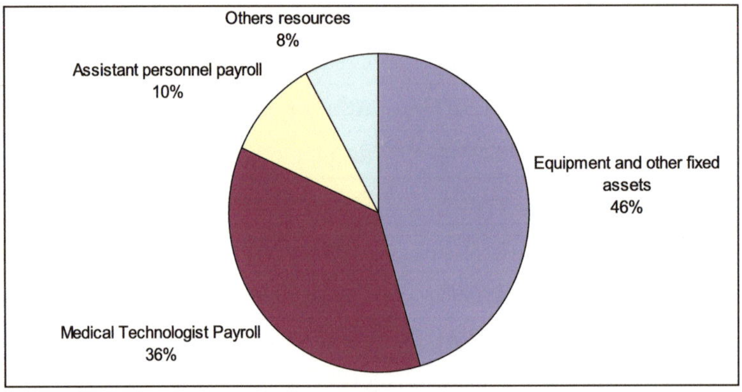


Fig. 4. Costs of resources - Activity take exams.

Considering that the resources employed in the activity of taking the exam are fixed, this says that if 1 x-ray or 1000 x-ray are made, the same fixed cost is incurred. Then, the manager of the MIC realizes that to generate value he must make decisions about the activity of taking the exam, for example, by increasing the production of X-rays the cost of that activity is amortized with more x-rays. Now, the manager wants to increase the production, but the analysis would consider this decision from a customer standpoint, that is, people need to get an X-Ray without long waiting times. In order to do this analysis, a value stream map (VSM) will be used.

From the standpoint of the VSM, there are three main activities: 1) the reception of patients in the reception area. 2) Proof of insurance or direct payment from the patient and 3) Taking the exam in the examination room. Figure 5 shows the VSM with the three main activities mentioned, and it can be seen that the bottleneck occurs in the examination room because the flow of patients, which in the previous stage was an average of 16.76 patients per hour, drops to 5.95 patients per hour.

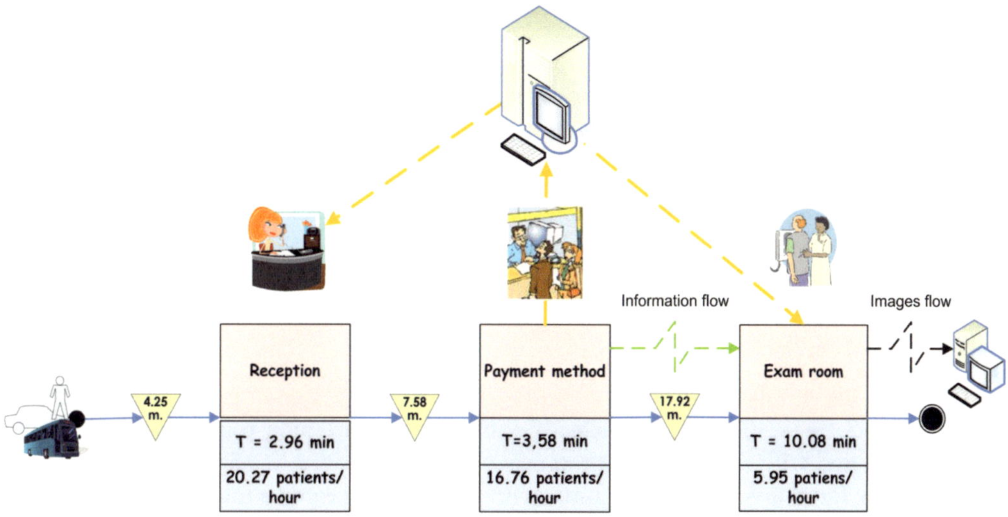


Fig. 5. Map of stream Value of the main processes in the X-ray area.

A more detailed analysis of what happens within the examination room, using the same tool again, established that the flow is leveled in the first three activities, having a capacity of 60 patients per hour. But the flow goes down in the last activity when the patient returns to the dressing room to put on his/her clothes, now, the capacity is to attend only 17.94 patients per hour, which is shown in Figure 6. This drives to the conclusion that as the dressing room is the bottleneck, by increasing the number of dressing rooms an increase in productivity will be achieved.

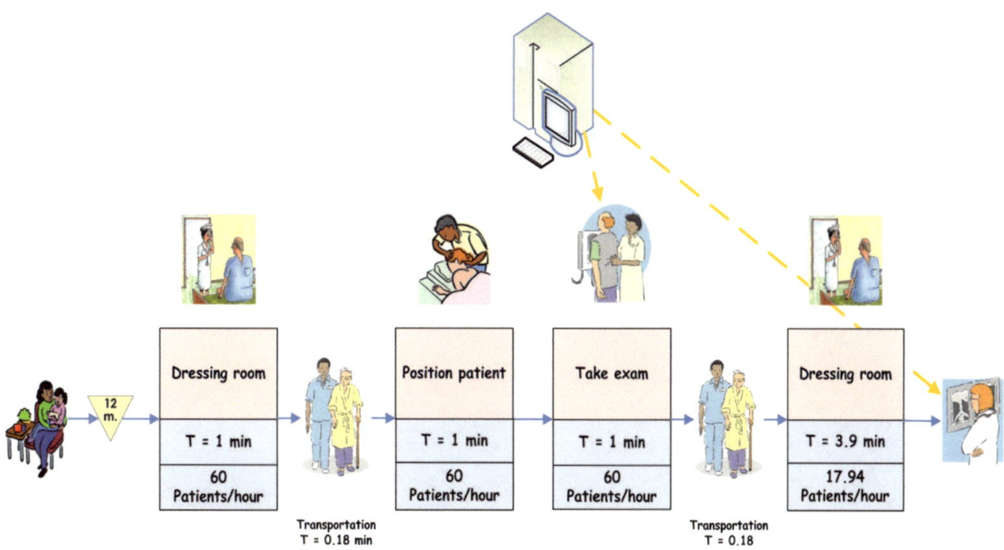


Fig. 6. VSM in the examination room.

## 5. Using simulation to test identified solutions

From the previous section it has been seen that the actual bottleneck is the dressing room, and then, by adding more rooms it should be improved the productivity of the x-ray section. To test this hypothesis, a simulation model was constructed, following the steps described to build a model and using the simulation package FlexsimHC.

The simplified model of the process is shown in figure 7. It is assumed that patients arrive and go directly to the service if the dressing room and the technician are idle; otherwise they go to the waiting room. Once the patient is ready, the technician will get him out of the dressing room, locate him/her into the table and take the image. Then, after some adjustments, the patient is taken back to the dressing room, where he/she gets dressed and then leaves ending the process.

As a result of the simulation it can be observed, by having one dressing room the technician is inactive about 65% of the time, instead by having two dressing rooms this figure goes down to 35%, and with three dressing rooms it sharply decreased to a 5% idle time. In terms of production, for a direct digital machine, with one dressing room a total of 50 patients will be attended, with two a total of 100 and with three dressing rooms a total of 125 patients per day. It is important to notice that increased productivity is achieved having the same resources, except for changing the number of dressing rooms.

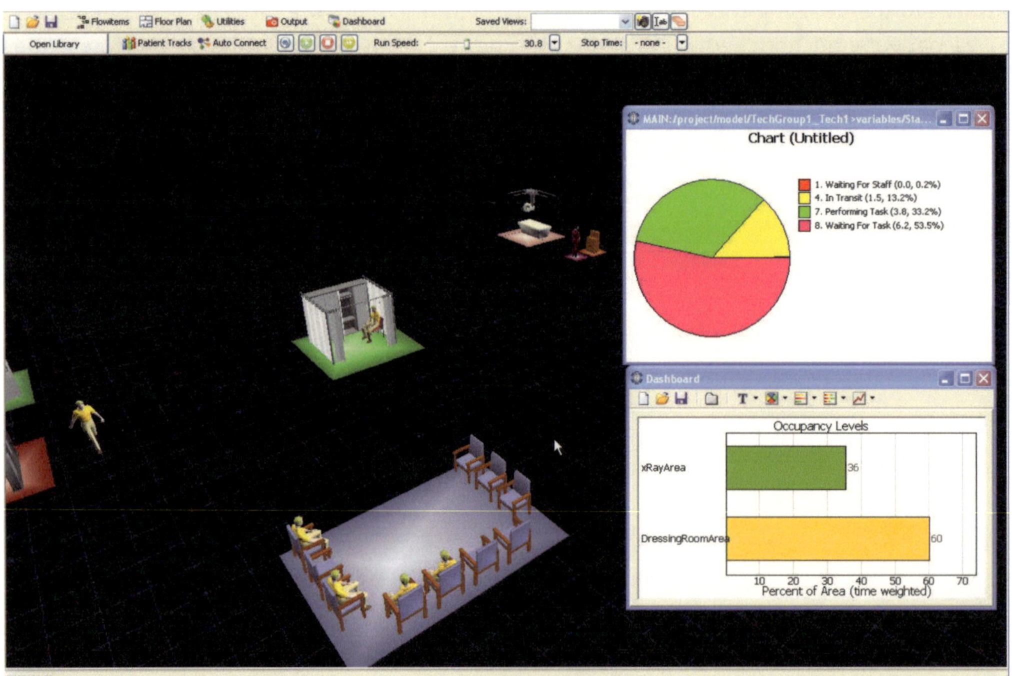


Fig. 7. Screen of simulation model.

## 6. Conclusions

This chapter shows the integration of three management tools, Activity Based Costing, Lean Healthcare and Process Simulation, to improve the waiting times and equipment rate of utilization at a clinical hospital. As a general conclusion we can say that:

1. Activity Based Costing is a valid tool for computing costs of products at healthcare institutions. ABC provides a powerful tool for Activity Based Management (ABM), because it shows the cost of the different activities involved in getting a given service/product.
2. Lean healthcare provides a focus on the wastes from the point of view of the customers, in this case, the waiting times.
3. Simulation is an appropriate tool for modeling in a healthcare environment, because of the complexity of the processes and the flexibility of the tool when modelling different situations. It was used to test solutions identified with ABC and Lean.

Specifically, we can conclude that, the bottleneck of the system is represented by the dressing rooms. By adding more of them in the X-ray section, the productivity was increased from 50 patients per shift to 125. Similarly, the average idle time of the technician taking the images decreased from 65% to 5%.

## 7. References

Canby, J. (1995). "Applying activity-based costing to healthcare settings". Healthcare Financial Management, 49, 2, 50-56.

Clevert, D. A., Stickel, M. Jung, E. M., Reiser, M. and Rupp, N. (2007). "Cost analysis in interventional radiology. A tool to optimize management costs". European Journal of radiology, 61, 144-149.

Cohen, M., Hawes, D., Hutchins, G., McPhee, W., LaMasters, M. and Fallon, R. (2000). "Activity-based cost analysis: A method of analyzing the financial and operating performance of academic radiology departments". Radiology, 215, 3, 708-716.

Eldabi, T., Paul, R. and Young, T. (2007). Simulation modelling in healthcare: reviewing legacies and investigating futures. Journal of the Operational Research Society, 58, 262-270.

Enzmann, D., Anglada, P. Haviley, C. and Venta, L. (2001). "Providing profesional mammography services: financial analysis". Radiology, 219, 2, 467-473.

Graban, M (2009), Lean Hospitals: Improving Quality, Patient Safety, and Employee Satisfaction. Taylor and Frances.

Gray, D., Hollingworth, W., Blackmore, C. B., Alotis, M., Martin, B., Sullivan, S., Deyo, R. and Jarvok, J. G. (2003). "Conventional Radiography, rapid MR imaging and conventional MR imaging for low back pain: Activity- based costs and reimbursement". Radiology, 227, 669-680.

Kaplan, R. and Cooper, R. (1997).Cost & Effect: Using Integrated Cost Systems to Drive Profitability and Performance. Harvard Business Press.

Laurila, J., Suramo, I., Brommels, M., Tolppanen, E-M., Koivukangas, P., Lanning, P., Standertskjöld-Nordenstam, C-G.(2000). "Activity-based costing in Radiology". ActaRadiologica 41, 189-195.

Laurila, J., Standertskjöld-Nordenstam, C-G., Suramo, I, Tolppanen, E-M., Tervonen, O., Korhola, O. and Brommels, M. (2001)."The Efficacy of a continuous quality improvement (CQI) method in a radiological department". Acta Radiologica 42, 96-100.

Law, A. (2007) Simulation Modeling and Analysis, Fourth Edition. New York. USA, McGraw-Hill

Monsef, Y (1997), "Modelling and simulation of complex systems," Society for computer simulation international. In. Jin, X., Kagioglou M., Aouad G. 2006, Towards a dynamic healthcare process: from requirement capture to simulation. Transactions of the SDPS JUNE 2006, Vol. 10, No. 2, pp. 1-19

NAE/IOM (2005), "Building a Better Delivery System", National Academy of Engineering and Institute of Medicine, USA.

Neriz, L., Ramis, F. and Sepulveda, J. (2011). "A New Approach for Healthcare Simulation", Proceedings Society of Health systems, SHS 2011, Orlando, USA

Poole, K., Hinton, J. and Kraebber K. (2010). "The gradual leaning of health systems". Industrial Engineer. April, 50-55.

Ramis, F., Neriz, L. and Sepúlveda, J. (2008). "A Simulator to Improve Waiting Times at an Emergency Unit". Industrial Engineering Research Conference, Vancouver, Canada.

Ramis, F., Concha, P. Neriz, L. and Sepúlveda, J. (2009). "Improving Services of a Hospital Imaging Center using ABC Costing, Lean and Simulation" .Simulation Solutions, IIE Annual Conference.

Suthummanon, S., Omachonu, V. and Akcin.M. (2005)."Applying activity-based costing to nuclear medicine unit". Health Services Magaement Research, 18, 141-150.

Wideman, C. and Gallet, J. (2006) "Analog to digital workflow improvement: A quantitative studt". Journal of Digital Imaging, 19 Suppl 1:29-34.

Womack, P. and D. T. Jones.(2005). Soluciones Lean. Gestión2000, Spain.

Young, T., Eatock, J., Jahangirian, M., Naseer, A. and Lilford, R. (2009)."Three critical challenges for modeling and simulation in healthcare". In Proceedings of the 2009 Winter Simulation Conference.

Flexsim user manual (2011), www.flexsim.com.

8

# High to Microwave Frequencies Imaging Techniques

George A. Kyriacou[1], Ilias N. Aitidis[1],
Dimitrios G. Drogoudis[1] and John N. Sahalos[2]
[1]*Department of Electrical and Computer Engineering, Democritus University of Thrace*
[2]*Department of Electrical & Computer Engineering, University of Nicosia*
[1]*Greece*
[2]*Cyprus*

## 1. Introduction

Microwave and high frequency tomography constitutes challenging electromagnetic inverse problems aiming at the reconstruction of its internal σ-, $\varepsilon_r$- and/or $\mu_r$- distributions. The object to be imaged is embedded in a lossy homogeneous background medium. This is surrounded by a fictitious (or real) surface preferably of canonical shape (circular, rectangular, cylindrical or spherical) over which a number of antennas (electrodes at lower frequencies) are evenly distributed. The hardware implementing the modality should be able to successively activate each one of them, while setting all the other antennas to a receive state operating as sensors. Instead of requiring all antennas to operate in both transmit and receive modes, a subset of antennas can be configured in transmit mode only (activated in turn) while a preferably larger subset is configured in receive only mode (passive sensors), all of them performing simultaneous measurements. In this manner the object is illuminated each time from a different angle creating a scattered field to all possible directions, which is sampled by the receiving antennas. The locations and number of transmit antennas should be designed to cover the required spatial illuminations (projection angles), while the number of the evenly distributed receiving antennas should fulfill the spatial sampling laws. An alternative configuration mimicking the one already used in X-Ray Computer Tomography (CT) and Magnetic Resonance Imaging (MRI) seems preferable and highly recommended for the microwave imaging. Spesifically, for two-dimensional imaging a single active antenna along with an array of sensing-passive antennas could be placed on a circular-colar possibly plastic platform surrounding the object to be imaged. In turn by rotating this supporting structure the object can be illuminated from all possible projection angles. For a three-dimensinal imaging the hosting platform could be a plastic cylinder holding multiple antenna ring arrays, each ring having one active and multiple passive antennas. Each antenna is activated successively in time while the whole cylinder is roteated providing all possible illuminations and data recording-sampling by all sensing antennas “simultaneously”. The information gathered by this measurement procedure constitutes the dataset to be exploited by the imaging algorithm to reconstruct the object’s internal properties distributions. This constitutes a challenging mathematical-computational and engineering problem since it is proved to be a highly non-linear and ill-posed inverse problem.

Analytical methods can be employed only for simple canonical geometries but these are valuable since they may serve as exact reference methods to validate numerical techniques. Hence, for the practical arbitrary shaped and inhomogeneous bodies numerical techniques are inevitable. It is on these approaches that the following chapter is elaborating.

For the reconstruction algorithm to be implemented a realistic as far as possible computer model of the practical structure is necessary. For this purpose the geometry is discretized including the appropriate antenna (or electrodes) modeling by following an engineering compromise between accurately reflecting the structure and the required computational resources. A usual approach is to consider a "virtual body area" of canonical shape large enough to contain the unknown irregularly shaped actual object with its unknown $\sigma$, $\varepsilon_r$, $\mu_r$ distributions. The properties of the background media outside this virtual surface are assumed known as it is practically selected as desired. The also virtual surface carrying the transmit/receive antennas is larger than the "virtual body area" but also embedded in the known background medium. Theoretically, this background media extends to infinity, however in order to implement a numerical technique a finite solution domain should be established. Hence, another fictitious surface enclosing the whole structure constituting the solution domain "truncation surface" is considered. In turn this truncation surface must not disturb the electromagnetic field solution or to be "transparent" to the impinging waves. The numerically discretized model includes everything within the truncation surface, but the inverse problem unknowns are only the constitutive parameters within the "virtual body area". By the aid of the discretization this "virtual body" is comprised of a number of pixels for two-dimensional (2-D) or voxels for three-dimensional (3-D) geometries. Each one ($i^{th}$) of them is assumed locally homogeneous with constant but unknown ($\sigma_i$, $\varepsilon_{ri}$, $\mu_{ri}$) properties which are in principle different for each pixel/voxel, forming the so-called piece-wise constant distribution. Now, the aim of the reconstruction is exactly the evaluation of these three vectors $[\sigma]=[\sigma_i]$, $[\varepsilon_r]=[\varepsilon_{ri}]$ and/or $[\mu_r]=[\mu_{ri}]$, by exploiting the dataset acquired from field measurements carried out on the real object. Numerous different approaches are established for the exploitation of this information. The most usual approach which is also elaborated herein is to formulate a cost function based on the least square method, which will be in turn minimized employing some type of optimization techniques. For this purpose an initial ($\sigma_i^o$, $\varepsilon_{ri}^o$, $\mu_{ri}^o$) distribution, usually simply a homogeneous one is assumed and the measurement procedure is mimicked through computer simulations. Namely, for each active antenna the **forward problem** corresponding to the solution of a vector wave equation or in general the numerical solution of Maxwell's equations, yields the field distribution all over the receiving antennas. Exactly the field calculated on the receiving antennas, when gathered from all illuminating active antennas, it setup a calculated dataset. On the other hand the field calculated all over the structure and particularly over the "virtual body area" is exploited within the methodology elaborated herein for the evaluation of a **"Sensitivity" or "Jacobian" matrix.** This is obtained through a closed form sensitivity equation established through a combination of an "Adjoint Network Theorem" following the Electromagnetics Reciprocity Theorem approach. Its entries exactly reflect the sensitivity of the calculated field at each sensing antenna with respect to a differential change of each pixel/voxel unknown parameter. With the availability of this information an algorithm minimizing the differences between measured and calculated fields (the complete datasets) based on a least square approach is established, which herein is efficiently implemented exploiting the sensitivity matrix in its closed form expression.

At this point two serious problems are introduced related to the inherent properties of the "sensitivity matrix". Firstly, its entries depend on the unknown properties ($\sigma_i$, $\varepsilon_{ri}$, $\mu_{ri}$), hence the system to be solved is a non-linear one. Secondly, this sensitivity matrix is usually an ill-posed one or a singular matrix. This latter means that if a singular value decomposition is performed (not eigenvalue since this is a rectangular MxN matrix, where the number of measurements M should be much greater than the number (N) of unknowns as M>>N in order to confront measurement errors, noise and ill-posedeness) the maximum singular value appears a few orders of magnitude larger than the minimum one. This inherent property is closely related to the measurement (generally the data collection) setup and can be significantly improved by intuitive techniques. Returning to the nonlinearity its direct consequence is that the resulting parameters ($\sigma_i$, $\varepsilon_{ri}$, $\mu_{ri}$) provided by the Minimization first iteration are not the true ones but only a better approximation, if the reconstruction process was successful. Hence, the whole procedure should be repeated again and again until the difference between the measured and the calculated dataset becomes comparable to the expected measurement error and/or the required convergence is achieved. Obviously, at each iteration a new sensitivity matrix and a new data set is evaluated and used.

In the following sections the reader will be introduced to the employed approaches from both the mathematical-computational as well as the electromagnetics point of view. But mostly the open research challenges will be pointed out motivating new research and paths toward RF-Microwave imaging practical implementation.

The forward and inverse problems general characteristics are discussed in the second section, after the introduction to high and microwave frequencies imaging modalities. The procedure to formulate and numerically solve the forward problem is given in the third section, for both the high (MHz) and microwave regimes. Within the foarth section the cost function is first setup and the Perturbation Methodology for its direct iterative solution is then introduced step-by-step from static to microwave imaging. The fifth section elaborates on the establishment of the "sensitivity Equation" based on the "Adjoint Network Theorem" for the microwave band and its equivalent "Electrical Networks Compensation Theorem" for the MHz range. Before presenting the forward and inverse problem numerical results (sixth section) the importance of the study of the sensitivity or Jacobian matrix is pointed out. This is a very promising research area especially when modern Principal Component Analysis (PCA) or its counterpart Proper Orthogonal Decomposition (POD) approaches are employed. Either PCA or POD are based on a Singular Value Decomposition of the sensitivity matrix (rectangular matrix) by an algebraic manipulation of its eigenvectors. These techniques present prospects for novel and computationally efficient methodologies for both the forward and the inverse problem solution.

The last section is devoted to numerical results. A series of successfully reconstructed conductivity and permittivity distributions for both the MHz and the microwave regimes will be presented. The algorithm performance will be discussed and possible improvements constituting future research areas will be suggested.

## 2. Forward problem & inverse problem characteristics

The first step in the course of establishing an imaging modality refers to the construction of the appropriate computer model, which should reflect the practical geometry as closely as possible. This model serves in twofold, first it should enable an approach which mimics the measurement procedure and secondly it should offer the ability to represent the unknown distribution ($\sigma$, $\varepsilon_r$ or both) as a set of successively improved-updated variables. Mimicking the measurement procedure refers to the solution of the governing differential equations, identified as a generalized Laplace or Poisson equation in MHz range, while the full wave Maxwell equations must be considered in the microwave regime. The practical bodies of interest are of arbitrary shape and present a complicated inhomogeneous internal structure in both $\sigma$ and $\varepsilon_r$.

In general, these objects should be represented as three dimensional (3-D) models, however in this case both the forward and the inverse problems become very complicated with high computational demands. Besides these, the data collection or measurement strategy is also complex. The possibility of a two-dimensional modeling even an approximate one could be very convenient, since it could simplify the forward problem solution, restricting the data collection approaches to just a few and overally resulting to a straightforward reconstruction algorithm. The question is when the involved approximations are acceptable and whether these introduce any fictitious mathematical or numerical complications? Let as elaborate next on the issue of a 3-D versus a 2-D modeling.

### 2.1 Non-linearity and Ill-conditioning of the inverse problem

The issue of two-dimensional modeling is not rhetorical, since it has been extensively exploited in most of the established imaging modalities like x-rays computerized tomography (CT). However, there is a significant difference between x-rays and electromagnetic tomography in that x-rays propagate along straight lines, but in contrary electric current and electromagnetic waves in general flow (stream-) lines are curved whenever they intercept an interface where the conductivity or permittivity changes [e.g. from ($\varepsilon_{r1}$, $\sigma_1$) to ($\varepsilon_{rz}$, $\sigma_z$)], as it usually happens in biological structures. This causes severe problems not only in worsening the option of a 2-D approximation but also in rendering a non-linear inverse electromagnetic problem. A fundamental reasoning for this difficulty is explained by the fact that current streamlines or wave propagation directions curvature strongly depends on the conductivity ($\sigma_z/\sigma_1$) and permittivity ($\varepsilon_z/\varepsilon_1$) contrast at these interfaces. But these contrasts are indeed the unknown quantities to be sought by the electromagnetic imaging algorithm. Namely, when the inverse problem is finally formulated into a discrete system of equations the stiffness matrix elements will depend on the unknown ($\sigma$, $\varepsilon_r$) distributions hence comprising a non-linear system. In general, this phenomenon can be identified as an internal scattering and/or diffraction which is equally present in Acoustical or Ultrasonic imaging.

Besides the non-linearity, the streamlines curvature appearing in bodies with very high $\sigma$ or $\varepsilon_r$ contrast (e.g. between blood and fat or bone tissues) results to regions with very high current densities (e.g. blood) while at others this is very low (in fat or bone). Similar high variations occur in the electric field intensities mainly due to the high $\varepsilon_r$ constrast. This is exactly what causes the high variation in the sensitivity of the measured quantity (voltage or electric field) with respect to the unknown $\sigma$ or $\varepsilon_r$ values. To understand this phenomenon assume a tissue (area) which is isolated from the current flowing through the body, this will in turn present a very low sensitivity as it cannot affect the injected current, which will not be able to "see" it. Hence, its $\sigma$ or $\varepsilon_r$ values cannot be reliably reconstructed. Mathematically, this high variation in the sensitivity over the body to be imaged is depicted as a high singularity or high ill-conditioning in the "Jacobian" matrix [J], which comprises the inverse problem matrix (as $[J][J]^T$). As will be explained latter the severity of ill-conditioning is defined by the ratio of the larger to the smaller singular value of the Jacobian matrix (singular instead of eigenvalue since the Jacobian matrix is rectangular due to the requirement of a number of measurements higher than the number of unknown $\sigma$, $\varepsilon_r$ degrees of freedom).

Summarizing the above, the imaging modality elaborated herein constitutes a highly non-linear and ill-conditioned (singular) inverse problem. The next issue to be discussed refers to the assumptions involved in a two-dimensional approximation.

## 2.2 Two-versus three-dimensional modeling

Theoretically an object can be represented by a two-dimensional model (2-D) if it is homogeneous and uniformly extends to "infinity" along a direction perpendicular to the modeled cross-section, which can be arbitrary shaped and inhomogeneous. The question is now, under what assumptions the current density, the electric potential or electric field intensity of a practical three-dimensional (3-D) object can be replicated over one of its cross-sections (2-D model)? Once again recall that this approach is very well suited for x-rays CT mainly because x-rays travel along straight lines and hence their measured intensity involves information relevant to the inhomogeneities (varying tissue) along the straight line from the transmiter to the receiving sensor. Thus by attaching an array of sensors in the same plane with the source as shown in Fig.1a, all measured intensities depend on the specific enclosed cross-section. Besides that the specific source location yields an illumination from a corresponding angle of view, called a "projection angle" from physical optics. It is, thus, found very convenient to locate the source and the receivers-sensors equidistantly along a circular bar (a plastic collar). Rotating this circular structure results to an illumination of the imaged cross-section from any possible angle of view, to be defined at the desired number enabling the image reconstruction.

A similar configuration could be in principle setup for the electrical impedance (EIT) or microwave tomography by planning an array of electrodes or antennas on a single plane around the desired cross-section as shown in Fig.1b and 1c respectively.

Focusing on EIT or MHz tomography the current density injected through the driven-active electrode (source) is curved around the objects of lower conductivity (Fig.1), but the same phenomenon occurs along the third dimension perpendicular to the cross-section under study. Consequently, the injected current density which offers the means to extract the information regarding the conductivity distribution to be imaged, cannot be restricted to flow only across the electrodes plane. Instead this current is spread in all directions around the active electrode and respectively it is collimated from all directions toward the current-sink active electrode. Thus, the coplanar voltage-sensing electrodes yield measurements infected by conductivity inhomogeneities above or below the studied cross-section. Additionally, it is impossible to estimate the total current flowing across the electrodes cross section. To explain the difficulty, assume that a 5mA current (I=5mA) is injected during the actual EIT measurements, the question is what is the current value to be applied to the active electrode in the 2-D model? This should be only the fraction of the 5mA actually flown through the electrode cross-section, otherwise by assuming a 5mA value yields overestimated calculated voltages at the electrodes. Besides this problem, by restricting the current to flow in a single plane in the 2-D model, its density becomes higher within the highly conducting areas. This phenomenon results to higher sensitivity related to these areas and causes the Jacobian matrix to be fictitiously more singular than its actual 3-D form. Exactly similar behavior is observed in MHz and microwave imaging where the role of high conductivity regions is also played by the high permittivity areas, especially as the source frequency is increased.

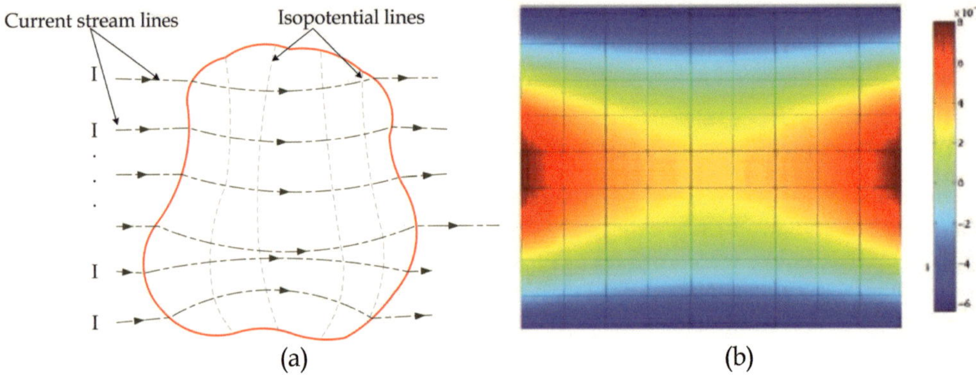


Fig. 1. (a) Current density distribution of an inhomogeneous 2-D model at low frequencies (b) Electric field distribution of an inhomogenous dielectric $(\varepsilon_r)$ at microwave frequency.

The above observation regarding the higher singularity of the 2-D model as compared to a 3-D model is very important and should be utilized as a guide toward the establishment of more robust imaging techniques. In particular, most of these complexities stems from the attempt to solve (simulate) the forward problem as a 2-D cross-sectional model, rather than caused from the 2-D inverse problem formulation. Hence, whenever the simplification of the 2-D setup is sought, it is a very good idea to adopt the corresponding electrode/antennas coplanar setup (e.g. Fig.2b, 2c) along with a uniform $(\sigma, \varepsilon_r)$ distribution in the axial direction, which yields a 2-D inverse problem formulation. However, a finite axial length is considered and a 3-D numerical technique is employed to solve the forward problem. The important benefit of this approach refers to the removal of the deviations between measured and calculated voltages or electric field intensities. Besides that, the fictitious higher sensitivity matrix singularity is reduced to the inherently existing as well.

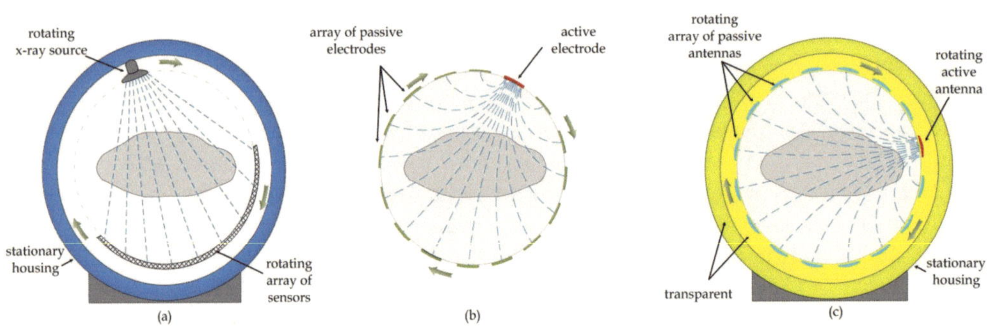


Fig. 2. a) An x-ray setup for cross-sectional imaging, different illumination by rotating the x-ray platform.
b) An electrode array for cross-sectional impedance tomography.
c) An antenna array for cross-sectional microwave imaging, that could be setup on a plastic "transparent to electromagnetic waves" collar just like the x-rays CT.

A more sophisticated trend toward singularity reduction or as sometimes assumed "toward optimal imaging setup" aims at the establishment of the optimum current density distribution for EIT or in the MHz range and respectively "optimal electric field intensity" distribution. As explained above all the involved complications stem from the current or field streamline curvature which depends on the unknown ($\sigma$, $\varepsilon_r$) discontinuities. But it is intuitively expected for EIT that these curvature may become smoother (or streamlines tending toward straight lines) when the active electrodes (both injecting and current sink) is increased. This phenomenon can be diaesthetically understood by realizing that all current (or field) streamlines are emanating from the source or converging toward the sink electrode, traveling toward all possible directions. Thus, their curvature becomes maximum for point electrodes and smooths down as its size is increased. This approach was forced to its limits in the EIT case by the groups of Isaacson [7] and Lionheart [8], where the active electrodes were increased at the limit of almost covering the entire object's surface, retaining only small gaps between them for isolation. This, voltage or electric field sensing electrode or antennas do not presume any large surface and they could retain a small size even almost infinitesimal (point sensing electrodes). Recall that the primary aim of this trend is to reduce the sensitivity or Jacobian matrix singularity, explicitly by reducing the ratio of its larger to the smaller singular value. Conversely means smoothing out the sensitivity over the body surface or volume by forcing more current to flow through low conductivity regions and lowering the current density within high conductivity areas. However, the Authors experience shows that one should not exaggerate in increasing the electrode or antenna surface, but the current should be allowed to follow its natural paths through the object, since this is indeed the mechanism of extracting information from the object interior. As a rule of thumb the electrode or antenna size could be increased only up to the point that the singularity becomes manageable by the reconstruction algorithm, which should withstand relatively high sensitivity variations. In turn the rotation of the active antenna illuminating the structure from all possible angles would ensure a higher overall-total information extraction.

### 2.3 Dual mesh discretization

Returning back to the different forward (3-D) and inverse 2-D model, another characteristic should be taken into account, which is related to the calculation accuracy and the desired imaging spatial resolution. Starting from the latter it depends on the available number of linearly independent measurements, which is in turn defined by the number of active and sensing electrodes/antennas, as it will be explained later on. Also, keep in mind that measured values are corrupted by noise and the measurement inaccuracies, including quantization noise introduced during the analog to digital conversion. Thus a reliable inversion scheme requires a quite higher number of measurements (M equal to the number of equations) than the number of unknowns (N) in order to cancel out these inaccuracies through minimization. As a rule of thumb the number of equations should be almost double than that of the unknowns ($M \geq 2N$). Conversely the number of electrodes/antennas corresponds to the achievable spatial voltage or filed intensity sampling, but it is actually defined by the practical setup as the electrode/antenna size and the hosting object dimensions on which these will be attached. Concluding the above parameters define an upper limit in the achievable number of unknowns (N) and hence the offered inverse problem spatial resolution-discretization. Thus the in principle continuous ($\sigma$, $\varepsilon_r$)

distribution should be discretized into N locally homogeneous elements comprising the so called piece-wise constant distribution ($\sigma_i$, $\varepsilon_{ri}$, i=1-N). This is actually formed by the "reconstruction-mesh", which is in general a 3-D one (Fig.3a), but it could also restricted to a 2-D assembly of bars with in general arbitrary cross-section (Fig.3b with brick bars).

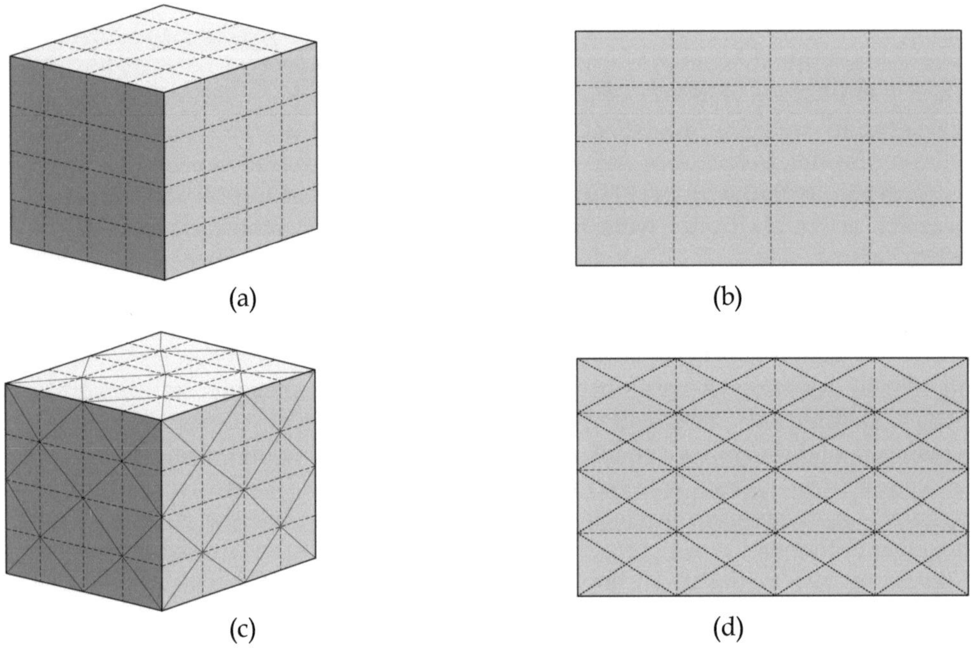


Fig. 3. Examples of reconstruction coarse meshes and forward fine meshes as: reconstruction (a) 3-D and (b) 2-D cases, forward: (c) 3-D and (d) 2-D cases corresponding to the structures (a) and (b) respectively.

The reasoning described above yields usually a coarse reconstruction mesh, which is always inappropriate for the forward problem solution. This one purpose is to ensure calculations providing an accuracy of the same order as the available measurements. In the low frequency EIT case it was proved by Barber and Seagar [9] that an accuracy of the order of 0.1% is necessary for a reliable reconstruction. On the other end, in the microwave regime it is widely understood that an acceptable simulation asks for a discretization with elements size smaller than one tenth of the wavelength ($\lambda/10$) for Moment Method (MoM) or Finite Element techniques (FEM), while the finest mesh of $\lambda/32$ is asked by Finite Difference Time Domain (FDTD) to ensure its stability. In any case trying to fulfill these requirements a very fine mesh is necessary for the forward problem solution, which also yields piece-wise constant ($\sigma$, $\varepsilon_r$) distributions. However, the inverse problem will be iteratively linearized first around the $(\sigma^0, \varepsilon_r^0)$ initial guess and subsequently around the most recently updated $(\sigma^k, \varepsilon_r^k)$ distribution at its k-th iteration. Multiple forward problem solutions are then required on this $(\sigma^k, \varepsilon_r^k)$ distribution, hence the "forward" and "reconstruction" meshes should be compatible. A very straight forward approach is to subdivide each of the reconstruction mesh into smaller forward mesh elements, as shown in Fig.3(c)-(d). Even though the forward mesh elements comprising each reconstruction cell have the same constitutive ($\sigma_i$, $\varepsilon_{ri}$) parameters, this subdivision in necessary in order to fullfill the voltage/field interpolation requirements. Explicitly, in most cases linear interpolation functions are considered within the established numerical techniques (MoM, FEM, FDTD). In turn the field variation especially around fine structures and around conductors are very high, thus asking either for highly non-linear interpolation functions or conversely very fine mesh of linearly interpolated elements ($\lambda/10$ up to $\lambda/32$).

Overally, up to now the basic configuration and limiting characteristics for the forward and inverse problems are explained. We are, thus, ready to proceed to the description of forward problem governing equations and their numerical solutions.

## 3. Forward problem

Electromagnetic problems are obviously governed by Maxwell equations in their full vector differential form, which in general include a temporal variation [10]. Even well-known, their solute, ion for complicated extremely inhomogeneous structures like the Human body constitutes a formidable task, especially when the conductivity anisotropy of skeletal and myocardial muscle is to be considered. Since, the inverse problem asks for multiple forward solutions (at least one for each illumination-projection angle) at each of its iterations, then a computationally efficient technique is inevitable. For this purpose a series of simplifications are necessary in order to reduce the involved complexity.

### 3.1 Excitation rationale

The temporal dependence could be employed in imaging modalities, since radar type techniques could be employed, but these are efficient for electrically large bodies (dimensions of multiple wavelengths) located at distances of at least a few wavelengths away from the illuminating source. Besides that pulsed-waveform excitation could be exploited for imaging in general, where the received pulse delay ($\Delta\tau$) in respect with the transmitted one provides the useful phase difference ($\Delta\varphi$). In turn based on $\Delta\varphi$ the ratio of imaginary to real part of the voltage or electric field is readily calculated, while the in principle required phase sensitive sensors are replaced by "scalar" measuring only their amplitude. As will be explained next, this information is directly proportional to ($\varepsilon_r/\sigma$) or inversely proportional to the dielectric loss tangent [$\tan\delta=\sigma/(\omega\varepsilon_0\varepsilon_r)$] of the media profile to be reconstructed. This imaging approach could be classified as a "multistatic phase" radar and it is very challenging as well as a promising modality, especially regarding the involved relative simplification of the sensing-measuring instrumentation. However, it has only received a very limited attention and to the Authors knowledge, there was only one Russian group working on that, [11]. Conversely, most of the research groups activated in the field in MHz and microwave imaging (including our own) assume time harmonic (sinusoidal) excitation due to its simplicity in the forward problem solution, thus the following analysis will be restricted to this case. Note that this excitation eliminates the temporal dependence but also avoids (dues not account for) the materials frequency dispersion $\sigma(\omega)$, $\varepsilon_r(\omega)$ which introduce more difficulties. In contrary this dispersion can be exploited as an additional degree of freedom enabling "dynamic imaging" or calibration purposes and even a spectral imaging by performing measurements and reconstructing the media profile at multiple frequencies ($\sigma(\omega_i)$, $\varepsilon_r(\omega_i)$) selected at appropriate steps ($\Delta\omega_i$).

### 3.2 Time harmonic fields & currents

Maxwell equations for the time harmonic excitation of the form $\propto e^{j\omega t}$ are significantly simplified since the temporal variation is substituted as $\partial / \partial t = j\omega$, while the actual field $\vec{\mathcal{E}}(t,\vec{r}), \vec{\mathcal{H}}(t,\vec{r})$ and source quantities $\vec{\mathcal{J}}(t,\vec{r})$ are replaced by the corresponding complex phasors $\vec{E}(\vec{r}), \vec{H}(\vec{r}), \vec{J}(\vec{r})$ as:

$$\vec{\mathcal{E}}(t,\vec{r}) = \mathrm{Re}\left(\vec{E}(\vec{r})e^{j\omega t}\right) \tag{1a}$$

$$\vec{\mathcal{H}}(t,\vec{r}) = \mathrm{Re}\left(\vec{H}(\vec{r})e^{j\omega t}\right) \tag{1b}$$

$$\vec{\mathcal{J}}(t,\vec{r}) = \mathrm{Re}\left(\vec{J}(\vec{r})e^{j\omega t}\right) \tag{1c}$$

In turn Maxwell equations for time harmonic fields read:

$$\vec{\nabla} \mathrm{x} \vec{\mathrm{E}} = \text{-j}\omega\mu_0\mu_r\vec{\mathrm{H}} \tag{2a}$$

$$\vec{\nabla} \mathrm{x} \vec{\mathrm{H}} = \mathrm{j}\omega\varepsilon_0\varepsilon_r\vec{\mathrm{E}} + \vec{\mathrm{J}} \tag{2b}$$

$$\vec{\nabla} \cdot \vec{\mathrm{D}} = \rho \Rightarrow \vec{\nabla} \cdot \varepsilon\vec{\mathrm{E}} = \rho \tag{2c}$$

$$\vec{\nabla} \cdot \vec{B} = 0 \Rightarrow \vec{\nabla} \cdot \mu\vec{H} = 0\Big|_{\mu=scalar} \rightarrow \vec{\nabla} \cdot \vec{H} = 0 \tag{2d}$$

Where the source quantities current ($\vec{J}$) and charge ($\rho$) densities should obey the continuity equation:

$$\vec{\nabla} \cdot \vec{J} = -\partial\rho / \partial t = -j\omega\rho \tag{3}$$

Additionally, for the conducting media assumed herein there is a conduction current ($\vec{J}_c$) flowing at any arbitrary point (movement of charges due to coulomb forces and the presence of electric field) as $\vec{J}_c = \sigma\vec{E}$. Thus, the current density $\vec{J}$ appearing in (2b) is comprised of the conduction current $\vec{J}_c$ and the current impressed by the source as $\vec{J}_{imp}$. Substituting in (2a) we may define an equivalent complex permittivity $\varepsilon_c$ or an equivalent complex conductivity $\sigma_c$ as:

$$\vec{\nabla} \mathrm{x} \vec{\mathrm{H}} = \mathrm{j}\omega\varepsilon_0\varepsilon_r\vec{E} + \sigma\vec{E} + \vec{J}_{imp} = \mathrm{j}\omega\varepsilon_0\varepsilon_{rc}\vec{E} + \vec{J}_{imp} = \sigma_c\vec{E} + \vec{J}_{imp} \tag{4}$$

where

$$\varepsilon_c = \varepsilon_0\varepsilon_{rc} = \varepsilon_0\varepsilon_r(1 - j\tan\delta) = \varepsilon_0\varepsilon_r\left(1 - j\frac{\sigma}{\omega\varepsilon_0\varepsilon_r}\right) \tag{5a}$$

$$\sigma_c = \sigma_{eff} = \sigma + j\omega\varepsilon_0\varepsilon_r \tag{5b}$$

Note that the term related to the actual permittivity *(ε)* is known as displacement current $\vec{J}_d = \partial\left(\varepsilon\vec{E}\right)/\partial t = j\omega\varepsilon_0\varepsilon_r\vec{E}$. A usual question regarding the body inherent bioelectric sources has actually no place herein since their spectral content is restricted to less than about 10KHz. Thus the impressed current in equation (4) is solely due to the source injecting current or illuminating the body. For safety reasons the injected current density should be less than 10mA/cm$^2$ according to recommendation included in [12]. Besides these, recall the possible anisotropy issue which only concerns the conductivity of skeletal muscular tissues and the myocardium. Both of them exhibit a fibrous structure, where each fiber has a high conductivity interior surrounded by a thin low conductivity membrane. It is this structure that causes the conductivity anisotropy where parallel (along) the fibers it is $\sigma_{//}$=7.3mS/cm while transverse to them it is only $\sigma_{\perp}$=0.49mS/cm. The question is how to include this anisotropy into the computer model. Mathematically the anisotropy is accounted for by a second rank tensor $\bar{\bar{\sigma}}$, but this could be only convenient if one of the coordinate axis could be oriented parallel to the muscle fibers. However, these fibers are curved and even twisted, hence they could be only represented by a full 3×3 tensorial $\bar{\bar{\sigma}}$. It is, indeed, very easy to model a diagonal tensor of either $\bar{\bar{\sigma}}$ or $\bar{\bar{\varepsilon}}_r$ parameters, but the mathematical and computational complexity of full tensor parameters is too high to be considered in most cases. Thus, herein the inherent muscles anisotropy will not be considered.

Returning back to Maxwell equations (2), it is well understood that the divergence equations (2c) and (2d) can be derived from the curl equations (2a) and (2b) by using continuity equation (3). Thus one may easily conclude that it is only necessary to solve the implicit pair of curl equations (2a), (2b) in conjunction with the boundary conditions for the tangential to the various media-tissue interfaces electric and magnetic field components. Recall that the latter are indeed obtained from the corresponding integral form laws resulting from the same curl equations, [10]. However, one should keep in mind that this conclusion is exactly valid only when an exact analytical solution is sought. In contrary when numerical solutions are adopted along with the internal structure discretization accompanied by approximate interpolation functions within each piece-wise homogeneous element, then the aforementioned "exact" conditions can be violated, resulting to field distributions not obeying the divergence conditions. Even though this could be kept in mind as a possible source of inaccuracies, usually their effects can be negligible. Thus there is indeed a very powerful method to discretized and solve the interdependent pair of vector curl differential equations (2a) and (2b), such as the Finite Difference Frequency Domain (FDFD) method established in our previous work, Lavranos [13] in two-dimensional curvilinear coordinates and currently been extended to 3-D structures as in Lavdas [14]. This approach can easily account for material anisotropy as well, within the usual FD limitations regarding the interfaces spatial resolution. Even though this is a promising approach we have not yet employed it within inverse problem solutions, but instead the Finite Element Method (FEM) is mostly employed for this purpose. Since FEM is formulated in an integral form, it is more convenient to decouple the two curl equations in order to formulate two separate vector wave equations for the electric and the magnetic field respectively as, e.g. Jin [15] or Volakis [16](p.5) :

$$\vec{\nabla}\mathrm{x}\left(\frac{1}{\mu_\mathrm{r}}\vec{\nabla}x\vec{E}\right)\text{-}\mathrm{k}_0^2\left(\varepsilon_\mathrm{r}-j\frac{\sigma}{\omega\varepsilon_0}\right)\vec{E}=-\mathrm{j}\omega\mu_0\vec{J}_{imp} \tag{6a}$$

$$\vec{\nabla}\text{x}\left(\frac{1}{\varepsilon_{\text{rc}}}\vec{\nabla}x\vec{H}\right)\text{-k}_0^2\mu_{\text{r}}\vec{H} = \nabla x\left(\frac{\vec{J}}{\varepsilon_{\text{rc}}}\right) \tag{6b}$$

Either wave equation could be solved employing FEM after constructing a functional (or weak form) to be minimized. This task is achieved utilizing either a variational approach or the Galerkin approach, e.g. Cangellaris [17]. The choice among the two wave equations is mainly undermined by the more convenient enforcement of boundary conditions. For the biomedical applications the media-tissues are non-magnetic ($\mu=\mu_0$) and the inhomogeneity is approximated by step changes in conductivity and permittivity. Thus the related boundary conditions are directly enforced to the electric field as Dirichlet type. Conversely, if ones solves for the magnetic field the same boundary condition would be translated into a Newmann type and a differentiation after the solution (prone to numerical errors) would be performed to evaluate the desired electric field. Hence, it is preferable to choose a straightforward solution of the electric field wave equation (6a).

Observing equation (6a) and following its solution in the next section one would realize that this is anything else but a trivial task, involving huge computational resources to solve over a Human body or just a Human torso. For this reason two simplifications will be presented next, a quasi-static approach valid for the frequency range up to a few MHz and a second approach with unidirectional dipole sources (aligned along the z-axis) and even a 2-D scalar Helmholtz wave equations excited by "line sources" which significantly reduce the involved complexity.

### 3.3 Quasi-static approach

Observing equations (2a) and (2b) one may recall the basic understanding that the electromagnetic waves are created and propagated due to the temporal variation of impressed current source which is inherited to the generated field. Explicitly, a time depended impressed current generates a temporally changing magnetic field through (2b). In turn the varying magnetic field $-\mu\partial\vec{H}/\partial t = -j\omega\mu\vec{H}$ produce an electric field with an identical time variation through (2a). This $\varepsilon\partial\vec{E}/\partial t = j\omega\varepsilon\vec{E}$ regenerates a changing magnetic field through (2b) and this cycle is infinitely repeated producing a propagating wave. However, this "chain" becomes very weak or breaks when either $j\omega\mu=j\omega\mu_0\mu_r$ or $j\omega\varepsilon=j\omega\varepsilon_0\varepsilon_r$ quantities become very small (where $\varepsilon_0=8.854\text{x}10^{-12}\text{F/m}$ and $\mu_0=4\pi\cdot10^{-7}\text{H/m}$). Biological tissues are non-magnetic $\mu_r=1$ while due to their high water content they present a very high dielectric constant which starts from about $\varepsilon_r\approx1000$ (or more) at 100KHz range and reduced to about $\varepsilon_r\approx80$ in the microwave (GHz) range. Based on this reasoning it was long ago realized, e.g. Price 1979 [18], that magnetic effects can be ignored for frequencies lower than about 10MHz. Namely, the electric filed generated by magnetic field temporal variations becomes negligible. From the wave propagation point of view the wavelength in a media $\varepsilon_r\approx100$ at f=10MHz is $\lambda_g = \lambda_0/\sqrt{\varepsilon_r} = 3m$ (and $\lambda_0=c/f$), which means that at a distance $d=\lambda_g/4=75\text{cm}$ the field or voltages changes due to wave propagation from its maximum value to zero and vice-versa. Hence for a thorax with larger dimension of about 40cm the 10MHz frequency constitutes indeed an upper limit.

In view of the above, the ignorant question asks then "from where comes the varying electric field and the desired electric potential"? Now we have to reconsider the divergence equation (2c) and the charge conservation law (3) as:

$$\vec{\nabla}\times\vec{E}\approx 0 \quad \Rightarrow \quad \vec{E}=-\vec{\nabla}V \tag{7a}$$

$$\vec{\nabla}\cdot\varepsilon\vec{E}=\rho \quad \Rightarrow \quad \vec{\nabla}\cdot\varepsilon\vec{\nabla}V=-\rho \tag{7b}$$

$$\vec{\nabla}\cdot\vec{J}=-j\omega\rho \Rightarrow \vec{\nabla}\cdot\sigma\vec{E}=-j\omega\rho \Rightarrow \vec{\nabla}\cdot\sigma\vec{\nabla}V=j\omega\rho \tag{7c}$$

Equations (7b) and (7c) seems to be in contradiction since, they call for different voltage definition or making V to voltage uniqueness. Here comes the original Maxwell observation, e.g. see Jackson [19]( p.238), that one could differentiate (2c) and substitute in charge conservation equation as:

$$\begin{matrix} (2c) & \Rightarrow & \vec{\nabla}\cdot\dfrac{\partial\vec{D}}{\partial t}=\dfrac{\partial\rho}{\partial t} \\ (3) & \Rightarrow & \vec{\nabla}\cdot J+\dfrac{\partial\rho}{\partial t}=0 \end{matrix} \left. \vphantom{\dfrac{\partial}{\partial}\dfrac{\partial}{\partial}} \right\} \begin{matrix} \vec{\nabla}\cdot\vec{J}+\vec{\nabla}\cdot\dfrac{\partial\vec{D}}{\partial t}=0 \\ or \ \vec{\nabla}\cdot\left(\vec{J}+\dfrac{\partial\vec{D}}{\partial t}\right)=0 \end{matrix} \tag{8a}$$

Substituting the constitutive relations $J=\sigma\vec{E}$ and $D=\varepsilon\vec{E}$ into (8a) and restricting ourselves to time harmonic fields we get:

$$\overline{\nabla}\cdot(\sigma+j\omega\varepsilon)\overline{E}=0 \tag{8b}$$

In turn utilizing (7a) the so called **generalized complex Laplace equation** is obtained:

$$\overline{\nabla}\cdot\varepsilon_c(\vec{r})\vec{\nabla}V=0 \tag{8c}$$

where:

$$\varepsilon_c(\rho)=\varepsilon(\vec{r})-j\sigma(\vec{r})/\omega \tag{9}$$

However, besides this classical approach, (8c) can be obtained by dividing (7c) with $j\omega$ and adding the result to (7b). Charge density at the operating frequency indeed exist over the metallic electrodes obeying (7c), but these can be taken into account through the **boundary conditions** to be enforced on the voltage distribution during the FEM formulation of the Newmann type:

$$-j\omega\varepsilon_c\frac{\partial V}{\partial n}=-j\omega\left(\varepsilon-j\frac{\sigma}{\omega}\right)\frac{\partial V}{\partial n}=\begin{cases} J & \text{on the electrode} \\ -j\omega\varepsilon_0\dfrac{\partial V}{\partial n} & \text{on the body air interface} \end{cases} \tag{10}$$

where $\partial V/\partial n$ denotes the normal derivative at the interface. At this point is important to note that (10) applies to both active-driven as well as passive (sensing) metallic electrodes, since current and charge density is induced on them. Most important is that the field and current singularity at metallic edges is a local phenomenon and thus it occurs at any frequency from DC to microwaves. Referring to a classical electromagnetics text book, e.g. Collin [10](p.25), field components normal to the edge as well as current density components parallel to the edge exhibit a singular behavior tending to infinity as $1/\sqrt{\rho}$, where ρ the distance from the edge. Conversely, field components parallel to the edge and current density normal to that vanish as ρ→0. This is an important behavior and it should be taken into account when an accurate modeling is sought. To clarify this behavior the current density on a patch electrode driven by a current 1 is shown in Fig.4a and the induced current density on a passive electrode is sketched in Fig.4b. Note that the corresponding integrals denote the total current I on the driven and zero on the passive electrode. Obeying equation (3) the charge density on the active or passive electrodes exhibits identical singular behavior.

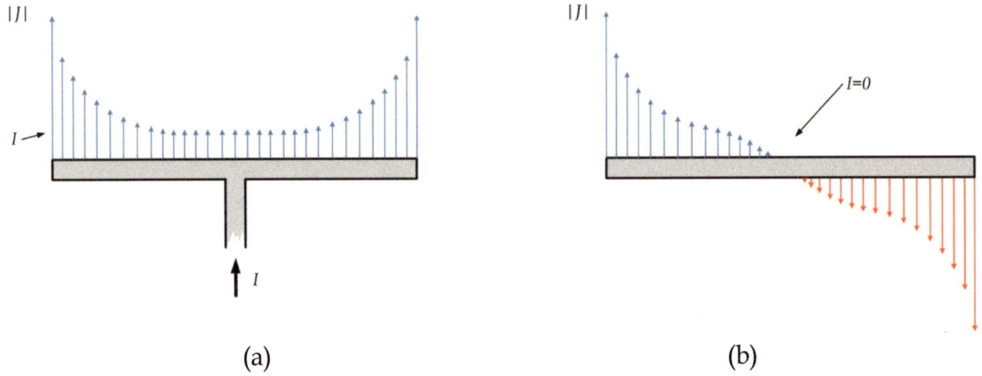


Fig. 4. Current density on metallic strip electrodes exhibiting the inherent singularity as a) emanating from an active electrode and b) induced on a passive electrode, e.g. [19](p.165)

### 3.4 Wave equation for microwave sources in biological media

The forward problem for the microwave imaging is governed by the wave equations (6a) or (6b). It was explained before that the electric field wave equation (6a) offers a straightforward enforcement of boundary condition at the different lossy dielectric interfaces as a rigid-Dirichlet type. Besides that, observing the first term of equation (6a) this could be significantly simplified for the non-magnetic biological media as $\mu=\mu_0=const$ or $\mu_r=1$. In contrary the corresponding first term of (6b) is complicated as it contains the spatially dependent complex $\varepsilon_{rc}=\varepsilon_{rc}(\vec{r})$. In view of this clarification the electric field wave equation (6a) can be simplified by utilizing the identity:

$$\vec{\nabla}\times\vec{\nabla}\times\vec{E}=\vec{\nabla}(\vec{\nabla}\cdot\vec{E})-\nabla^2\vec{E} \tag{11}$$

For the divergence of $\vec{E}$ we may again exploit the original Maxwell observation [19](p.238) as given in equation (8c) which is generally valid and using the symbolism (5a) $\varepsilon_c=\sigma+j\omega\varepsilon$, then (8c) reads:

$$\vec{\nabla}\cdot\left(\varepsilon_c(\vec{r})\vec{E}(\vec{r})\right)=0 \;\rightarrow\; \varepsilon_c(\vec{r})\vec{\nabla}\cdot\vec{E}(\vec{r})+\vec{E}(\vec{r})\cdot\vec{\nabla}\varepsilon_c(\vec{r})=0 \tag{12a}$$

or

$$\vec{\nabla}\cdot\vec{E}(\vec{r})=-\frac{\vec{E}(\vec{r})\cdot\vec{\nabla}\varepsilon_c(\vec{r})}{\varepsilon_c(\vec{r})} \tag{12b}$$

Substituting equation (12b) into (11) and the resulting expression back into (6a) the desired electric field wave equation for biological media is obtained:

$$\vec{\nabla}^2\vec{E}+k_0^2\mu_r\left(\varepsilon_r-j\frac{\sigma}{\omega\varepsilon_0}\right)\vec{E}+\vec{\nabla}\left(\frac{\vec{E}\cdot\vec{\nabla}(\sigma+j\omega\varepsilon)}{\sigma+j\omega\varepsilon}\right)=j\omega\mu_0\mu_r\vec{J}_{imp} \tag{13}$$

It is now convenient to define a complex inhomogeneous wavenumber $\vec{K}(\vec{r})$ in the usual form as:

$$K^2(\vec{r})=k_0^2\mu_r\left(\varepsilon_r(\vec{r})-j\frac{\sigma(\vec{r})}{\omega\varepsilon_0}\right) \tag{14}$$

With the aid of (14) the electric wave equation reads

$$\nabla^2\vec{E}(\vec{r})+K^2(\vec{r})\vec{E}(\vec{r})+\vec{\nabla}\left(\frac{\vec{E}(\vec{r})\cdot\vec{\nabla}K^2(\vec{r})}{K^2(\vec{r})}\right)=j\omega\mu_0\mu_r\vec{J}_{imp}(\vec{r}') \tag{15}$$

where $(\vec{r}')$ denotes the source spatial vector.

### 3.5 Two dimensional structure-inhomogeneous cross-section

The convenience offered by a two dimensional imaging are already explained in section II.2 along with the necessity of solving a three-dimensional forward problem. The geometry considered in this case is a cylindrical structure with an arbitrary shaped cross-section but uniform along its axial $\hat{z}$ -direction. Likewise the material complex permittivity to be sought is inhomogeneous in the (xy) cross section but uniform along the z-direction, like an assembly of different dielectric bars, as $\varepsilon_c(\vec{r})=\varepsilon_c(x,y)$ . Due to the uniformity in the axial $\hat{z}$ -direction the structure can be considered as an inhomogeneously loaded lossy dielectric open waveguide of arbitrary cross-section which is excited-illuminated by different type of sources. In view of this uniformity the electromagnetic field within and outside this open waveguide could be expressed as a superposition (expansion) of an in general infinite number of modes either propagating or evanescent just as classically done in the mode-Matching technique. Even though this is a very promising approach to our knowledge it has not yet being exploited for imaging purposes. Let us give a formal description of such a methodology. For each one of the possibly excited modes the field dependence in the $\hat{z}$ -direction can be denoted as:

$$\vec{E}_i(x,y,z)=\vec{e}_i(x,y)e^{-j\beta_i z} \tag{16a}$$

$$\vec{H}_i(x,y,z)=\vec{h}_i(x,y)e^{-j\beta_i z} \tag{16b}$$

where $\beta_i$ is the $i^{th}$ mode complex propagation constant. When β is real or exhibits a small imaginary part due to losses, then it represents a propagating wave. Conversely, when β is purely imaginary then it represents an evanescent or non-propagating wave which can be excited by the source but is exponentially attenuated away from that. Namely, it exists only around the source, it does not transfer energy but it only stores electric and magnetic energy in its neighborhood, thus contributing only to the reactive part of the source (antenna) input impedance. In order to utilize the eigenmode expansion approach the characteristics of every possible mode, its eigenfunctions $\vec{e}_i(x,y), \vec{h}_i(x,y)$ and the complex propagation ($\beta_i$) constant should be estimated first. The corresponding expansion formally reads:

$$\vec{E} = \sum_{i=1}^{\infty} w_{ei}\vec{E}_i = \sum_{i=1}^{\infty} w_{ei}\vec{e}_i(x.y)e^{-j\beta_i z} \tag{17a}$$

$$\vec{H} = \sum_{i=1}^{\infty} w_{mi}\vec{H}_i = \sum_{i=1}^{\infty} w_{ei}\vec{h}_i(x.y)e^{-j\beta_i z} \tag{17b}$$

Where $w_{ei}$ and $w_{mi}$ represent the modal amplitudes or weighting factors which depend on the source type and its location, see for example our work [20]. These can be estimated through a power conservation low which is the basis of a mode matching technique. Explicitly, each specific source can be enclosed inside a fictitious box inside which the field is described with the aid of a numerical technique on a fine mesh exploiting the knowledge of source modeling, e.g. Volakis [16](p.238). Outside the fictitious surface the eigenfunctions (17) is considered and the weighting factors $w_{ei}$ and $w_{mi}$ are evaluated through field continuity conditions across this psudo surface. It is important to keep in mind that the power conservation low should be enforced, which is preferably formulated in conjunction with the modes orthogonality properties, e.g. [21].

The above mode matching approach pressumes the knowledge of the eigenvalues *($\beta_i$)* and the eigenfunctions $\vec{e}_i, \vec{\mathrm{h}}_i$ which for the considered inhomogeneous cross-section can only be acquired numerically. For this purpose the wave equation (6a) shall be formulated as an eigenvalue problem and the usual approach is based on the separation of both the electric field $\vec{e}$ and the nabla $(\vec{\nabla})$ differential operator into axial ($\hat{z}$) and transverse *(t)* components as:

$$\vec{e} = \vec{e}_t + \hat{z}e_z \quad and \quad \vec{e}_t = e_x\hat{x} + e_y\hat{y}, \qquad \vec{h} = \vec{h}_t + \hat{z}h_z \tag{18a}$$

$$\vec{\nabla} = \vec{\nabla}_t + \hat{z}\frac{\partial}{\partial z} = \vec{\nabla}_t - j\beta\hat{z}, \qquad \vec{\nabla}_t = \hat{x}\frac{\partial}{\partial x} + \hat{y}\frac{\partial}{\partial y} \tag{18b}$$

The detailed procedure given in a lot of textbooks, e.g. Volakis et al [16](p.98) is summarized as follows:

$$\vec{\nabla} \times \vec{e} = \vec{\nabla}_t \times \vec{e}_t + (\vec{\nabla}_t e_z + j\beta\vec{e}_t) \times \hat{z} \tag{19}$$

Which can be substitute into (6a) to yield a pair of differential equations for the axial ($e_z$) and transverse ($\vec{e}_t$) field components as:

$$\vec{\nabla}_t \times \left(\frac{1}{\mu_r}\vec{\nabla}_t \times \vec{e}_t\right) - j\frac{\beta}{\mu_r}\left(\vec{\nabla}_t e_z + j\beta\vec{e}_t\right) - k_0^2\varepsilon_{rc}\vec{e}_t = 0 \tag{20a}$$

$$\vec{\nabla}_t \times \left( \frac{1}{\mu_r} (\vec{\nabla}_t e_z + j\beta \vec{e}_t) \times \hat{z} \right) - k_0^2 \varepsilon_{rc} e_z \hat{z} = 0 \tag{20b}$$

The pair of equations (20) constitutes the eigenproblem to be solved numerically. Observing that the transverse component $\vec{e}_t$ mainly occurs a product jβ $\vec{e}_t$, the eigenproblem in further simplified by letting $j\beta\vec{e}_t \to \vec{e}_t'$ and multiplying (20a) by jβ yields:

$$\vec{\nabla}_t \times \left( \frac{1}{\mu_r} \vec{\nabla}_t \times \vec{e}_t' \right) + \beta^2 \frac{1}{\mu_r} \left( \vec{\nabla}_t e_z + \vec{e}_t' \right) = k_0^2 \varepsilon_{rc} \vec{e}_t' \tag{21a}$$

$$\beta^2 \vec{\nabla}_t \times \left( \frac{1}{\mu_r} (\vec{\nabla}_t e_z + \vec{e}_t') \times \hat{z} \right) = \beta^2 k_0^2 \varepsilon_{rc} \cdot e_z \hat{z} \tag{21b}$$

Equations (21) constitute the desired eigenproblem for the $\beta$ eigenvalue. The interested reader may contact our previous work [22] on open waveguides which was carried out within Dr. Allilomes doctoral thesis [23] also available online (in Greek).

Even though the above 2-D analysis offered some simplification the forward problem still remains complicated and computationally demanding. A truly two-dimensional approach presumes the sources to be two dimensional, i.e. tending to infinity along the z-axis, just as in the case of an "infinite line source".

### 3.6 Two dimensional object excited by infinite line sources

The field of an infinite electric line source embedded in a homogeneous media is well studied and can be found in any classical electromagnetics textbook, e.g. Balanis [24]( p.571). Since the line source is infinite its current density must be constant and if it is considered aligned along the z-axis, then:

Line Source:

$$\bar{J}(\vec{r}') = J_{2L} \hat{z} = \frac{I}{A} \delta(\vec{\rho} - \vec{\rho}') \hat{z} \tag{22}$$

where I is a sinusoidal current ($I = I_0 e^{j\omega t}$) and ρ the polar radial coordinate transverse to $\hat{z}$, as A let the line source cross section assumed very small.

For a homogeneous medium the field generated by an infinite line source is a Transverse Magnetic ($TM^z$), $H_z=0$ with only and axial electric field $\vec{E} = E_z \hat{z}$ and its transverse eigenfunction is identical to a cylindrical Hankel function of the second type $H_0^{(2)}(k\rho)$ assuming that the line source is at ρ=0, for details in [24]( p.571). For the case of the inhomogeneous cross-section the TM nature of the wave is exactly preserved, thus $\vec{E} = E_z \hat{z}$ and $E_x=E_y=0$. Besides that the two-dimensional complex dielectric profile is uniform along the z-axis or $d\varepsilon_c(\vec{r}) / dz = 0$ and consequently from equation (14) it is $\partial K(\vec{r}) / \partial z = 0$. In view of the above simplifications the third term of equation (15) vanishes as also explained by Fang [25] :

$$\left.\begin{array}{l} E_x = E_y = 0 \\ \partial^2 K^2(\vec{r}) / \partial z = 0 \end{array}\right\} \quad \vec{E}(\vec{r}) \cdot \nabla^2 K^2(\vec{r}) = 0 \tag{23}$$

Consequently, the wave equation (15) is reduced to a scalar Helmholtz equation:

2-D & Line Source:

$$\vec{\nabla}^2 E_2(\vec{r}) + K^2 E_2(\vec{r}) = j\omega\mu_0\mu_r J_{ZL} \tag{24}$$

A more practical structure to be considered herein is comprised by the same lossy dielectric profile $\varepsilon_c(x,y)$ but with a finite extend in the z-direction and illuminated by a circular array of infinitesimal $\hat{z}$-directed dipoles located at the mid z-plane and encircle the object to be imaged. Even though this can again be classified as a 2-D inverse problem and solved accordingly, the corresponding forward problem is governed by the 3-D wave equation (6a) or (15) and it will be solved with the aid of a 3-D finite element method.

### 3.7 Variational formulation

The finite element will be employed for the numerical solution of either the generalized Laplace equation (8c), the scalar wave equation (24) or the general vector wave equation (6a). For each case the structure will be discretized with the aid of the appropriate forward fine mesh. The first step of this procedure refers to the formulation of the differential equation into an appropriate integral functional or weak formulation which will, in turn, be minimized to obtain the numerical solution. Let us start from the simpler case.

#### 3.7.1 Functional for the generalized laplace equation

For these relatively simple scalar problems the variational formulation is usually adopted. According to the approach, e.g. Jin [15]( p.72), the differential equation (8c) along with its boundary conditions yields the functional to be minimized. These are as follows:

1. Neumann boundary conditions at the active current electrodes and along the body-surrounding air interface:

$$-j\omega\varepsilon_c \frac{\vartheta V}{\vartheta n} = \begin{cases} J, & \text{on driven electrodes} \\ -j\omega\varepsilon_0 \dfrac{\vartheta V}{\vartheta n}, & \text{on body-air interface} \end{cases} \tag{25}$$

   where $\vartheta V / \vartheta n$ is the potential derivative in the direction normal to the unknown object surface.

2. Mixed Dirichlet and Neumann boundary conditions between different media regions-object elements (i,j) as:

$$V_i = V_j \text{ and } \varepsilon_{ri}^* \frac{\vartheta V_i}{\vartheta n} = \varepsilon_{rj}^* \frac{\vartheta V_j}{\vartheta n} \tag{26}$$

These are natural boundary conditions which are an inherent property of the differential equation (8c). Namely, these are automatically imposed through the FEM solution of (8c). Note that the above does not include any Dirichlet condition, namely only the derivatives are defined (delta change), hence the resulting solution will be floating and thus non-unique. To avoid this problem at least one point must be grounded (V=0)

**Absorbing boundary conditions**

At this point recall that the Generalized Laplace equation solution domain is basically infinite, since for high frequency sources (i.e. in the MHz range) the electric field $(\vec{E})$ and the related scalar potential (V) extends in the air to "infinity" obeying in general the Sommerfeld radiation condition. Explicitly, for very low frequencies the static potential in the air surrounding the structure vanishes since the conduction current $\vec{J}_c = \sigma\vec{E}$ is zero and $\sigma = 0$ in the air. However, as frequency (ω) is increased a significant displacement current $\vec{J}_d = j\omega\varepsilon_o\vec{E}$ flows in the air around the structure and this phenomenon must be taken into account. But, for a numerical solution the analysis domain must be finite and restricted if possible to the actual body of interest. For this purpose the solution domain is enclosed within a fictitious closed surface of canonical shape on which "transparent Absorbing Boundary Conditions (ABC)" are enforced. Transparent ABCs means that they should not disturb the field distribution but conversely to behave like perfect absorbers (if possible), absorbing any wave incident on them without any reflection, just like a termination load. For the two dimensional forward mesh of Fig.5a enclosed within a fictitious circular contour-C, the quasi-static potential ABCs read [15](p.97):

$$\frac{\vartheta V}{\vartheta \rho} \approx \frac{1}{\rho ln\rho} V \text{ on circle } \rho = \rho_c \tag{27}$$

where $\rho = \sqrt{x^2 + y^2}$ the radial polar coordinate.

The three dimensional structure of Fig.6b is enclosed within a fictitious cylindrical surface on which the appropriate ABCs should be imposed. In order to understand the ABCs in both 2-D and 3-D structures it worths to recall that these are extracted from a generalized type of boundary conditions, [15](p137). For this purpose let us write the generalized Laplace (8c) or Poisson equation in the general form of:

$$-\frac{\partial}{\partial x}\left(\varepsilon_{cx}\frac{\partial V}{\partial x}\right) - \frac{\partial}{\partial y}\left(\varepsilon_{cy}\frac{\partial V}{\partial y}\right) - \frac{\partial}{\partial z}\left(\varepsilon_{cz}\frac{\partial V}{\partial z}\right) + \beta V = f \tag{28a}$$

Considering the solution domain enclosed within a closed surface $S = S_1 + S_2$ on which two type of boundary conditions can be imposed as:

Dirichlet Boundary Condition:

$$V = \rho \text{ on } S_1 \tag{28b}$$

General (mixed Dirichlet & Newmann) Boundary Condition

$$\left(\varepsilon_{cx}\frac{\partial V}{\partial x} + \varepsilon_{cy}\frac{\partial V}{\partial y} + \varepsilon_{cz}\frac{\partial V}{\partial z}\right)\cdot\hat{n} + \gamma V = q \text{ on } S_2 \tag{28c}$$

where $\hat{n}$ the outward unit normal vector. Besides these the field and consequently the scalar electric potential should obey the Sommerfeld radiation condition at infinity which reads, [15](p.8) or [16]( p.8):

$$\text{3-D: } \lim_{r\to\infty} r\left\{\nabla\times\left(\vec{\Psi}\right)+jk_o\hat{r}\times\left(\vec{\Psi}\right)\right\}=0 \tag{29a}$$

where $\vec{\Psi}=\vec{E}$ or $\vec{H}$ and $r=\sqrt{x^2+y^2+z^2}$ ,which states that the field is comprised of an outgoing wave with dependence $e^{-jk_or}$ as $r\to\infty$. For a two-dimensional case (29a) where $\vec{E}=E_z\hat{z}$ (e.g. $TM_z$ modes) or $\vec{H}=H_z\hat{z}$ (for $TE_z$ modes) equation (29a) reduces to:

$$\lim_{r\to\infty}\rho\left\{\frac{\partial}{\partial\rho}(\Psi_z)+jk_o\times(\Psi_z)\right\}=0 \tag{29b}$$

where $\Psi_z=E_z$ or $H_z$. The question is now how to express (29b) in the general form of (28c) to be applied on the fictitious boundary truncating the solution domain, by keeping in mind that $\vec{E}=-\vec{\nabla}V$. Additionally it has been proved that for a 2-D case the potential (the static or the quasi-static approximation) asymptotically behaves as [15](p.97):

$$\text{2-D: } V=A\ln\rho \text{ as } \rho\to\infty \tag{30a}$$

where A is a constant.

For a three-dimensional domain the potential in the homogenous background (i.e. air) and at a large distance from its sources behaves as [15](p150):

$$a\approx\frac{A}{r} \tag{30b}$$

where $r=\sqrt{x^2+y^2+z^2}$.

For the two dimensional case let $\partial V/\partial z=0$ and the 2-D ABC (27) is obtained from (28c) by letting $q=0$ and $\gamma=1/(\rho\ln\rho)$. Note, that inside the fictitious surface-S there is always an air layer ($\varepsilon_{rx}=\varepsilon_{ry}=\varepsilon_{rz}=1$), hence (28c) reads:

$$\left(\frac{\partial V}{\partial x}+\frac{\partial V}{\partial y}\right)\hat{n}=-\frac{1}{\rho\ln\rho}V \tag{31a}$$

For a circular fictitious surface it is $\hat{n}=\hat{\rho}$ and for a large enough radius the left hand side of (29) is reduced to $\partial V/\partial\rho$ to yield the ABCs of (27), (the related vector identities see e.g. Balanis [24] (appendix II)

Likewise, for the three dimensional domain eq.(28c) yields the absorbing boundary conditions.

For a spherical fictitious surface with radius $r_c$ large enough the absorbing boundary conditions take the form:

$$\frac{\partial V}{\partial r}\approx-\frac{1}{r}V \tag{31b}$$

which, in turn, can be expressed through (28c) by letting $\gamma=1/r$, $q=0$ and $\hat{n}=\hat{\rho}$.

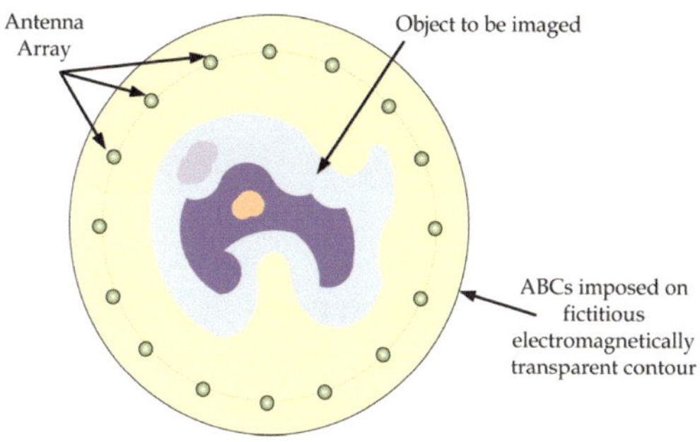


(a)

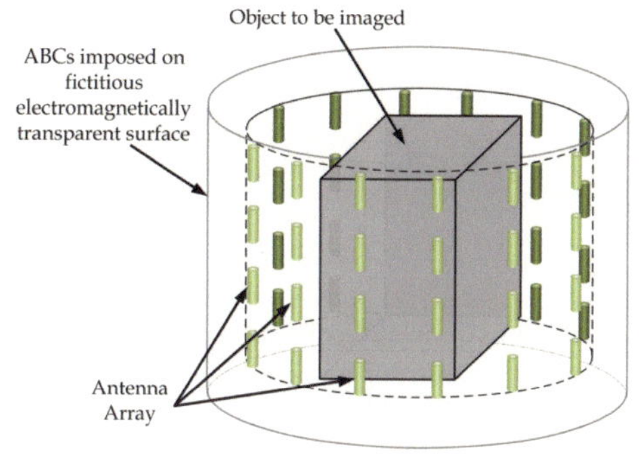


(b)

Fig. 5. The object to be imaged is surrounded by the illumintating or sensing antennas array and is enclosed within a fictitious surface "transparent" to electromagnetic waves on which ABCs are imposed: (a) 2-D and (b) 3-D configuration.

For the scalar microwave case where $\psi = E_z$ or $H_z$ equation (29a) yields the absorbing boundary condition along a cruved fictitious surface as,

$$\frac{\partial \psi_z}{\partial \rho} = \left( -jk_o - \frac{1}{2\rho} \right) \psi_z \tag{31c}$$

### 3.7.2 Functional for generalized Laplace equation

With the aid of the variational technique the generalized Laplace equation (8c) along with the boundary conditions (25), (26) or their general form (28) and the corresponding ABCs in (27), are found to be equivalent to the minimization of the following functional:

$$F(V) = \frac{1}{2} \sum_{e=1}^{M} \varepsilon_c \int\int_{\Omega_e} \left[ (\frac{\vartheta V}{\vartheta x})^2 + (\frac{\vartheta V}{\vartheta y})^2 \right] dxdy + \oint JV d\ell = \sum_{e=1}^{M} F^e(V^e) \tag{32}$$

where M is the total number of elements and $\Omega_e$ is the area of each e-element. Note that the variational formula (32) is valid for either real or complex quantities according to [15](p.76) and the references therein. For *F(V)* to be minimized, its partial derivatives with respect to the elements nodal voltages must be zero, namely:

$$\frac{\vartheta F(V)}{\vartheta V_i} = 0 \quad for \quad i = 1, 2, \ldots, n \tag{33}$$

where n is the total number of nodes.

### 3.7.3 Functional for the vector and scalar wave equations

A variational technique can be employed to formulate the microwave functional for the vector wave equation (6a) along with the appropriate boundary conditions and the corresponding Absorbing Boundary Conditions. The resulting functional reads [15]:

$$\text{3-D: } F(\vec{E}) = \frac{1}{2}\iiint_V \left[ \frac{1}{\mu_r}(\vec{\nabla}\times\vec{E})\cdot(\vec{\nabla}\times\vec{E}) - k_o^2\varepsilon_{rc}\vec{E}\cdot\vec{E} \right] dV + \oiint_S \left[ \underbrace{\frac{jk_o}{2}(\hat{r}\times\vec{E})\cdot(\hat{r}\times\vec{E})}_{ABCs} \right] dS$$
$$+ \iiint_V \underbrace{j\omega\mu_o \hat{J}_s \cdot \vec{E}}_{source}\, dV \tag{34}$$

Likewise, the scalar wave equation (24) when a 2-D structure is illuminated by a line source results to the functional:

$$\text{2-D: } F(\vec{E}) = \frac{1}{2}\iint_S \left[ \left(\frac{\partial E_z}{\partial x}\right)^2 + \left(\frac{\partial E_z}{\partial y}\right)^2 - k_o^2\varepsilon_{rc}E_z \right] dS + \frac{1}{2}\underbrace{\oint_{\Gamma_s}\left(jk_o + \frac{1}{2r}\right)E_z^2 dl}_{ABCs} + \iint_S \underbrace{j\omega\mu_o J_z E_z}_{source}\, dS \tag{35}$$

The surface integral in eq.(34) is defined over the fictitious cylinder truncating the solution domain. Likewise the line integral in eq. (35) is defined along a fictitious circle ($\Gamma_S$) terminating the 2-D mesh. Both these integrals express the absorbing boundary condition.

### 3.7.4 Finite element solution of the forward problem

For both the quasi static and the microwave approach the structure must be discretized utilizing a dual mesh. A fine one for the forward problem and a coarse mesh for the inverse problem, as shown in Fig.3. The coarse mesh is defined only over the object to be imaged (Fig.6), while the fine-forward mesh covers the whole solution domain up to the fictitious line or surface enclosing all constituents including antennas of electrodes. Besides that every coarse element is subdivided in a number of smaller fine mesh elements. The nodal FEM approach is employed for the MHz potential estimation as well as the 2-D scalar Helmholtz equation involving only Ez component referred bellow as scalar FEM. Conversely, the edge elements technique is adopted for the 3-D vector wave equation. Since, for the reconstruction mesh the body under consideration is split into cubic (or rectangular) elements with constant $\sigma$ and $\varepsilon_r$, so a piecewise homogeneous model is constructed as:

$$\varepsilon_c(x,y) = \sum_{k=1}^{E} \varepsilon_{ck}\psi_k, \qquad \psi_k = \begin{cases} 1 & \text{within k-th element} \\ 0 & \text{elsewhere} \end{cases} \tag{36}$$

Even though FEM is well described in numerous textbooks, e.g. [15], [16] and [17] for multigrid approaches, a short description of the basic interpolation functions and the related element matrices is given next, since they are necessary for the definition and evaluation of the Jacobian-Sensitivity matrix.

### 3.7.5 Scalar nodal 2-D approach

Either the potential in the functional (32) or the $E_z$ component of (35) are discretized employing first order linear triangular elements with the unknowns (degrees of freedom) defined on their nodes as:

$$\text{2-D triangular: } \psi^e = \sum_{i=1}^{3} N_i^e \psi_i^e \tag{37}$$

where $\psi^e = V^e$ or $E_z^e$ respectively. The scalar interpolation or basis function are given by:

$$N_i^e = \frac{1}{2\Delta^e}\left(a_i^e + b_i^e x + c_i^e y\right),\ i = 1,2,3 \tag{38}$$

$\Delta^e$ = area of the e-th element, $a_1^e = x_2^e y_3^e - y_2^e x_3^e$, $b_1^e = y_2^e - y_3^e$, $c_1^e = x_3^e - x_2^e$, $a_2^e, a_3^e, b_2^e, b_3^e, c_2^e, c_3^e$ can be found by cyclic interchange. The above interpolation functions include unknown coefficients related to the element geometry and its material constitutive parameters. These are estimated by applying the interpolation functions at the points where the field or potential is sampled, in this case the element nodes. The resulting system of equations is analytically solved for these unknowns in terms of the potential or field values at the nodes. These are, then, substituted back into the interpolation function. In turn, this can be readily exploited in the conditions minimizing the FEM functional like that of equation (33) through an analytical evaluation of the derivatives with respect to the unknown potentials ($V_i$) or field components $E_{zi}$. Observe at this point that the involved surface integrals over the solution domain (e.g. (32) or (35)) are discriminated into a sum of integrals over each element. The latter yields a system of equations of the form:

$$\left[Y^e\left(\varepsilon_c^e\right)\right]\left[V^e\right] = \left[I^e\right] \tag{39}$$

or respectively:

$$\left[K^e\left(\varepsilon_c^e\right)\right]\left[E_z^e\right] = \left[B(J_z)\right] \tag{40}$$

Within the classical FEM the above element equations are assembled to from a unified system matrix representing the whole solution domain. Hence, this matrix should include all boundary conditions along with the illuminating sources and passive substructures like sensing electrodes or antenna models as well. The latter is useful and it should be accounted at least when the methodology is matured, but it is for now neglected. Regarding the important absorbing boundary conditions these are usually imposed through the closed contour integral over $\Gamma_S$ in equations (32) and (35). For this purpose the contour $\Gamma_S$ is discretized into line segments coinciding with the corresponding edge of the peripheral triangles (as depicted in Fig.6)

The corresponding line element matrices are as follows:

$$\text{Quasi-static ABCs: } K_s = -j\omega\varepsilon_o \int_{\partial\Gamma_s} \frac{V^2}{\rho \ln \rho} dl \tag{41}$$

$$\text{2-D microwave ABCs: } \left[K_s\right] = \oint_{\partial\Omega} \left(jk_o + \frac{1}{2r}\right) N_i N_j d\Gamma_s \tag{42}$$

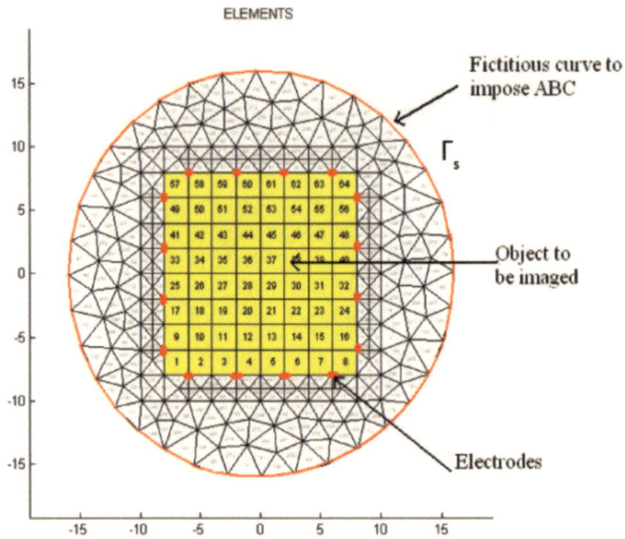


Fig. 6. Example of coarse mesh overlapping a fine mesh, for 2-D rectangular object enclosed in a fictitious circle *($\Gamma_S$)*. The contour $\Gamma_S$ is discretized using line segments which coincide with the corresponding edge of the peripheral triangles

The last term to be included here is the feeding sources contribution through the corresponding terms of equations (32) and (35). Herein the simplest possible sources are considered, i.e. infinitesimal electrodes or dipoles respectively. In both cases the current density is approximated as uniform ignoring the field/current singularity at the edges (a phenomenon which should be included in a most complete version), thus given by the ratio of the feeding current (I) to the antenna or electrode cross section (A) like *J=I/A*. The related integrals over the source yield the right hand side *[I]* or $B(J_z)$ respectively. The resulting FEM system of equations takes the form:

$$\text{Quasi static FEM: } \left[Y(\varepsilon_c)\right]\left[V\right]=\left[I\right] \tag{43}$$

$$\text{2-D microwave FEM: } \left[K(\varepsilon_c)\right]\left[E_z(\varepsilon_c)\right]=\left[B(J_z)\right] \tag{44}$$

Classical numerical techniques can be employed to solve systems (43) or (44), but it is useful to keep in mind that multiple solutions are necessary (for each inverse problem iteration), one for each illuminating antenna or active electrodes pair position. Hence a technique based on the inversion of the system matrix like the LU decomposition is very convenient, since the solution for each k$^{th}$-right hand side is obtained by a simple multiplication as $\left[V^k\right]=\left[Y^{-1}\right]\left[I^k\right]$.

### 3.7.6 Vector edge elements FEM

For the volume integral of the electric field vector in the functional of (34) first order tetrahedral vector-edge elements are employed. The electric field $\vec{E}$ within each tetrahedral is expanded in terms of the FEM basis functions as, [15]:

$$\text{3-D: } \vec{E}^e = \sum_{i=1}^{6} \vec{N}_i^e E_i^e \tag{45}$$

$E_i^e$ denotes the tangential field values along the i-th edge and $\vec{N}_i^e$ is the vector interpolation or basis function given by:

$$\vec{N}_i^e = W_{i_1 i_2} l_i^e = \left( L_{i_1}^e \vec{\nabla} L_{i_2}^e - L_{i_2}^e \vec{\nabla} L_{i_1}^e \right) l_i^e \tag{46}$$

The edge numbers and the associated nodes $i_1$ and $i_2$ are defined in Table 1 and in Fig.7. For a detailed definition of the quantities involved in (46) one may consult [15, 17]

| Edge $i$ | Node $i_1$ | Node $i_2$ |
|---|---|---|
| 1 | 1 | 2 |
| 2 | 1 | 3 |
| 3 | 1 | 4 |
| 4 | 2 | 3 |
| 5 | 4 | 2 |
| 6 | 3 | 4 |

Table 1. Edge definition for a tetrahedral element

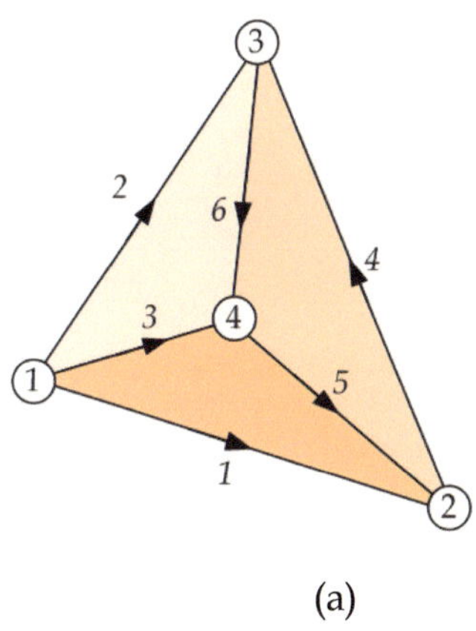


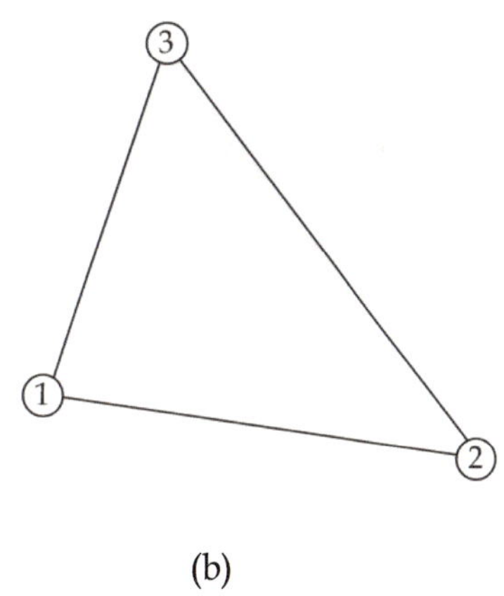


Fig. 7. Finite elements employed for the discretization, (a) tetrahedral edge element for 3-D and (b) triangular node element for 2-D.

Following an approach similar (but more complicated) to that for the 2-D case the resulting volume element matrix reads:

$$\text{vector-tetrahedral: } \left[ K^e \right] = \iiint_V \left[ \frac{1}{\mu_r^e} \left\{ \vec{\nabla} \times \vec{N}_i^e \right\} \cdot \left\{ \vec{\nabla} \times \vec{N}_j^e \right\}^T - k_o^2 \varepsilon_c^e \left\{ \vec{N}_i^e \right\} \cdot \left\{ \vec{N}_j^e \right\} \right] dV \tag{47}$$

The absorbing boundary conditions stem from (29a) and take the form of the corresponding term in (34) through an asymptotic approximation. In order to evaluate this integral, the closed fictitious surface (S) is discretized into triangles coinciding with the outer surface of the peripheral tetrahedrals as shown if Fig.8. The resulting element matrix reads:

$$\text{3-D ABCs: } \left[K^s\right] = \oiint_S \left[\frac{jk_o}{2}\left(\hat{r}\times\vec{N}_i\right)\cdot\left(\hat{r}\times\vec{N}_j\right)\right]dS \tag{48}$$

where $\hat{r}$ is the outward unit normal vector. Note that the above involved triangular edge elements shape functions are not trivial, since each triangle has a different orientation in a 3-D space. The most convenient way to extract them is through the degeneration of the corresponding peripheral tetrahedral into a surface triangle. Regarding the source modeling an infinitesimal dipole approximation is again considered as for the 2-D case.

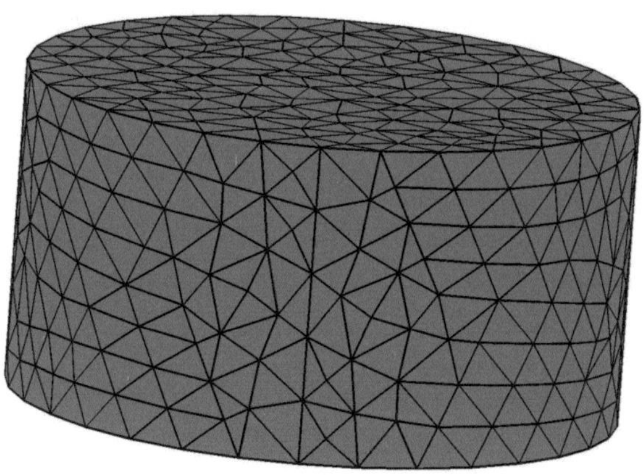

Fig. 8. Triangles coinciding with the outer surface of the peripheral tetrahedrals

The linear system solution in the 3-D case constitutes a major difficulty due to the large number of unknowns. Thus the performance of direct inversion methods like LU decomposition becomes questionable and iterative techniques are also tried herein. Specifically, in the 3-D case the inversion of the matrix K will consume all the system memory due to the size of the matrix, so an iterative solver is preferred with the appropriate preconditioner. The Generalized Minimum Residual method (GMRES) is used for the solution of the linear system with a symmetric successive over-relaxation-vector (SSOR-vector) preconditioner.

Solving this system the electric fields (or the potential) on the receiving antennas (or electrodes) and at all the internal edges or nodes is calculated and stored, to be used latter within the reconstruction algorithm. An example of the electric field distribution when one of the infinitesimal dipole or a line-source antenna is activated is shown in Fig. 9.

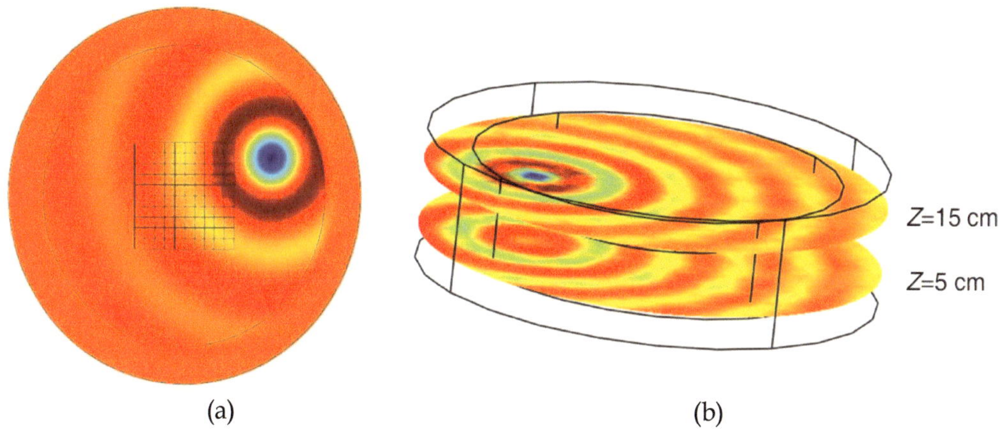


Fig. 9. (a) Electric field distribution when a 2D structure is illuminated by an infinitesimal dipole operated at 800MHz and (b) electric field distribution at two planes when a 3D structure is illuminated by an infinitesimal dipole operated at 1 GHz.

## 4. Inverse problem

The reconstruction algorithm is based on the modified perturbation method that was initially developed for the conductivity imaging in Electrical Impedance Tomography [26] and later on extended to higher frequencies (up to 10MHz),[27]. This research was carried out within the doctoral thesis of D. Drogoudis [28], which was primarily focused to extend MPM and prove its validity in the microwave regime. Indeed this proof of concept was achieved and published in [29] and [30]. For the introduction of the reader to the inverse problem approach but also to provide him with the knowledge to proceed further and ultimately achieve its practical implementation, the reasoning behind its implementation and the logical steps for its extension will be given next. Thus, let us start by reviewing the static MPM and proceed to its extension to the MHz and finally the microwave range.

### 4.1 Review of the static MPM algorithm

First a review of the static algorithm will be given and based on that the steps towards its present time harmonic formulation will be described. According to [26] the σ-imaging algorithm reads:

$$\sigma_j^n = \sigma_j^{n-1} + k_1 \frac{\sum_{i=1}^{M} \frac{V_{mi} - V_{ci}}{V_{mi}} \frac{\vartheta V_i}{\vartheta \sigma_j}}{\sum_{k=1}^{M} \left| \frac{\vartheta V_k}{\vartheta \sigma_j} \right|} \sigma_j^{n-1} \tag{49}$$

where M is the total number of linearly independent measurements, $V_{mi}$ and $V_{ci}$ are the measured and calculated voltage differences at the i$^{th}$ port (electrodes pair) and $k_1$ is the relaxation factor to be chosen in the range $0<k_1<2$ in order to provide faster convergence. The partial derivatives $\vartheta V_i / \vartheta \sigma_j$ or $\vartheta V_k / \vartheta \sigma_j$ constitute the elements of the Jacobian matrix. These are calculated from the voltage distributions all over the object cross section through a closed form expression given by Yorkey et al. [31]. The latter is based on the electrical circuit compensation theorem as applied on a resistor network equivalent for each σ-element, as shown in Fig.10. In turn these expressions are given in [31] as:

$$J_{ij} = \frac{\vartheta V_i}{\vartheta \sigma_j} = -\frac{1}{I_i} \sum_{\ell=1}^{L} S_\ell V_{ij(\ell)} V_{kj(\ell)} \tag{50}$$

where $V_{ij(\ell)}$ and $V_{kj(\ell)}$ are the voltages developed across the $l_{th}$ branch of the $j_{th}$ element Fig.10 when a sinusoidal current with amplitude $I_i = I_k$ is successively injected through the ports -i and -k respectively. The constants $S_\ell$ are the normalized geometrical weights arising from the finite element formulation. $S_\ell$ are actually given by the non-diagonal entries of the $[Y]_e$ -element matrix as: $[Y]_e = \sigma_j [K_e]$ and $[S_\ell]_e =$ non-diagonal entries of $[K_e]$.

An indicative example of these branch admittance values is through the definition of the resistance network for the rectangular element (Fig.10) and its related element matrix:

*static triangular element*

$$[Y]_3 = \begin{bmatrix} G_{11} & -G_{12} & -G_{13} \\ & G_{22} & -G_{23} \\ symmetric & & G_{33} \end{bmatrix} = \sigma_j \cdot [K]_3 \tag{50a}$$

$$[K]_3 = \frac{1}{4\Delta} \begin{bmatrix} b_1^2 + c_1^2 & b_1 b_2 + c_1 c_2 & b_1 b_3 + c_1 c_3 \\ & b_2^2 + c_2^2 & b_2 b_3 + c_2 c_3 \\ symmetric & & b_3^2 + c_1^3 \end{bmatrix} \tag{50b}$$

*static rectangular element*

$$[Y]_4 = \begin{bmatrix} G_{11} & -G_{12} & -G_{13} & -G_{14} \\ & G_{22} & -G_{23} & -G_{24} \\ & & G_{33} & -G_{34} \\ symetric & & & G_{44} \end{bmatrix} \tag{50c}$$

$$[K]_4 = \begin{bmatrix} 2a^2 + 2b^2 & a^2 - 2b^2 & -a^2 - b^2 & -a^2 - b^2 \\ & 2a^2 + 2b^2 & -a^2 - b^2 & -a^2 - b^2 \\ & & 2a^2 + 2b^2 & a^2 - 2b^2 \\ symetric & & & 2a^2 + 2b^2 \end{bmatrix} \tag{50d}$$

and $$\Delta = \frac{1}{2} \begin{vmatrix} 1 & x_1 & y_1 \\ 1 & x_2 & y_2 \\ 1 & x_3 & y_3 \end{vmatrix} = \frac{1}{2}(b_1 c_2 - b_2 c_1) \quad \begin{matrix} a_1 = x_2 y_3 - y_2 x_3, \; b_1 = y_2 - y_3, \; c_1 = x_3 - x_2 \\ a_2 = x_3 y_1 - y_3 x_1, \; b_2 = y_3 - y_1, \; c_2 = x_1 - x_3 \\ a_3 = x_1 y_2 - y_1 x_2, \; b_3 = y_1 - y_2, \; c_3 = x_2 - x_1 \end{matrix}$$

A detailed derivation of the Compensation theorem can be found in Yorkey et al. [31] as well as in Sahalos et al. [32](p.229). Guidelines for its implementation are also given therein.

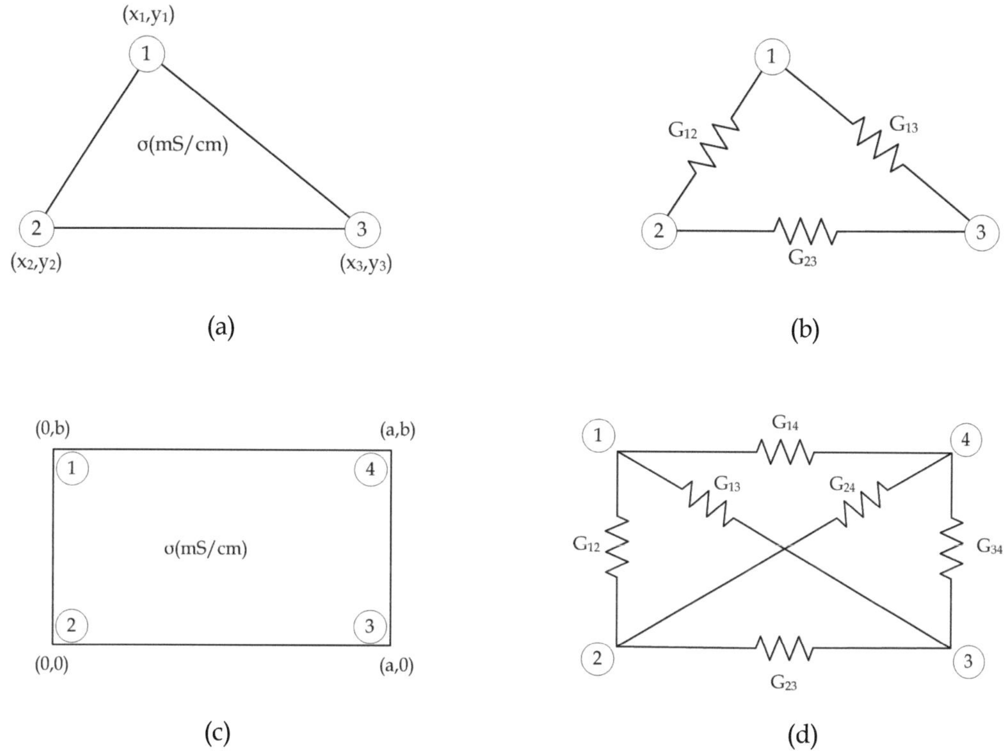


Fig. 10. Equivalent resistor network for each $j_{th}$ element with locally homogenous conductivity $\sigma_j$: (a) Triangular element defined by its coordinates *(x<sub></sub>i,yi)*, (b) equivalent network of (a) (c) Rectangular element of dimensions a×b, (d) equivalent network of (c).

### 4.2 MPM extension to high frequencies

Working on the extension of the algorithm toward complex permittivity imaging, equations (49) and (50) should be modified for complex voltages and complex admittances.

*Analyzing the constituents of MPM algorithm:* Let us clarify equation (49) starting from each term in the numerator sum which runs over all i=1, to M voltage measurement ports. The i-th term corresponds to the i-th port where the difference between measured $(V_{m,i})$ and calculated $(V_{c,i})$ voltages $(V_{m,i} - V_{c,i})$ is normalized by the measured value and this term is multiplied by the sensitivity of the i-th port with respect to the j-th pixel conductivity $\sigma_j$ (being currently updated), namely $\delta V_i / \delta\sigma_j = \vartheta V_i / \vartheta\sigma_j$. As for the denominator sum in (49) it is just a term normalizing the sensitivities to unity. It is exactly the same as saying that that the infinite integral of a probability density function is equal to unity. From a different point of view, each measurement port contribute to the total updating summation by its normalized voltage deviation from the measured value weighted by the port's normalized sensitivity. The same principle can be readily applied to the complex or two variables $(\sigma_j^e, \varepsilon_{rj}^e)$ update (this could be even generalized to multiple variables) scheme, provided that the corresponding sensitivities are available.

*Extending MPM to complex quantities:* Recall that when Laplace equation is solved only for a conductivity distribution the calculated voltage will be real or in-phase with the injected sinusoidal current (source), just as injecting a current in its equivalent network in Fig.10. In contrary, when permittivity is included in the model a $90^{\circ}$ phase shifted (quadrature) component appears in the developed voltage as well. This is in turn equivalent to injecting a sinusoidal current on a complex admittance network (Fig.11) and measuring the complex voltage across any i[th] admittance, which reads:

$$V_i = V_i^{re} + jV_i^{im} = V_i^{re}(\sigma,\varepsilon_r) + jV_i^{im}(\sigma,\varepsilon_r) \tag{51}$$

In view of the above a complex sensitivity $J_{ij} = \partial V_i / \partial \varepsilon_{cj}$ is required in order to establish an algorithm similar to (49). For this purpose a complex derivative can be defined as [33-36]:

$$J_{ij} = \frac{\partial V_i}{\partial(\omega\varepsilon_{cj})} = \frac{\partial V_i}{\partial \sigma_j} + j\frac{\partial V_i}{\partial(\omega\varepsilon_j)} \tag{52}$$

with:

$$j\omega\varepsilon_{cj} = j\omega\varepsilon_j + \sigma_j \text{ or } j\omega\varepsilon_0\varepsilon_{crj} = j\omega\varepsilon_0\varepsilon_{rj} + \sigma \text{ or } \omega\varepsilon_{cj} = \omega\varepsilon_j + j\sigma_j \tag{53}$$

This complex derivative definition has already been employed by many researchers, e.g Franchois et al. [33] and Rekanos et al. [34-36], for the definition of a complex gradient (complex Jacobian matrix) working toward the establishment of a complex permittivity microwave imaging. The definition of (52) is exploited herein in order to identify the complex Jacobian matrix $J_{ij}$ into four real submatrices as presented by Polydorides [37]

$$J_{ij} = \begin{bmatrix} J_{ij}^{RR} & J_{ij}^{RI} \\ J_{ij}^{IR} & J_{ij}^{II} \end{bmatrix} = \begin{bmatrix} \dfrac{\vartheta V^{re}}{\vartheta \sigma_j} & \dfrac{\vartheta V^{re}}{\vartheta(\omega\varepsilon_j)} \\ \dfrac{\vartheta V^{im}}{\vartheta \sigma_j} & \dfrac{\vartheta V^{im}}{\vartheta(\omega\varepsilon_j)} \end{bmatrix} \tag{54}$$

An alternative approach, instead of using a complex derivative is to expand the problem into two real functions $V^{re}(\sigma,\varepsilon_r)$ and $V^{im}(\sigma,\varepsilon_r)$ each one depended on two real unknown variables $(\sigma,\varepsilon_r)$. In turn the basic MPM algorithm (49) can be employed four times for each one of the sensitivities just as those occurring in (54). As explained above this is possible not only for two but even for any arbitrary number of variables. Attention must be paid to the normalized contributing terms (summations) similar to that of (49), since all terms referring to the same variable $(\sigma,\varepsilon_r)$ must be added together after being weighted by an appropriate relaxation factor k. Hence, measurements at each i[th] port along with the solutions of the complex generalized Laplace equation yields complex voltages which are separated into real $(V_i^{re})$ and imaginary parts $(V_i^{im})$. These numerical solutions yield complex voltage distributions at the FEM nodes all over the model of the body to be imaged. Before proceeding to the complex MPM algorithm, the analytical expressions for the evaluation of the above four sensitivities must be extracted.

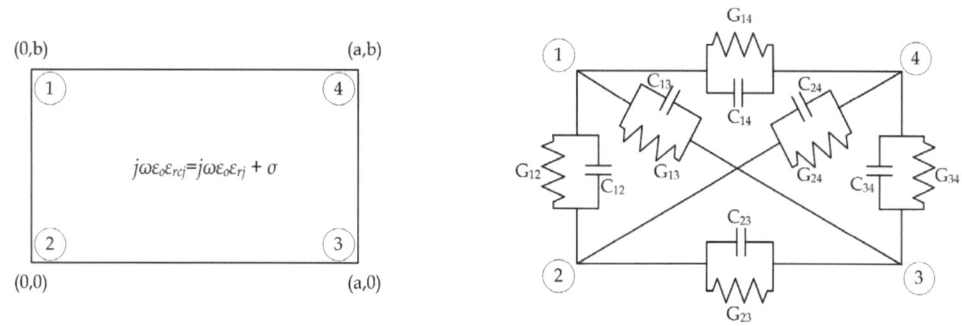


(a) (b)

Fig. 11. Equivalent admittance network for complex permittivity elements, (a) Rectangular and (b) its equivalent networks.

### 4.3 Complex MPM formulation for the MHz range

The complex derivative of equation (52) presents the important decoupling of its real and imaginary parts, thus actually providing separate real and imaginary sensitivities. Specifically its real part constitutes the sensitivity of the measured complex voltage with respect to the conductivity $\sigma_j$. Respectively, the imaginary part comprises the sensitivity with respect to the j[th] element permittivity $\varepsilon_{rj}$. Additionally each one of them can be discriminated into two terms by substituting the complex $V_i$ from (51). Consequently, the complex permittivity imaging is readily provided by applying the basic MPM algorithm (49) for each one of the four sensitivity terms. Specifically, considering the conductivity $\sigma_j$ update we may set-up a summation like that of (49) comprised of the contributions of the real voltage part $V_i^{re}$ weighted by the sensitivities $\vartheta V_i^{re} / \vartheta\sigma_j$. But, now the imaginary part of the voltage $V_i^{im}$ weighted by its sensitivity $\vartheta V_i^{im} / \vartheta\sigma_j$ comprises another sum similar to (49). The real and imaginary voltage contributions are summed together and multiplied by the proper relaxation factor to form the formula for σ-imaging. Likewise, the real and imaginary voltages are weighted with the corresponding sensitivities with respect to permittivity $\vartheta V_i^{re} / \vartheta(\omega\varepsilon_j)$ and $\vartheta V_i^{im} / \vartheta(\omega\varepsilon_j)$ to formulate the ε-imaging algorithm. These two could be given either separately or combined together in a complex $\varepsilon_c$ imaging algorithm as:

$$j\omega(\varepsilon_{cj})^n = \sigma_j^n + j\omega\varepsilon_0\varepsilon_{rj}^n = j\omega\varepsilon_0(\varepsilon_{rcj})^n = \left[\sigma_j^{n-1} + k_1 W_1 \sigma_j^{n-1}\right] + j\omega\varepsilon_0\left[\varepsilon_{rj}^{n-1} + k_2 W_2 \varepsilon_{rj}^{n-1}\right] \quad (55)$$

$$W_1 = \frac{\sum_{i=1}^{M} \frac{V_{mi}^{re} - V_{ci}^{re}}{V_{mi}^{re}} \frac{\vartheta V_i^{re}}{\vartheta\sigma_j}}{\sum_{k=1}^{M} \left|\frac{\vartheta V_k^{re}}{\vartheta\sigma_j}\right|} + \frac{\sum_{i=1}^{M} \frac{V_{mi}^{im} - V_{ci}^{im}}{V_{mi}^{im}} \frac{\vartheta V_i^{im}}{\vartheta\sigma_j}}{\sum_{k=1}^{M} \left|\frac{\vartheta V_k^{im}}{\vartheta\sigma_j}\right|} \quad (56)$$

$$W_2 = \frac{\displaystyle\sum_{i=1}^{M} \frac{V_{mi}^{re} - V_{ci}^{re}}{V_{mi}^{re}} \frac{\vartheta V_i^{re}}{\vartheta(\omega\varepsilon_0\varepsilon_{rj})}}{\displaystyle\sum_{k=1}^{M} \left| \frac{\vartheta V_k^{re}}{\vartheta(\omega\varepsilon_0\varepsilon_{rj})} \right|} + \frac{\displaystyle\sum_{i=1}^{M} \frac{V_{mi}^{im} - V_{ci}^{im}}{V_{mi}^{im}} \frac{\vartheta V_i^{im}}{\vartheta(\omega\varepsilon_0\varepsilon_{rj})}}{\displaystyle\sum_{k=1}^{M} \left| \frac{\vartheta V_k^{im}}{\vartheta(\omega\varepsilon_0\varepsilon_{rj})} \right|} \tag{57}$$

M is the total number of linearly independent measurements, $V_{mi}$ and $V_{ci}$ are the measured and calculated voltage differences at the $i^{th}$ port (electrodes pair) and $k_1, k_2$ are the relaxations factors that may provide faster convergence.

The optimum values of $k_1, k_2$ can be obtained through a numerical investigation. If these are not known then is preferable to set $k_1 = k_2 = 1$ (no relaxation). Even though a relaxation factor could in general speed up convergence, however in all performed numerical experimentation the best performance was obtained without relaxation.

#### 4.4 MPM for microwave imaging

Working toward the extension of MPM algorithm to microwave imaging we simply need to substitute the complex voltage by the complex electric field. Indeed, the expressions of equations (55)-(57) are readily applicable for the 2-D microwave imaging when the electric field is comprised of only one component $\vec{E} = E_z\hat{z}$ or it is a complex scalar function. However, the proposed procedure is general and applies for the arbitrary 3-D imaging where the electric field is a complex vector quantity. Restricting ourselves to the 2-D case we may repeat the definition of the complex derivative just for clarity as:

$$J_{ij} = \frac{\partial E_i}{\partial \varepsilon_{cj}} = \frac{\partial E_i}{\partial \varepsilon_{cj}^{real}} + j\frac{\partial E_i}{\partial \varepsilon_{cj}^{imag}} \tag{58}$$

In turn, by following exactly the same rationale as for the MHz imaging the microwave reconstruction algorithm reads:

$$\varepsilon_{ck}^{n} = \left[\varepsilon_{ck}^{real(n-1)} + k_1 W_1 \varepsilon_{ck}^{real(n-1)}\right] + j\left[\varepsilon_{ck}^{imag(n-1)} + k_2 W_2 \varepsilon_{ck}^{imag(n-1)}\right] \tag{59}$$

$$W_1 = \frac{\displaystyle\sum_{i=1}^{M} \frac{E_{mi}^{real} - E_{ci}^{real}}{E_{mi}^{real}} \frac{\partial E_i^{real}}{\partial \varepsilon_{ck}^{real}}}{\displaystyle\sum_{i=1}^{M} \left| \frac{\partial E_k^{real}}{\partial \varepsilon_{ck}^{real}} \right|} + \frac{\displaystyle\sum_{i=1}^{M} \frac{E_{mi}^{imag} - E_{ci}^{imag}}{E_{mi}^{imag}} \frac{\partial E_i^{imag}}{\partial \varepsilon_{ck}^{real}}}{\displaystyle\sum_{i=1}^{M} \left| \frac{\partial E_k^{imag}}{\partial \varepsilon_{ck}^{real}} \right|} \tag{60a}$$

$$W_2 = \frac{\displaystyle\sum_{i=1}^{M} \frac{E_{mi}^{real} - E_{ci}^{real}}{E_{mi}^{real}} \frac{\partial E_i^{real}}{\partial \varepsilon_{ck}^{imag}}}{\displaystyle\sum_{i=1}^{M} \left| \frac{\partial E_k^{real}}{\partial \varepsilon_{ck}^{imag}} \right|} + \frac{\displaystyle\sum_{i=1}^{M} \frac{E_{mi}^{imag} - E_{ci}^{imag}}{E_{mi}^{imag}} \frac{\partial E_i^{imag}}{\partial \varepsilon_{ck}^{imag}}}{\displaystyle\sum_{i=1}^{M} \left| \frac{\partial E_k^{imag}}{\partial \varepsilon_{ck}^{imag}} \right|} \tag{60b}$$

where M is the total number of linear independent measurements, $E_{mi}$ and $E_{ci}$ are the measured and calculated fields at the $i^{th}$ antenna and $k_{1,2}$ are the relaxations factors that may provide faster convergence. The optimum values of $k_1$, $k_2$ can be obtained through a numerical investigation. Observing the MPM reconstruction equations e.g. (59) to (60) or even the original static MPM in (49) one may discuss on the expected robustness or the immunity of the method to the problem of ill-posedness. As it is well understood the ill posedness is due to very large variations (of the order of $10^6$) of the sensitivity. For example very large sensitivity values $(\partial E_i / \partial \varepsilon_{ck})$ may be observed for the voxels-k around the transmitting antenna and along the axis of transmit-receive antenna pairs. But the sensitivity away from these object regions become very small and may be even lower than the measurement or calculations inaccuracies. When exact inverse problem formulations are employed these large variations in sensitivity yields an ill posed Hessian matrix accompanied by a lot of difficulties during its required inversion. Actually, the very large variation in sensitivity corresponds to very large variation in the Hessian matrix eigenvalues which reflects to a high singularity degree. In contrary, these very low sensitivities occur as very small weighting factors in the summations involved in MPM, e.g. (60). Thus, the very small sensitivity has negligible contribution in the complex permittivity update, which from a different point of view is shadowed by the higher sensitivities. This is equivalent to discarding very small singular values of the Jacobian (or Hessian), or using relatively large regularization parameter. Hence, the resulting reconstruction algorithm is expected to be robust during the first few iterations and it was indeed proved to converge always in our previous works, e.g. [26-30, 38]. The observed monotonous convergence was independent of the electrodes or antenna locations which greatly affects the sensitivity distribution. This is in turn a clear evidence of the MPM immunity against the problem of ill-posedness. Based on these observations MPM ensures convergence without the sophistication of regularization techniques. However, the penalty paid by MPM for its robustness is the absence of any control of the implicitly involved regularization. Instead, an exact method may involve a controllable regularization parameter which is gradually reduced from one iteration to the next. The reduction of the regularization parameter allows for the small eigenvalues or low sensitivities to be exploited.

According to Meaney et al. [39], most regularization methods require the use of a varying degree of a priori information in order to ensure convergence. In contrary MPM ensures convergence without any a priory information, but its accuracy is compromised by its inability to exploit the hidden low sensitivities. Thus, a logical hypothesis toward accuracy improvement is to formulate an exact inverse problem (e.g., a Gauss-Newton scheme) and exploit the final image provided by MPM as an initial guess (a priori information). The regularization parameter within this scheme can be gradually set to zero or to a very small value, uncovering the very low sensitivities (exploiting the very small eigenvalues) which are expected to fine tune the image within a few iterations. The proof of this hypothesis constitutes one of our next tasks.

Observing the above MPM reconstruction expression it is obvious that the Jacobian-sensitivity matrix constitutes the fundamental basis of the proposed method. Its accurate and computationally efficient calculation is of primary importance in ensuring successful imaging. For this purpose the next section elaborates on an Adjoint network for the microwave imaging and its counterpart network compensation theorem for the MHz range, both resulting in closed form expressions for the Jacobian matrix entries.

## 5. Jacobian or sensitivity matrix

As explained in the introductory section the current paths following through the object depend on the unknown $\sigma$ and $\varepsilon_r$ profiles. Also the current density (or field intensity) is very high around the active electrodes (or antennas). These two phenomena make the $\sigma$- and $\varepsilon_r$-imaging a strongly non-linear inverse problem by creating zones with very high and others with very low sensitivity. This severe singularity presents ratios of maximum to minimum singular values $\sigma_{max}/\sigma_{min}$ as high as $10^6$. Mathematically this reflects to a strongly non-linear Jacobian function $J_{ij}(\sigma,\varepsilon_r)$. The present method handles the non-linearity, since it calculates the Jacobian matrix at each n-th iteration, namely for each $(\sigma,\varepsilon_r)$ distribution. The additional computation cost of this task is negligible, since the Jacobian is calculated from closed form expressions from already available voltage or electric field distribution data.

Let us proceed to the presentation of the methodologies resulting the closed form expressions for the Jacobian matrix.

### 5.1 Compensation theorem on an admittance network

The sensitivities of the MHz range imaging can be obtained by extending the resistive network compensation theorem (50) originally given by Yorkey et al. [31] and later on reviewed in detail by Sahalos et al. [32](p 229). This is equivalent to the application of the circuits compensation theorem on an admittance network. For this purpose an equivalent admittance network is considered for each triangular or rectangular element $(\sigma_j,\varepsilon_{rj})$ as shown in Fig.11. The admittance values are obtained from the non-diagonal entries of the corresponding element matrix as: $[Y]_e = (\sigma_j + j\omega\varepsilon_j)[K]_e$ where as defined $[S_\ell]_e =$ non-diagonal entries of $[K]_e$.

For a triangular element (Fig.11a-b)

$$[Y]_3 = \begin{bmatrix} Y_{11} & -Y_{12} & -Y_{13} \\ & Y_{22} & -Y_{23} \\ symmetric & & Y_{33} \end{bmatrix} = (\sigma_j + j\omega\varepsilon_j)\cdot[K]_3 \tag{61}$$

For a rectangular element (Fig.11c-d):

$$[Y]_4 = \begin{bmatrix} Y_{11} & -Y_{12} & -Y_{13} & -Y_{14} \\ & Y_{22} & -Y_{23} & -Y_{24} \\ & & Y_{33} & -Y_{34} \\ symmetric & & & Y_{44} \end{bmatrix} = (\sigma_j + j\omega\varepsilon_j)\cdot[K]_4 \tag{62}$$

Where $[K]_3$ and $[K]_4$ are defined in (50) and $Y_{ij} = G_{ij} + j\omega C_{ij}$

According to the network compensation theorem, a differential change of the $l$-th branch admittance $Y_l$ by $\Delta Y_l$ causes a differential variation $\Delta V_i$ at the $i$-th port voltage as:

$$\Delta V_{i\ell} = -\frac{1}{I_i}\cdot\Delta Y_\ell\cdot V_{ij\ell}\cdot V_{kj\ell} \tag{63}$$

Assuming that the *l*-th branch belongs to the equivalent network of the j-th element, then:

$$\Delta Y_{\ell} \rightarrow \Delta Y_{\ell j} = S_{\ell} \cdot (\Delta\sigma_j + j\omega\Delta\varepsilon_j) \tag{64}$$

Since the voltage is linearly dependent on the network admittances then the superposition principle can be applied in two-fold. Summing over all element branches (Fig.11) one may obtain the total variation of the i-th port voltage $\Delta V_i$. Additionally, in order to evaluate the four Jacobian submatrices, the above approach can be applied once when only the conductivity of the jth element is varied $(\Delta Y_{\ell j} = S_{\ell} \cdot \Delta\sigma_j)$ and again when only the permittivity is varied ($\Delta Y_{\ell j} = S_{\ell} \cdot j\omega\Delta\varepsilon_j$). Applying (62) for each case and separating into real and imaginary parts one may end up to the desired Jacobian submatrices as:

$$J_{ij}^{RR} = \frac{\vartheta V_i^{re}}{\vartheta \sigma_j} = -\frac{1}{I_i} \sum_{\ell=1}^{L} S_{\ell} \cdot V_{RI} \tag{65a}$$

$$J_{ij}^{IR} = \frac{\vartheta V_i^{im}}{\vartheta \sigma_j} = -\frac{1}{I_i} \sum_{\ell=1}^{L} S_{\ell} \cdot V_{II} \tag{65b}$$

$$J_{ij}^{RI} = \frac{\vartheta V_i^{re}}{\vartheta (\omega\varepsilon_j)} = +\frac{1}{I_i} \sum_{\ell=1}^{L} S_{\ell} \cdot V_{II} \tag{65c}$$

$$J_{ij}^{II} = \frac{\vartheta V_i^{im}}{\vartheta (\omega\varepsilon_j)} = -\frac{1}{I_i} \sum_{\ell=1}^{L} S_{\ell} \cdot V_{RI} \tag{65d}$$

where

$$V_{RI} = V_{ijl}^{re} V_{kjl}^{re} - V_{ijl}^{im} V_{kjl}^{im} \tag{66a}$$

$$V_{II} = V_{ijl}^{re} V_{kjl}^{im} + V_{ijl}^{im} V_{kjl}^{re} \tag{66b}$$

As a point of interest showing the potential of extending this method to microwave imaging, it is proved that the employed Network Compensation Theorem constitutes a particular case of the more general ``Adjoint Network Theorem'', which is in turn a direct consequence of the electromagnetism ``Reciprocity Theorem''.

### 5.2 Sensitivity equation based on Adjoint Network Theorem

Regarding the microwave sensitivity a more general approach is employed based on the electromagnetic field of a particular illuminating antenna combined with an adjoint configuration field (herein that for a different transmitting antenna location) through the Reciprocity Theorem. Explicitly the components of the Jacobian are the partial derivatives (or the sensitivities) of the electric field $\vec{E}_r$ measured at the r-th antenna to the complex permittivity $\varepsilon_c^e$ of the e-th element-pixel, when the s-th antenna is activated. As explained below this is in turn evaluated through closed form expressions resulting from the reciprocity theorem and the employment of an adjoint problem. For this purpose an approach similar to that given by Oldenburg [40] and the original research cited therein is adopted. Namely, the two Maxwell Curl equations are written for the source $\left(\vec{J}_s\right)$ at s-th antenna and the involved fields $\left(\vec{E},\vec{H}\right)$ are differentiated with respect to the e-th complex permittivity. For the adjoint fields $\left(\vec{E}^a,\vec{H}^a\right)$ these two curl equations are written considering a source $\left(\vec{J}_r\right)$ at the r-th antenna (Fig.12). The four curl equations are in turn combined following the reciprocity theorem procedure. Specifically, for a dipole antenna at the s-th location the curl equations reads:

$$\vec{\nabla}\times\vec{E} = -j\omega\mu\vec{H} \tag{67a}$$

$$\vec{\nabla}\times\vec{H} = j\omega\varepsilon_c\vec{E} + \vec{J}_s \tag{67b}$$

Taking the derivatives of (67a) and (67b) with respect to $\varepsilon_{ck}$ defined in Eq. (36):

$$\vec{\nabla}\times\frac{\partial\vec{E}}{\partial\varepsilon_{ck}} = -j\omega\mu\frac{\partial\vec{H}}{\partial\varepsilon_{ck}} \tag{68a}$$

$$\vec{\nabla}\times\frac{\partial\vec{H}}{\partial\varepsilon_{ck}} = j\omega\varepsilon_c\frac{\partial\vec{E}}{\partial\varepsilon_{ck}} + j\omega\psi_k\left(\vec{r}\right)\vec{E} \tag{68b}$$

Consider an auxiliary (adjoint) Maxwell problem with a dipole source $\left(\vec{J}_r\right)$ located at the observation point $\vec{r} = \vec{r}_r$ as shown in Fig.12.

$$\vec{\nabla}\times\vec{E}^a = -j\omega\mu\vec{H}^a \tag{69a}$$

$$\vec{\nabla}\times\vec{H}^a = j\omega\varepsilon_c\vec{E}^a + \vec{J}_r \tag{69b}$$

For the application of the Reciprocity theorem procedure to (68a), (68b) and (69a), (69b) according to Balanis [24](p. 324), lets take the inner product of $\vec{H}^a\cdot$ (68a) and $\frac{\partial\vec{E}}{\partial\varepsilon_{ck}}\cdot$ (69b) and subtract:

$$\vec{H}^a\cdot\vec{\nabla}\times\frac{\partial\vec{E}}{\partial\varepsilon_{ck}} - \frac{\partial\vec{E}}{\partial\varepsilon_{ck}}\cdot\vec{\nabla}\times\vec{H}^a = -j\omega\mu\vec{H}^a\cdot\frac{\partial\vec{H}}{\partial\varepsilon_{ck}} - j\omega\varepsilon_c\frac{\partial\vec{E}}{\partial\varepsilon_{ck}}\cdot\vec{E}^a - \frac{\partial\vec{E}}{\partial\varepsilon_{ck}}\cdot\vec{J}_r \tag{70}$$

Making use of the identity:

$$\vec{\nabla}\cdot\left(\vec{A}\times\vec{B}\right) = \vec{B}\cdot\left(\vec{\nabla}\times\vec{A}\right) - \vec{A}\cdot\left(\vec{\nabla}\times\vec{B}\right) \tag{71}$$

For $\vec{B} = \vec{H}^a$ and $\vec{A} = \frac{\partial\vec{E}}{\partial\varepsilon_{ck}}$ the left hand side of (70) can be written as $\vec{\nabla}\cdot\left(\frac{\partial\vec{E}}{\partial\varepsilon_{ck}}\times\vec{H}^a\right)$.

In turn, one may take a volume integral of (70) over a domain enclosed by a sphere with a radius tending to infinity and apply the divergence theorem on the left side.

$$\iiint_V \left(\vec{\nabla}\cdot\vec{F}\right)du = \oiint_S \vec{F}\cdot d\vec{S} \tag{72}$$

to get:

$$\oiint_S \left(\frac{\partial\vec{E}}{\partial\varepsilon_{ck}}\times\vec{H}^a\right)\cdot d\vec{S} = \iiint_V \left(-j\omega\mu\vec{H}^a\cdot\frac{\partial\vec{H}}{\partial\varepsilon_{ck}} - j\omega\varepsilon_c\frac{\partial\vec{E}}{\partial\varepsilon_{ck}}\cdot\vec{E}^a - \frac{\partial\vec{E}}{\partial\varepsilon_{ck}}\cdot\vec{J}_r\right)dV \tag{73}$$

Likewise, dot-multiplying $\vec{E}^a\cdot$(68b) and subtracting $-\left(\partial\vec{H}/\partial\varepsilon_{ck}\right)\cdot$ (69a) yields:

$$\vec{\nabla}\cdot\left(\frac{\partial\vec{H}}{\partial\varepsilon_{ck}}\times\vec{E}^a\right) = \vec{E}^a\cdot\vec{\nabla}\times\frac{\partial\vec{H}}{\partial\varepsilon_{ck}} - \frac{\partial\vec{H}}{\partial\varepsilon_{ck}}\cdot\vec{\nabla}\times\vec{E}^a = j\omega\varepsilon_c\vec{E}^a\cdot\frac{\partial\vec{E}}{\partial\varepsilon_{ck}} + j\omega\psi_k(\vec{r})\vec{E}^a\cdot\vec{E} + j\omega\mu\frac{\partial\vec{H}}{\partial\varepsilon_{ck}}\cdot\vec{H}^a \tag{74}$$

Adding (74) and (70) the similar terms are canceled, then the use of vector identities $\vec{A}\cdot\vec{B}=\vec{B}\cdot\vec{A}$ and $\vec{A}\times\vec{B}=-\vec{B}\times\vec{A}$ results to:

$$\vec{\nabla}\cdot\left(\frac{\partial\vec{H}}{\partial\varepsilon_{ck}}\times\vec{E}^a\right)+\vec{\nabla}\cdot\left(\frac{\partial\vec{E}}{\partial\varepsilon_{ck}}\times\vec{H}^a\right)=\vec{\nabla}\cdot\left(\frac{\partial\vec{E}}{\partial\varepsilon_{ck}}\times\vec{H}^a-\vec{E}^a\times\frac{\partial\vec{H}}{\partial\varepsilon_{ck}}\right)=-\frac{\partial\vec{E}}{\partial\varepsilon_{ck}}\cdot\vec{J}_r+j\omega\psi_k(\vec{r})\vec{E}^a\cdot\vec{E} \tag{75}$$

Taking the volume integral over a domain enclosed within a sphere of an infinite radius and applying the divergence theorem ends up to:

$$\oiint_S \left(\frac{\partial\vec{E}}{\partial\varepsilon_{ck}}\times\vec{H}^a - \vec{E}^a\times\frac{\partial\vec{H}}{\partial\varepsilon_{ck}}\right)d\vec{S} = \iiint_V \left(-\frac{\partial\vec{E}}{\partial\varepsilon_{ck}}\cdot\vec{J}_r + j\omega\psi_k(\vec{r})\vec{E}^a\cdot\vec{E}\right)dV \tag{76}$$

The left hand side is identically zero, since both fields intensities tend to zero at infinity by simply considering artificially small unbounded medium losses. Hence, (76) finally gives the so called sensitivity equation as:

$$\iiint_V \frac{\partial\vec{E}}{\partial\varepsilon_{ck}}\cdot\vec{J}_r dV = \iiint_V j\omega\psi_k(\vec{r})\vec{E}^a\cdot\vec{E}dV \tag{77}$$

The sensitivity equation (77) can be further simplified to yield a closed form for the Jacobian matrix entries $\left(\partial\vec{E}/\partial\varepsilon_{ck}\right)$ by first introducing the FEM basis functions and by considering the specific receiving- sensing antennas. Starting from the integrals of (77), these are in general over the whole solution domain. But, actually the left hand side is restricted over the current carrying volume ($V_r$) of the r-th antenna. In turn, considering the definition (36) for the complex dielectric expansion the right hand side integral of (77) is obviously restricted over the volume ($V_k$) of the k-th element. Further a closer look at the dot product of (77) left hand side reveals that the involved electric field is that produced by a radiating antenna at the $\vec{r}=\vec{r}_s$ position (Fig. 12) illuminating the receiving antenna at $\vec{r}=\vec{r}_r$ position (sensing port) with only the field component parallel to its current $\vec{J}_r$ producing a net effect. Hence, the derivative $\left(\partial\vec{E}/\partial\varepsilon_{ck}\right)$ can be identified as the sensitivity of the r-th receiving antenna (r-th sensing port) with respect to the k-th element complex permittivity $(\varepsilon_{ck})$ when the s-th antenna illuminates the structure, or specifically the (*s, r, k*) entry of the Jacobian matrix, $J_{s,r,k} = \left(\partial \vec{E} / \partial \varepsilon_{ck}\right)$.

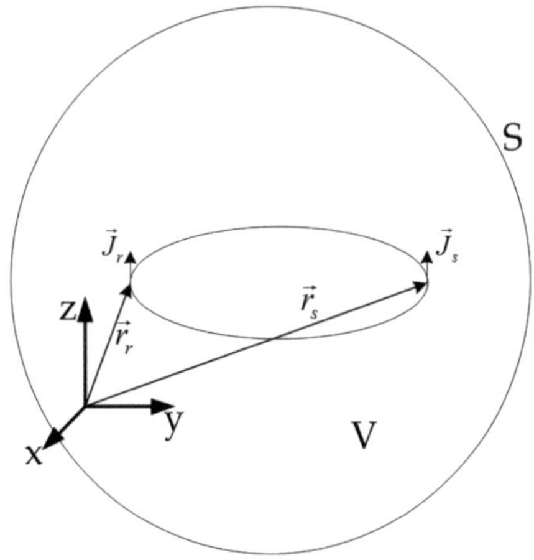


Fig. 12. Geometry for the application of the reciprocity theorem

Since the integration is restricted over the k-th element volume *($V_k$)*, then the fields $\vec{E}$ and $\vec{E}^a$ can be expanded into the FEM basis (shape) functions according to (45). In view of the above description (77) can be rewritten in the form:

$$\iiint_{V_k} \frac{\partial \vec{E}}{\partial \varepsilon_{ck}} \cdot \vec{J}_r dV_r = j\omega \iiint_{V_k} \vec{E}^a \cdot \vec{E} dV_k = j\omega \iiint_{V_k} \sum_i E_i^k \cdot N_i^k \sum_j E_j^{ak} \cdot N_j^k dV_k \tag{78}$$

Working toward a closed form expression for the Jacobian matrix, the next step is to consider specific antenna types. For the two-dimensional (2-D) case when the complex permittivity is assumed homogeneous in the z-direction, along which the structure is assumed infinite, it is convenient to employ infinitely extending thin line sources as illuminating antennas with current density defined by:

Line source: $\vec{J}_r = I\delta(\vec{r} - \vec{r}_r)\hat{z}$ where $I$ is a constant current (79)

In this case the sensitivity entries are readily simplified as:

$$\text{2-D: } J_{((s,r),k)} = \frac{\partial \vec{E}(\vec{r})}{\partial \varepsilon_{ck}} = \frac{j\omega}{I} \oiint_{S_k} \sum_i E_i^k \cdot N_i^k \sum_j E_j^{ak} \cdot N_j^k dS_k \tag{80}$$

For a three dimensional structure (3-D) illuminated by thin elementary dipoles of length *($\Delta l$)* the current density reads:

$$\text{z-oriented elementary dipole: } \vec{J}_r = I\delta\left(\rho - \rho'\right)\hat{z} \tag{81}$$

where $\rho = \sqrt{x^2 + y^2}$. Similarly, the sensitivity equation becomes:

$$\text{3-D: } J_{((s,r),k)} = \frac{\partial \vec{E}(\vec{r})}{\partial \varepsilon_{ck}} = \frac{j\omega}{I\Delta l} \iiint_{V_k} \left( \sum_i E_i^k \cdot N_i^k \right) \cdot \left( \sum_j E_j^{ak} \cdot N_j^k \right) dV_k \tag{82}$$

The above z-oriented current excitations yields a primarily z-polarized electric field which is expected to interact mainly with the $\varepsilon_{zz}$ component of a possibly anisotropic complex permittivity. In general, the orientation of the radiating dipoles could be exploited as an additional degree of freedom to extract information from dielectrically anisotropic structures, e.g. [41, 42].

The above sensitivity expressions can be written in matrix form as:

$$J_{((s,r),k)} = \gamma \left[ E^k \right] \cdot \left[ F^k \right] \cdot \left[ E^{ak} \right] \tag{83}$$

where $\gamma = j\omega / I$ or $j\omega / I\Delta l$ is the constant term for the line source and elementary dipole excitations and

$$\left[ F_{ij}^k \right] = \iiint_{V_k} \left\{ N_i^k \right\} \cdot \left\{ N_j^k \right\} dV_k \tag{84}$$

Matrices (vectors) $[E^k]$, $[E^{ak}]$ represent the tangential electric fields along the edges of the k-th tetrahedral element in three dimensional case or the $E_z$ electric field on the nodes of the k-th triangular element for the two dimensional case. These fields are already computed during the multiple forward problem solutions performed during the setup of the calculated data-set (once for each illuminating antenna). The matrix $\left[ F_{ij}^k \right]$ is a 6 ×6 matrix in 3D or a 3 ×3 matrix in 2D and its entries can be constructed from the FEM element matrices, [15].Recall at this point that FEM is applied on a fine mesh of tetrahedral or triangular elements while the image reconstruction is carried out on a coarse rectangular (pixels) or cubical (voxels) mesh. Each reconstruction element consists of a number of forward elements and similarly a number of nodes or edges that belong to these forward elements. Equation (83) results to a partial Jacobian matrix for each triangular or tetrahedral forward element. However, the desired Jacobian is that of the rectangular-pixel or cubical-voxel reconstruction element. For each evaluation the Fk matrices are assembled together according to a classical FEM procedure to yield a m×m matrix $M^e$, where $e$ the global number of the reconstruction element and m the number of edges or nodes that are inside the e-th element. Note that this matrix depends only on the geometry (independent of $\varepsilon_{rc}$ distribution) and its calculated only once and stored for multiple usage. Consequently, the Jacobian matrix of the e-th element reads:

$$J_{((s,r),e)} = \gamma \left[ E^e \right] \cdot \left[ M^e \right] \cdot \left[ E^{ae} \right] \tag{85}$$

where $\left[ E^e \right] = \left[ E_1^e, E_2^e, ..., E_m^e \right]$ and $\left[ E^{ae} \right] = \left[ E_1^{ae}, E_2^{ae}, ..., E_m^{ae} \right]$.

### 5.3 Sensitivities and features of the Jacobian matrix

The Jacobian matrix is a rectangular one with dimensions M>N where M the number of linearly independent measuring points and N the number of unknown $(\sigma_i, \varepsilon_{ri})$ pairs. The study of tis characteristics is quite important especially in the course toward inventing the best data collection strategy, i.e. active and sensing antenna or electrode pairs locations and their subsequent activation. Additionally, the sensitivity matrix study with the aid of the recently revisited Proper Orthogonal Decomposition [43] techniques constitutes an interesting research challenge. Even though our group is already working on this subject it will not be considered herein as it requires a separate chapter of its own. For some preliminary results regarding the SVD analysis of the Jacobian matrix please contact our previous work [30] and wait for al follow up publication.

## 6. Numerical results & discussions

The proposed algorithm was applied for the imaging of numerous conductivity and permittivity distributions for both circular and rectangular models and satisfactory reconstructions are obtained. The background and anomaly conductivity and permittivity values resemble these of typical human tissues.

Before proceeding to the presentation of reconstructed images the convergence criteria should be first defined.

### 6.1 Inverse problem convergence criteria

*Computer Test Approach:* The so called "computer test" was employed in all cases throughout this chapter. First a "target model" is considered and the forward problem is solved for each illumination position. Namely, the first antenna is activated and the forward problem is solved to calculate and store the electric field at all the remaining-receiving antennas. Each one antenna is activated in turn and the received electric fields are stored to form a complete dataset labeled as "measurements". The reconstruction algorithm starts from a homogeneous model and the desired complex permittivity profile is sought.

*Convergence Criteria:* Two convergence criteria are adopted. The more general concerns the "available information", which is determined by the difference between fields "measured" on the target model ($E_m$ or $V_m$) and fields calculated at the n-th iterative solution of the forward problem. As in every minimization approach, the sum of squares (SSQ) is the appropriate figure taking signs in to account. Hence the summation over all measurements ports (M) gives:

$$SSQ = \sum_{i=1}^{M} \left( V_{meas_i} - V_{calc_i} \right)^2 \tag{86}$$

or

$$SSQ = \sum_{i=1}^{M} \left( E_{meas_i} - E_{calc_i} \right)^2 \tag{87}$$

For comparison purposes it is more convenient to present its normalized value *($SSQ_N$)* with respect to its maximum *($SSQ_{max}$)* occurring at the first iteration of the inverse problem as:

$$SSQ_N = \frac{SSQ}{SSQ_{\max}} \tag{88}$$

While SSQ is general and can be calculated in all cases, it is only an indirect indication of convergence. Namely, its minimization ensure $\varepsilon_c$ convergence when a unique solution is safeguarded. But, this condition may be disturbed by the problem singularity degree, which in turn depends on the data collection strategy. For this purpose the well- posedeness or the singularity degree, of the sensitivity-Jacobian matrix should be preliminary examined. However a further elaboration is required. Besides this for the particular case of the "computer test" the target or true *($\sigma$,$\varepsilon_r$)* distributions are available. Hence, the estimated normalized deviations of $\left(\sigma_{calc}^{n}, \varepsilon_{calc}^{n}\right)$ from their true values at the n-th iteration can be defined as a norm of relative error:

$$\sigma - error = \left( \sum_{i=1}^{P} \left( \sigma_{true}^{i} - \sigma_{calc}^{i} \right)^2 \Big/ \sum_{i=1}^{P} \left( \sigma_{true}^{i} - \bar{\sigma}_{true} \right)^2 \right) \tag{89}$$

$$\varepsilon_r - error = \left( \sum_{i=1}^{P} \left( \varepsilon_{r-true}^{i} - \varepsilon_{r-calc}^{i} \right)^2 \Big/ \sum_{i=1}^{P} \left( \varepsilon_{r-true}^{i} - \bar{\varepsilon}_{r-true} \right)^2 \right) \tag{90}$$

where $\bar{\sigma}_{true}$ and $\bar{\varepsilon}_{r-true}$ are the average values of the target profiles and P is the number of elements of the reconstruction mesh. We should keep in mind that the $\sigma$-error, $\varepsilon_r$-error criteria are not applicable for practical in-vivo or even for the "laboratory test" cases where the objects $(\sigma, \varepsilon_r)$ distributions are unknown.

### 6.2 Quasi-static MHz reconstruction

The algorithm was applied for the circular cross-section of Fig.13a and for the rectangular cross-section of Fig.13b. A total number of 32 electrodes were used, where only two of them are active in each projection angle. An indicative example with a double anomaly is presented herein. The target $\sigma$- and $\varepsilon_r$-profiles are shown in Fig.14a. The values for conductivity are $\sigma_1 = 21mS/cm$ and $\sigma_2 = 14mS/cm$ and for permittivity $\varepsilon_{r1} = 300$ and $\varepsilon_{r2} = 150$, in a homogeneous background of $\sigma_o = 7mS/cm$ and $\varepsilon_{ro} = 100$. The frequency of the injected current was $f = 8MHz$. The relaxation factors $k_1, k_2$ are set equal to unity. The reconstructed image after 15 iterations are shown in Fig.14b

The algorithm was also tested for the rectangular model of Fig.6. An anomaly with conductivity $\sigma_1 = 20mS/cm$ and permittivity $\varepsilon_{r1} = 300$ was introduced in a homogeneous background of $\sigma_o = 7mS/cm$ and $\varepsilon_{ro} = 150$. The frequency of the injected current is now $f = 9MHz$. The relaxation factors are set equal to unity. The target model and the reconstructed image after 15 iterations are shown in Fig. 15.

For details on the algorithm convergence rate and its performance, please wait for a follow up publication which is now in preparation.

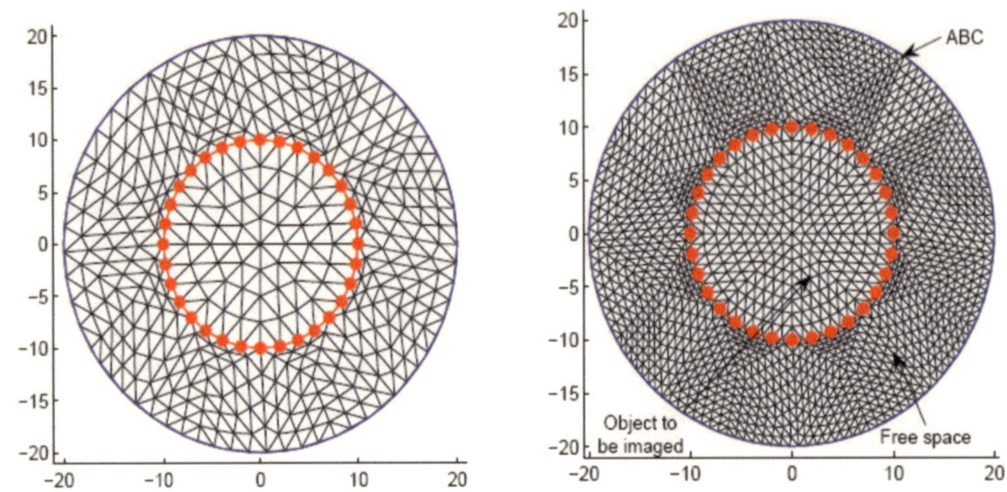


(a) (b)

Fig. 13. The FEM meshes: (a) fine forward mesh and (b) coarse reconstruction mesh.

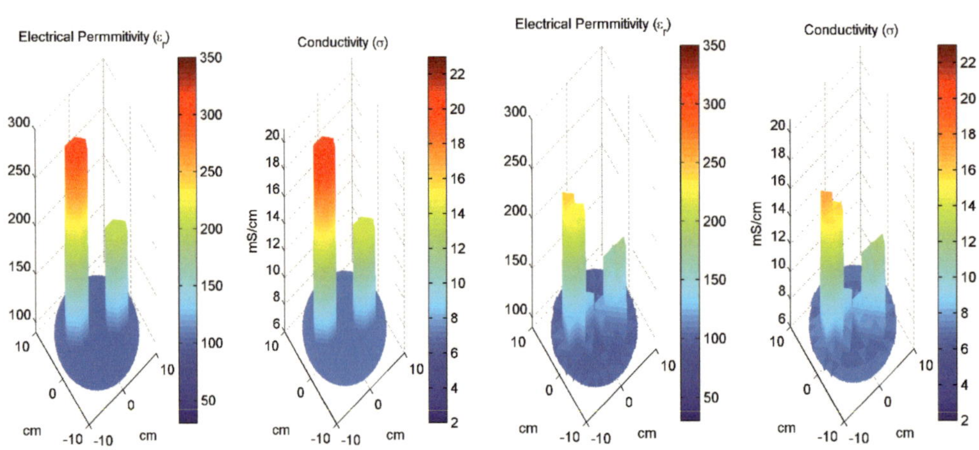


(a) (b)

Fig. 14. Computer phantom with two anomalies in both $\varepsilon_r$ and $\sigma$. (a) The target model and (b) the reconstructed $\sigma$- and $\varepsilon_r$-profiles after 15 iterations.

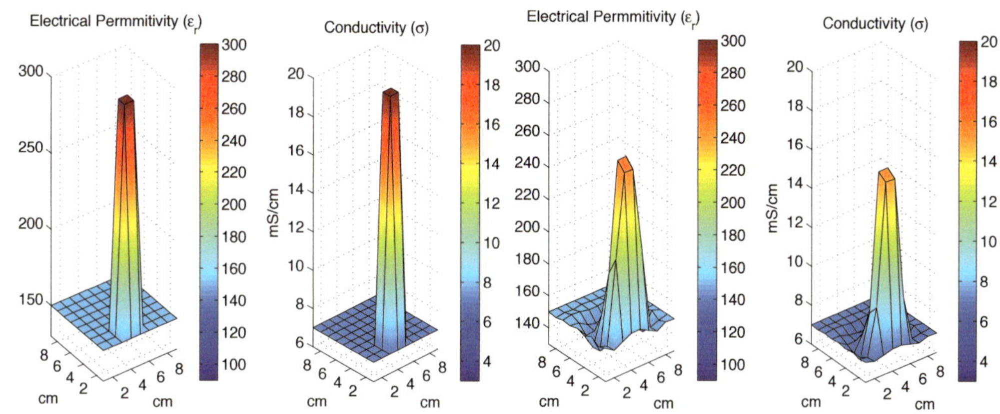


(a) (b)

Fig. 15. (a) The target model and (b) the reconstructed σ and $\varepsilon_r$ -profiles after 15 iterations for the rectangular model.

### 6.3 2-D microwave reconstruction

The target model simulated as a computer phantom is presented in Fig.16. A total number of 32 antennas (line sources) were used, where only 28 are exploited as receivers for each projection angle. A single offset anomaly with conductivity $\sigma_1 = 0.15\ S/m$ and permittivity $\varepsilon_{r1} = 15$ was introduced in a homogeneous background of $\sigma_o = 0.3\ S/m$ and $\varepsilon_{ro} = 30$. The frequency of operation was assumed at $f = 1.1GHz$. The image reconstructed after 9 iterations is presented in Fig.17 for the conductivity and the permittivity profile respectively. The correct location of the anomaly as well as its $\sigma$ and $\varepsilon_r$ peak values are obtained, but some artifacts are caused.

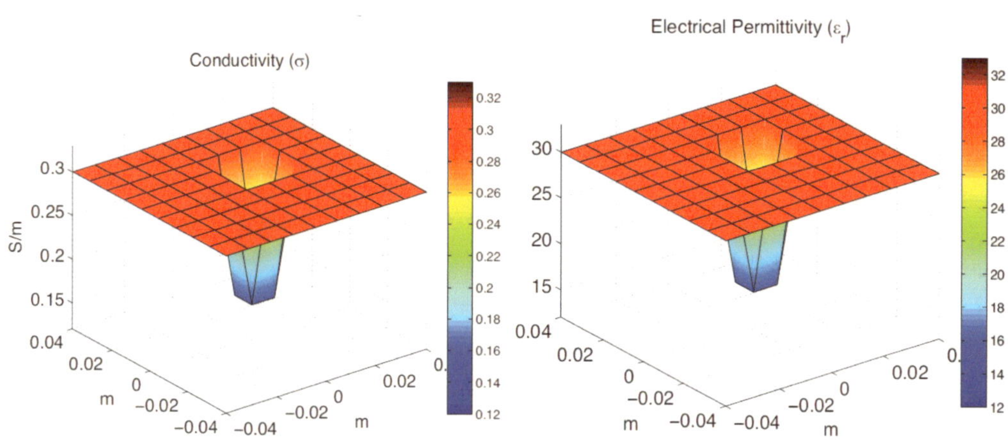


(a) (b)

Fig. 16. Target model (a) conductivity profile, (b) permittivity profile.

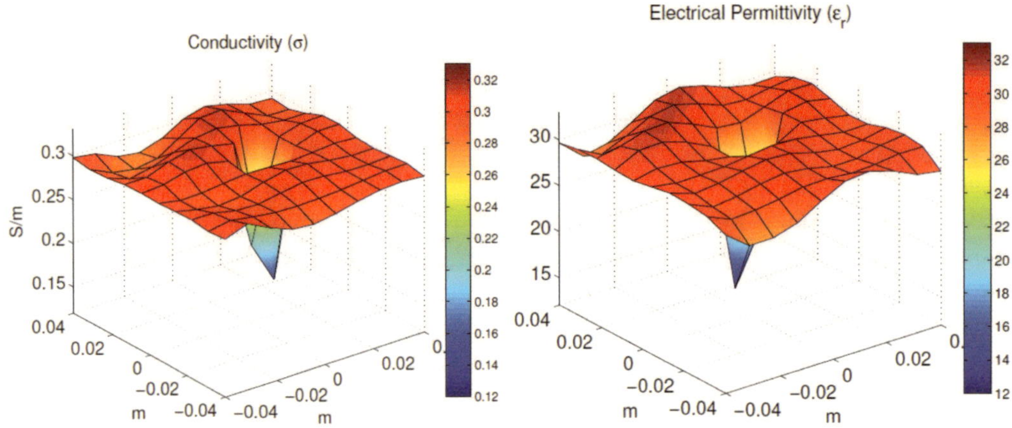


(a) (b)

Fig. 17. Reconstructed profiles for the example of Fig.16, (a) conductivity and (b) permittivity distributions after 9 iterations. The object is discretized into 100 pixels and is illuminated by 32 line sources at a frequency of 1.1 GHz.

### 6.4 3-D microwave reconstruction

The target model comprised of 4 layers as showin in Fig.18. A total number of 48 antennas arranged in three rings of 16 antennas (elementary dipoles) were used, where only 39 are exploited as receivers for each projection angle. A single offset anomaly with conductivity $\sigma_1 = 0,15\ S/m$ and permittivity $\varepsilon_{r1} = 15$ was introduced at $z = -0.5\ cm$ (only at the second layer) in a homogeneous background of $\sigma = 0.6\ S/m$ and $\varepsilon_r = 60$. The frequency of operation was assumed at $f = 1.4GHz$. The image reconstructed after 9 iterations is presented in Fig.19 for the conductivity and the permittivity profiles respectively.

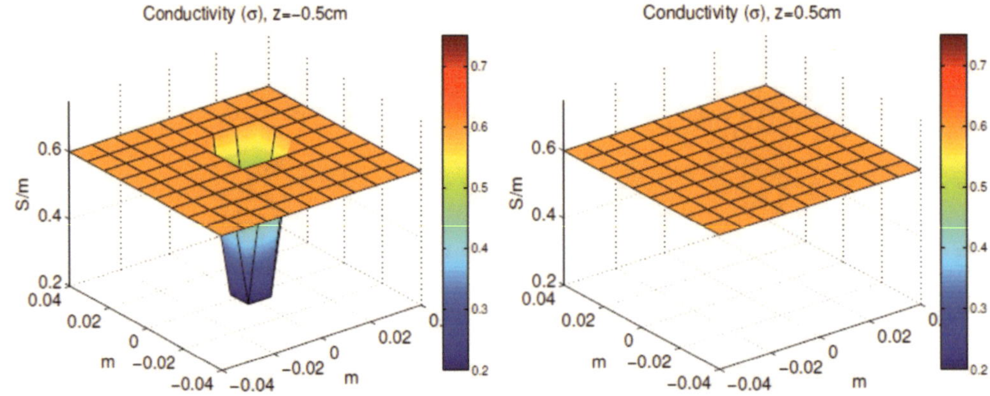


(a) (b)

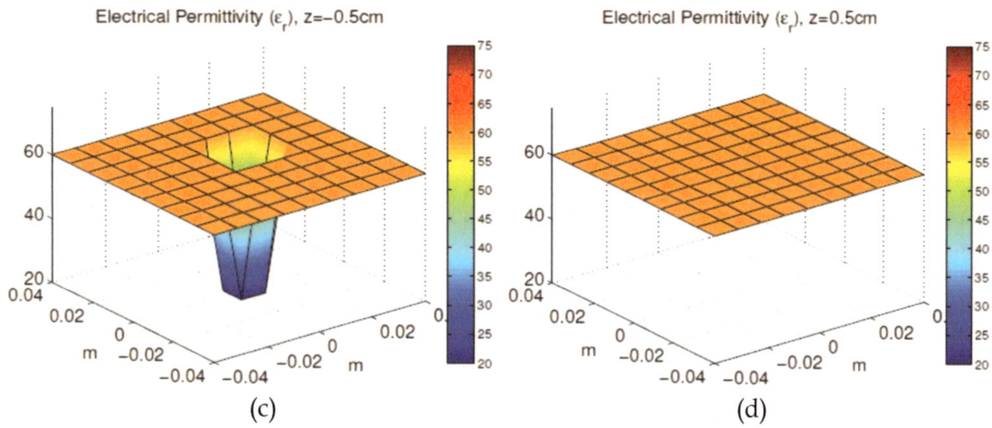


Fig. 18. Target model comprised of 4 layers to test the 3-D microwave imaging.

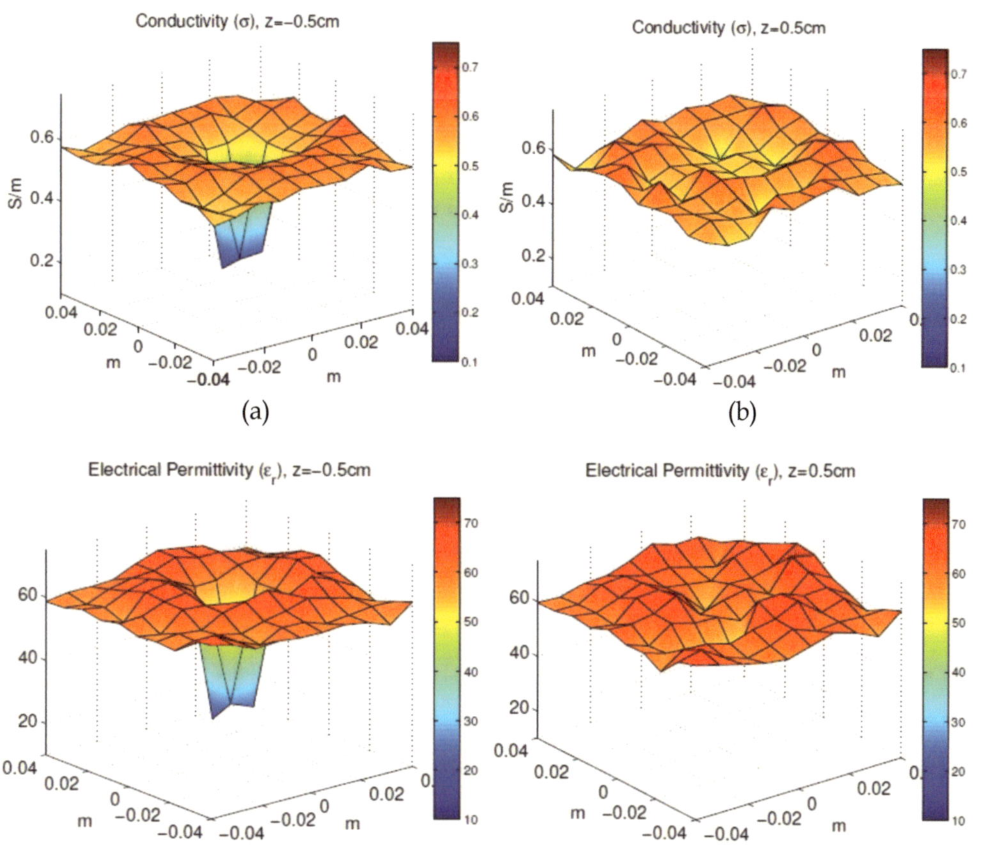


Fig. 19. Reconstructed profiles for the 3-D model of Fig.18 (a) 2nd layer, (b) 3rd layer conductivity, (c) 2nd layer, (d) 3rd layer permittivity distributions, after 9 iterations. The object is discretized into 400 voxels and is illuminated by 48 dipole sources at a frequency of 1.4 GHz.

For details on the 3-D algorithm performance and its convergence characteristics please contact our work [30].

## 7. Conclusions

A modified perturbation method reconstruction algorithm for MHz and microwave tomography is successfully established at a computer test level. The key constituent of this algorithm is a close form evaluation of the sensitivity or Jacobian matrix based on an adjoint network and reciprocity theorem approach. For the MHz frequency range th Jacobian is based on an extension of the electrical networks compensation theorem but it can be obtained as a particular case fo the general Adjoint network approach. The established algorithm is proved robust and able to withstand a large amount of inverse problem ill-posedeness. Despite its simplicity this algorithm is able to successfully localize the target anomalies reaching conductivity and permittivity patterns very close to the expected global minimum at about the 6th iteration. The penalty paid for this simplicity and robustness is a compromise in the finally achieved solution mostly appearing as artefacts around the target anomalies. A further improvement, which also constitutes our next task, refers to the formulation of an exact inverse problem, which may start from the finally obtained image herein and iteratively fine tune it. This can be readily formulated exploiting the exact Jacobian matrix established herein.

## 8. References

[1] G. V. Keller, "Electrical properties of rocks and minerals", *Handbook of Physical Constants (S.P. Clark, ed.),N.Y., Geological Society of America*, pp. 553-770, 1988

[2] R. Pethig, "Dielectric properties of biological materials: Biophysical and medical applications", *IEEE Transactions on Electrical Insulation*, vol. EI, pp. 453-474, Oct.1984

[3] C. Gabriel, S. Gabriel, and E. Corthout, "The dielectric properties of biological tissues: Part I, II and III", *Phys. Med. Biol.*, vol. 41, 1996

[4] Q. Fang, P. M. Meaney, S. D. Geimer, A. V. Streltsov, and K. D. Paulsen, "Microwave image reconstruction from 3-D fields coupled to 2-D parameter estimation", *IEEE Trans. Medical Imaging*, vol. 23, pp. 475-484, 2004

[5] P. M. Meaney, K. D. Paulsen, A. Hartov, and R. K. Crane, "Microwave imaging for tissue assessment: initial evaluation in multi-target tissue-equivalent phantoms", *IEEE Trans. Biomed. Eng.*, vol. 43, pp. 878-890, 1996

[6] S. H. Zainud-Deen, W. M. Hassen, E. E. D. ali, and K. H. Awadalla, "Breast cancer detection using a hybrid finite difference frequency domain and particle swarm optimization techniques", *Progress in Electromagnetics Research B*, vol. 3, pp. 35-46, 2008

[7] J. Goble and D. Isaacson, "Optial current patterns for three-dimensional computed tomography," in *Proc. Int. conf. IEEE Trans. Eng. in medicine & biology soc.*, 1989, pp. 463-464,

[8] W. R. B. Lionheart, J. Kaipio, and C. N. McLeond, "Generalized optimal current patterns and electrical safety in EIT", *IOP publ, Physiological Meas.*, vol. 22, pp. 85-90, 2001

[9] D. C. Barber and A. D. Seagar, "The Sheffiled data collection system", *Clin. Phys. & Physiol. Meas.*, vol. 8, pp. 91-97, 1987

[10] R. E. Collin, *Filed Theory of Guided Waves*, 2nd ed.: IEEE Press, 1991.

[11] A. V. Korzhnenevskii, V. N. Kornienko, M. Y. Kultiasov, Y. S.Kultiasov, and V. A. Cherepenin, "Electrical Impedance Computerized Tomography for Medical Applications", *Instruments for Experimental Tech.*, vol. 40, pp. 415-421, 1997

[12] B. H. Brown, "Tissue impedance methods," in *Imaging with non-ionizing radiations*, Ann. of the NYAS, 1983,
[13] C. S. Lavranos and G. A. Kyriacou, "Eigenvalue analysis of curved waveguides employing an orthogonal curvilinear frequency domain finite difference method", *IEEE Microwave Theory and Techniques,*, vol. 57, pp. 594-611, March 2009, http://ieeexplore.ieee.org/stamp/stamp.jsp?arnumber=04783093
[14] S. Lavdas, C. Lavranos, and G. A. Kyriacou, "A finite difference frequency domain method for the eigenanalysis of anisotropically loaded curved periodic structures," in *32nd Antenna Workshop on Antennas for Space Applications*, ESA/ESTEC, Noordwijk, 2010,
[15] J. Jin, *The finite element method in electromagnetics*: John Wiley & Sons, 1993.
[16] J. L. Volakis, A. Chatterjee, and L. C. Kempel, *Finite Element Method for Electromagnetics*: IEEE Press, 1998.
[17] Y. Zhu and A. C. Cangellaris, *Multigrid Finite Element Methods for Electromagnetic Field Modeling*: IEEE Press, 2006.
[18] L. R. Price, "Electrical Impedance Computed Tomography (ICT): A New CT Imaging Technique", *IEEE Transactions on Nuclear Science,* vol. 26, pp. 2736-2739, 1979
[19] J. D. Jackson, *Classical Electrodynamics*, 3rd ed.: Wiley, 1999.
[20] C. Zekios, P. Allilomes, and G. Kyriacou, "Eigenfunction expansion for the analysis of closed cavities," presented at the Loughborough Antennas and Propag. Conf., 2010, http://ieeexplore.ieee.org/xpls/abs_all.jsp?arnumber=5666915
[21] S. G. Diamantis, A. P. Orfanidis, G. A. Kyriacou, and J. N. Sahalos, "Horn Antennas Analysis Using a Hybrid Mode Matching-Auxiliary Sources Technique " in *Proc. of PIERS* PISA March 2004, pp. 457-460,
[22] P. C. Allilomes and G. A. Kyriacou, "A Nonlinear Finite-Element Leaky-Waveguide Solver", *IEEE Transactions on Microwave Theory and Techniques,* vol. 55, pp. 1496-1510, July 2007, http://ieeexplore.ieee.org/xpls/abs_all.jsp?arnumber=4268422&tag=1
[23] P. Allilomes, "Electromagnetic Simulation of open-radiating structures using the Finite Element method," Ph.D. Thesis, Dept. of El. & Comp. Eng, Democtirus University of Thrace, Xanthi, 2007,
[24] C. A. Balanis, *Advanced Engineering Electromagnetics*: John Wiley & Sons, 1989.
[25] Q. Fang, "Computational methods for microwave medical imaging," Ph.D. Thesis, Dartmouth College Hanover, New Hampshire, 2004,
[26] G. Kyriacou, C. Koukourlis, and J. Sahalos, "A reconstruction algorithm of electrical impedance tomography with optimal configuration of the driven electrodes", *IEEE Trans. Medical Imaging,* vol. 12, pp. 430-438, Sept. 1993
[27] D. Drogoudis, G. Trichopoulos, and G. A. Kyriacou, "A modified pertubation method for three-dimensional time harmonic impedance tomography", *PIERS Online,* vol. 1, pp. 151-155, 2005
[28] D. Drogoudis, "The inverse electromagnetic problem in high frequency tomography," Ph.D. Thesis, Democritus University of Thrace, Dec. 2009 (in Greek), http://thesis.ekt.gr/thesisBookReader/id/18153#page/4/mode/2up
[29] D. Drogoudis, G. A. Kyriacou, and J. N. Sahalos, "A three dimensional microwave tomography exploiting an adjoint network theorem based sensitivity matrix", *IEEE Trans. Magnetics,* vol. 45, pp. 1686-1689, 2009,

http://piers.org/piersonline/pdf/Vol3No8Page1217to1221.pdf
[30] D. G. Drogoudis and G. A. Kyriacou, "Microwave Tomography Employing an Adjoint Network Based Sensistivity Matirx," presented at the Progress in Electromagnetic Research, 2009, http://www.jpier.org/PIER/pier94/13.09060808.pdf
[31] T. J. Yorkey, J. G. Webster, and W. J. Tompkins, "Using the GRID to improve the computation speed of electrical impedance tomography (EIT) reconstruction algorithms", *Transactions on Biomedical Engineering,* vol. 26, pp. S209-S215, 1987a
[32] J. N. Sahalos, G. A. Kyriacou, and C. Koukourlis, "Techniques in Electrical Impedance Tomography (EIT)," ed, 1997.
[33] A.Franchois and A. G. Tijhuis, "A quasi-Newton reconstruction algorithm for a complex microwave imaging scanner environment", *Radio Science,* vol. 38, pp. 8011-8016, 2003
[34] I. T. Rekanos, M. Efraimidon, T. Yioultsis, C. Antonopoulos, T. Tsiboukis, and E. Kriezis, "Antennas, Propagation and EM Theory, ISAPE 2000," in *5th International Symposium on* 2000, pp. 187-190,
[35] I. T. Rekanos, M. Efraimidon, and T. Tsiboukis, "Microwave imaging: Inversion of scattered near-field measurements", *IEEE Trans. Magnetics,* vol. 37, pp. 3294-3297, 2001
[36] I. T. Rekanos and T. Tsiboukis, "A finite element based technique for microwave imaging of two-dimensional objects", *IEEE Transactions on Instrumentation and Measurement,* vol. 49, pp. 234-239, 2000
[37] N. Polydorides, "Image reconstruction algorithms for soft field Tomography," Ph.D. thesis, University of Manchester, 2002,
[38] D. Drogoudis, G. A. Kyriacou, and J. N. Sahalos, "A sensitivity matrix based microwave tomography exploiting an adjoint network theorem", *PIERS Online,* vol. 3, pp. 1217-1221, 2007
[39] P. M. Meaney, K. D. Paulsen, B. W. Progue, and M. I. Miga, "Microwave image reconstruction utilizing log-magnitude and unwrapped phase to improve high-contrast object recovery", *IEEE Trans. Medical Imaging,* vol. 20, pp. 104-116, 2001
[40] D. Oldenburg, "Practical strategies for the solution of large-scale electromagnetic inverse problems", *Radio Science,* vol. 29, pp. 1081-1099, 1994
[41] J. J. Shyu, C. H. Chan, M. W. Hsiung, P. N. Yang, H. W. Chen, and W. C. Kuo, "Diagnosis of articular cartilage damage by polarizations sensitive optical coherence tomography and extracted optical properties", *Progress in Electromagnetics Research,* vol. PIER 91, pp. 365-376, 2009
[42] P. Mauriello and D. Patella, "Resistivity tensor propability tomography", *Progress in Electromagnetics Research B,* vol. 8, 2008
[43] M. Scherg, "Functional imaging and localization of electromagnetic brain activity", *Brain Tomography,* vol. 5, pp. 103-111, 1992

9

# A Mutual Information-Based Image Quality Metric for Medical Imaging Systems

Du-Yih Tsai, Eri Matsuyama and Yongbum Lee
*Niigata University*
*Japan*

## 1. Introduction

Information on physical image quality of medical images is important for imaging system assessment in order to promote and stimulate the development of state-of-the-art imaging systems. In this chapter, we present a method for quantifying overall image quality of digital imaging systems using mutual information (MI) metric. The MI which is a concept from information theory is used as a measure to express the amount of information that an output image contains about an input object. The MI value is considered that it can be used to express combined physical properties of image noise, resolution and contrast of an imaging system. The higher the MI value, the better the image quality. The advantages of using the MI metric are: (1) simplicity of computation, (2) simplicity of experimentation, and (3) combined assessment of image contrast, noise and resolution.

The structure of this chapter is as follows. Section **.2 provides a basic overview of factors that affect medical image quality. Section **.3 describes the mutual information-based evaluation framework utilized in this work. An example of how to calculate MI is also given to provide a deep understanding of applying MI to the evaluation of medical imaging systems. Section **.4 shows a series of computer simulations, followed by investigating the utility and superiority of MI method by evaluating the performance of two imaging-plate detectors. Section **.5 presents the results that were obtained. Section **.6 ends with a discussion and conclusions.

## 2. Background

In medical imaging, image quality is determined by at least five factors: contrast, resolution, noise, artifacts, and distortion. Of these factors, resolution and noise are the most commonly used physical characteristics. As is well known, they are described by the modulation transfer function (MTF) and noise power spectrum (NPS), respectively. The MTF describes the ability of an imaging system to reproduce the frequency information contained in the incident x-ray signal. The NPS describes the frequency content of the noise of an imaging system. However, one of the dilemmas in medical radiography is the extent to which theses characteristics affect image quality. In comparison of two imaging systems, for example, an imaging system may only be superior in one physical characteristic while being inferior to another in the other characteristic. To deal with this issue, the noise equivalent quanta or detective quantum efficiency (DQE), which can be calculated if the MTF, NPS, and the input signal-to-noise ratio of the x-ray beam used to measure the NPS are known, is used as a single parameter to describe the general quality of the system. Measurements of the MTF and NPS are conceptually straightforward but difficult to carry out experimentally and accurately. Moreover, the results of these measurements vary with the methods employed. Therefore, a simple and synthetic method for measuring image quality has been desirable.

In this chapter, we present a simple and straightforward method for synthetically evaluating digital radiographic images using MI. MI originating from information theory has been used as an effective similarity metric in medical image registration tasks and template matching schemes, and used as a feature selection criterion in computer-aided detection (Last et al., 2001; Pluim et al., 2003; Saunders et al., 2003; Tourassi et al., 2007). From the diversity of modalities (for example, computed tomography, magnetic resonance, and positron-emission tomography) and objects (the imaged anatomy) found in the literature, it is clear that MI has become a generally applicable measure. Here, the difference between the MI employed in image fusion and that employed in the present work needs to be clarified. In image fusion, MI is a similarity measure and usually serves as a criterion of alignment between two images. MI reaches its maximum value when two images are well aligned. In contrast, in the current work, MI is a physical measure of image quality and serves as a metric of overall physical quality of the imaging system being investigated. MI reaches its maximum value when the detected image (output of the transmission channel) completely corresponds to the image object (input of the transmitted channel).

Several studies have been published on the relation between MI and image quality. Using two Lucite step-wedges as phantoms to study the relations between MI and image noise as well as image blurring was made (Tsai et al., 2008) . However, the study did not examine the effect of image contrast on MI. Moreover, it did not make a comparison of MI with the MTF, NPS, and DQE. Investigating the combined effect of noise and resolution degradation on MI value by employing two imaging plates used for computed radiography was also conducted (Matsuyama et al., 2008). These pervious studies concluded that MI has close correlation with both image noise and image blurring. However, the study has not taken into account the effect of image contrast on MI. Furthermore, it did not make a direct comparison of MI with other image quality metric such as DQE.

The current study includes the following contents: (1) investigating individual and combined effects of contrast, noise and blur on images obtained from medical imaging systems; (2) conducting various simulation studies with a parametric model to verify the relationship of MI among the three major physical factors affecting image quality in medical imaging systems; and (3) comparing the evaluation results obtained using the MI metric to that using the DQE metric. In addition, two imaging plates for computed radiography were used for verification of the potential usefulness of the MI metric. The verification was made by showing clinical images with discussion.

## 3. Mutual information-based evaluation framework

MI is briefly described as follows.

Given events $S_1, \ldots.. S_n$ occurring with probabilities $p(S_1), \ldots\ldots p(S_n)$, then the average uncertainty associated with each event is defined by the Shannon entropy as

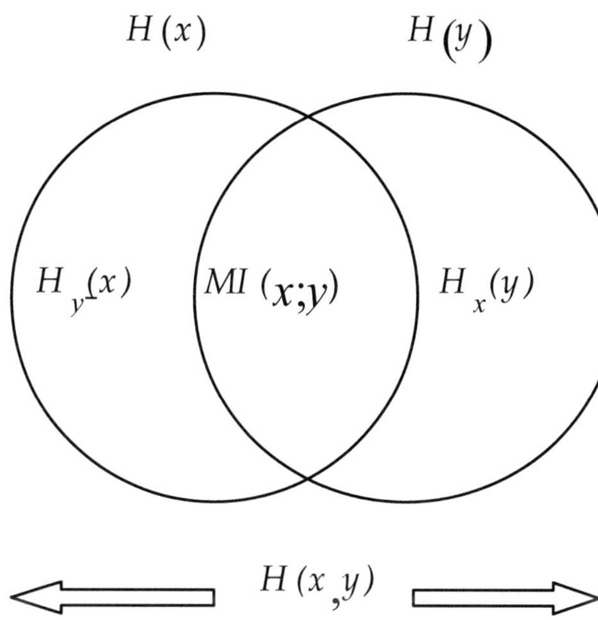


Fig. 1. Relationship among $H(x)$, $H(y)$, $H(x,y)$, $H_x(y)$, $H_y(x)$, and $MI(x;y)$.

$$H(S) = -\sum_{i=1}^{n} p(S_i) \cdot \log_2 p(S_i) \tag{1}$$

Considering $x$ and $y$ as two random variables corresponding to an input variable and an output variable, the entropy for the input and that for the output are denoted as $H(x)$ and $H(y)$, respectively. For this case the joint entropy, $H(x,y)$, is defined as

$$H(x,y) = H(x) + H_x(y) = H(y) + H_y(x) \tag{2}$$

where $H_x(y)$ and $H_y(x)$ are conditional entropies. They are the entropy of the output when the input is known and that of the input when the output is known, respectively. In this situation, we can compute MI, $MI(x;y)$, as:

$$\begin{aligned} MI(x;y) &= H(x) - H_y(x) = H(y) - H_x(y) \\ &= H(x) + H(y) - H(x,y) \end{aligned} \tag{3}$$

A useful way of visualizing the relationship between these entropies is provided by a Venn diagram as shown in Fig.1. Consider an experiment in which every input has a unique output belonging to one of various output categories. In this study, for simplicity, the inputs may be considered to be a set of subjects (e.g., phantoms in simplicity) varying in composition, while the outputs may be their corresponding images varying in optical density or gray level. An orderly system is employed in the present study to calculate the entropies of input, output, and their joint entropies (Attneave, 1959). With this orderly system, the amount of MI is easily computed. The frequency with which each output is made to each input is recorded in Table 1.

| | Input $x$ | | | | | | |
|---|---|---|---|---|---|---|---|
| Output $y$ | $x_1$ | $x_2$ | $\cdots$ | $x_i$ | $\cdots$ | $X$ | Frequency |
| $y_1$ | $n_{11}$ | $n_{21}$ | $\cdots$ | $n_{i1}$ | $\cdots$ | $n_{X1}$ | $n_{j=1}$ |
| $y_2$ | $n_{12}$ | $n_{22}$ | $\cdots$ | $n_{i2}$ | $\cdots$ | $n_{X2}$ | $n_{j=2}$ |
| $y_3$ | $n_{13}$ | $n_{23}$ | $\cdots$ | $n_{i3}$ | $\cdots$ | $n_{X3}$ | $n_{j=3}$ |
| … | … | … | … | … | … | … | … |
| $y_j$ | $n_{1j}$ | $n_{2j}$ | $\cdots$ | $n_{ij}$ | $\cdots$ | $n_{Xj}$ | $n_{j=j}$ |
| … | … | … | … | … | … | … | … |
| $Y$ | $n_{1Y}$ | $n_{2Y}$ | $\cdots$ | $n_{iY}$ | $\cdots$ | $n_{XY}$ | $n_{j=Y}$ |
| Frequency | $n_{i=1}$ | $n_{i=2}$ | $\cdots$ | $n_{i=i}$ | $\cdots$ | $n_{i=X}$ | $n$ |

Table 1. A data matrix of occurrence frequency for Y outputs to X inputs.

The columns and lows of this table represent various inputs and outputs. The various inputs, $x_1$, $x_2$......$x_i$.....$X$, are assumed to take discrete values of input variables $x$. Likewise, the various outputs, $y_1$, $y_2$......$y_j$....$Y$ are discrete values of output variables $y$. The upper-case $X$ and $Y$ stand for the number of input and output categories, respectively. Note that the subscript $i$ refers to any particular but unspecified input, whereas the subscript $j$ refers to any particular but unspecified output. The number of times input $x_i$ is presented will be symbolized by $n_i$, the frequency of output, $y_j$, by $n_j$, and the frequency, with which the input $x_i$ corresponds to the output $y_j$, is given by $n_{ij}$. The total of all frequencies is given by $n$. It is apparent from Table 1 that

$$\sum_j n_{ij} = n_i \tag{4}$$

$$\sum_i n_{ij} = n_j \tag{5}$$

$$\sum_{ij} n_{ij} = \sum_i n_i = \sum_j n_j = n \quad . \tag{6}$$

Referring to the definition of information entropy as shown in Equation (1), three informational quantities, namely, $H(x)$, $H(y)$, and $H(x,y)$, can be calculated from Table 1.

$$H(x) = \sum_i p_i \log_2(1/p_i) \tag{7}$$

$$H(y) = \sum_j p_j \log_2(1/p_j) \tag{8}$$

$$H(x,y) = \sum_{ij} p_{ij} \log_2(1/p_{ij}) \tag{9}$$

where $p_i=n_i/n$, $p_j=n_j/n$, and $p_{ij}=n_{ij}/n$. For simplicity, we can rewrite the above equations as follows:

$$H(x) = \log_2 n - (1/n)\sum_i n_i \log_2 n_i \tag{10}$$

$$H(y) = \log_2 n - (1/n)\sum_j n_j \log_2 n_j \tag{11}$$

$$H(x,y) = \log_2 n - (1/n)\sum_{ij} n_{ij} \log_2 n_{ij} \tag{12}$$

Then, the MI $MI(x;y)$ can be obtained from Equation (3) together with Equations (10), (11), and (12). The MI conveys the amount of information that "$y$" has about "$x$".

Table 2 gives an example of how to calculate MI. Assume that a subject (e.g., a step-wedge) having five steps with different thickness was used for the experiment. The five steps correspond to five inputs present equiprobably. The gray-scale pixel values of 100 pixels in each step after imaging were measured randomly. The distributions of the pixel values are considered as the corresponding outputs and their respective frequencies are given in the table. The frequencies will be referred to by means of the symbols given in Table 1; for example: $n_{12}$=60, $n_{j=3}$=118, $n_{i=2}$=100, $n$=500, and so on. Now, there are three information quantities, namely, $H(x)$, $H(y)$, and $H(x,y)$, that can be calculated directly from Table 2 by using equations (10), (11), and (12).

| | Input x | | | | | |
|---|---|---|---|---|---|---|
| Output y | 1 | 2 | 3 | 4 | 5 | Frequency |
| 1 | 20 | | | | | 20 |
| 2 | 60 | 4 | | | | 64 |
| 3 | 20 | 88 | 10 | | | 118 |
| 4 | | 8 | 76 | 14 | | 98 |
| 5 | | | 12 | 80 | 2 | 94 |
| 6 | | | 2 | 6 | 8 | 16 |
| 7 | | | | | 90 | 90 |
| Frequency | 100 | 100 | 100 | 100 | 100 | 500 |

Table 2. An example of how to calculate the mutual information. The frequencies shown in the table is referred to by means of the symbols given in Table 1, for example, $n_{23}$=88, $n_{j=2}$=64, $n_{i=1}$=100, $n$=500, and so on.

For the data given in Table 2,

$$H(x) = \log_2 n - (1/n)\sum_i n_i \log_2 n = \log_2 5 = 2.323 \quad \text{(since inputs are equiprobable)}$$

$$H(y) = \log_2 500 - (1/500) \times (20\log_2 20 + 64\log_2 64 + 118\log_2 118 \ldots\ldots etc.) = 2.575$$

$$H(x,y) = \log_2 500 - (1/500) \times (20\log_2 20 + 60\log_2 60 + 4\log_2 4 \ldots\ldots etc.) = 3.235$$

Applying Equation (3) to the values calculated above, we have

$$MI(x;y) = H(x) + H(y) - H(x,y) = 2.323 + 2.575 - 3.235 = 1.663\,.$$

This is the estimate of the amount of information transmitted by the subject from input to output: 1.633 bits, out of a possible of 2.323 bits.

If the output is identical to the input, then knowing the output provides complete information about the input. In this case, the MI is maximized and equal to the input entropy, and the uncertainty of the input is reduced to 0. It means that knowing (or viewing) the image of an object (subject) receives complete information about the object (subject). Thus the quality of the obtained image reaches to a maximum in terms of the MI. If, on the other hand, the output and the input are independent, then knowing the output does not help make any conclusions about the input. In this case, MI value is zero, and therefore the uncertainty about the input remains unchanged. This means that the obtained image has the lowest quality from the point of view of the MI.

## 4. Materials and methods

### 4.1 Image simulation

Simulation studies were designed, and the framework is as follows. In mathematical terms, a simulated image $g(x,y)$ is the convolution of a uniformly distributed signal (an object) $f(x,y)$ and the blurring function $B$. If the noise $u(x,y)$ is also taken into consideration, the simulated image may be represented by the following formula:

$$g(x,y) = \sum_{k=1}^{5} \{[k \times f(x,y)] * B + u(x,y) \times W\} \qquad (13)$$

where the symbol * represents the convolution operation, and $k$ is an integer representing the number of steps of the simulated image ($k$=1,2, ….5). In the simulation studies, the input signal is a five-step wedge or a five-gray-level grid pattern with a specific intensity or pixel value on each step. The term of $W$ is a weighting coefficient used to adjust the extent of noise, and $u(x,y)$ is a zero-mean Gaussian noise with a standard deviation of 0.5.

An image of a simulated step-wedge generated by using Equation (13) is shown in Fig.2(a). Five regions of interests (ROIs) indicated with rectangles near the boundaries of two adjacent steps were chosen for calculation of MI. The five steps of the image are numbered from the right as step 1, step 2, and so on. The left band without a rectangular box is considered as the background of the image. The corresponding pixel-value distributions measured from the ROIs are given in Fig.2(b). The area of each ROI used in this study was

50×200 pixels. As a result, a total of 10,000 data for each step was obtained. As shown in Fig.2(a), the number of inputs is five, and the number of outputs is the range of gray levels shown on the horizontal axis of the pixel-value distributions [see Fig.2(b)].

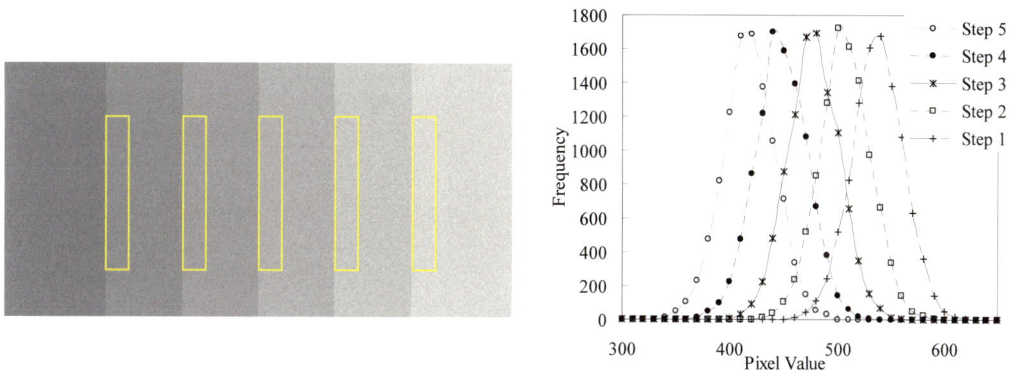


(a) (b)

Fig. 2. (a) Computer-simulated step-wedge. A region of interest (ROI) shown with a rectangle at each step of the step-wedge was chosen for entropy computation. (b) The corresponding pixel-value distributions measured from the ROIs shown in (a).

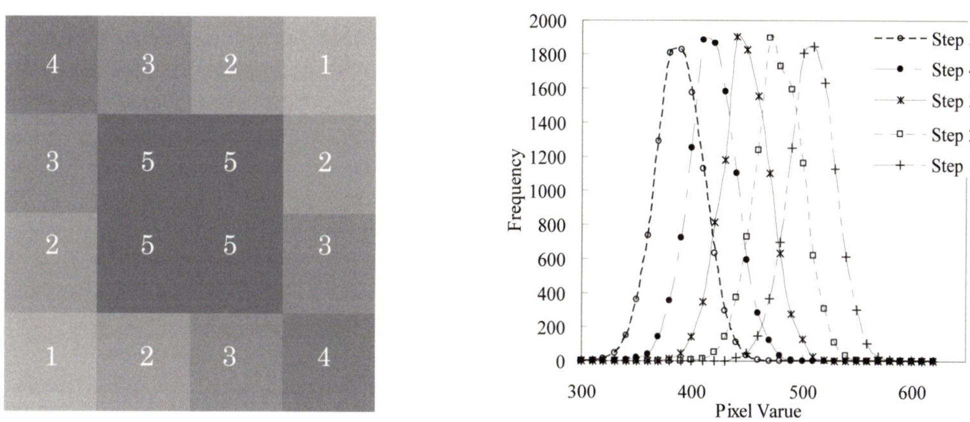


(a) (b)

Fig. 3. (a) Simulated grid-pattern image with five different gray levels. (b) The corresponding pixel-value distributions measured from the ROIs of (a).

Grid-pattern images with various noise levels and different size of blur were also generated using Equation (13) for another simulation study. A simulated grid-pattern image is illustrated in Fig.3(a). Five different gray levels were used to construct the grid-pattern image. The image consists of 16 blocks and is symmetric with respect to the main diagonal. An ROI with a size of 50×50 was selected from the central area of the blocks numbered 2, 3, and 5, while two nonoverlapped ROIs near the central area of the blocks numbered 1 and 4 (at the four corners) were chosen for MI measurement. As a result, a total of 10,000 data for a specific gray level could be obtained. Fig.3(b) illustrates the corresponding pixel-value distributions measured from the ROIs of the simulated image [Fig.3(a)].

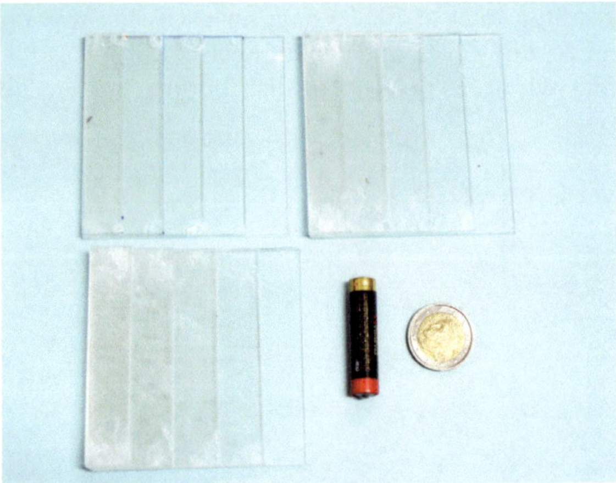

Fig. 4. Photograph of the three step-wedges (phantoms A, B, and C) used in the experiments.

Three different simulations were performed using the simulated step-wedge and grid pattern. The first simulation was carried out to investigate the relationship between image contrast and MI for various noise levels and different extent of blurring. In this study, we defined image contrast as the difference of the mean pixel values between two adjacent steps of a simulated step-wedge [Fig.2(a)] or the difference between two consecutive numbers of gray-level steps [Fig.3(a)]. We employed signal-to-noise ratio (SNR) to describe the extent of noise level. The signal and noise used for SNR calculation were $f(x,y)$ and $u(x,y)\times W$, respectively, as given in Equation (13). As a blurring function, we used a Gaussian filter with a size of $d\times d$ ($d$ is an odd integer). The extent of blurring was adjusted by varying the filter size. The second simulation was performed to investigate the relationship between the image noise and MI for different extent of blurring and various levels of contrast. The third simulation was conducted to investigate the relationship between the blurring and MI for various levels of noise and contrast.

### 4.2 Real images of step wedges

In addition to the simulation studies, phantom studies were also conducted (Matsuyama et al., 2009). Three Lucite step-wedges with 0, 0.5, 1.0, 1.5, 2.0, and 2.5 mm (phantom A); 0, 1, 2, 3, 4, and 5 mm (phantom B); and 0, 1.5, 3.0, 4.5, 6.0, and 7.5 mm (phantom C) in thickness were used as objects for experiments (see Fig.4). Two imaging plates (IPs) for computed radiography (standard resolution type ST and high resolution type HR, Fuji Film Inc., Tokyo, Japan) were used as detectors to record x-ray intensities for performance evaluation. It is known that the intensity of the transmitted x-ray beam is reduced when the thickness of the step-wedge increases. The area of each ROI and the number of data used for calculation of MI were the same as those used in the step-wedge simulation studies.

### 4.3 Detective quantum efficiency measurement

In order to connect MI to the commonly used image quality metric, the DQE that is usually obtained from presampling MTF and NPS was measured. As is well known, the presampling MTF and NPS are used to describe the spatial resolution properties (blur) and noise properties of imaging systems, respectively. The presampling MTF of IPs was measured with an angled-edge method (Samei et al., 1998). The edge is made of a 100-μm-thick sharp-edged-tungsten plate, and its dimension was 10×10 $cm^2$. After the image of the edge was acquired, the digital image data were transferred to a computer for computation. The details of the processing method are given elsewhere (Flymn & Samei, 1999). NPS measurements were made by exposing IPs to a uniform beam of radiation. For the calculation, the central portion of each obtained uniform image was divided into multiple non-overlapping regions, 256×256 in size. A total of 25 regions were used. The details of the methodology are reported elsewhere (Monnin et al., 2007; Samei & Flynn, 2002).

The DQE is a spatial frequency-based measurement of the ability of the imaging device to convert the spatial information contained in the incident x-ray fluence to useful image information (Fetterly & Hangiandreou, 2001; Neitzel et al., 2004; Spahn, 2005). It is defined as

$$DQE = SNR^2{}_{out} \,/\, SNR^2{}_{in} \tag{14}$$

where $SNR_{out}$ and $SNR_{in}$ are the spatial frequency-dependent signal-to-noise ratios of the imaging device at the output and input, respectively. It was calculated using the following formula (Fettery & Schueler, 2006).

$$DQE = MTF^2 \,/\, (q \times NNPS) \tag{15}$$

where $q$ is the x-ray photon fluence density ($mm^{-2}$) used for the uniform exposure image, and *NNPS* is the normalized *NPS*. For a perfect imaging detector, DQE can reach a maximum value of 1.0.

As can be seen from Equation (15), three quantities must be measured to obtain DQE. It is obvious from the equation that DQE value would be high when any of the following situations occurs: (1) high MTF value (high spatial resolution), (2) low NNPS value ( low noise level), and (3) low x-ray photon fluence density. Because the calculation of DQE includes a complicated set of measurements, there is thus a need to provide an easier and less complicated methodology for the use of assessing overall image quality. The present work was just motivated by this need.

## 5. Results

Simulations were performed to investigate individual effects of contrast, noise and blur on MI. Fig.5(a) shows the relationship between the contrast and MI for different levels of SNR, when the filter size (FS) of blurring function was 1×1 (FS=1). On the left is the result obtained from the simulated step-wedges, while on the right is that obtained from the simulated grid patterns. Fig.5(b) illustrates the relationship between the contrast and MI for various levels of blur, when the SNR was fixed at 35 dB.

As a whole, the results show that MI increases with the increase of image contrast at constant levels of noise and blur. It is seen from Fig.5(a) that the MI at low noise levels (high level of SNR) shows remarkable increase as compared to high noise levels (low level of SNR). For example, the MI value at SNR of 31 is considerably lower than that at SNR of 40.

This means that the MI value is greatly influenced by the noise level. As shown in Fig.5(b), the MI curves of different levels of blur (filter size; FS) are similar in shape. The difference in MI values at low contrast level is not obvious, even if the filter sizes change. However, the difference becomes notable at high contrast levels. The results demonstrate that the effect of blur on MI value is more obvious at higher contrast levels as compared to that at lower contrast levels. It is noted that the results obtained by using the simulated step-wedges and that by the grid patterns have a similar tendency.

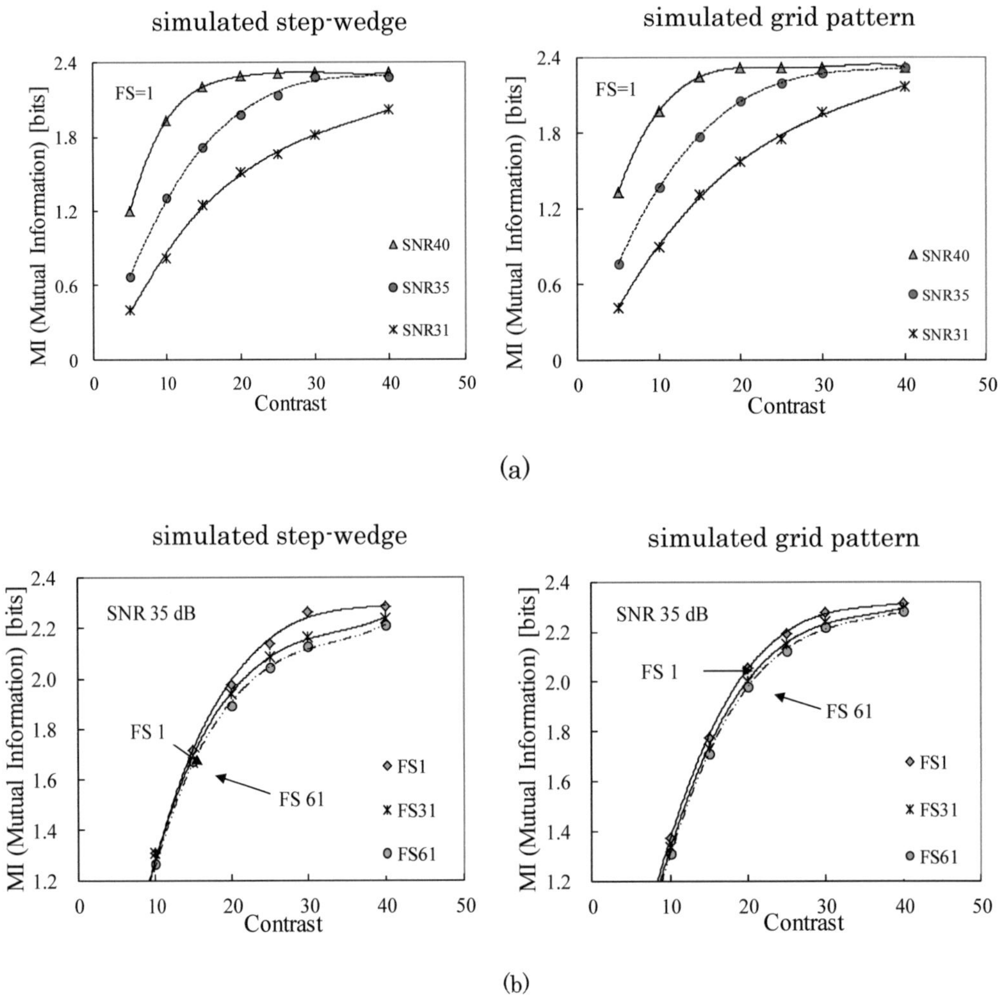


Fig. 5. Relationship between the contrast and MI. Left column: simulated step-wedge. Right column: simulated grid pattern. (a) For various levels of SNR at a size of blurring function FS of 1. (b) For various levels of blur at an SNR of 35dB.

Figs.6(a) and 6(b) illustrate MI as a function of SNR for various levels of blurring at image contrast of 20 and for different contrast levels at FS=1, respectively. The results from the figures indicate that the MI value increases with the increase of SNR (decrease in noise level). The figures on the left were the results from the simulated step-wedges, while those on the right were from the simulated grid patterns. It is seen from Fig.6(a) that the difference in MI values among various filter sizes at low SNR levels (high noise levels) is not significant. Similar results were obtained at high SNR levels (low noise levels). MI reaches to its maximum when SNR is higher than 45 dB. This implies that MI could be almost the same value when noise level is lower than a certain level. As illustrated in Fig.6(b), the MI curves for different contrast levels are in similar shape. MI reaches to the maximum when SNR is approximately 38 dB at contrast of 30, and similarly, when SNR is 40 dB at contrast of 20. This means that the two images would provide the same image quality in terms of MI metric. It is noted that the results obtained from the simulated step-wedge and those from grid patterns have the same tendency.

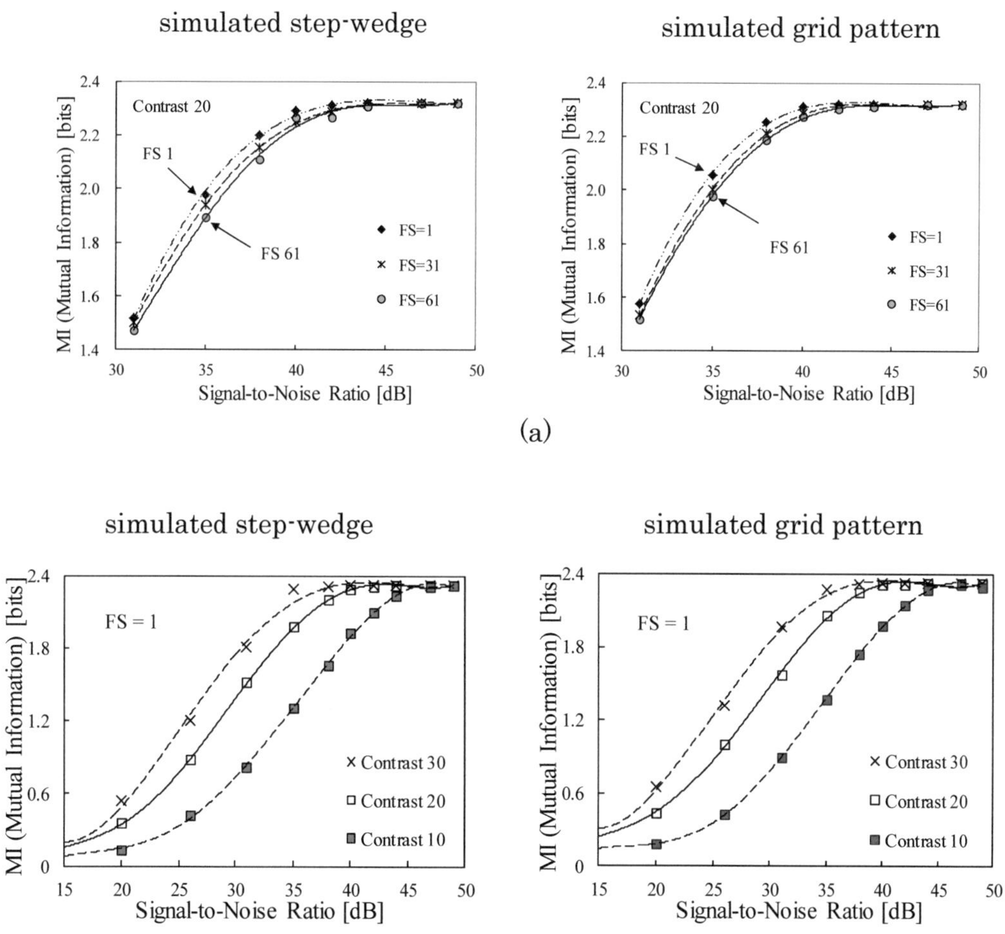


Fig. 6. Relationship between the SNR and the MI. Left column: simulated step-wedge. Right column: simulated grid pattern. (a) For various levels of blur at an image contrast of 20. (b) For various levels of contrast at a size of blurring function (FS) of 1.

Fig.7(a) shows MI as a function of filter size of blurring function for various levels of SNR at image contrast of 20 for the simulated step-wedges (left) and grid patterns (right). Fig.7(b) shows MI as a function of filter size of blurring function for various contrast levels at SNR of 35 dB for the two various simulated images. The results from the figures show that MI value decreases when filter size of the blurring function increases, although the decrease is relatively small. This means that the effect of the level of blur on the MI is not so obvious in comparison to noise and contrast. Fig.8 illustrates images of the simulated step-wedges and grid patterns with different sizes of blurring (FS=7, 21, and 41), while the SNR and image contrast were kept constant at 30 and 20, respectively. The images demonstrate that image resolution degrades with the increase of filter size of blurring function. Therefore, MI values decrease with the increase of filter size.

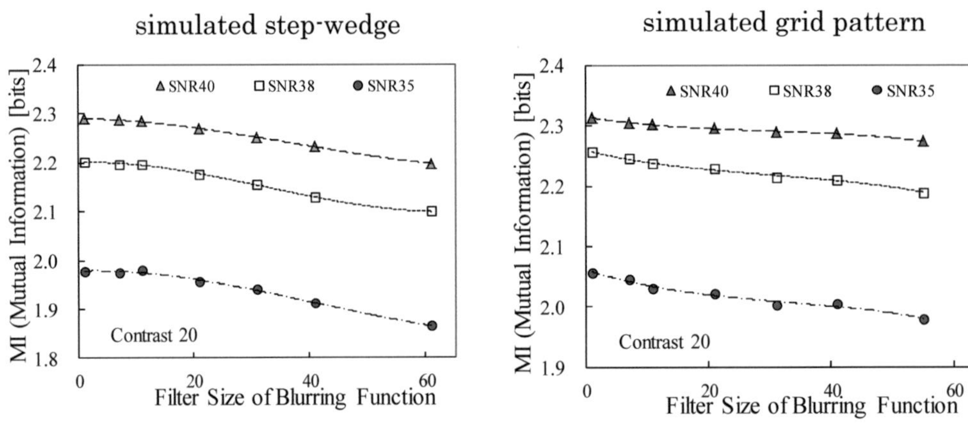


(a)

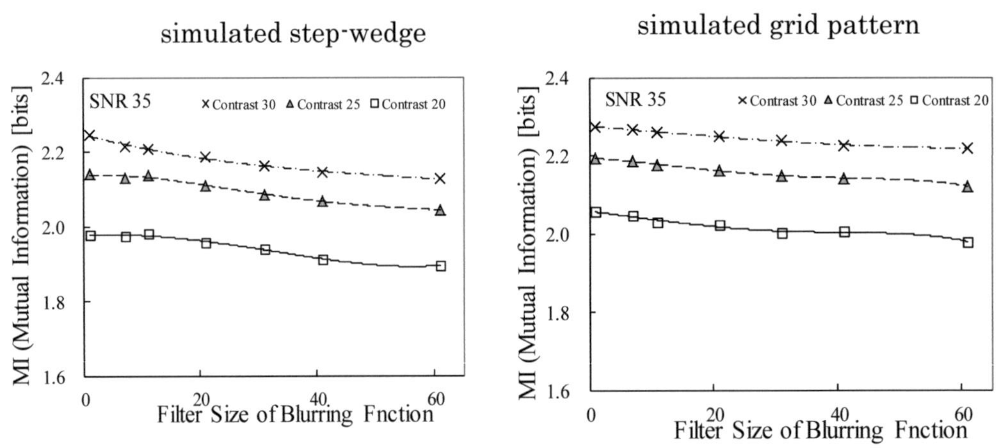


(b)

Fig. 7. Relationship between the filter size of blurring function and the MI. Left column: simulated step-wedge. Right column: simulated grid pattern. (a) For various levels of SNR at an image contrast of 20. (b) For various levels of image contrast at a SNR of 35 dB.

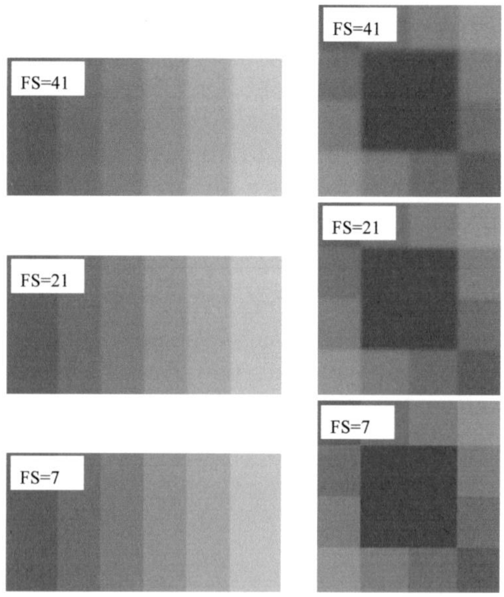


Fig. 8. Images of the simulated step-wedge and grid pattern with different sizes of blurring (FS=7, 21, and 41), while the SNR and image contrast were kept constant at 30 and 20, respectively.

Fig.9 shows MI as a function of exposure dose for the images of a Lucite step-wedge (phantom B) obtained with ST and HR IPs for computed radiography. The results illustrate that MI increases with the increase of exposure dose. The rise of MI value might be mainly due to the decrease of noise, resulting from the increase of radiation dose. The trend of the

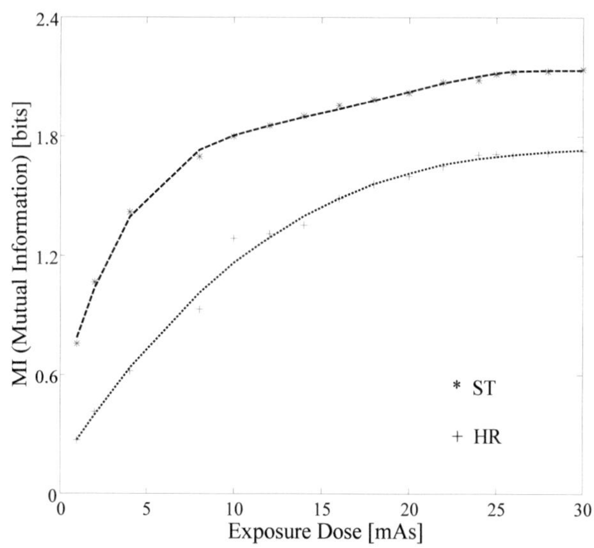


Fig. 9. Mutual information as a function of exposure dose for the images of a Lucite step-wedge (phantom B) obtained with ST and HR imaging plates.

MI curves is similar to that shown in Fig.6(b), although the two figures are plotted with different units: one is the exposure dose, and the other is the SNR. However, it is reasonable to say that the two units are associated with noise levels and are closely correlated. As shown in the figure, the MI value for the ST plate is higher than that for the HR plate at the same exposure dose. This can be explained by the fact that combined effects of blur and noise lead to a higher MI value for the ST plate at a given image contrast. This suggests that the image obtained with the ST plate transmits more information in comparison to that with the HR plate under the same exposure conditions.

Fig.10(a) illustrates the measured presampling MTFs of the two IPs at 42 kV. The result indicates that the HR plate has higher MTF as compared to the ST plate. This is mainly due to the difference in the spatial resolution of the two IPs: HR is a high-resolution plate, while ST is a standard one.

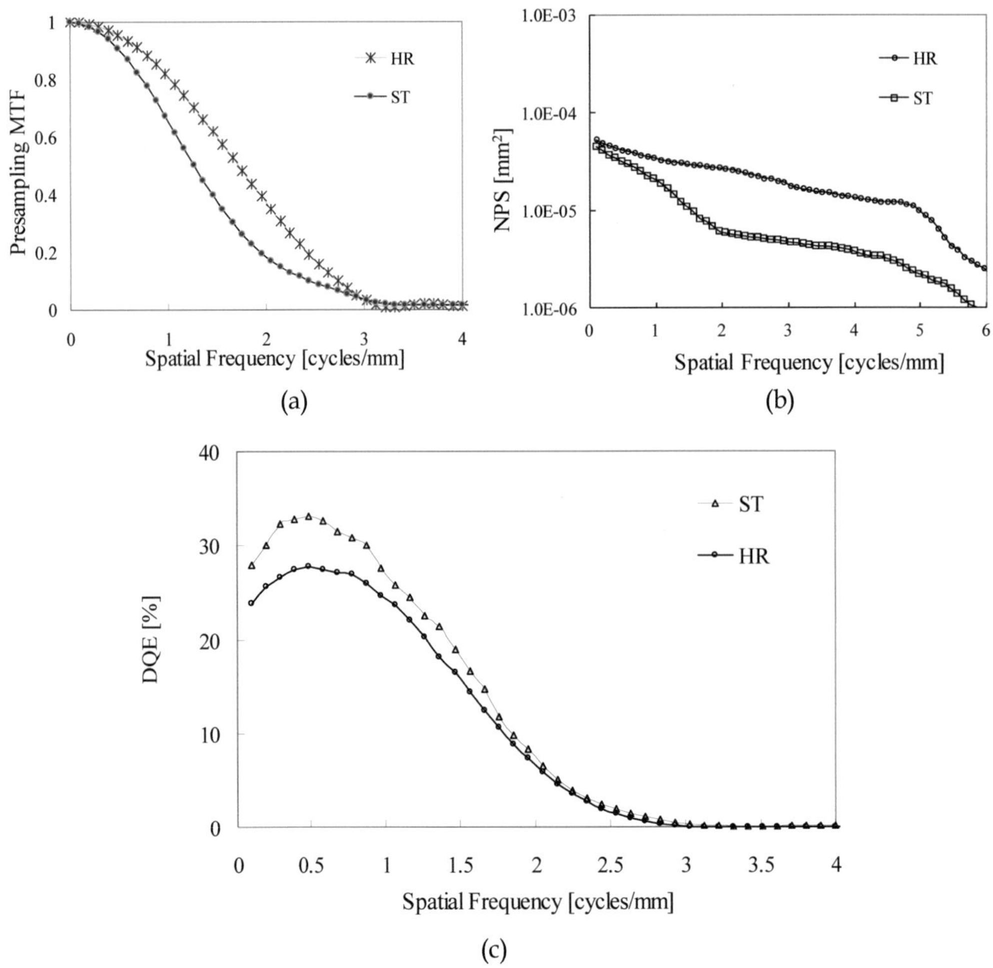


Fig. 10. (a) Experimental results for the presampling MTF measurement with the edge method for the two imaging plates. (b) NPS versus spatial frequency for the two imaging plates. (c) DQE versus spatial frequency at 76-μGy exposure level for the two imaging plates.

In Figs.11 and 12, we display the real images of the femur and metacarpus acquired with ST and HR IPs under the same exposure conditions. In these two figures, the left column illustrates the original images, while on the right are the magnified images of the white squares indicated in the original images. It is clear from the magnified images of Fig.11 that the lesser trochanter (with a white arrow) obtained with HR plate shows better resolution as compared to ST plate. Similarly, the magnified images of Fig.12 (the carpal bone indicated by white arrows) obtained with HR plate shows better resolution as compared to ST plate. The experimental validation provides confirming evidence for the MTF results.

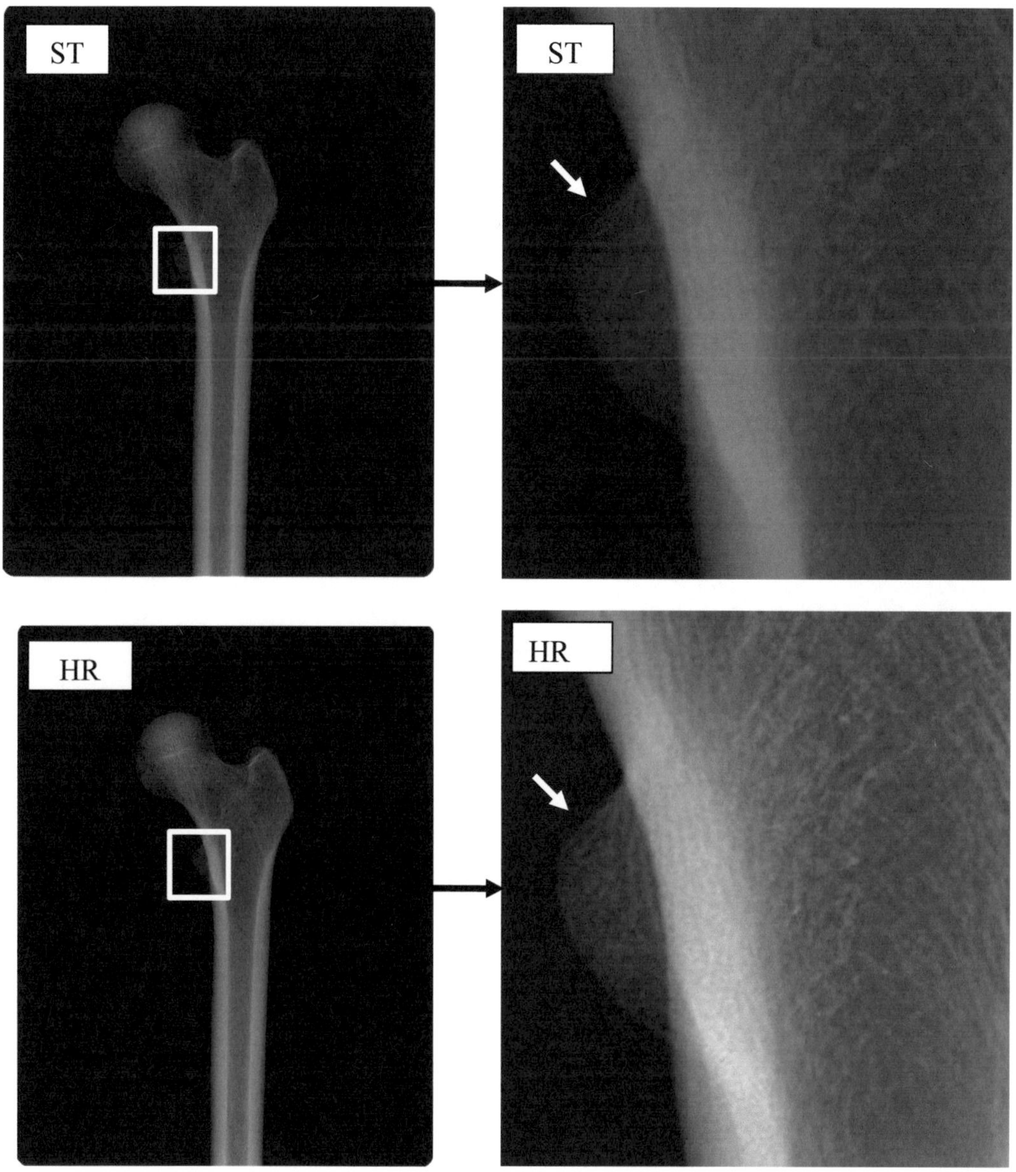


Fig. 11. Clinical images of the femur acquired with ST and HR image plates.

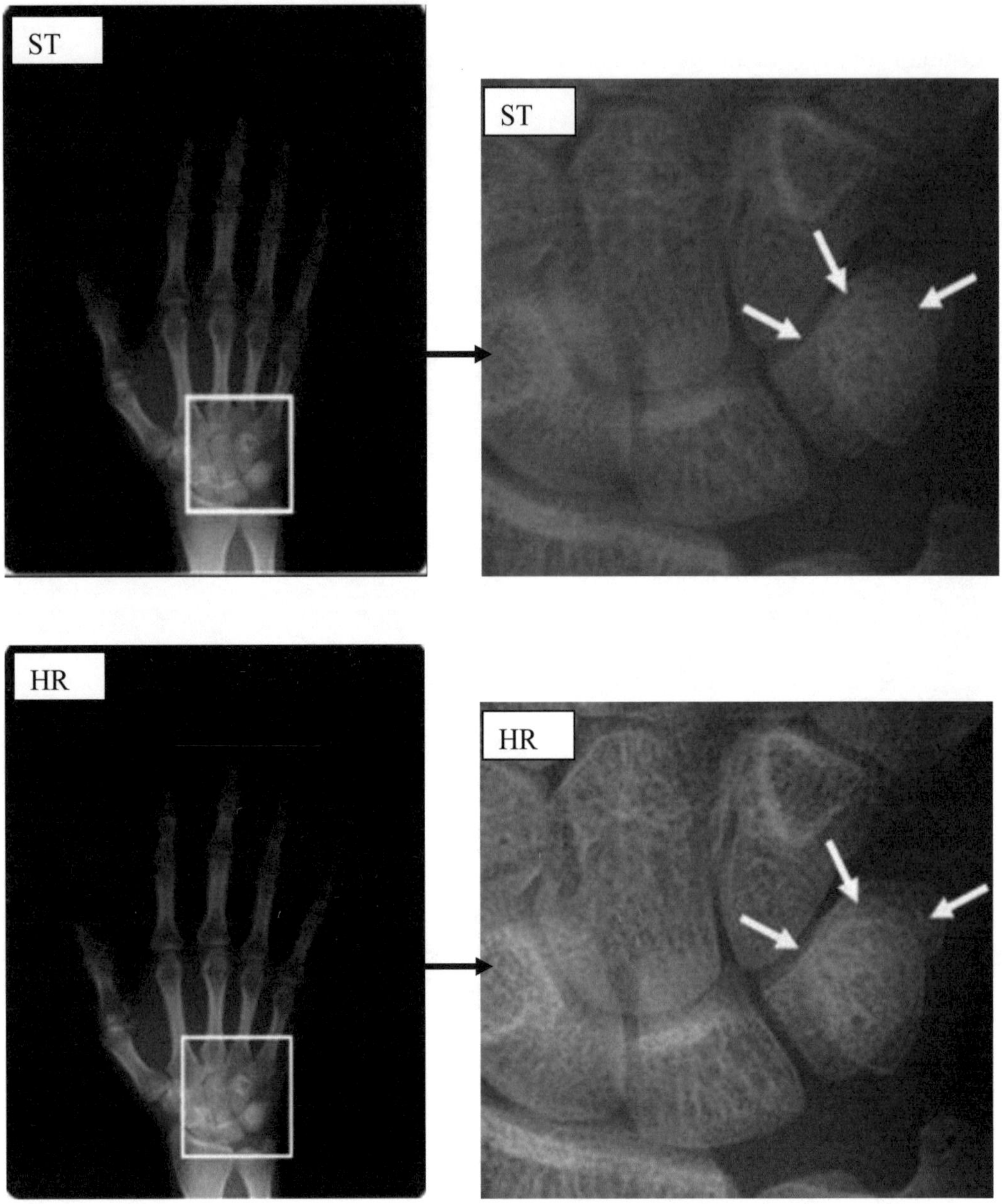


Fig. 12. Clinical images of the metacarpus acquired with ST and HR image plates.

Fig.10(b) illustrates the NPS versus spatial frequency at 42 kV acquired with ST and HR IPs. As shown in the figure, the NPS of the HR IP is higher than that of the ST plate at the same radiation dose. It can be seen from the magnified images of Figs.11 and 12 that the images acquired with HR plates show higher noise levels. The perceptual results correctly reflect the outcome of the NPS shown in Fig.10(b).

The DQEs of ST and HR IPs versus spatial frequency at 76-μGy exposure level are presented in Fig.10(c). In the present study, the DQEs were assessed using Equation (15) — in order words, the results of Fig.10(c) were obtained from the measured results shown in Figs.10(a) and 10(b). It is known that the MTF values are generally independent of exposure levels. Thus the MTF values shown in Fig.10(a) were used for calculating the DQEs of IPs at different exposure doses. In spite of having lower MTFs, the DQEs for the ST plates are higher than those for the HR plates at the same exposure level. The higher value in DQE might be attributed to the better noise performance of ST plates. In other words, as compared to resolution, noise greatly affects overall performance of the imaging systems.

When looking at Fig.9 and Fig.10(c), the performance ranking of MI values for ST and HR IPs and those of DQE values for the two IPs are the same, *i.e.*, the MI value and DQE value for the ST plate are higher than those for the HR plate. The experimental results may confirm that MI and DQE metrics are highly correlated.

## 6. Discussion and conclusions

In our simulation studies, we demonstrated that MI increases with the increase of contrast and decreases with the increase of noise and blur. Therefore, it is considered that MI could be used as a simple metric for evaluation of overall imaging performance. In this study, we applied the MI metrology to evaluate the performance of two IPs for computed radiography. The measured MI shown in Fig.9 is consistent with the DQE shown in Fig.10(c), although they are described in different domains: one is in the spatial domain scalar metric, and the other is in the spatial frequency domain metric. The results suggest the usefulness of the proposed MI metric.

There are several advantages of using the MI metric to evaluate the performance of imaging systems. First, computation of MI is much easier in comparison to that of spatial frequency domain measures such as MTF, NPS and DQE. Second, the experiment setup is simple. For example, a step-wedge or an equivalent test device is sufficient for conducting experiments. Third, three of the most important image quality factors, *i.e.*, contrast, noise, and blur, can be integrated for overall evaluation. However, it should be stated clearly that our proposed MI metric is not intended for replacing the conventionally used metrics. The main objective of the present work is to provide a scalar metrology based on simple image statistics for image quality evaluation.

In conclusion, we have described an information-theoretic method for quantifying overall image quality in terms of MI. We demonstrated by way of image simulation that MI increases with contrast, decreases with noise, and increases with resolution. We investigated the utility of this method by applying it to evaluating the performance of two imaging detectors. We also compared evaluation results in terms of MI against those in terms of the commonly used DQE metric. Our simulation and experimental results demonstrate that the proposed method is simple to implement and has potential usefulness for evaluation of overall image quality.

## 7. Acknowledgment

This work was supported in part by the Ministry of Education, Culture, Sports, Science and Technology of Japan (Tokyo, Japan) through a grant-aid for Scientific Research (23602004).

## 8. References


Attneave, F. (1959). *Applications of Information Theory to Psychology.* Holt, Rinehart and Winston, New York

Fetterly, K.A. & Hangiandreou, N.J. (2001). Effect of x-ray spectra on the DQE of a computed radiography system. *Medical Physics,* Vol.28, pp. (241-249)

Fettery, K.A. & Schueler, B.A. (2006). Performance evaluation of a computed radiography imaging device using a typical front side and novel dual side readout storage phosphors. *Medical Physics.* Vol.33, pp. (290-296)

Flynn, M. & Samei, E. (1999). Experimental comparison of noise and resolution for 2k and 4k storage phosphor radiography systems. *Medical Physics,* Vol.26, pp. (1612-1623)

Last, M.; Kandel, A. & Maimon, O. (2001). Information-theoretic algorithm for feature selection. *Pattern Recognition Letters,* Vol.22, pp. (799-811)

Matsuyama, E.; Tsai, D.Y. & Lee, Y. (2009). Mutual information-based evaluation of image quality with its preliminary application to assessment of medical imaging systems. *Journal of Electronic Imaging,* Vol.18, pp. (033011-1-11)

Matsuyama, E.; Tsai, D.Y.; Lee, Y.; Sekiya, M. & Kojima, K. (2008). Physical characterization of digital radiological images by use of transmitted information metric. *Proceedings of SPIE Medical Imaging,* Vol.6913, pp. (69130V1-8)

Monnin, P.; Gutierrez, D.; Bulling, S.; Guntern, D. & Verdun, F.R. (2007). A comparison of the performance of digital mammography systems. *Medical Physics,* Vol.34, pp. (906-914)

Neitzel, U.; Gunther-Kohfahl, S.; Borasi, E. & Samei, E. (2004). Determination of the detective quantum efficiency of a digital x-ray detector: comparison of three evaluations using a common image data set. *Medical Physics,* Vol.31, pp. (2205-2211)

Pluim, J.P.M.; Maintz, J.M.A. & Viergever, M.A. (2003). Mutual-information-based registration of medical images: A survey. *IEEE Transactions on Medical Imaging,* Vol.22, pp. (986-1004)

Samei, E. & Flynn, M.J. (2002). An experimental comparison of detector performance for computed radiography systems. *Medical Physics,* Vol.29, pp. (447-459)

Samei, E.; Flynn, J. & Reimann, D.A. (1998). A method for measuring the presampled MTF of digital radiographic systems using an edge test device. *Medical Physics,* Vol.25, pp. (102-113)

Saunders, Jr R.S. & Samei, E. (2003). A method for modifying the image quality parameters of digital radiographic images. *Medical Physics,* Vol.30, pp. (3006-3017)

Spahn, M. (2005). Flat detectors and their clinical applications. *European Radiology,* Vol.15, pp(1934-1947)

Tourassi, G.D.; Harrawood, B.; Singh, S. & Lo, J.Y. (2007). Information-theoretic CAD system in mammography: Entropy-based indexing for computational efficiency and robust performance. *Medical Physics,* Vol.34, pp. (3193-3204)

Tsai, D.Y,; Lee, Y. & Matsuyama, E. (2008). Information-entropy measure for evaluation of image. *Journal of Digital Imaging,* Vol.21, pp. (338-347)

# Part 3

# Applications in Clinical Settings

# 10

# Diagnostic Imaging in Oral and Maxillofacial Pathology

Hasan Ayberk Altug[1] and Aydin Ozkan[2]
*[1]Gulhane Military Medical Academy*
*Department of Oral and Maxillofacial Surgery*
*[2]Diyarbakir Military Hospital, Dental Service*
*Turkey*

## 1. Introduction

During the diagnosis of oral and maxillofacial diseases, clinical and radiological data play a major role. In this region, only a good clinical diagnosis along with a radiological examination may lead to a successful diagnosis. A successful diagnosis and evaluation of clinical examination are generally up to a profound knowledge of the normal anatomy of the region.

## 2. Radiographic anatomy of oral and maxillofacial region

X-rays (invisible rays) were discovered by W. Conrad Roentgen in 1895. They are a form of electromagnetic radiation with high energy and are part of electromagnetic spectrum. In order to create X-ray, a target tissue is bombardized with energized electrons and then they are suddenly brought to rest. The entire process takes place in a small evacuated glass envelope which is called X-ray tube (Whaites, 2002).

### 2.1 Periapical radiography

Periapical radiography is a projection of radiographs including interoral radiographs which depict 3-4 teeth and the tissue around them (Whaites, 2002). There are two projection techniques for periapical radiography:

- The paralleling technique (Long-cone technique): The periapical film is stood parallel to the long axis of the teeth and the central is aimed at the right angles of the teeth and the film (Fig. 1A).
- The bisecting-angle technique: The periapical film is stood as close as possible to the palatal/lingual surface of the teeth. The film and the teeth form an angle with its apex at the point where the film is in contact with the teeth. Central ray is directed at apex of the teeth (Fig. 1B) (White & Pharoah, 2004).

In order to create a high-quality radiograph, the central ray beam must pass through root apex or alveolar crest. Radiolucent/radioopaque images which were obtained with periapical radiography may not only depict pathological conditions which require treatment but also normal anatomic variations. Therefore, achieving a good differential diagnosis has an utmost importance. 10 periapical radiographs, 5 of them for the upper jaw and 5 of them for the lower jaw, are applied for kids, whereas 14 periapical radiographs, 7 of them for the upper jaw and 7 for the lower jaw, are applied for the adolescents, performed using the paralleling technique (Fig. 2). It needs to different projection angle to capture third molar. During the creation of periapical radiographs, film holders might be used in order to comply with standardization. However, free-handed positioning may also be preferred (Wood et al. 1997; Pasler, 1993).

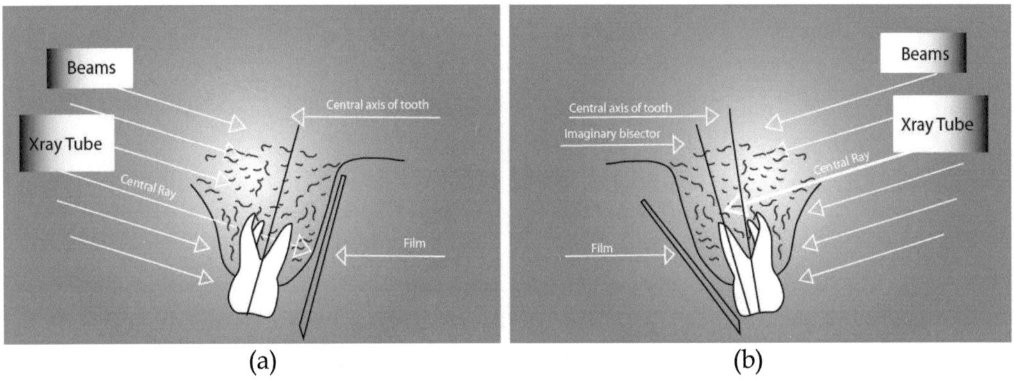


Fig. 1. (a) The paralleling technique; (b) The bisecting-angle technique.

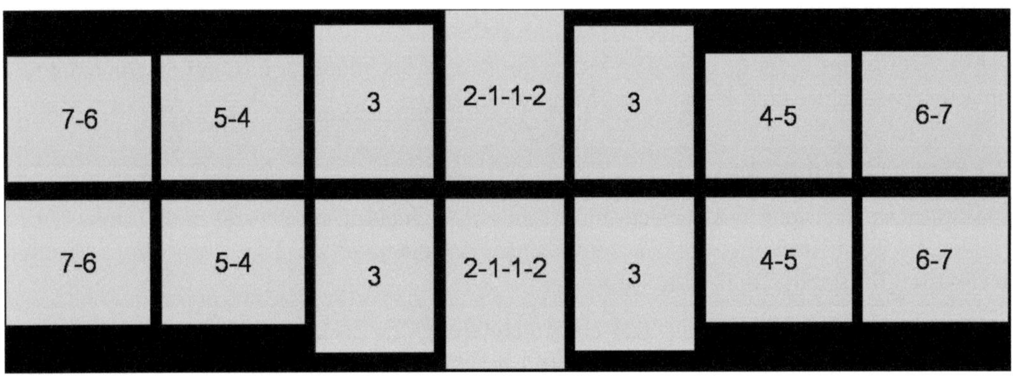


Fig. 2. Periapical radiographic survey for adolescents.

Indications:

- Evaluation of periapical and periodontal tissue health
- Before, during and/or after surgical and endodontic treatments
- Assessment of the teeth and adjacent tissue after trauma
- Evaluation of apical pathology within the alveolar bone
- To clarify of the presence/absence of unerupted teeth (Whaites, 2002).

### 2.1.1 Anatomic landmarks of periapical radiograph

#### 2.1.1.1 Maxilla

**Maxillary anterior region**

Cervical dentin of the anterior teeth is penetrated in its lateral aspects by the X-ray beam. It is seen in the radiograph as a radiolucent image which is known as "burn-out effect". The anterior portions of the nose and the median suture can also be seen clearly in the radiographs taken from maxillary anterior region (Fig.3A).

**Maxillary canine region**

This projection exhibits a nasal process of the maxilla and the nasal soft tissues. Nasopalatine canal, incisive foramen and anterior lobe of the maxillary sinus can also be visible in this projection (Fig.3B).

**Maxillary premolar region**

The radiographs which were taken from premolar region exhibit the floor of the nasal cavity and maxillary sinus, usually separated from septum above the root tip of the second premolar (Fig.3C).

**Maxillary molar region**

The radiographs which were taken from premolar region exhibit maxillary sinus, maxillary tuberosity, and usually the body of the zygoma. Sometimes the process of the palatal bone, the pterygoid process and coronoid process of the mandible, so-called "radix relicta" appear in the radiograph (Fig.3D) (Pasler,1993; Pasler&Visser, 2003).

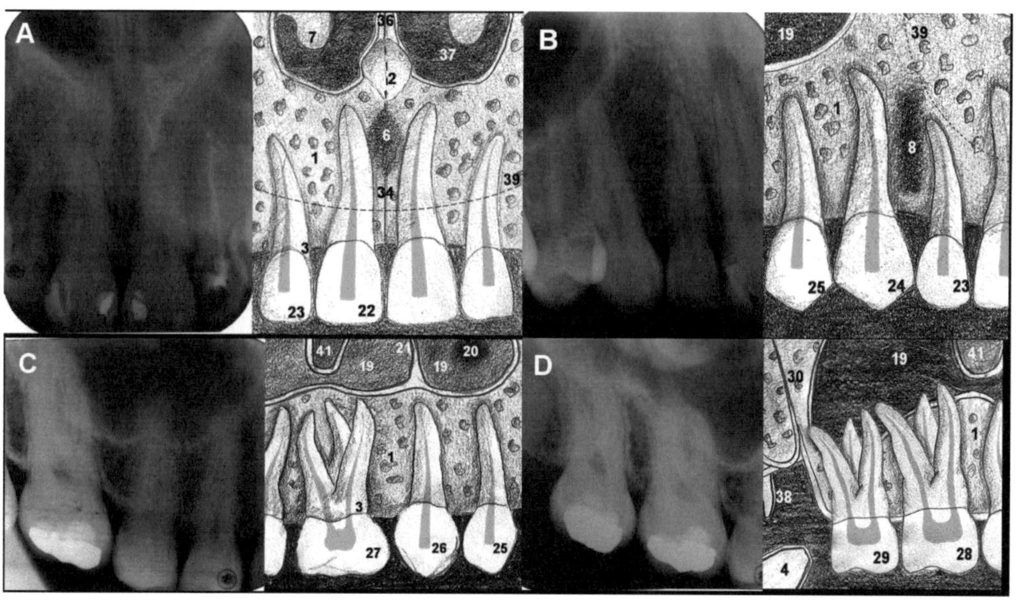


Fig. 3. A: Periapical view and schematic drawing of maxillary anterior region B: Periapical view and schematic drawing of maxillary canine region C: Periapical view and schematic drawing of maxillary premolar region D: Periapical view and schematic drawing of maxillary molar region

### 2.1.1.2 Mandible

**Mandibular anterior region**

The radiographs which were taken from the anterior region exhibit 4 mandibular incisor teeth, mental fovea which shows a radiolucent outfit, vascular canals and the chin prominence. Burn-out effect may also be observed in this radiograph just like in the radiographs which were taken from the maxillary region (Fig. 4A).

**Mandibular canine region**

The radiographs which were taken from this region do not exhibit any important anatomic formation. Depending on the radiographic angle, mental foramen and enostosis surrounding it can be seen (Fig.4B).

**Mandibular premolar region**

The radiographs which were taken from premolar region exhibit mental foramen between the roots of the premolar, course of mandibular canal and sublingual fovea. Depending on the radiographic projection angle, mental foramen may lead to diagnostic problem. It may be seen as a periapical lesion (Fig.4C).

**Mandibular molar region**

The radiographs which were taken from molar region exhibit mandibular canal, mylohyoid line, external and internal oblique line (Fig.4D) (Pasler,1993; Pasler&Visser, 2003).

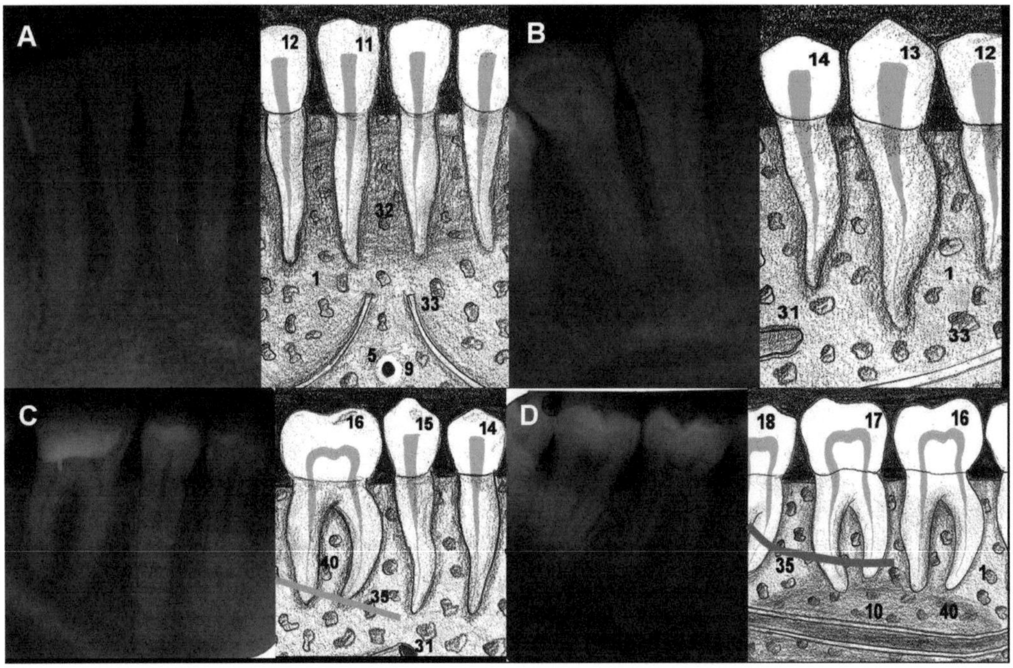


Fig. 4. A: Periapical view and schematic drawing of mandibular anterior region B: Periapical view and schematic drawing of mandibular canine region C: Periapical view and schematic drawing of mandibular premolar region D: Periapical view and schematic drawing of mandibular molar region

Legends for Figure 3-4:

1. Alveolar bone
2. Anterior nasal spine
3. Burn-out effect
4. Coronoid process
5. Genial tubercle
6. Incisive foramen
7. Infeior nasal concha
8. Lateral fossa
9. Lingual foramen
10. Mandibular canal
11. Mandibular tooth 1, central incisor
12. Mandibular tooth 2, lateral incisor
13. Mandibular tooth 3, canine
14. Mandibular tooth 4, first premolar
15. Mandibular tooth 5, second premolar
16. Mandibular tooth 6, first molar
17. Mandibular tooth 7, second molar
18. Mandibular tooth 8, third molar
19. Maxillary sinus
20. Maxillary sinus recession
21. Maxillary sinus septum
22. Maxillary tooth 1, central incisor
23. Maxillary tooth 2, lateral incisor
24. Maxillary tooth 3, canine
25. Maxillary tooth 4, first premolar
26. Maxillary tooth 5, second premolar
27. Maxillary tooth 6, first molar
28. Maxillary tooth 7, second molar
29. Maxillary tooth 8, third molar
30. Maxillary tuberosity
31. Mental foramen
32. Mental fossa
33. Mental ridge
34. Middle suture of hard palate
35. Mylohyoid ridge
36. Nasal septum
37. Nasal cavity
38. Processus hamularis
39. Soft tissue of nose
40. Submandibular fossa
41. Zygomatic arch

### 2.2 Panoramic radiography

Panoramic radiography, also known as an orthopantomogram, is a panoramic scanning dental X-ray of the two-dimensional view of the jaws and their supporting structures from ear to ear. It is obtained with patient, whose head stands between X-ray generator and the film. The main advantage of panoramic radiography is the fact that it is clinically useful for diagnostic problems associated with maxilla and mandible. One of the disadvantages of it is that the images do not exhibit a fine anatomically detailed outfit gained from periapical radiographs. Another problem related to orthopantomogram includes unequal magnification (Lurie, 2004).

Indications of panoramic radiographies are included in the following cases:

- Detection of the presence/absence of unerupted teeth
- Evaluation of relationship of the upper posterior teeth with maxillary sinus
- Evaluation of relationship of the lower posterior teeth with canalis alveolaris inferior
- Suspicion of asymptomatic swellings
- Radiographic examination of temporomandibular joint disturbances
- Examination of odontogenic, nonodontogenic cysts and tumors
- Evaluation of alveolar crest for insertion dental implants
- Evaluation of maxillomandibular region following trauma
- Examination of maxillary/mandibular surgical interventions

### 2.2.1 Anatomic landmarks of panoramic radiograph

While evaluating panoramic radiographs, first of all, normal anatomic structure of the region must be known well. Complicated structure of the regions, superposition of these structures and variations of the projection orientations may lead to problems during the evaluation process.

There are four diagnostic regions in the panoramic radiography:

- Dentoalveolar Region
- Maxillary Region
- Mandibular Region
- Temporomandibular, Retromaxillary and Cervical Region.

**Dentoalveolar region**

It is surrounded by maxillary sinus and inferior border of the nasal cavity from above and mandibular canal from below. Frontal side of ramus takes place on its left and its right. The teeth which are located in the upper and lower jaws and alveolus supporting them are seen in this region. Caries, fillings and prostheses are evaluated for the teeth whereas periodontal problems and intraalveolar pathologies related to the teeth are evaluated for alveolus (Fig.5).

**Maxillary region**

It is surrounded by orbita from above and maxillary sinus and the inferior border of the nasal cavity from below. Coronoid processus of the mandible and zygoma take place on its left and its right. Maxillary sinuses, zygomatic complex, nasal cavity and conchae, sphenoid, ethmoid, palate, frontal bones and pterygomaxillary fissure can be observed in this region. Lefort fractures and maxillary sinus pathologies are evaluated in this region (Fig.5).

**Mandibular region**

It is comprised of the mandibular teeth and mandibula rather than alveolus. Condylar and coronoid processes, ramus, body and angle and symphysis take place in this region. Mandibular canal, mental foramen, submandibular fossa, superimposed shadow of cervical vertebrae, external oblique ridge, posterior surface of tongue, soft palate and uvula, floor of nasopharynx and hyoid bone can also be observed in this region. Internal bone lesions and fractures are evaluated (Fig.5).

**Temporomandibular, retromaxillary and cervical region**

It is surrounded by temporal bone from above, and hyoid bone from below. Anterior of the ramus of the mandible takes place in its anterior. Cervical vertebra takes place in its posterior. The most important anatomic formation in this region is temporomandibular joint (TMJ). TMJ is comprised of glenoid fossa, articular eminence and articular process of mandibular condyle. Cervial vertebra, ear lobe, soft palate and uvula, posterior pharyngeal airway, floow of nasopharynx, zygomatic arch, styloid process of temporal bone, pterygomaxillary fissure and maxillary tuberosity can be observed in this region. Fractures in this region are evaluated (Fig.5) (Lurie, 2004).

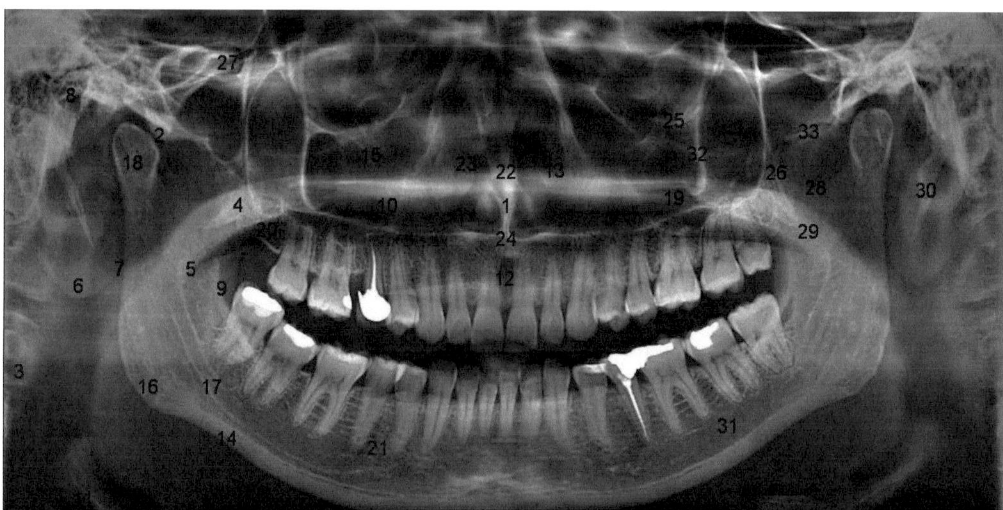


Fig. 5. Panoramic radiograph with marked anatomic structures

Legends for Figure 5:

1. Anterior nasal spine
2. Articular tubercle of the temporal bone
3. Cervical vertebra
4. Coronoid process
5. Dorsum of tongue (Shadow)
6. Ear lobe
7. Epipharynx

8. External auditory canal
9. External oblique ridge
10. Hard palate
11. Hyoid bone
12. Incisive foramen
13. Inferior nasal concha
14. Inferior border of mandible
15. Infraorbital canal
16. Mandibular angle
17. Mandibular canal
18. Mandibular condyle
19. Maxillary sinus
20. Maxillary tuberosity
21. Mental foramen
22. Nasal septum
23. Nasal cavity
24. Nasopalatine canal
25. Orbital rim
26. Pterygoid process of sphenoid bone
27. Pterygopalatine fossa
28. Sigmoid notch
29. Soft palate
30. Styloid process
31. Submandibular fossa
32. Zygoma
33. Zygomatic arch

### 2.3 Dental computed tomography

Computed tomography was discovered by Hounsfield in 1974. After improvements, nowadays, dental computed tomography is performed for diagnosis of oral and maxillofacial pathology in most patients. Its advantage over 2D radiography is the fact that it can eliminate the superimposition of images of adjacent tissues. Since it provides bone images at the highest quality, it is the most widely used imaging technique (Curtain et al., 1998; Karjodkar,2006). Tomographic images are taken as trans-axial cross sections. These images are stored on the computer and then recreated from the cross sections passing through the surfaces which are desired to be observed. This is called multiplanar reformation. This way, axial, sagittal and coronal planes of the material that was imaged can be obtained. When these planes are combined by means of a software application, a 3D image may also be obtained. The images are obtained with the patient supine and during quite respiration. Contrast agent injection may be needed to evaluate soft tissues. When taking a computed tomography of oral and maxillofacial region, images are acquired from the top of the frontal sinus to the sub mental region (Hermans et al., 2006). Computerized tomography is used in maxillofacial surgery, reconstructive surgery, orthognatic surgery, dental implant applications, and detection of lesions like cyst/tumor, trauma and temporomandibular joint diseases.

Dental computed tomography has a number of advantages over other conventional radiography:

- Undesired superimposition of other tissues in the region is eliminated.
- Thanks to the high-resolution of computerized tomography, differences between the tissues with different physical densities can be distinguished better.
- It is possible to obtain images of the tissues which are located on axial, coronal sagittal planes.
- It is especially a very useful tool for the planning of dental implant insertion.
- It has no magnification and no distortion.
- In the presence of formations like cysts/tumors, it can be determined whether this formation has a solid or a liquid structure by means of density measurements (Frederiksen, 2004).

Dental computed tomography has also disadvantages over other conventional radiography:

- Administration of contrast agent is necessary for imaging soft tissue
- More radiation exposure
- Degradation of image quality by metallic objects, like as dental crown, fillings

### 2.3.1 Anatomic landmarks of dental tomography

This chapter presents the imaging of normal anatomic structures by dental tomography on axial, coronal, sagittal planes and in 3D view (Fig.6,7,8).

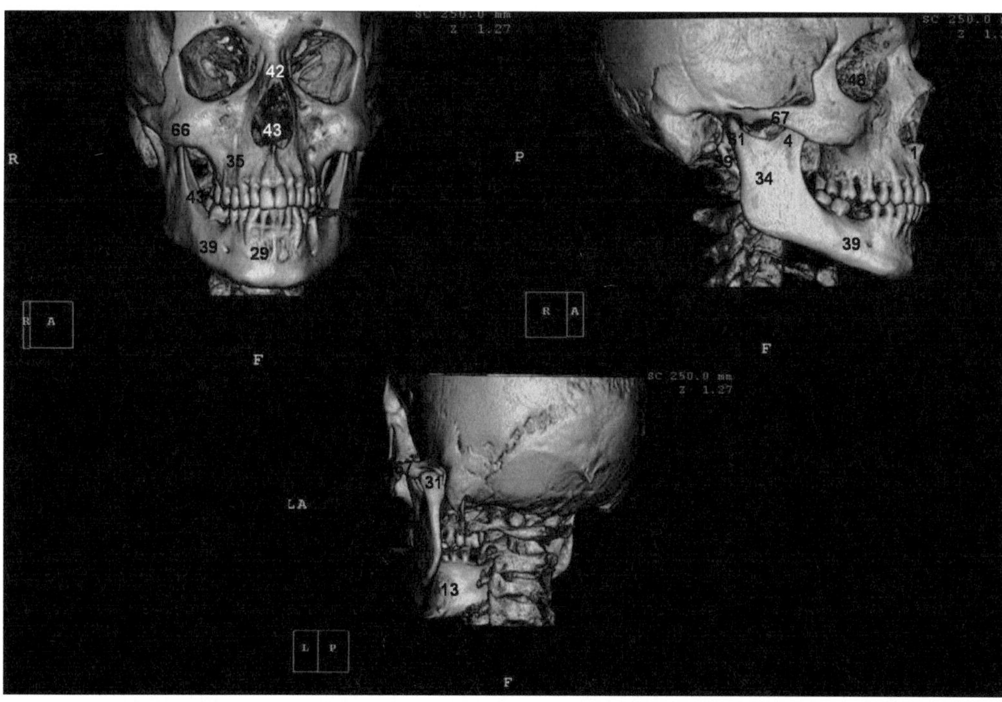


Fig. 6. 3D CT anatomy of the facial skeleton

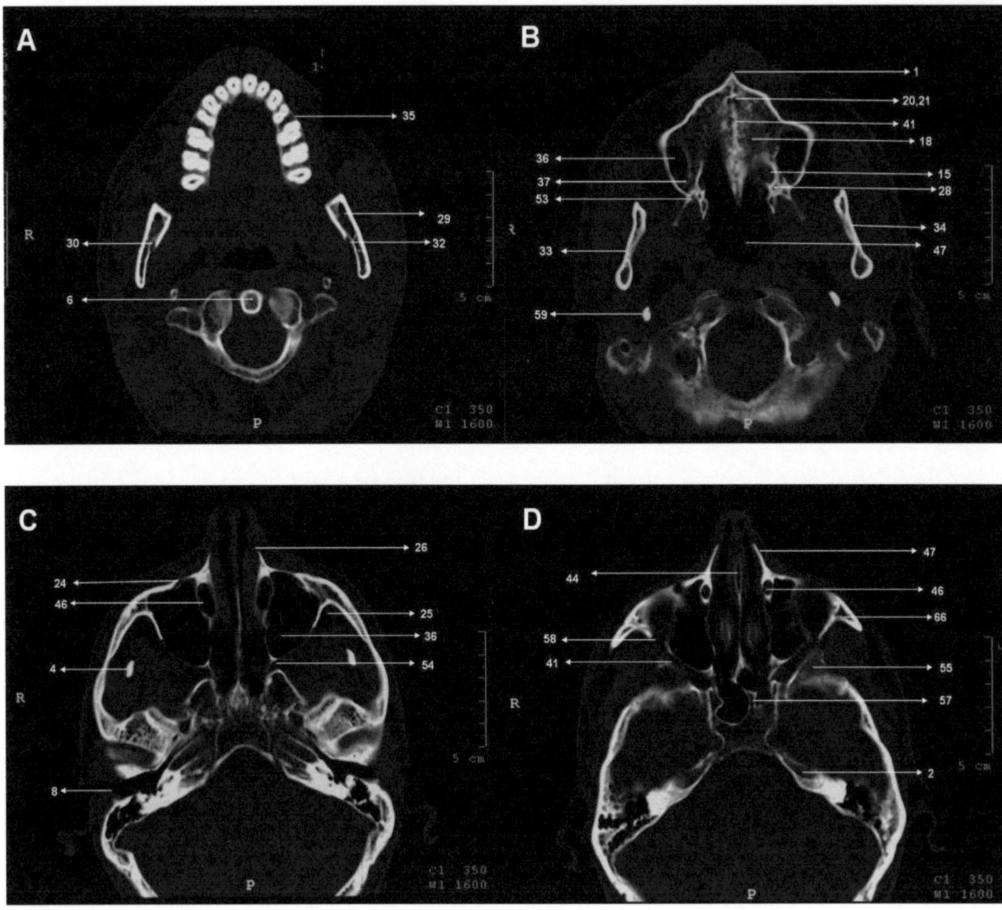


Fig. 7. (A,B). Axial CT anatomy of the facial skeleton; (C,D). Axial CT anatomy of the facial skeleton

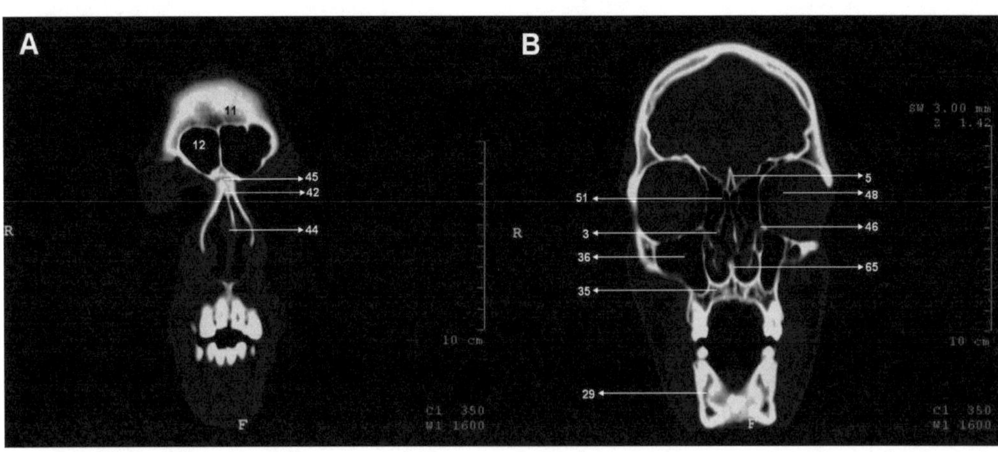

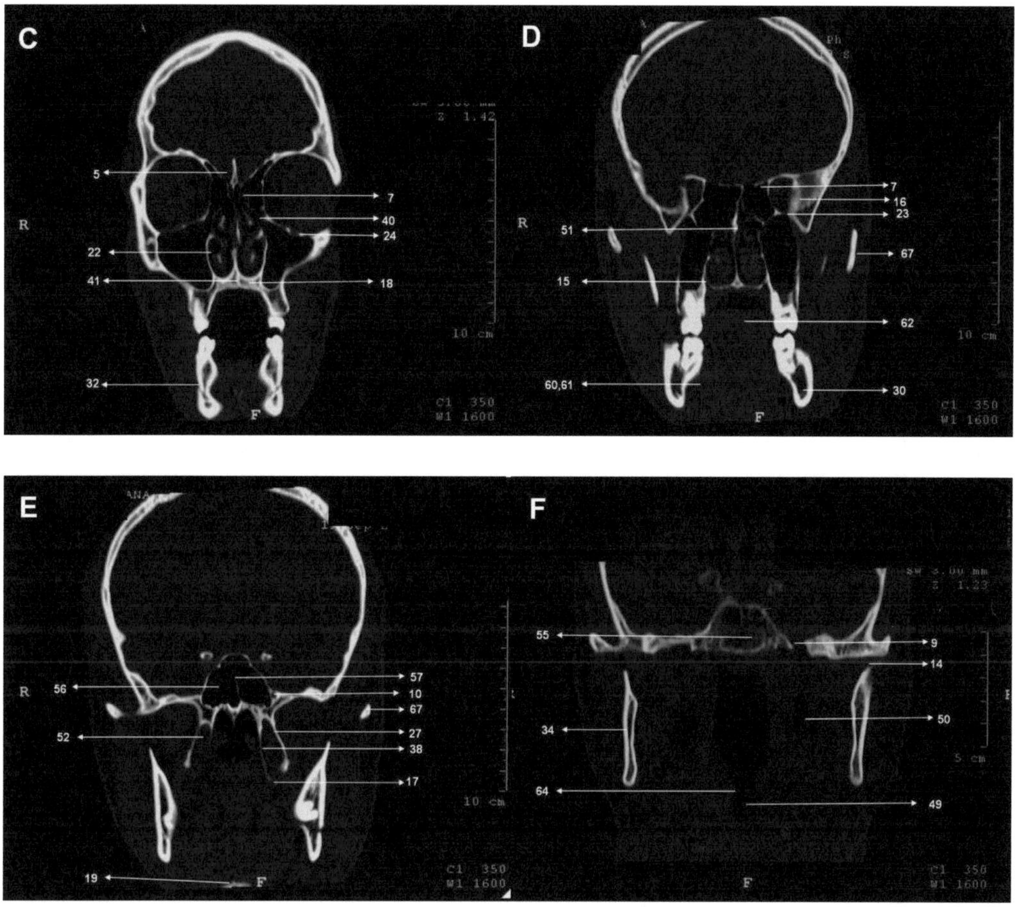


Fig. 8. (A,B). Coronal CT anatomy of the facial skeleton; (C,D). Coronal CT anatomy of the facial skeleton; (E,F). Coronal CT anatomy of the facial skeleton

Figure legends for figure 6,7,8:

1. Anterior nasal spine
2. Carotid canal
3. Concha bullosa
4. Coronoid process
5. Crista galli
6. Dens axis
7. Ethmoid sinus
8. External auditory canal
9. Foramen ovale
10. Foramen rotundum
11. Frontal bone
12. Frontal sinus
13. Genial tubercle of mandible
14. Glenoid fossa
15. Greater palatine canal

16. Greater wing of sphenoid bone
17. Hamulus of medial pterygoid plate
18. Hard plate
19. Hyoid bone
20. Incisive canal
21. Incisive foramen
22. Inferior meatus
23. Inferior orbital fissure
24. Infraorbital canal
25. Infratemporal fossa
26. Lacrimal bone
27. Lateral pterygoid plate
28. Lesser palatin canal
29. Mandible
30. Mandibular canal
31. Mandibular condyle
32. Mandibular foramen
33. Mandibular notch
34. Mandibular ramus
35. Maxilla
36. Maxillary sinus
37. Maxillary tuberosity
38. Medial pterygoid plate
39. Mental foramen
40. Middle meatus
41. Middle suture of hard palate
42. Nasal bone
43. Nasal cavity airway
44. Nasal septum
45. Nasofrontal suture
46. Nasolacrimal canal
47. Nasopharynx
48. Orbit
49. Oropharynx
50. Parapharyngeal space
51. Perpendicular plate of ethmoid bone
52. Pterygoid fossa
53. Pterygoid process of sphenoid bone
54. Pterygopalatine fossa
55. Sphenoid bone
56. Sphenoid sinus
57. Sphenoid sinus septum
58. Sphenozygomatic suture
59. Styloid process
60. Submandibular space
61. Submandibular gland
62. Tongue
63. Trigomun retromolare
64. Uvula

65. Vomer
66. Zygoma
67. Zygomatic arch

## 3. Radiographic description of oral and maxillofacial pathology

### 3.1 Radiolucent/radiopaque lesions of the jaws

Odontogenic cysts and tumors present problems of diagnosis, radiology and histopathology. In general, their differential diagnosis requires radiographic clinical data, since many of them possess similar histological characteristics. Radiologic appearance of jaw cysts and odontogenic tumors varies considerably. The common lack of physical findings and the development of most of these lesions within the confines of the bone make radiologic investigation and interpretation uniquely important. Radiographs are also important in treatment planning for surgical removal. They can evaluate encroachment on vital structures, extent into soft tissue, size of the lesion, and requirements for reconstruction. Radiography allows for creation of a radiologic differential diagnosis. (Escobar et al.,2007)

#### 3.1.1 Radiolucent lesions of the jaws

- Dental granuloma
- Radicular cyst
- Dentigerous cyst
- Keratocystic odontogenic tumor
- Ameloblastoma
- Incisive canal cyst
- Simple bone cyst
- Central giant cell granuloma
- Odontogenic myxoma

#### 3.1.2 Radiopaque lesions of the jaws

- Odontoma
- Torus
- Osteoma
- Osteochondroma
- Cementoblastoma
- Fibrous dysplasia (late stage)

#### 3.1.3 Mixed radiolucent/radiopaque lesions of the jaws

- Fibrous dysplasia (early stage)
- Ossifying fibroma
- Cemento-osseous dysplasia
- Chronic osteomyelitis
- Osteosarcoma
- Metastasis

**Dentigerous cyst**

Dentigerous cysts are the second most common odontogenic cysts after radicular cysts. It surrounds the crown of an impacted tooth, caused by fluid accumulation between the reduced enamel epithelium and the enamel surface, resulting in a cyst in which the crown is located within the lumen and roots outside. It is usually asymptomatic but produces some swelling or pain when become large or inflamed. It is associated clinically with impacted tooth most commonly an unerupted 3rd molar (mandibular- more than maxillary), then maxillary canines, rarely involve deciduous teeth. Radiographically, the dentigerous cyst appears as a unilocular radiolucency of variable size with well-defined sclerotic borders, associated with the crown of an unerupted tooth. In an infected cyst the borders may be ill-defined. The radiographic appearance of such a cyst, though quite typical, is not diagnostic (Daley&Wysocki, 1995). The treatment of dentigerous cysts is determined by the size of the lesion. Small lesions should be removed by surgery; larger cysts are treated by marsupialization or decompression. The possible complications of the dentigerous cysts are the permanent bony deformation from its expansive destruction of bone, loss of essential permanent dentition or its innervation of the mandibular nerve. Dentigerous cysts with long evolution can present areas with keratin or dysplasic changes of its epithelial revetment with development of an ameloblastoma or an epidermoid carcinoma (Fig.9) (Weber, 1993).

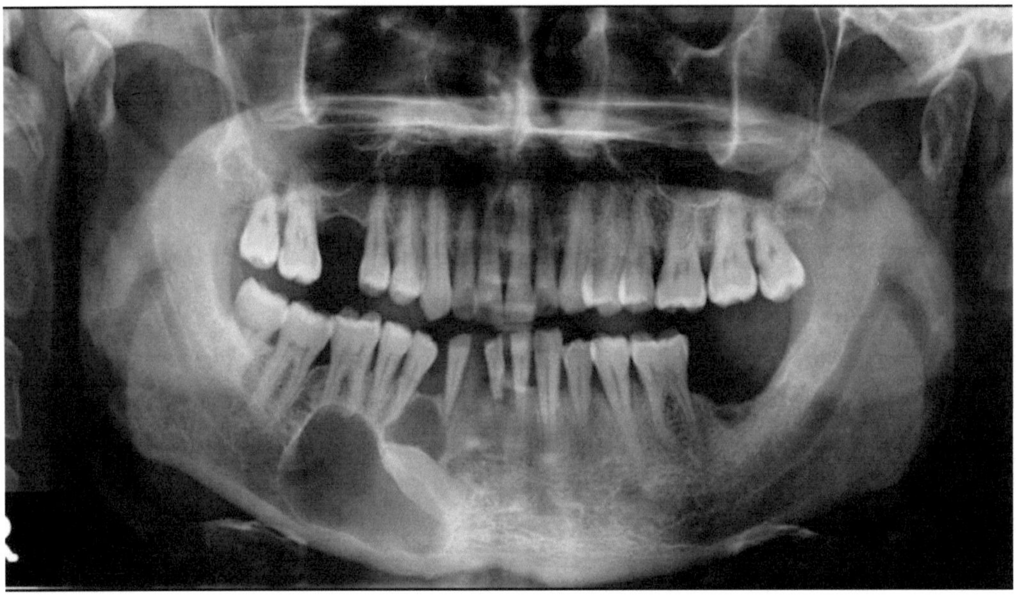

Fig. 9. Panoramic radiograph shows a well-defined expansile radiolucent lesion in the right mandible and unerupted right canine.

**Radicular cyst**

Radicular cysts are the most common cyst of the jaws. They are most frequent between the ages of 20 and 60 years. Radicular cysts may cause slowly progressive painless swellings, with no symptoms until they become expansion of the cortical plates. If the infection enters, the tooth and swelling develop all the painful symptoms of an abscess. Initially, the swelling is rounded and hard. Later they are caused the demolition of cortical plate, than the swelling is rubbery and fluctuant because of the cyst fluid. Large cysts may involve a complete quadrant with some of the teeth occasionally mobile and some additional pulps nonvital. Radiographically, radicular cyst appears well defined radiolucent area. Infection of a cyst causes resorption of the surrounding tissue. If the cyst extends slowly, a condensed radiopaque periphery is present. Enucleation is usual method for the treatment of radicular cyst. Larger cysts are treated by marsupialization (Fig.10) (Cawson&Odell, 2002; Wood et al.,1997; Sahin et al., 2009).

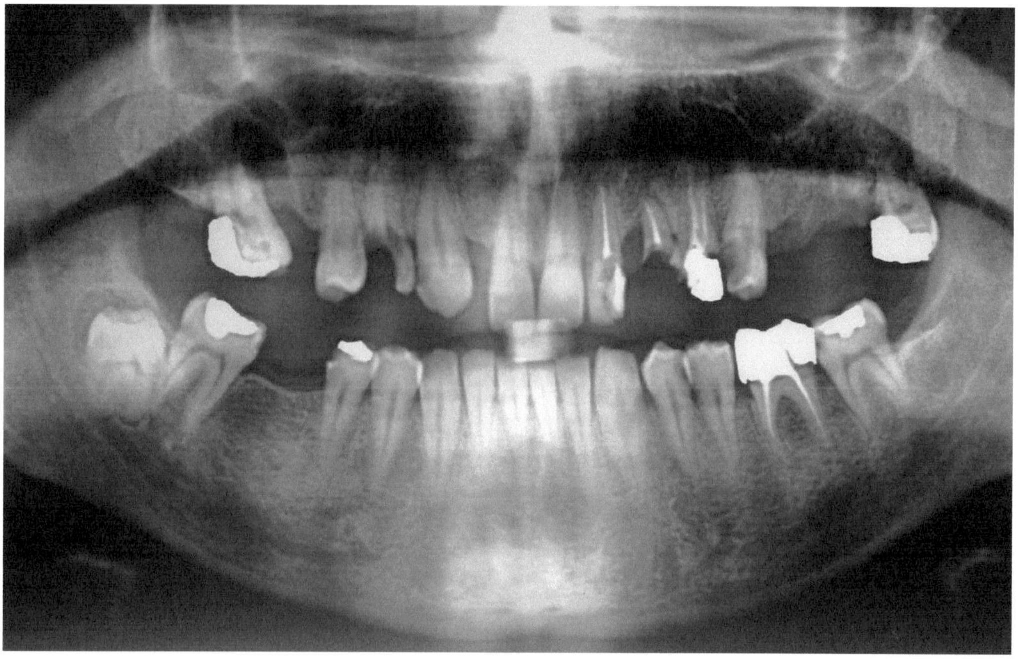

Fig. 10. Radiographic appearance of the radicular cyst (maxillary right second molar region) on the panoramic radiograph

**Keratocystic odontogenic tumor**

The most recent classification of the World Health Organization (WHO) reallocated keratocyst (keratinized primordial cyst) within the classification of odontogenic tumours under the term "keratocystic odontogenic tumor." It has specific histopathological features and clinical behavior, it makes up to 10- 20% of all developmental odontogenic cyst (Barnes et al.,2005). Keratocystic odontogenic tumor occurs more in mandible 80% (posterior body and ascending ramus). It grows in anterior-posterior direction within medullary cavity of the bone without causing obvious bone expansion. This is useful to differentiate clinical and radiographic dentigerous and radicular cyst of similar size which produce bone expansion. Multiple keratocystic odontogenic tumor is seen in nevoid basal cell carcinoma (gorlin syndrome). Radiographically, it is well defined radiolucent area with smooth corticated margin. Large lesions in posterior body and ascending ramus of the mandible appear as multilocular radiolucency. An unerupted tooth is involved in the lesion in 25-40 % of cases. The treatment of keratocystic odontogenic tumor is complete removed by enucleation and curettage it has tendency to recurred because of friable nature of cyst wall that result in fragment or due to formation of new cysts from dental lamina (daughter cysts). Marsupialization has been effective in reducing the size of the cyst (Fig.11) (Mendes RA et al., 2010)

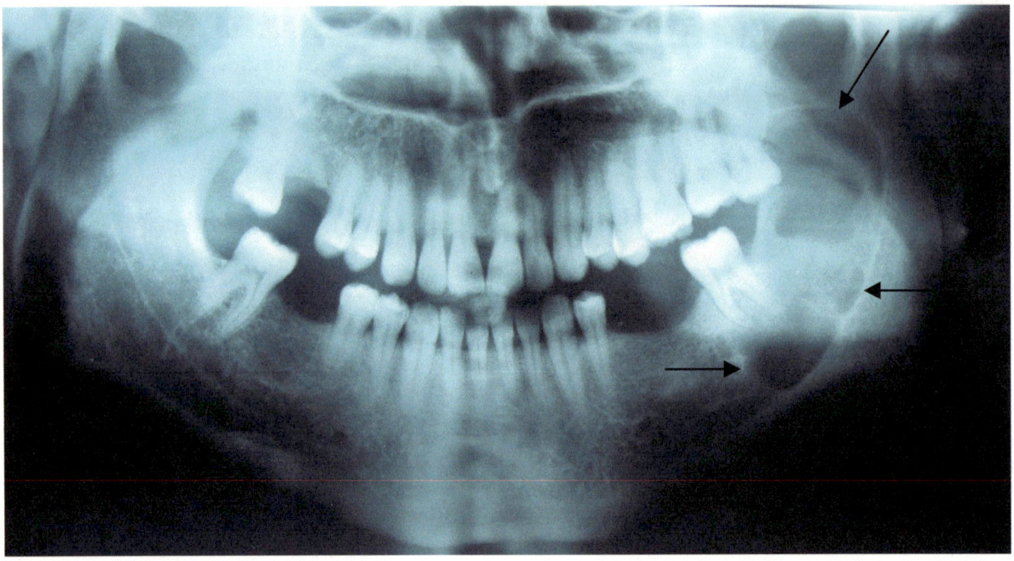

Fig. 11. Panoramic radiograph shows an ellipsoid, expansile, well-corticated, radiolucent lesion in left mandibular body and ascending ramus.

**Lateral periodontal cyst**

Lateral periodontal cyst is rare asymptomatic lesion, mainly in mandible in canine-premolar region. It is usually seen by chance in routine radiographs. Radiographically, it appears as a well circumscribed radiolucent area located laterally to the roots of vital tooth. Occasionally this cyst appears as multilocular (poly cystic) named botryoid odontogenic cyst. The radiographical picture is not diagnostic. Lateral periodontal cyst should be enucleated. If the affected tooth is healthy, it can be retained (Fig.11) (Cawson&Odell, 2002).

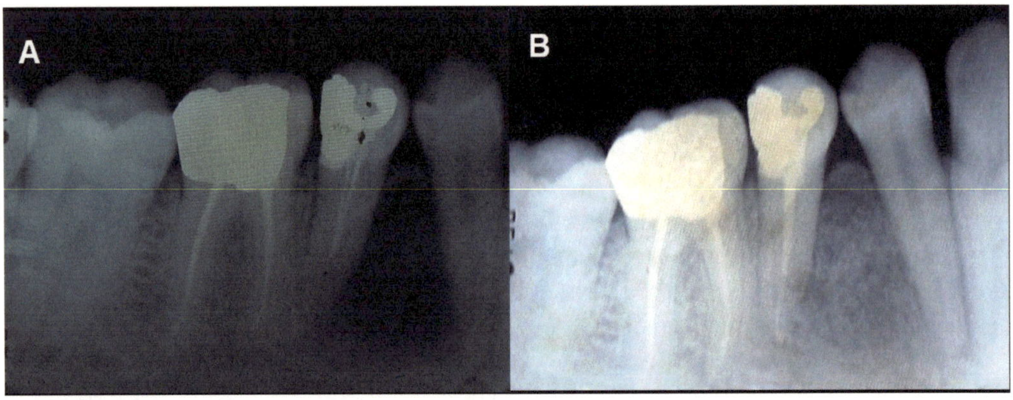


Fig. 12. Periapical view of lateral periodontal cyst A. Pre-treatment B. Post-treatment

**Ameloblastoma**

Ameloblastoma are most common tumors of jaws. The majority of ameloblastoma are benign, with less than 1% showing malignant behavior. The most common site of ameloblastoma is the ascending ramus and proximal body of the mandible (80%). Based on radiological appearance, ameloblastomas are divided into two subtypes. Multicystic ameloblastomas account for approximately 85% of all ameloblastomas and occur in the third to seventh decades of life. On radiographs, it is typically form rounded, cyst-like, radiolucent area appear multilocular. There is marked buccolingual cortical expansion with internal osseous septae, giving rise to a "soap bubble" appearance. Tooth displacement or root resorption may occur. Unicystic ameloblastomas occur in a younger age group and tend to be non-invasive. They present as a well-circumscribed, unicystic, radiolucent lesion, mostly in the region of the mandibular third molar (DelBalso, 1998). Treatment is by wide excision, preferably taking up to 2 cm of apparently surrounding normal tissue. Unicystic ameloblastomas can be enucleated with low risk of recurrence (Cawson&Odell, 2002).

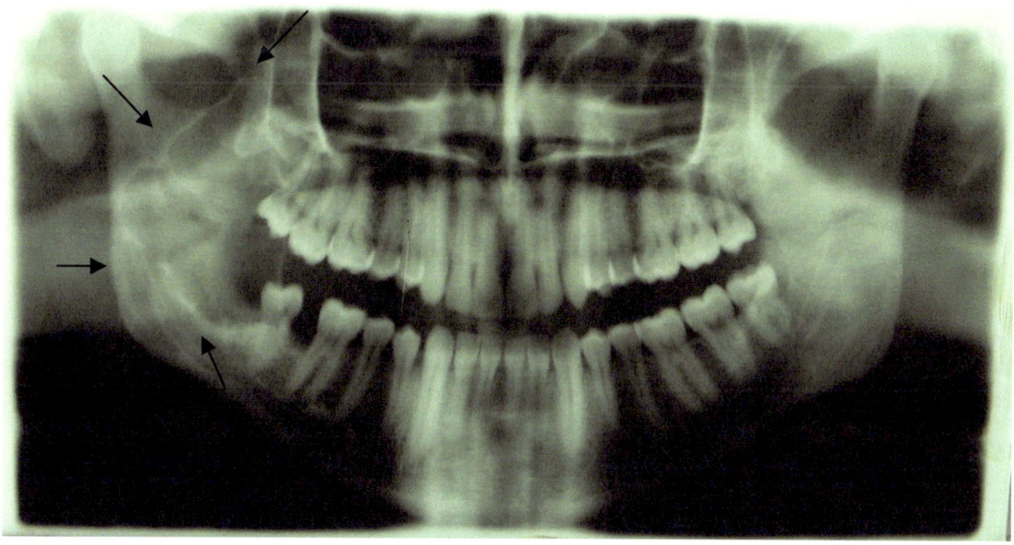

Fig. 13. Panoramic radiographic view of ameloblastoma of mandibular ramus.

**Central giant cell granuloma**

Central giant cell granulomas (CGCG) typically occur in patients younger than 30 years of age, more often in females. The lesion is more common in the anterior part of mandible with a tendency to cross the midline. In the early stage, the lesion manifests as a small unilocular lucent lesion. However, with development, it appears multilocular with fine trabeculae. They may cause a variable degree of bony expansion, divergence of roots and root resorption. Brown tumour of hyperparathyroidism can mimic CGCGs radiologically as well as pathologically; however, the patient's age, radiological changes in other bones, and biochemical findings help in differentiation (Altug et al., 2011b).

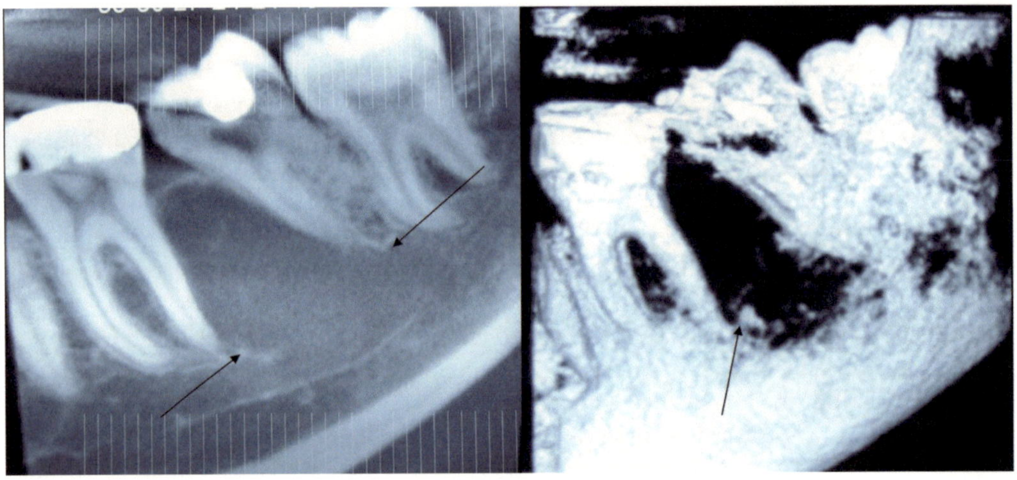

Fig. 14. Panoramic radiographic view of CGCG of mandibula.

**Odontoma**

Odontomas are considered to be a hamartomatous lesion rather than a neoplasm. Most cases are diagnosed in the second decade of life, and are usually associated with an impacted tooth. Radiologically, it is seen as a radiopaque mass surrounded by thin radiolucent space. The compound odontomas are composed of multiple well-formed teeth whereas the complex odontomas appear as an irregular calcified tissue. A related but very rare lesion is ameloblastic fibro-odontoma. Most cases occur in young males involving posterior jaws and may expand into the ramus. The amount of radiolucent internal structure exceeds the odontomas component (Weber et al., 1993; Altug et al, 2010b).

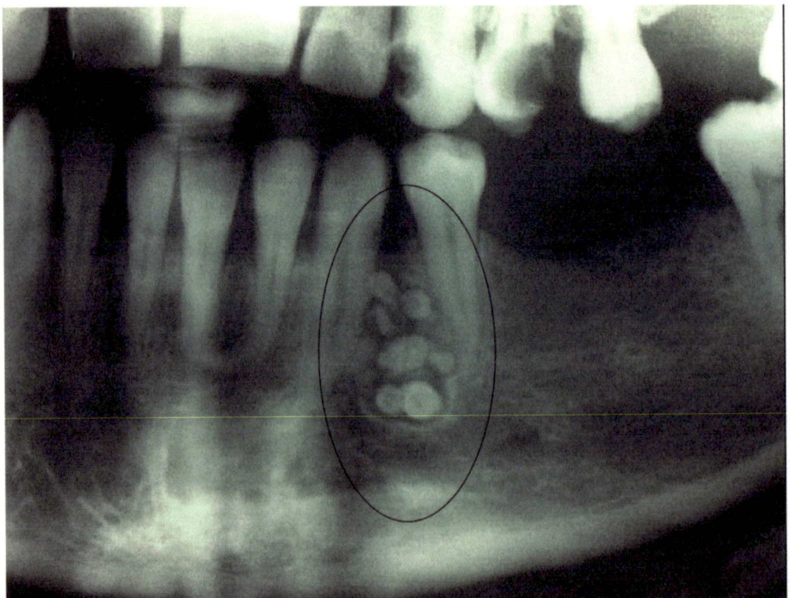

Fig. 15. Panoramic radiographic view of odontoma of mandibular canine region.

### Ossifying fibroma

Ossifying fibroma is rare. It is slow expansile growth and it can expand the cortices and displace adjacent structures. True benign tumors of mesenchyme are with strong predilection for tooth-bearing sections of jaw. Patients are usually females in 20-40s. Radiographically, early lesion is radiolucent with varying degrees of calcification and has well circumscribed margins. If the lesion is more opaque shows that the lesion is mature. The patterns of calcifications have no effect on the lesions behavior. Small lesions should be removed by enucleation and curettage. However, large lesions (5mm margin) which have distorted the jaw require local resection. Recurrence is rare (Fig. 16) (Cawson & Odell, 2002; Ortakoğlu et al., 2006).

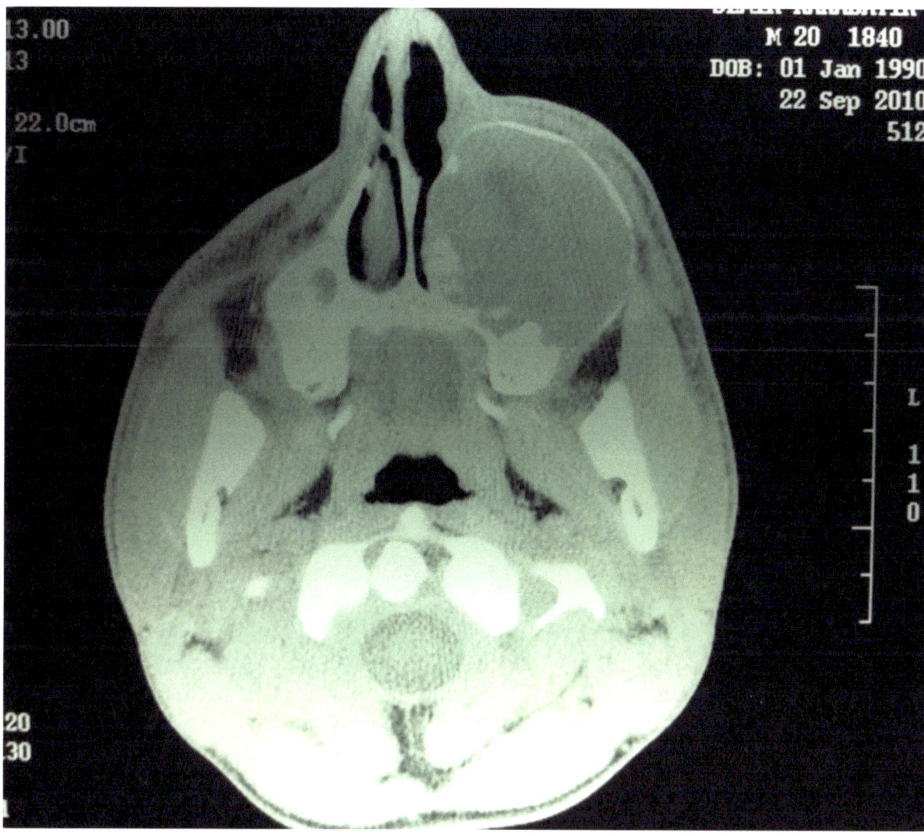


Fig. 16. Axial CT view of maxillary ossifying fibroma

### Cementoblastoma

Cementoblastoma is a benign neoplasm and forms a mass of cementum and cementum-like tissue on roots of teeth. It is usually affect of posterior region of mandible, especially mandibular first molar. Clinically, cementoblastoma mainly affects young adults, particularly males. It is slow-growing and usually asymptomatic; but pain and swelling have been reported in a number of cases. Radiographically, there is typically a radiopaque mass with a thin radiolucent margin with the root of the tooth. The mass may be rounded or irregular in shape. Resorption of related tooth's roots is common, but the tooth remains vital (Fig.17) (Sumer M et al., 2006).

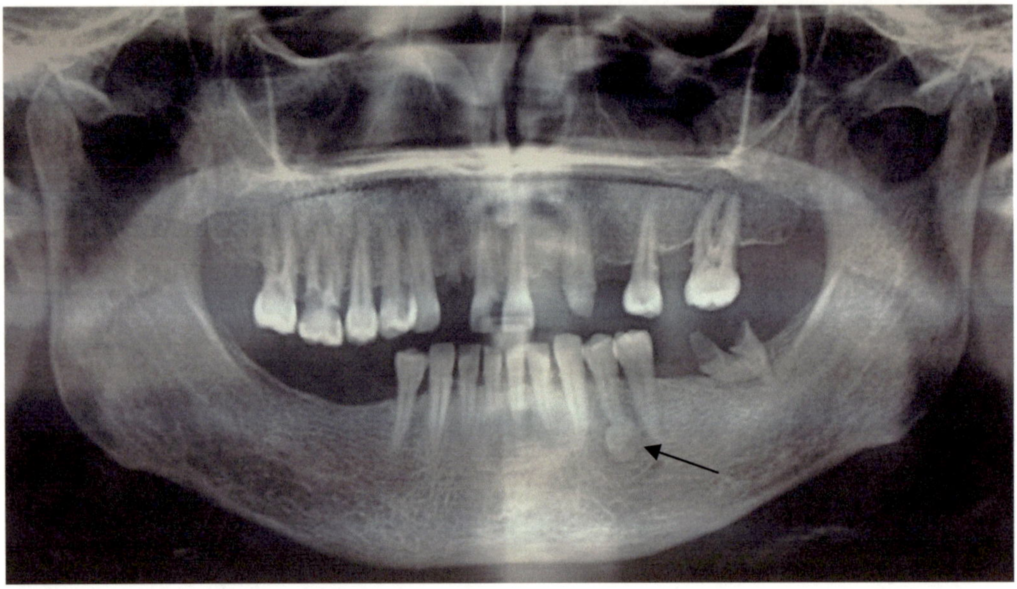

Fig. 17. Panoramic radiographic view of cementoblastoma related to mandibular premolar tooth.

**Focal osseous-dysplasia**

The current classification of fibro-osseous lesions, released in 2005 by the World Health Organization (Barnes et al.,2005), is based on age, sex and histopathologic, radiographic and clinical characteristics, as well as location of the lesion. Focal osseous dysplasia is an asymptomatic benign malformation and belonging to the group of fibro-osseous lesions. Although the etiology and pathogenesis of focal osseous-dysplasia are unknown, histogenetically it is believed that it originated from periodontal ligament. It usually appears in dentate and/or edentulous posterior mandibular region. Radiographically, the lesion is well defined by radiolucent borders and an unilocular dense radiopaque appearance. No treatment is necessary for focal osseous dysplasia and follow-up is essential to confirm the diagnosis. Some authors have suggested that the transformation into florid cemento-osseous dysplasia is possible and should be considered at recall visits (Fig.18) (Summerlin &Tomich, 1994).

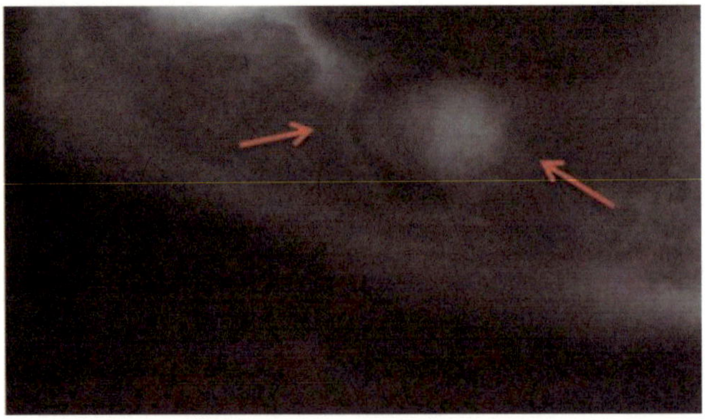

Fig. 18. Periapical radiographic view of focal osseous dysplasia in mandible

**Odontogenic myxoma**

Odontogenic myxoma derives from dental mesenchyme and generally affects the young persons (of average age 15 years). It usually affects in the mandible, and typically appears in the mandibular angles. It has benign behaves but can infiltrate widely. Due to the inadequate surgical excision, it may recur. Radiographically, the odontogenic myxoma may produce several types: unicystic, multilocular, pericoronal and radiolucent-radiopaque and it is close resemblance to soap bubble-like picture of ameloblastoma. The lesion gives rise to fusiform swelling and radiolucent area with scalloped margins. The treatment of odontogenic myxoma is required wide excision but some cases have been seen over 30 years after the first intervention (Fig.19) (Cawson & Odell, 2002; Wood et al., 1997; Altug et al., 2011a).

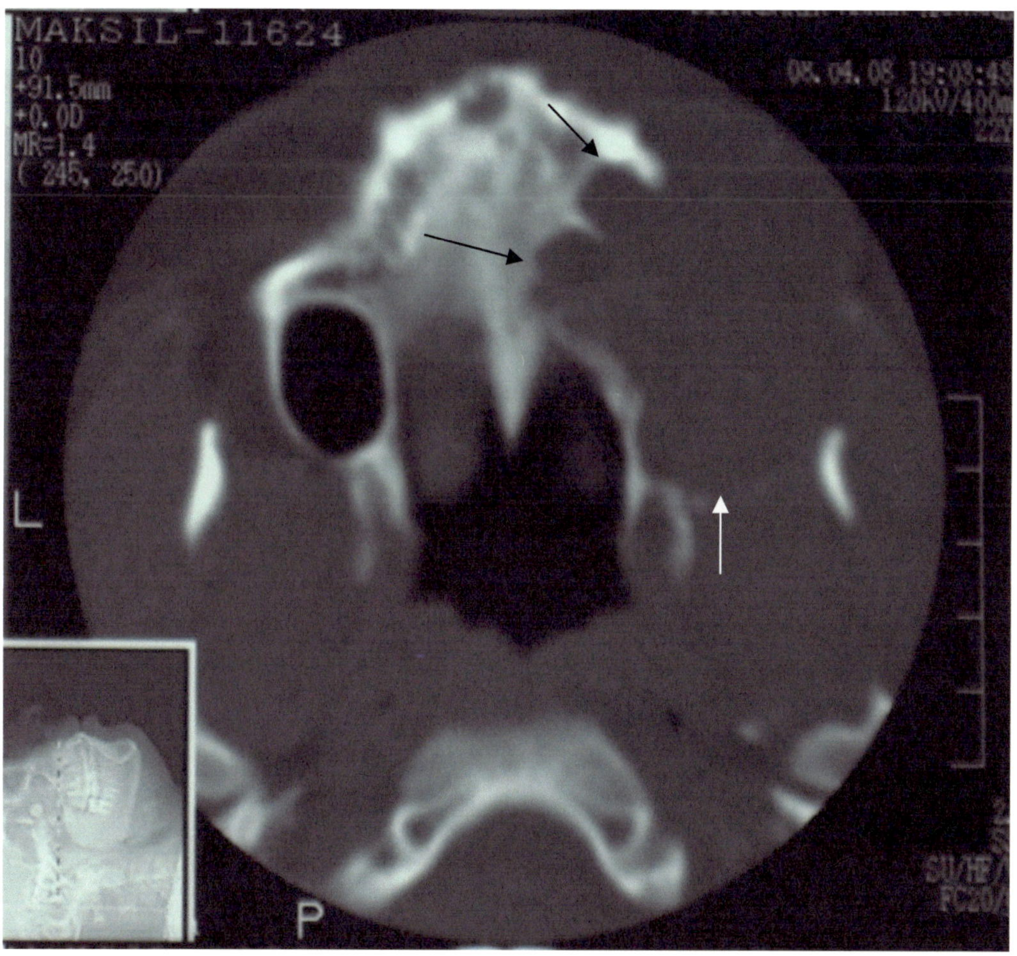


Fig. 19. Axial CT view of maxillary odontogenic myxoma.

**Solitary eosinophilic granuloma**

Solitary eosinophilic granuloma of the jaws belongs to the group of langerhan's cell histiocytosis and causes restricted bone destruction with swelling and pain. It generally occurs in child and young adults. Eosinophilic granuloma can affect almost any bone but, when the jaws are affected mandible is commonly. Radiographically, the lesion has rounded radiolucency and an appearance of teeth floating air. The treatment of eosinophilic granuloma curettage is sufficient and some localize cases spontaneous regression are possible (Fig.20) (Cawson & Odell , 2002; Altuğ et al.,2010a)

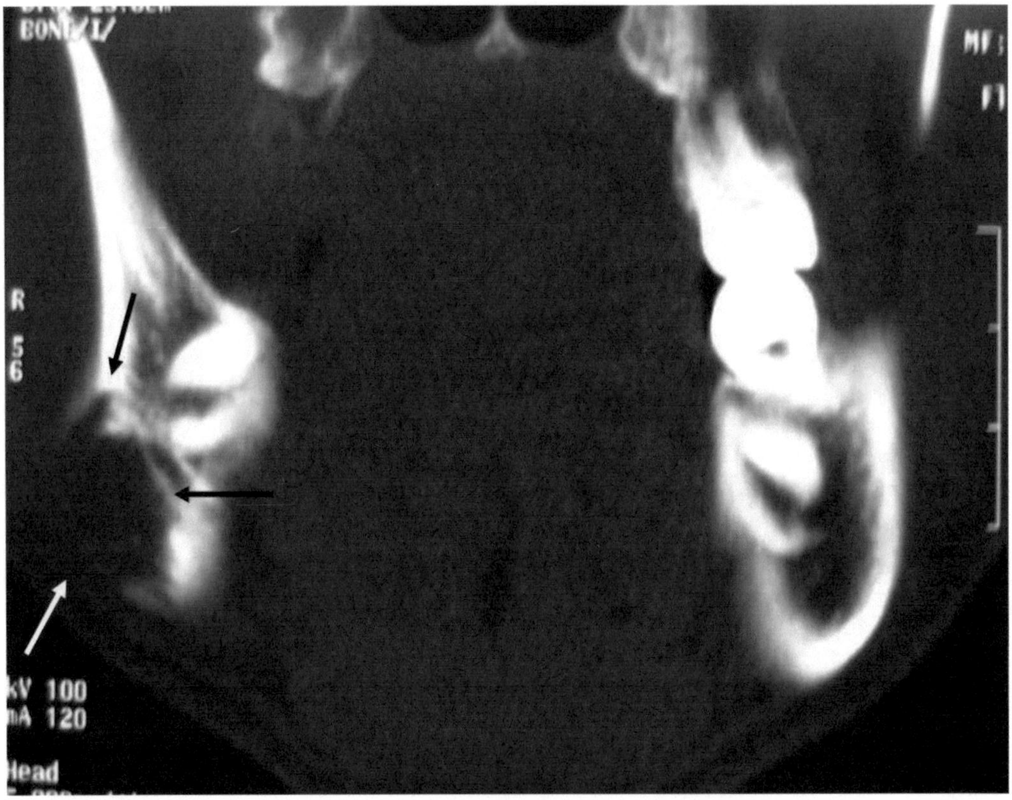


Fig. 20. Coronal CT view of mandibular eosinophilic granuloma.

## 4. Conclusion

Although oral radiology is the precious member of oral diagnosis procedures, only one imaging modality can provide us to wrong diagnosis in maxillofacial region. Especially in cysts/tumors differential diagnosis, it is recommended that combination of different imaging modalities.

## 5. Acknowledgment

We are grateful to Mrs. Muge Unlukoc, has provided invaluable help throughout including providing us with periapical radiographic illustrations. We would like to thank Mr. Hakan Yamanyar, for English proof-reading.

## 6. References

Altuğ, HA, Alömeroğlu, M, Şahin, S, Şençimen, M, Doğan, N. & Krıshnan, DG. (2010a). Incidental discovery asymptomatic radiolucent lesion of the posterior mandible. *J Oral Maxillofac Surg,* Vol.68. pp:845-848 ISSN 0278-2391

Altug, HA, Altug, H, Sari, E, Sencimen, M. & Altun C. (2010b). Diagnosis and surgically management of supernumerary teeth in both the primary and the permenant dentitions. *The Journal of Gazi University Faculty of Dentistry.* Vol.27. pp:77-82 ISSN 1300-3100

Altuğ, HA, Gülses, A & Şençimen M. (2011a). Clinico-radiographic Examination of Odontogenic Myxoma with Displacement of Unerupted Upper Third Molar: Review of the Literature. Int J Morphol 29(3):930-933 ISSN 0717 9367

Altuğ, HA, Şençimen, M, Altun, C & Guven G. (2011b). Computed tomography and magnetic resonance imaging of giant cell granuloma of the mandible. Int J Comp Asist Radiol Surg. 6:s384-s385 ISSN 1861 6410

Barnes, L, Eveson, JW, Reichart, P. & Sidransky, D. (2005). Classification of Tumors In: *Pathology & Genetics Head and Neck Tumours.* IARCPress, ISBN 92 832 2417 5, Lyon, France

Cawson, RA. & Odell, EW. (2002). Hard Tissue Pathology, In: *Cawson's Essentials of Oral Pathology and Oral Medicine.* Seventh edition, 102-158, ISBN 0 443 071055, Spain

Curtin, HD., Ishwaran, H., Mancuso, AA., Dalley, RW., Caudry, DJ. & McNeil, BJ. (1998). Comparison of CT and MR imaging in staging of neck metastases. *Radiology,* Vol.207(1):123–130, ISSN 0033-8419

Daley, TD. & Wysocki, GP. (1995). The small dentigerous cyst. A diagnostic dilemma. *Oral Surg Oral Med Oral Pathol Oral Radiol Endod,* Vol.79, pp:77-81,101-120 ISSN 1079-2104

DelBalso, AM. (1998). An approach to the diagnostic imaging of jaw lesions, dental implants, and the temporomandibular joint. *Radiol Clin North Am.* Vol. 36, pp:855-90 ISSN 0033 8389

Escobar, E, Godoy, L. & Peñafiel, C. (2007). Odontogenic Cysts: Analysis of 2.944 cases in Chile Germán Ochsenius. *Med Oral Pathol Oral Cir Bucal,* Vol.12,pp:E85-91, eISSN 1698-6946

Frederiksen, NL. (2004). Specialized Radiographic Techniques, In: *Oral Radiology: Principles and Interpratation,* White, SC.&Pharoah, MJ, (Ed), 245-250, Mosby, ISBN 978-0-323-02001-5, China

Hermans, R., De Keyzer, F.& Vandecaveye V. (2006). Imaging Tecqnique, In: *Medical Radiology, Diagnostic Imaging,* A.L. Baert, K.Sartor, (Ed),31-43, Springer-Verlag, ISBN 3-540-22027-5, Germany

Karjodkar, FR. (2006). History of Radiology, In: *Textbook of Dental and Maxillofacial Radiology,*1-11, Jaypee Brothers Medical Publishers, ISBN 81-8061-854-4, India

Lurie, AG. (2004). Panoramic Imaging, In: *Oral Radiology: Principles and Interpratation*, White, SC.&Pharoah, MJ, (Ed), 191-195, Mosby, ISBN 978-0-323-02001-5, China

Mendes, RA, Carvalho, JF. &Van der Waal, I. (2010). Characterization and management of the keratocystic odontogenic tumor in relation to its histopathological and biological features. *Oral Oncol.* Vol.46, No.4, pp:219-225, ISSN 1368 8375

Ortakoğlu, K, Aydıntuğ, YS, Altug, HA, Okçu, KM. & Günhan Ö. (2006). Benign fibroosseous lesions. *The Turkish J Dentistry* Vol.65. pp:132-136 ISSN 1304-6071 Pasler, FA& Visser, H. (2003). Radiographic Anatomy in Intraoral Radiographs, In : *Pocket Atlas of Dental Radiology*, 70-80, Thieme, 978-3-13-139801-7, USA

Pasler, FA. (1993). Radiographic Anatomy of Special Region, In: *Color Atlas of Dental Medicine.Radiology*, K.H. Rateitschak, H.F. Wolf, (ed),71-80,Thieme, ISBN 3-13-78901-6,USA.

Şahin, S, Saygun, NI, Çanakçı, CF, Öngürü, Ö. & Altug HA. (2009). Root canal treatment failure mediated lateral radicular cyst: Case report. *T Klin J Dental Sciences*, Vol.15. pp: 214-219 ISSN 1300-7734

Scholl, RJ, Kellett, HM, Neumann, DP. & Lurie, AG. (1999). Cysts and cystic lesions of the mandible: clinical and radiologic-histopathologic review. *Radiographics* Vol.19. pp:1107-24 ISSN 0271 5333

Sumer, M, Gunduz, K, Sumer, AP. & Gunhan O. (2006). Benign cementoblastom A case report. *Med Oral Patol Oral Cir Bucal.* Vol. 11. pp:e483-4855. ISSN 1698-6946

Summerlin, DJ. & Tomich, CE. (1994). Focal cemento-osseous dysplasia: a clinico-pathologic study of 221 cases. *Oral Surg Oral Med Oral Patho Oral Radiol Endod,* Vol. 78. pp:611–20, ISSN 1079-2104

Weber, AL. (1993). Imaging of the cyst and odontogenic tumors of the jaw. Definition and classification. *Radiol Clin North Am*, Vol.31,pp:101-120, ISSN 0033 8389

Whaites, E. (2002). Periapical Radiograph, In: *Essential of Dental Radiograhy and Radiology,* 75-100, Harcourt Publihers Limited, ISBN 0443-07027-X, China

White, SC.& Pharoah, MJ. (2004). Intraoral Radiographic Examinations, In :*Oral Radiology : Principles and Interpratation,* 121-126, Mosby, ISBN 978-0-323-02001-5, China

Wood, NK., Goaz PW., Jacobs MC. (1997). Periapical Radiolucencies, In : *Differential Diagnosis of Oral and Maxillofacial Lesions,* N.K. Wood, P.W. Goaz, (Ed), 252-279,Mosby, ISBN 0-8151 9432-3, St Louis, USA

# 11

# Fast MRI Methods for the Clinical Evaluation of Skeletal Disorders

Renato Toffanin[1], Giuseppe Guglielmi[2,3] and Maria A. Cova[4]
[1]*Advanced Research Centre for Health, Environment and Space (ARCHES)*
[2]*Dept. of Radiology, Casa Sollievo della Sofferenza, IRCCS*
[3]*Dept. of Radiology, University of Foggia*
[4]*Dept. of Radiology, University of Trieste*
*Italy*

## 1. Introduction

Evaluation of specific magnetic resonance (MR) parameters of the skeletal system holds great potential for the accurate clinical assessment of degenerative changes occurring in bone and soft tissues at different anatomical sites. MR imaging of the water in a joint can provide anatomical information about all the soft tissues within the synovial sac (articular cartilage, meniscus, ligaments, synovial fluid) and surrounding it (muscles, tendons, vascular structures). Importantly too, MRI of the water-plus-fat can provide information pertaining both to the bone density and trabecular architecture. Recent developments have led to combinations of scan protocols and image-measurement software such that MRI can be used to evaluate the spatial distribution of specific relaxation parameters and thus detect, assess, and quantify the many pathologic processes affecting the skeletal tissues. In the articular cartilage of knee, for example, gradual deterioration of the chondral tissue leads to progressive increases in the transverse relaxation time (T2) of the water protons (David-Vaudey, 2004; Dunn et al., 2004; Apprich et al., 2010). Similarly, bone loss in the calcaneus of patients with varying degrees of osteopenia and osteoporosis causes a prolongation of the effective transverse relaxation time (T2*) of the bone marrow protons (Wehrli et al., 1995; Damilakis et al, 2004). Nonetheless, standard scan protocols for quantitative MRI are relatively slow and, therefore, not suitable for routine clinical applications. Faster methods would highly enhance their applicability in the clinical evaluation of skeletal disorders.

The purpose of this chapter is to provide a perspective on fast MRI methods for the non-invasive assessment of the skeletal status and their relevance to the diagnosis of osteoporosis and osteoarthritis, two major public health burdens (Hannan et al., 2001; Theis et al., 2007). The emphasis lies on echo-planar imaging (EPI)-based sequences (Tsao, 2010) for the accurate evaluation of pathologic processes affecting bone marrow and cartilage at different anatomical locations. A multi-shot EPI sequence is proposed for the fast T2* mapping of the lumbar bone marrow while a gradient- and spin-echo (GRASE) sequence is suggested for the fast T2 mapping of patellar articular cartilage. The description of these fast acquisition techniques is followed by a presentation of two in vivo feasibility studies on a clinical 1.5 T MRI scanner. These investigations demonstrate that the proposed MRI methods can produce relaxation maps of specific skeletal sites in just a few minutes, and with mean values comparable with data obtained using conventional sequences. Their potential application in the clinical evaluation of osteoporosis and osteoarthritis is also discussed.

## 2. Fast MRI techniques

Transverse relaxation is the result of random interactions at the atomic and molecular levels (Abragam, 1961). This physical phenomenon is primarily related to the intrinsic field caused by adjacent protons (spins) and hence is called spin-spin relaxation. Transverse relaxation causes irreversible dephasing of the transverse magnetization. There is also a reversible bulk field dephasing effect caused by local field inhomogeneities, and its characteristic time is referred to as T2* relaxation. These additional dephasing fields come from the main magnetic field inhomogeneity, the differences in magnetic susceptibility among various tissues or materials, chemical shift, and gradients applied for spatial encoding (Mugler, 2006). This dephasing can be eliminated by using a 180° pulse, as in a spin-echo sequence. Therefore, in a spin-echo sequence, only the 'true' T2 relaxation is seen. In gradient-echo sequences, there is no 180° refocusing pulse, and these dephasing effects are not eliminated. Hence, transverse relaxation in gradient-echo sequences (i.e., T2* relaxation) is a combination of 'true' T2 relaxation and relaxation caused by magnetic field inhomogeneities.

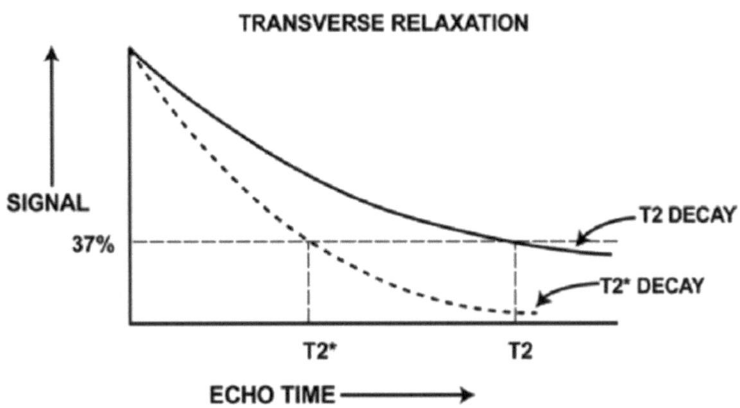


Fig. 1. A diagram showing the T2 and T2* relaxation decay curves

In order to obtain an accurate estimate of the transverse relaxation decay curves several images obtained at different echo times are generally required. The gold standard for T2 acquisition is likely to be a single slice single echo sequence (*i.e.* spin-echo sequence), repeated at several echo times, with long TR. A major improvement of the spin-echo technique is represented by the turbo spin-echo (TSE) sequence, of which a simplified diagram is depicted in Fig. 2.

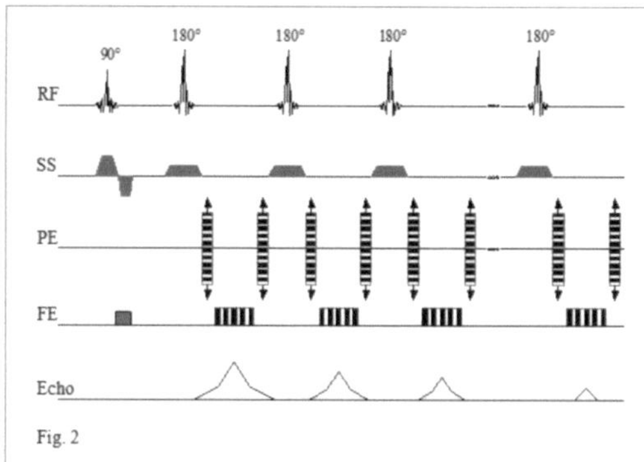


Fig. 2. A simplified diagram for the turbo spin-echo pulse sequence. RF: radiofrequency pulse, SS: slice selection gradient, PE: phase encoding gradient, FE: frequency encoding gradient

This sequence is based on multi-echo multi-shot (MEMS) (Mehlkopf et al., 1984) and rapid acquisition with relaxation enhancement (RARE) (Hennig et al., 1986) sequences and provides T2-weighted images at fractions of the acquisition time of the conventional spin-echo images. By applying multiple refocusing 180° RF pulses after the first echo, additional spin echoes can be generated. Between each successive echo, the phase-encoding gradients can be used to prepare the spins for different lines in k-space. Thus, multiple lines in k-space can be sampled per excitation. Each echo in the readout train is progressively weaker, as defined by the T2 decay.

Another method of decreasing image acquisition time is by echo-planar imaging (EPI) (Mansfield, 1977). In EPI multiple lines of k-space are acquired through a multiple-echo readout. However, in EPI signals are produced by rapid switching of gradient polarity in place of the slower selective 180° RF pulses. In this way, EPI can produce an image in less than 100 ms. However, in EPI sequences, since the multiple echoes are refocused by gradients and not by 180° pulses, there is more effect of T2* decay and other artefacts. Therefore, both spin-echo and gradient-echo EPI sequences may be applied for the fast evaluation of the T2* relaxation.

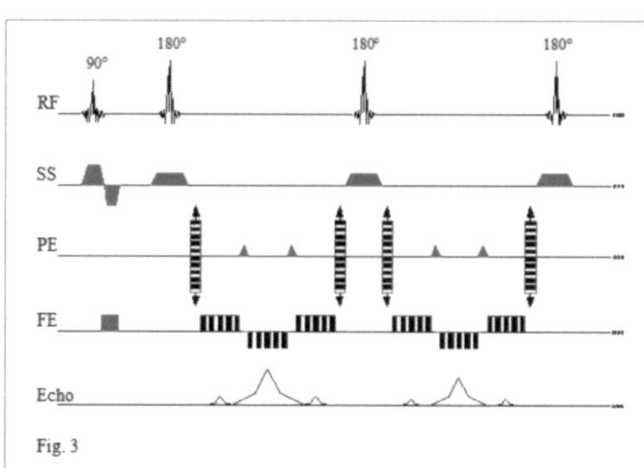


Fig. 3. A simplified diagram for the GRASE (gradient- and spin-echo) pulse sequence

By combining the TSE and EPI methods, the GRASE (gradient- and spin-echo) sequence (Fig. 3) uses a train of refocusing 180° pulses, but for each spin-echo of the readout, there are additional gradient recall echoes (Feinberg & Oshio, 1991; Oshio & Feinberg, 1991). In this sequence, each successive spin-echo is progressively weaker, as defined by T2 decay whereas the strength of the gradient recalled echoes surrounding the spin-echo is defined by the T2* decay envelope. By combining spin-echoes and short gradient-echo trains, the GRASE technique overcomes several potential problems of EPI, including large chemical shift, image distortions and signal loss from field inhomogeneity.

## 3. MRI of trabecular bone

Even though bone cannot be evaluated with most of the available MRI techniques in that they are unable to generate sufficient signal, new quantitative MRI approaches are used to study trabecular bone density and structure (Wehrli et al., 2006; Majumdar, 2008). MRI can be used to evaluate trabecular bone in a number of skeletal sites, indirectly via the protons of the bone marrow. Indeed, the presence of the trabecular bone matrix affects the signal intensity of bone marrow, an effect that is particularly pronounced with certain MRI sequences. With respect to gradient-echo acquisitions, static magnetic field inhomogeneities produced by the difference between trabecular bone and neighbouring bone marrow cause a more rapid decay of the MRI signal, which can be quantified by measuring T2*. Pioneering studies have shown that T2* is correlated with trabecular bone density (Davis et al., 1986; Rosenthal et al., 1990), and therefore, the effective transverse relaxation (T2*) is shorter in normal trabecular bone than in the less dense trabecular structures of osteoporotic bone tissue. It has also been shown that bone marrow T2* reflects the orientation of the trabeculae and correlates with their mechanical strength (Chung et al., 1993; Jergas et al., 1995). These characteristics make MRI a fundamental tool in evaluating the quality of spongy bone and increase the ability of the technique not only in identifying occult fractures but also in making possible a more accurate prediction of fracture risk.

T2* relaxometry has been conducted at several sites of both axial and peripheral skeleton (Funke et al., 1994; Grampp et al., 1995; Link et al., 1998). The preferred site for quantitative MRI studies is the calcaneus in that it is mostly composed of spongy bone (95%). Therefore quantitative MRI of the calcaneus is extremely sensitive in identifying changes in bone quality that are not revealed by bone mineral densitometry. In one MRI study at 1.5 T that examined 68 women with different degrees of vertebral deformity (Wehrli et al., 2002), it was demonstrated that of the various areas of the calcaneus examined, the subtalar region was best able to discriminate patients with fracture from those without. The authors of this study also demonstrated that the R2* (1/T2*) is sensitive to changes in bone quality that were not identified with BMD.

Trabecular bone is also prominent in the vertebral body (up to 90%). The spine certainly represents the most critical skeletal site for quantitative MRI since vertebral fractures are the most common type of osteoporotic fractures (Wasnisch, 1999). In one MRI investigation done at 1.5 T on a group of 54 postmenopausal women, T2* mapping of the lumbar spine was shown to be capable of differentiating between healthy subjects and subjects with low energy fractures (Damilakis et al., 2004).

The use of T2* relaxometry can certainly promote the application of quantitative MRI in the diagnosis of osteoporosis. Nonetheless, MRI protocols commonly applied to estimate T2* in bone marrow are relatively slow and, therefore, not suitable for routine clinical application. In one recent study on the calcaneus of six healthy volunteers, Toffanin et al. (2006) demonstrated the possibility of ultrafast T2* mapping of the bone marrow both at 1.5 and 3 T. To obtain an accurate estimate of T2* at 3.0 T or higher magnetic fields, corrective measures may be required during postprocessing to minimise local field variations ($\Delta B0$) responsible for signal loss and consequent overestimation of the R2* relaxation rate (1/T2*). In the method proposed by Dahnke and Schaeffter (2005), the main field heterogeneity is derived from T2* calculated on more than one slice and is used as an initial value for interactive optimisation, with which the relaxation signal is corrected for each voxel.

### 3.1 Fast T2* mapping of the lumbar bone marrow

The feasibility of a multi-shot gradient-echo EPI sequence for the fast T2* mapping of the lumbar bone marrow was evaluated by our research team on a commercial clinical 1.5 T MRI scanner located in the Department of Radiology of the Cattinara Hospital at the University of Trieste. The MRI trial was performed on 21 subjects (8 males and 13 females) referred to the hospital for low back pain. Five slices were acquired to image the lumbar spine in the sagittal plane and the L2 vertebral body in the axial plane. In both cases, a fast field-echo (FFE) multi-shot EPI sequence was applied with removed blip gradients in order to apply the same phase encoding to all gradient echoes The overall examination time was approximately 5 minutes. The main acquisition parameters are summarised in Table 1.

| | Sagittal plane | Axial plane |
|---|---|---|
| TR | 400 ms | 400 ms |
| TEmin | 2.0 ms | 2.0 ms |
| TEmax | 15.8 ms | 15.8 ms |
| EPI factor | 25 | 25 |
| Flip angle | 30° | 30° |
| FOV | 300 mm × 300 mm | 200 mm × 200 mm |
| Matrix | 320 × 320 | 224 × 224 |
| Slice thickness | 5 mm | 5 mm |
| No. of slices | 5 | 5 |

Table 1. Acquisition parameters of the fast field-echo multi-shot EPI sequence used for fast T2* mapping of the lumbar bone marrow at 1.5 T

Estimation of the T2* relaxation time was performed on one manually-defined region drawn on the entire L2 vertebral body as shown in Fig. 4. The multi-shot EPI sequence produced T2* maps with mean values comparable with previous data obtained with conventional sequences (Fig. 5). The mean T2* measured in the sagittal plane (14.2 ± 3.9 ms) was slightly lower than that measured in the axial plane (14.7 ±3.9 ms) but no statistically significant difference was observed ($P < 0.05$).

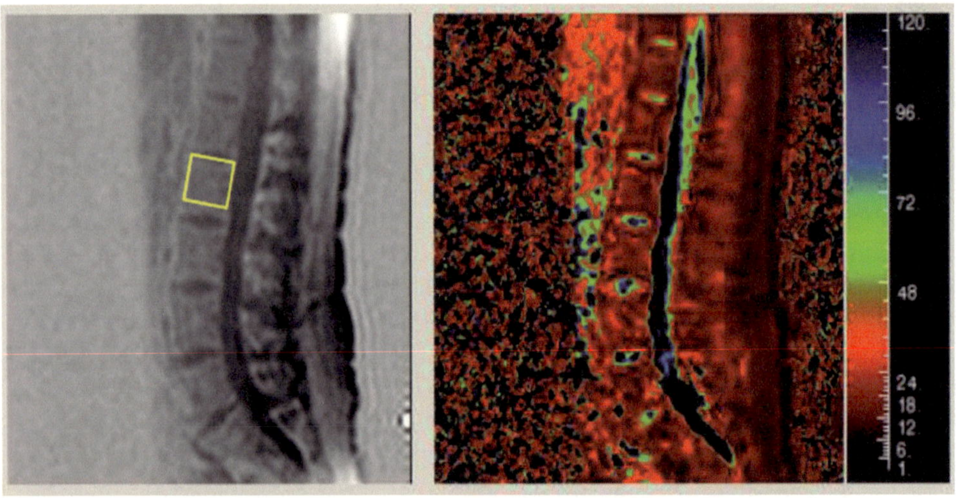


(a)

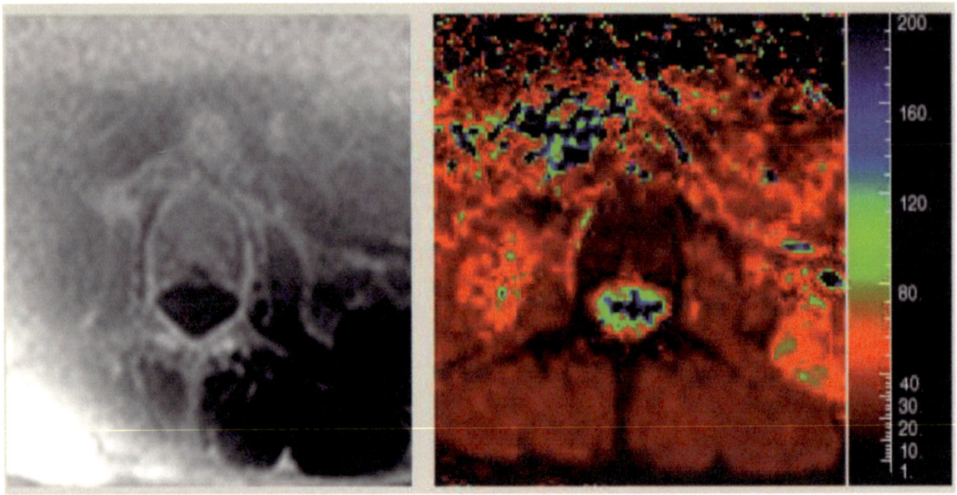


(b)

Fig. 4. T2* maps of the central slice of the L2 vertebra generated from sagittal (a) and axial (b) images by means of a monoexponential fitting algorithm as described by Dahnke & Schaeffter (2005). The mean T2* was measured over the entire vertebral body excluding the cortical bone

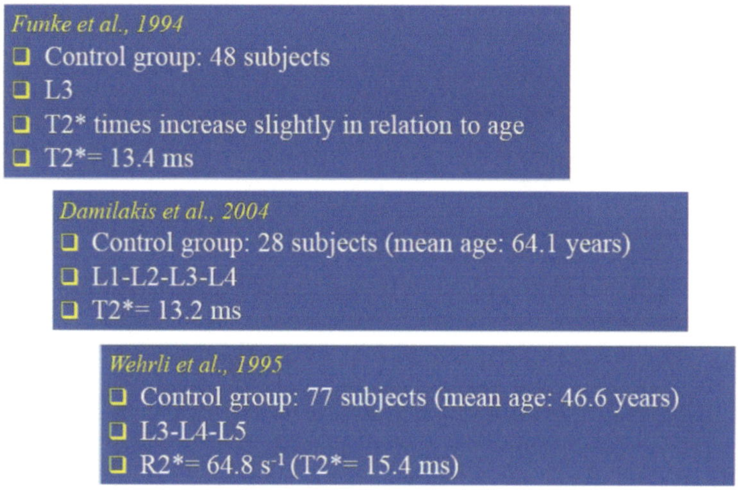


Fig. 5. Overview of the T2* data previously obtained with conventional sequences

These results indicate that fast T2* mapping of the lumbar bone marrow is feasible on a 1.5 T scanner. However, further studies are required to investigate the full potential of the proposed approach in the clinical evaluation of osteoporosis.

## 4. MRI of articular cartilage

Articular cartilage, is one of the types of hyaline cartilage that persists throughout adult life. Basically, it comprises chondrocytes incorporated in an extracellular matrix composed mainly of water, collagen II fibrils and proteoglycans (Seibel et al., 2004). Despite its simple appearance, this tissue hides various modifications in respect of the original cartilage that make it a singular structure. The articular cartilage is, in fact, stratified and classically, four distinct layers are described from the surface to the interior: tangential, transitional, radial and calcified, respectively (Fig. 6). Both morphological and biochemical information can be obtained by MRI, which is probably the most accurate imaging modality in evaluating the state of hyaline cartilage (Disler et al., 2000; Cova & Toffanin, 2002). Apart from clinical MRI protocols that depict cartilage morphology, there is a growing interest in developing quantitative MRI approaches that are sensitive to its early structural changes (Burstein et al., 2000; Mosher & Dardzinski, 2004).

Over the past years, quantification of the human articular cartilage has been performed using T1, T1ρ and T2 relaxation time constants as well as the magnetization transfer ratio (Toffanin et al., 2001; Menezes et al., 2004; Wheaton et al., 2005). One of the magnetic parameter that is currently evaluated for studying cartilage damage is the transverse relaxation time (T2), whose relaxation mechanism results dominated by the dipolar interaction between water molecules and collagen (Mlynárik et al., 2004) In this regard, dual-echo or multi-echo sequences are typically employed for quantitative T2 mapping. Nonetheless, faster quantitative MRI techniques are required in order to allow the introduction of T2 mapping in routine clinical protocols.

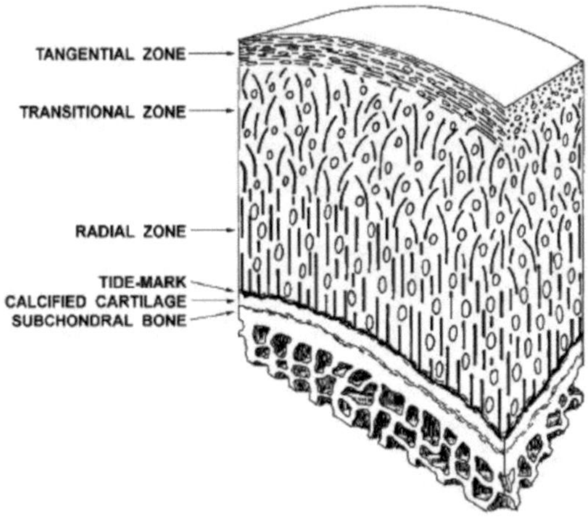


Fig. 6. Histological zones in hyaline cartilage. Collagen fibres are parallel to the surface in the superficial (tangential) zone, curved in the intermediate (transitional) zone and perpendicular to subchondral bone in the deep (radial) zone (From Cova & Toffanin, 2002. Reprinted with permission).

### 4.1 Fast T2 mapping of the patellar articular cartilage

Recently, we have devoted particular attention to optimising specific quantitative MRI protocols for the fast T2 mapping of knee cartilage. The focus was on the gradient- and spin-echo (GRASE) sequence able to produce a set of T2-weighted images in less than 2 minutes. Also this research study was conducted on a commercial clinical 1.5 T MRI scanner located in the Department of Radiology of the Cattinara Hospital at the University of Trieste. The feasibility of the proposed approach was assessed on 35 patients (21 males and 14 females) with moderate degree of patellar osteoarthritis. (Quaia et al., 2008).

For each patient, transverse GRASE and TSE images of patellar cartilage were acquired using the scan protocols summarised in Table 2.

| | GRASE | TSE |
|---|---|---|
| TR | 3,000 ms | 3,000 ms |
| $TE_{min}$ | 15 ms | 15 ms |
| $TE_{max}$ | 120 ms | 120 ms |
| EPI factor | 3 | - |
| Turbo factor | 8 | 8 |
| FOV | 80 mm × 80 mm | 80 mm × 80 mm |
| Matrix | 128 × 128 | 128 × 128 |
| Slice thickness | 3 mm | 3 mm |
| No. of slices | 10 | 10 |
| Total scan time | 1 min 51 s | 5 min 52 s |

Table 2. Acquisition parameters of the GRASE and TSE sequences used for fast T2 mapping of the patellar articular cartilage at 1.5 T

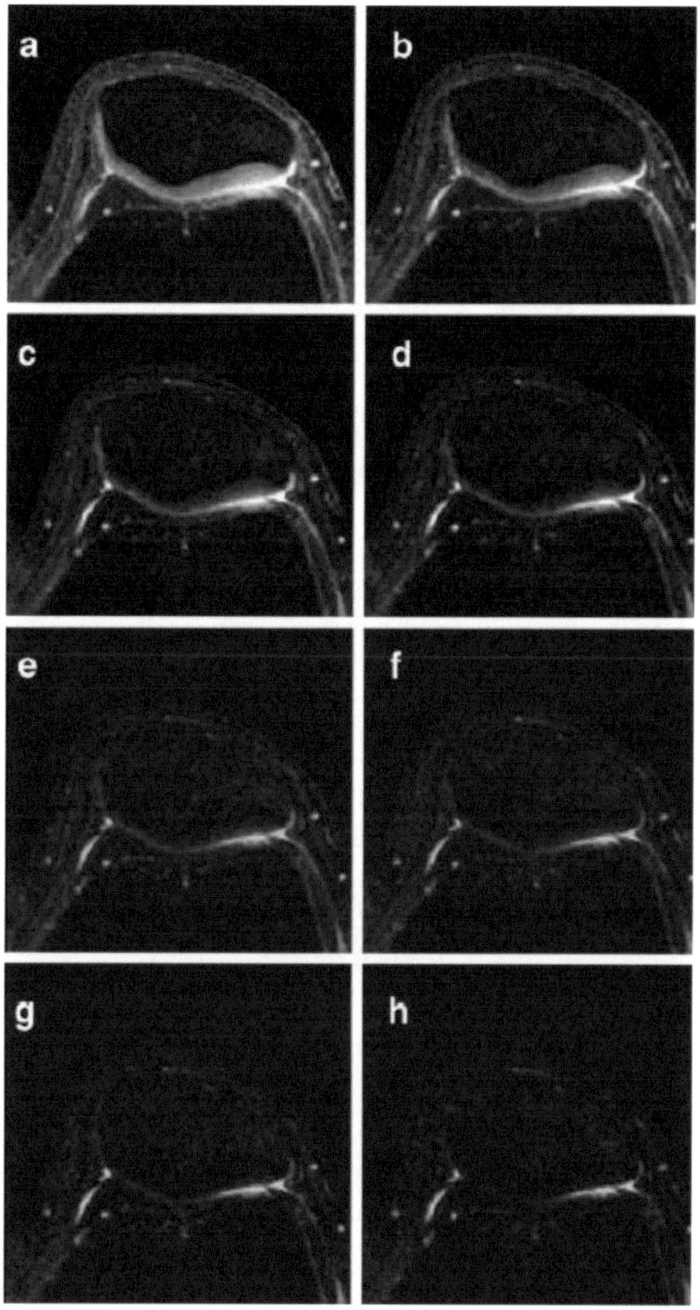


Fig. 7. a–h. Axial GRASE images of patella cartilage (TR/$TE_{min}$-$TE_{max}$: 3,000/15–120 ms); a: 15 ms, b: 30 ms, c: 45 ms, d: 60 ms, e: 75 ms, f: 90 ms, g: 105 ms, h: 120 ms. There is a clear decay in the signal intensity of the patellar articular cartilage at longer TE, which can be visually observed. The T2 relaxation time constant was calculated from a linear least-square fit to the logarithm of the image intensity data (From Quaia et al., 2008. Reprinted with permission).

Estimation of T2 was performed on one manually-defined region drawn on the entire patella cartilage as shown in Fig. 8.

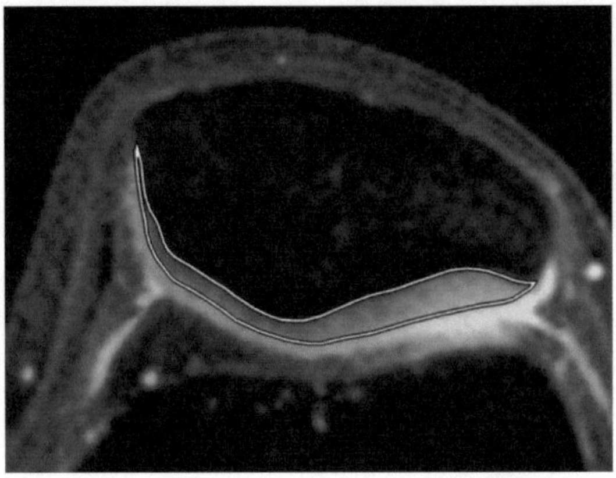

Fig. 8. Axial GRASE image of patella cartilage (TR/TE: 3,000/15 ms). A manually defined ROI is drawn on the entire patellar articular cartilage for the quantification of the global T2 relaxation time. The ROI includes the entire cartilage, encompassing both the deep cartilage close to the subchondral bone and the superficial cartilage, and the edges of the joint surface (From Quaia et al., 2008. Reprinted with permission).

| Patient No. | GRASE | TSE | Arthroscopic grading |
|---|---|---|---|
| 1 | 44.0±10.0 | 43.5±8.0 | 2B |
| 2 | 48.3±8.0 | 47.2±6.0 | 2B |
| 3 | 25.5±9.0 | 26.3±7.5 | 0 |
| 4 | 38.1±7.0 | 38.4±6.0 | 1 |
| 7 | 45.2±6.0 | 46.3±7.0 | 3A |
| 12 | 30.5±8.0 | 31.0±6.0 | 2A |
| 18 | 35.5±8.0 | 37.2±8.0 | 1 |
| 20 | 39.2±7.0 | 38.5±6.0 | 2A |
| 27 | 28.5±6.0 | 29.0±9.0 | 0 |
| 28 | 58.2±6.0 | 57.2±11.0 | 3A |
| 35 | 61.2±11.0 | 64.3±10.0 | 3B |

Table 3. Mean T2 values for patellar articular cartilage obtained from the GRASE and TSE images of the patellar articular cartilage of selected patients together with the corresponding arthroscopic grading[1].

[1] Osteoarthritis from anteroposterior radiographs was graded according to the Kellgren–Lawrence scoring system (0=no osteoarthritic features; 1=minute osteophytes of doubtful importance; 2=definite osteophytes without reduction of the joint space; 3=reduction of the joint space; 4=greatly reduced joint space and sclerosis of the subchondral bone) (Kellgren & Lawrence, 1957).

In our series the GRASE sequence provided T2 values slightly lower than those obtained by the TSE sequence in most patients. This may relate to T2* decay present in the GRASE sequence. Indeed, a potential drawback of the GRASE sequence is the possible presence of artefacts due to the echo-planar imaging readout module that may lead to pronounced chemical shift, image distortion, and signal loss from magnetic field inhomogeneity. Nonetheless, differences in T2 values within deep and superficial cartilage were in line with those observed with other MR sequences (Van Breuseghem et al., 2004). They are related to cartilage T2 anisotropy determined by the different direction of the collagen fibres in the superficial and deep cartilage with respect to the static magnetic field (Mosher et al., 2001).

## 5. Conclusion

The above MRI methods can drastically reduce the scan time for measuring the spatial distribution of specific relaxation parameters in bone and cartilage. They may become more widely adopted, being applied either with other imaging techniques or in isolation, to better evaluate skeletal disorders, identify early tissue degeneration, tailor therapeutic interventions and follow treatment response.

## 6. Acknowledgment

This work was supported in part by a grant from the Italian Ministry for Education, University and Research (5 per mille 2009).

## 7. References

Abragam, A. (1983). *The Principles of Nuclear Magnetism* (2nd edition), Oxford University Press, ISBN 978-0-19-852014-6, New York

Apprich, S.; Welsch, G.H.; Mamisch, T.C.; Szomolányi, P.; Mayerhoefer, M.; Pinker, K. & Trattnig, S. (2010). Detection of degenerative cartilage disease: comparison of high-resolution morphological MR and quantitative T2 mapping at 3.0 Tesla. *Osteoarthritis and Cartilage*, Vol.18, No.9, pp. 1211-1217, ISSN 1063-4584

Burstein, D.; Bashir, A. & Gray, M.L. (2000). MRI techniques in early stages of cartilage disease. *Investigative Radiology*, Vol.35, No.10, pp. 622-638, ISSN 0020-9996

Chung, H.; Wehrli, F.W.; Williams, J.L. & Kugelmass, S.D. (1993). Relationship between NMR transverse relaxation, trabecular bone architecture, and strength. *Proceedings of the National Academy of Sciences U.S.A.*, Vol.90, No.21, pp. 10250-10254, ISSN 0027-8424

Cova, M. & Toffanin, R. (2002). MR microscopy of hyaline cartilage: current status. *European Radiology*, Vol.12, No.4, pp. 814-823, ISSN 0938-7994

Dahnke, H. & Schaeffter, T. (2005). Limits of detection of SPIO at 3.0 T using T2* relaxometry. *Magnetic Resonance in Medicine*, Vol.53, No.5, pp 1202-1206, ISSN 0740-3194

Damilakis, J.; Maris, T.; Papadokostakis, G.; Sideri, L. & Gourtsoyiannis, N. (2004). Discriminatory ability of magnetic resonance T2* measurements in a sample of postmenopausal women with low-energy fractures. A comparison with phalangeal speed of sound and dual X-ray absorptiometry. *Investigative Radiology*, Vol.39, No.11, pp. 706-712, ISSN 0020-9996

David-Vaudey, E.; Ghosh, S.; Ries, M. & Majumdar, S. (2004). T2 relaxation time measurements in osteoarthritis. *Magnetic Resonance Imaging*, Vol.22, No.5, pp. 673–682, ISSN 0730-725X

Davis, C.A.; Genant, H.K. & Dunham, J.S. (1986). The effects of bone on proton NMR relaxation times surrounding liquids. *Investigative Radiology*, Vol.21, No.6, pp. 472–477, ISSN 0033-8419

Disler, D.G.; Recht, M.P. & McCauley, T.R. (2000). MR imaging of articular cartilage. *Skeletal Radiology*, Vol.29, No.7, pp. 367-377, ISSN 0364-2348

Dunn, T.C.; Lu, Y.; Jin, H.; Ries, M.D. & Majumdar, S. (2004). T2 relaxation time of cartilage at MR imaging: comparison with severity of knee osteoarthritis. *Radiology*, Vol.232, No.2, pp. 592–598, ISSN 0033-8419

Feinberg, D.A. & Oshio, K. (1991). GRASE (Gradient- and spin-echo) MR imaging: a new fast clinical imaging technique. *Radiology*, Vol.181, No.2, pp. 597-602, ISSN 0033-8419

Funke, M.; Bruhn, H.; Vosshenrich, R.; Rudolph, O. & Grabbe, E. (1994). The determination of the T2* relaxation time for characterizing trabecular bone. *Rofo-Fortschritte auf dem Gebiet der Röntgenstrahlen und der Bildgebenden Verfahren*, Vol.161, No.1, pp. 58-63, ISSN 1438-9029

Grampp, S.; Majumdar, S.; Jergas, M. Lang P, Gies, A. & Genant, H.K. (1995). MRI of bone marrow in the distal radius: in vivo precision of effective transverse relaxation times. *European Radiology*, Vol.5, No.1, pp. 43-48, ISSN 0938-7994

Guglielmi, G.; Biccari, N.; Mangano, F. & Toffanin, R. (2010). 3 T magnetic resonance imaging of the musculoskeletal system. *La Radiologia Medica*, Vol.115, No.4, pp. 571-584, ISSN: 0033-8362

Hannan, H.L.; Magaziner, J.; Wang, J.J.; Eastwood, E.A.; Silberzweig, S.B.; Gilbert, M.; Morrison, R.S.; McLaughlin, M.A.; Orosz, G.M. & Siu, A.L. (2001). Mortality and locomotion 6 months after hospitalization for hip fracture: risk factors and risk-adjusted hospital outcomes. *JAMA*, Vol.285, No.21, pp. 2736-2742, ISSN 00987484

Hennig, J.; Nauerth, A. & Friedburg, H. (1986). RARE imaging: a fast imaging method for clinical MR. *Magnetic Resonance in Medicine*, Vol.3, No.6, pp. 823-833, ISSN 0740-3194

Jergas, M.D.; Majumdar, S.; Keyak, J.H.; Lee, I.Y.; Newitt, D.C.; Grampp, S.; Skinner, H.B. & Genant, H.K. (1995). Relationship between young modulus of elasticity, ash density, and MRI derived effective transverse relaxation T2* in tibial specimens. *Journal of Computed Assisted Tomography*, Vol.19, No.3, pp. 472–479, ISSN 0363-8715

Kellgren, J. & Lawrence, J. (1957). Radiological assessment of osteoarthritis. *Annals of the Rheumatic Diseases* Vol.16, No.4, pp. 494–502, ISSN 00034967

Link, T.; Majumdar, S.; Augat, P.; Lin, J.C.; Newitt, D.; Lane, N.E. & Genant, H.K. (1998). Proximal femur: assessment for osteoporosis with T2* decay characteristics at MR imaging. *Radiology*, Vol.209, No.2, pp. 531-536, ISSN 0033-8419

Majumdar, S. (2008). Magnetic resonance imaging for osteoporosis. *Skeletal Radiology*, Vol.37, No.2, pp. 95–97, ISSN 0364-2348

Mansfield, P. (1977). Multi-planar imaging formation using NMR spin-echo. *Journal of Physics C: Solid State Physics*, Vol.10, pp. L55-L58, ISSN 0022-3719

Mehlkopf, A.F.; van der Meulen, P. & Smidt, J. (1984). A multiple-echo and multiple-shot sequence for fast NMR-Fourier imaging. *Magnetic Resonance in Medicine*, Vol.1, No.2, pp. 295-297, ISSN 0740-3194

Menezes, N.M.; Grey, M.L.; Hartke, J.R. & Burstein, D. (2004). T2 and T1(rho) MRI in articular cartilage systems. *Magnetic Resonance in Medicine*, Vol.51, No.3, pp. 503–509, ISSN 0740-3194

Mlynárik, V.; Szomolányi, P.; Toffanin, R.; Vittur, F. & Trattnig, S. (2004). Transverse relaxation mechanisms in articular cartilage. *Journal of Magnetic Resonance*, Vol.169, No.2, pp. 300-307, ISSN 1090-7807

Mosher, T.J.; Smith, H.; Dardzinski, B.J.; Schmithorst, V.J. & Smith, M.B. (2001). MR imaging and T2 mapping of femoral cartilage: in vivo determination of the magic angle effect. *AJR American Journal of Roentgenology*, Vol.177, No.3, pp. 665–669, ISSN 0361-803X

Mosher, T.J. & Dardzinski, B.J. (2004). Cartilage MRI T2 relaxation time mapping: overview and applications. *Seminars in Musculoskeletal Radiology*, Vol.8, No.4, pp. 355-368, ISSN 1089-7860

Mugler, J.P. III. (2006). Basic principles. In: *Clinical Magnetic Resonance Imaging*, Edelman, R.R.; Hesselink, J.R.; Zlatkin, M.B.; Crues, J.V., Editors, pp. 23–57, Elsevier, ISBN 978-0721603063, Philadelphia

Oshio, K. & Feinberg, D.A. (1991). GRASE (Gradient- and Spin-Echo) imaging: a novel fast MRI technique. *Magnetic Resonance in Medicine*, Vol.20, No.2, pp. 344-349, ISSN 0740-3194

Quaia, E.; Toffanin, R.; Guglielmi, G.; Ukmar, M.; Rossi, A.; Martinelli, B. & Cova, M.A. (2008). T2 mapping of the patellar articular cartilage with gradient and spin-echo magnetic resonance imaging at 1.5 T: validation and initial clinical experience in patients with osteoarthritis. *Skeletal Radiology*, Vol.37, No.6, pp. 511-517, ISSN 0364-2348

Rosenthal, H.; Thulborn, K.R.; Rosenthal, D.I.; Kim, S.H. & Rosen, B.R. (1990). Magnetic susceptibility effects of trabecular bone on magnetic resonance bone marrow imaging. *Investigative Radiology*, Vol.25; No.2, pp. 173–178, ISSN 0020-9996

Seibel, M.J.; Robins, S.P. & Bilezikian, J.P. (Eds.). (2004). *Dynamics of Bone and Cartilage Metabolism*, Academic Press, ISBN 978-0-12-088562-6, San Diego, USA

Theis, K.A.; Murphy, L.; Hootman, J.M.; Helmick, C.G. & Yelin, E. (2007). Prevalence and correlates of arthritis-attributable work limitation in the US population among persons ages 18-64: 2002 National Health Interview Survey Data. *Arthritis & Rheumatism*, Vol.57, No.3, pp. 355-363, ISSN 1529-0131

Toffanin, R.; Mlynárik, V.; Russo, S.; Szomolányi, P.; Piras, A. & Vittur, F. (2001). Proteoglycan depletion and MR parameters of articular cartilage. *Archives of Biochemistry and Biophysics*, Vol.390, No.2, pp. 235–242, ISSN 0003-9861

Toffanin, R.; Cadioli, M.; Scotti, G. & Cova, M.A. (2006). Ultrafast T2* mapping of bone marrow at 1.5 Tesla and 3.0 Tesla. *Proceedings of the 14th Annual Meeting of the International Society for Magnetic Resonance in Medicine*, p. 3631, Seattle, Washington, USA, May 6-12, 2006, ISSN 1545-4428

Tsao, J. (2010). Ultrafast imaging: principles, pitfalls, solutions, and applications. *Journal of Magnetic Resonance Imaging*, Vol.32, No.2, pp. 252-266, ISSN 1053-1807

Van Breuseghem, I.; Bosmans, H.T.; Elst, L.V.; Maes, F.; Pans, S.D.; Brys, P.P.; Geusens, E.A. & Marchal, G.J. (2004). T2 mapping of human femorotibial cartilage with turbo mixed MR imaging at 1.5 T: feasibility. *Radiology*, Vol.233, No.2, pp. 609–614, ISSN 0033-8419

Wasnich, R.D. (1999). Incidence Rates for Vertebral, Wrist & Hip Fractures in Women after Age 50. In: *Primer on the Metabolic Bone Diseases and Disorders of Mineral Metabolism.*

(4th edition), Murray, F.J., Editor, pp. 257–259, Lippincott, Williams & Wilkins, ISBN 978-0781720380, Philadelphia

Wehrli, F.W.; Hilaire, L.; Fernández-Seara, M; Gomberg, B.R.; Song, H.K.; Zemel, B.; Loh, L. & Snyder, P.J. (2002). Quantitative magnetic resonance imaging in the calcaneus and femur of women with varying degrees of osteopenia and vertebral deformity status. *Journal of Bone Mineral Research*, Vol.17, No.12, pp. 2265–2273, ISSN 0884-0431

Wehrli, F.W.; Ford, J.C. & Haddad, J.G. (1995). Osteoporosis: clinical assessment wit quantitative MR imaging in diagnosis. *Radiology*, Vol.196, No.3, pp. 631-641, ISSN 0033-8419

Wehrli, F.W.; Song, H.K.; Saha, P.K. & Wright, A.C. (2006). Quantitative MRI for the assessment of bone structure and function. *NMR in Biomedicine*, Vol.19, No.7, pp. 731–776, ISSN 0952-3480

Wheaton, A.J.; Dodge, G.R.; Borthakur, A.; Kneeland, J.B.; Schumacher, H.R. & Reddy, R. (2005). Detection of changes in articular cartilage proteoglycan by T1(rho) magnetic resonance imaging. *Journal of Orthopaedic Research*, Vol.23, No.1, pp. 102–108, ISSN 0736-0266

12

# Determination of Cardiac Ejection Fraction by Electrical Impedance Tomography

Franciane C. Peters[1], Luis Paulo da S. Barra[2] and Rodrigo W. dos Santos[2]
[1]*Federal University of Rio de Janeiro*
[2]*Federal University of Juiz de Fora*
*Brazil*

## 1. Introduction

Cardiac ejection fraction is a clinical parameter that infers the efficiency of the heart as a pump. The ejection fraction of left ventricle (EFLV) and right ventricle (EFRV) are determined separately. However, the clinical use of EFLV is more common and it is frequently called ejection fraction (EF). By definition, the ejection fraction is calculated in the following way:

$$EF = \frac{PV}{EDV} = \frac{EDV - ESV}{EDV}, \tag{1}$$

where $PV$ is the volume of blood pumped, that is given by the difference between the end-diastolic volume ($EDV$) and the end-systolic volume ($ESV$). Cardiac ejection fraction is a relevant parameter because it is highly correlated to the functional status of the heart. To determine the EF, different non-invasive techniques can be used, like echocardiography, cardiac magnetic resonance and computed tomography. However, they are not suitable for continuous monitoring. In this work, we numerically evaluate a new method for the continuous estimation of cardiac ejection fraction based on Electrical Impedance Tomography (EIT).

EIT is a technique that reconstructs an image of the electrical resistivity inside a domain based on protocols of current injection and potential measurement on the external boundary of the domain. Detailed description about the development of this technique can be found, for instance, in Cheney et al. (1999) and Holder (2005). The EIT has a large utilization on geophysics and monitoring of industrial activities (Kim et al., 2004; Park et al., 2008), as non-destructive technique to evaluate structures (Karhunen et al., 2009; Peters et al., 2010) and on biomedical engineering (Barber & Brown, 1984; Brown et al., 1985; Mello et al., 2008; Trigo et al., 2004). In this last area, the EIT has been developed to detect breast and other kinds of cancer (Choi et al., 2007; Seo et al., 2004) and to monitor lung ventilation (Adler et al., 1997; Lima et al., 2007), brain activity (Polydorides et al., 2002), heart activity (Peters et al., 2009; Zlochiver et al., 2006), among others.

The special interest of the biomedical engineering in the development of the EIT is due to its safety for monitoring long periods, since it is not based on ionizing radiation. On the other hand, the EIT spacial resolution is not as high as the traditional imaging methods.

Nevertheless, its portability, low cost and time resolution are the main advantages of the technique.

Mathematically, the EIT is classified as a non-linear inverse problem. Inverse because one wants to find the electrical resistivity of the body using measures of electrical potential on the boundary excited by known electrical current. The forward (or direct) problem related to the inverse one is to compute the electrical potential with known body resistivity and injected current. The inverse problem is non-linear, what means that there is not a linear relation between electrical resistivity and the electrical potential on the boundary. So, in general, the solution process starts with an estimated resistivity distribution and such estimative is iteratively adjusted in order to achieve an acceptable approximation for the actual resistivity distribution.

Furthermore, the inverse problem is ill-posed and ill-conditioned. In general, the number of parameters needed to represent the resistivity distribution is greater than the number of potential measures. So, in order to treat the ill-posedness of the problem, some strategies of regularization should be implemented. For instance, via the inclusion of previously known information about the resistivity distribution in the solution of the inverse problem. The problem is considered ill-conditioned because small perturbations in the measures can cause a large change in the found resistivity distribution. So, the process of image generation by EIT is very sensible to noise in the potential measures.

It is possible to see that many aspects are involved in the solution of the EIT problem and some of them were discussed in previous works of the same authors. Barra et al. (2006a) and Barra et al. (2006b) treat some computational aspects of the solution process. Peters & Barra (2009) treats the special kind of regularization also adopted here. Peters & Barra (2010) compares different measurement protocols and addresses the sensitivity of the process in the presence of noisy measures. Peters et al. (2009) presents the viability analysis of a biomedical application of the EIT. So the aim of this work is to revisit this particular biomedical application, describing all the procedures involved in the generation of a computational model based on cardiac magnetic ressonance images that allows the determination of the cardiac ejection fraction by the EIT. Preliminary results are presented and the potentialities and limitations of the proposed technique are discussed. The results suggest the proposed technique is a promising diagnostic tool that offers continuous and non-invasive estimation of cardiac ejection fraction.

## 2. Methods

Usual strategies to generate the EIT image is based on the discretization of the body in small parts (Borsic et al., 2001). Each part has an unknown parameter, its resistivity. So, to get a good image resolution, a great number of parameters is needed and the problem becomes ill-posed. In this strategy, regularization techniques are applied and after solving the inverse problem, the image obtained is modified by a limiarization process in order to get the final image.

In this work we adopted a different strategy to generate the EIT images. In order to monitor the cardiac ejection fraction, we assume that recent magnetic resonance images of the patient are available. So, this previous information allows the use of a different kind of parameterization in which the number of parameters is greatly reduced.

In this section, all the methods used to solve the EIT problem will be described. First, the parameterization based on magnetic resonance images will be explained, as well as the resistivity model of the thorax. Second, the governing equations of the forward problem will be introduced in addition to the numerical methods used to solve it. Third, the inverse problem will be formulated as a minimization problem and the adopted optimization method will be presented. Finally, the computational experiments will be reported.

### 2.1 Two-dimensional models based on magnetic resonance images

#### 2.1.1 Parameterization

From magnetic resonance (MR) images, the regions of interest, in this case the two ventricles, were manually segmented in two different phases: end of the systole and the end of diastole. Each curve of the segmentation was parameterized by a spline, with a minimum number of points. The left ventricle spline has 7 control points and the right one 8 points. The external boundary of the thorax and the boundaries of the lungs were also segmented. For simplicity, the shape and size of the thorax and the lungs are assumed constant during the heart cycle. Figure 1 shows a segmentation example.

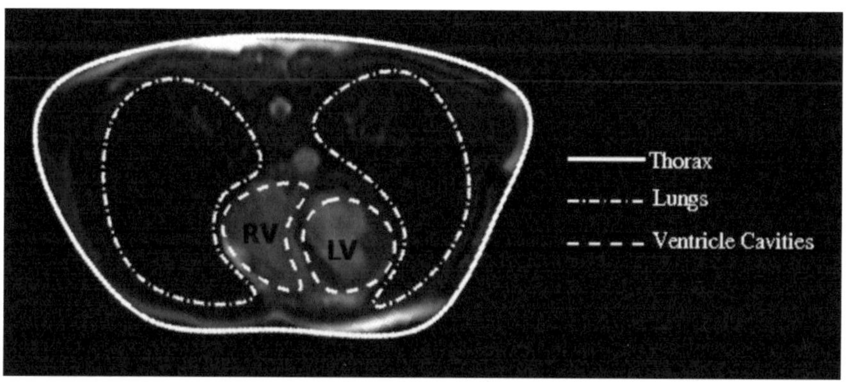


Fig. 1. Manual segmentation of an MR image. The boundaries of the lungs, ventricle cavities and thorax are represented by splines. LV and RV denotes left ventricle and right ventricle, respectively.

The goal of our method is to recover the shape of the internal cavities of the heart, presently considered in two dimensions, from electric potential measures. Therefore, with two coordinates for each control point of the spline, the methods would need to estimate a total of 30 ($(7 + 8) \times 2$) parameters. To reduce the number of parameters in half, another parameterization is used. In this, only one parameter defines the position of each control point.

During MRI segmentation we have used the same number of control points for the splines in both systolic and diastolic phase. This allows us to restrict the search space forcing that each control point $i$ belongs to a line that connects its position at systole and diastole, as shown in Fig. 2.

A linear interpolation, parameterized by a scalar $t_i$, is used between the values of the coordinates of each control point $i$. The spline relative to the end of systole can be obtained

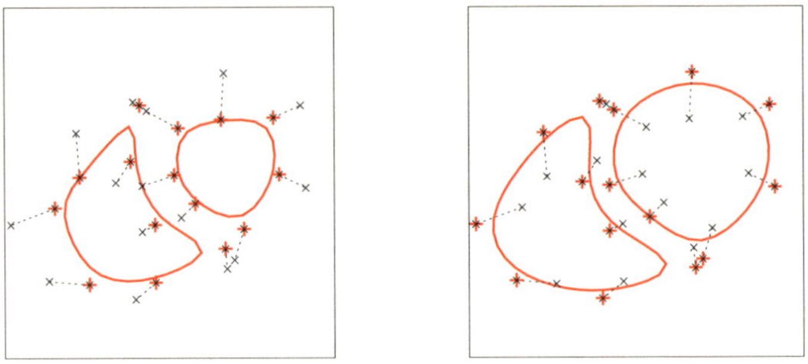

(a) Systole (b) Diastole

Fig. 2. The control points are represented by red crosses. The dashed lines are the search space.

with $t_i = 0$ for all $i$, and the one relative to the end of diastole with $t_i = 1$ for all $i$. Doing so, the method goal is to recover the shape of the ventricular cavities via the estimation of the 15 parameters $t_i$, with $i = 1, 2, ..., 15$.

### 2.1.2 Splines

Splines are mathematical models that associate a curve with a set of points named control points. Here we use a special type of spline called Extended Cross-Splines or Extended X-Splines (Blanc & Schlick, 1995), for short. In this model, each control point $i$ has the coordinates $(x_i, y_i)$ and an additional parameter $s_i \in [0,1]$ that allows the curve $C(t)$ approximates ($0 < s_i \leq 1$) or sharp interpolates ($s_i = 0$) the control point. This feature is very interesting because it allows the definition of smooth or sharp curves. In this work, just smooth curves are represented.

Considering an Extended X-Spline model in which each segment depends on four control points, a segment $C(t)$ on the parameter range $(t_{k+1}, t_{k+2})$ is defined as follows:

$$\mathbf{C}(t) = F_0\mathbf{P}_k + F_1\mathbf{P}_{k+1} + F_2\mathbf{P}_{k+2} + F_3\mathbf{P}_{k+3}\,, \tag{2}$$

where the blending functions $F_k$ are obtained by the normalization of the blending functions $A_k(t)$ as follows:

$$F_k(t) = \frac{A_k(t)}{A_0(t) + A_1(t) + A_2(t) + A_3(t)} \tag{3}$$

and their non null part can be divided in two parts, $F_k^-$, defined between $T_k^-$ and $T_k$, and $F_k^+$, defined between $T_k$ and $T_k^+$.

The functions $A_k(t)$ are obtained by the generic quintic polinomial $f_p(u)$, whose coefficients were determined in order to satisfy the constraints of the model, resulting the following expression:

$$f_p(u) = u^3\left(10 - p + (2p - 15)\,u + (6 - p)\,u^2\right)\,. \tag{4}$$

Hence, for the non null parts of the functions $A_k(t)$, we have:

$$A_0(t) = f_{p_{k-1}}(u_0)\;,\; A_1(t) = f_{p_k}(u_1)\;,\; A_2(t) = f_{p_{k+1}}(u_2)\;,\; A_3(t) = f_{p_{k+2}}(u_3) \tag{5}$$

with

$$u_0 = \frac{t - T_k^+}{t_k - T_k^+}, \; u_1 = \frac{t - T_{k+1}^+}{t_{k+1} - T_{k+1}^+}, \; u_2 = \frac{t - T_{k+2}^-}{t_{k+2} - T_{k+2}^-}, \; u_3 = \frac{t - T_{k+3}^-}{t_{k+3} - T_{k+3}^-} \tag{6}$$

and

$$p_{k-1} = 2\left(t_k - T_k^+\right)^2, \; p_k = 2\left(t_{k+1} - T_{k+1}^+\right)^2, \tag{7}$$

$$p_{k+1} = 2\left(t_{k+2} - T_{k+2}^-\right)^2, \; p_{k+2} = 2\left(t_{k+3} - T_{k+3}^-\right)^2. \tag{8}$$

The flexibility of the model is improved by the introduction of new degree of freedom $s_k$. In each control point $\mathbf{P}_k$ this new parameter affects the values $T_{k-1}^+$ e $T_{k+1}^-$ as follows:

$$T_{k-1}^+ = t_k + s_k, \; T_{k+1}^- = t_k - s_k \tag{9}$$

In other words, one can say that the parameter $s$ controls the distance between the curve and the control point, what allows the approximation or the interpolation of these points, as shown in Fig. 3.

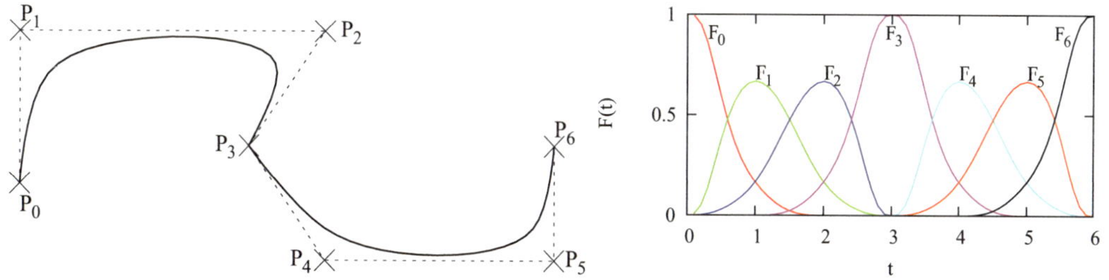

(a) Shape of the curve (b) Blending functions

Fig. 3. The values of the parameters of each control point are: $s_0 = 0, s_1 = 1, s_2 = 0, s_3 = 0, s_4 = 0, s_5 = 1, s_6 = 0$. These figures were inspired by the work of Blanc & Schlick (1995).

Although the expressions used to implement the Extended X-spline were rewritten above, detailed description about this and other types of splines can be found in Blanc & Schlick (1995).

### 2.1.3 Resistivity model

The proposed 2D model splits the domain in regions that represent different biological tissues, heart cavities, lungs and torso, each one associated with a different electrical resistivity.

Grimnes (2008) presents the main factors that influence the properties of biological tissues. Although they may be classified in only four groups ( epithelium, muscle, connective tissue and nervous tissue), the tissues can be divided in thirty kinds in accordance to their electrical properties (Gabriel, 1996). In addition, the value of the resistivity of each tissue depends on the frequency of the electrical current, on the temperature, on the presence of water, among other issues.

In this work, we assume the resistivity of each tissue as known, constant and isotropic. These are all simplified assumptions, since biological tissues are usually heterogeneous and anisotropic. However, biological tissues are difficult to characterize, and the reported values vary substantially in the literature. Table 1 presents some resistivity values for blood, heart and lung found in the literature.

| Tissue | Resistivity ($\Omega cm$) |
|---|---|
| Blood | 150 (Barber & Brown, 1984) |
| | 150 (Yang & Patterson, 2007) |
| | 100 (Schwan & Kay, 1956) |
| Heart | 400 (Patterson & Zhang, 2003) |
| | 250 (Yang & Patterson, 2007) |
| | 400 - 800 (Baysal & Eyuboglu, 2000) |
| Lung | 727 - 2363 (Barber & Brown, 1984) |
| | 1400 (Patterson & Zhang, 2003) |
| | 600 - 2000 (Baysal & Eyuboglu, 2000) |

Table 1. Resistivity values of biological tissues that are found in the literature.

For the remaining tissues that compose the section of the thorax, called here torso region, Bruder et al. (1994) proposes a mean resistivity of $500\Omega cm$. The resistivity of the air is $10^{20}\Omega cm$, but the resistivity of the lung filled of air is difficult to determine. Rush et al. (1963) presents a very simplified resistivity distribution model of the thorax characterized by the presence of cavities filled of blood, surrounded by homogeneous material with resistivity ten times greater. The same scheme, properly extended to include the lung regions, is used in this work. Preliminarily, the resistivity of the blood is here taken as $100\Omega cm$ and the torso to be $1000\Omega cm$. Two different values were tested for the resistivity of the lungs: $20000\Omega cm$ (Ratio of Lung to Torso resistivity, RLT = 20) and $50000\Omega cm$ (RLT = 50).

### 2.2 Forward problem

The forward problem consists on calculating the electrical potential on the external boundary of the torso that is generated by the current injection on a pair of electrodes. Figure 4 presents the simplified model of the thorax.

Given that our 2D model has three regions with different but constant and isotropic conductivities (heart cavities full of blood, $\Omega_B$, lungs, $\Omega_L$, and torso, $\Omega_T$) the electrical potential $u$ at each point of the regions must satisfy Laplaces' equation:

$$\nabla^2 u(\mathbf{x}) = 0\,, \quad \mathbf{x} \in \Omega\,, \tag{10}$$

the following boundary conditions:

$$\frac{1}{\rho_T}\frac{\partial u}{\partial \mathbf{n}} = J_i\,, \quad \mathbf{x} \in \Gamma_3^{ie} \tag{11}$$

$$\frac{\partial u}{\partial \mathbf{n}} = 0\,, \quad \mathbf{x} \in (\Gamma_3 - \Gamma_3^{ie}) \tag{12}$$

and these compatibility equations:

$$\rho_L \nabla u = \rho_T \nabla u \,, \quad \mathbf{x} \in \Gamma_1 \tag{13}$$

$$\rho_B \nabla u = \rho_T \nabla u \,, \quad \mathbf{x} \in \Gamma_2 \tag{14}$$

where $\Omega = \Omega_L + \Omega_B + \Omega_T$, $\Gamma_1$ is the interface between the lung and torso region, $\Gamma_2$ is the interface between the blood and the torso region, $\Gamma_3$ is the external boundary of the thorax, $\Gamma_3^{ie}$ is the part of $\Gamma_3$ where the ith electrode is, $J_i$ is the electrical current injected on the i-*th* electrode and $\rho_L$, $\rho_B$ and $\rho_T$ are the resistivities of the lung, blood and torso, respectively.

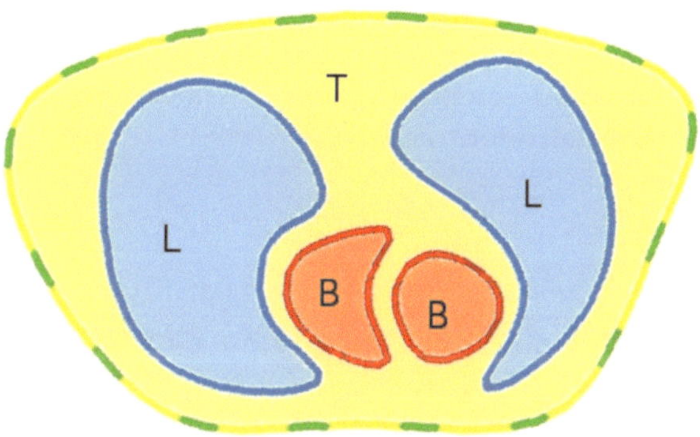


Fig. 4. The simplified thorax model. Here, the electrodes are represented in green. The regions **L** represent the lungs, **B** the blood and **T** the torso.

### 2.2.1 Numerical solution of Laplace's equation

In order to solve Equation 10 for each subregion the Boundary Element Method (BEM) is used. Further details about this technique can be found in Brebbia et al. (1984). The integral equation of BEM for this problem is

$$c(\xi)u(\xi) + \int_\Gamma p^*(\xi;\mathbf{x})u(\xi;\mathbf{x})d\Gamma(\mathbf{x}) = \int_\Gamma u^*(\xi;\mathbf{x})p(\xi;\mathbf{x})d\Gamma(\mathbf{x}) \,, \tag{15}$$

where $\xi$ is the collocation point, $\Gamma$ is the boundary of the sub-domain, $u$ is the electrical potential, $p$ is its derivative, $u^*$ and $p^*$ are the fundamental solutions for the potential and its normal derivative, respectively, and $c(\xi)$ is a function of the boundary shape, whose value is 0 if $\xi$ is outside of the domain, 1 if $\xi \in \Omega$ and $\beta/2\pi$ if $\xi \in \Gamma$. The parameter $\beta$ is the angle between the left and right tangents at the collocation point $\xi$.

To obtain a numerical solution for Equation 15, the boundary of the body is discretized. The external boundary is divided in $N_0$ elements and each subregion boundary in $N_k$ elements. In this work, the element adopted approximates the geometry linearly and the value of the electrical potential is considered constant in each element. In this case, the parameter $\beta = \pi$ and then $c(\xi) = 0.5$ if $\xi \in \Gamma$. Each boundary element has two nodes for the geometrical definition and a centered node, called functional node, where the potential and its derivative are computed. Thus, the discretized form of Equation 15 for each subregion $k$ allows evaluating the potential at each functional node as follows

$$c(\xi_i)u(\xi_i) + \sum_{j=1}^{N_k} u_j \int_{\Gamma_j} p^* d\Gamma_J = \sum_{j=1}^{N_k} p_j \int_{\Gamma_j} u^* d\Gamma_J \,, \tag{16}$$

where $u_j$ and $p_j$ represent the potential and its normal derivative at the $j$-th functional node. The regular integrals are computed numerically by the usual Gauss Quadrature scheme and the singular ones are computed analytically.

The application of Equation 16 for each sub-domain $\Omega_k$, in addition to the boundary and compatibility conditions (Equations 11 to 14) for the potential and its normal derivative at the functional nodes of the interface elements at $\Gamma_{0k}$, yields a linear system of algebraic equations that can be expressed in the matrix form as follows:

$$\mathbf{Hu} = \mathbf{Gp} \,, \tag{17}$$

where $\mathbf{u}$ and $\mathbf{p}$ are vectors that store the values of potential and its derivative, respectively, at the functional nodes of the boundary elements. The matrices $\mathbf{H}$ and $\mathbf{G}$ store the respective computed coefficients.

The number of unknowns is the number of the external boundary elements, in which the potential or the flux is unknown, in addition to the double of interface elements, in which the potential and the flux are unknowns. After collect all of them at the vector $\mathbf{y}$, Equation 17 can be rewritten as

$$\mathbf{Ay} = \mathbf{b} \,, \tag{18}$$

where $\mathbf{A}$ is the matrix of coefficients and $\mathbf{b}$ is the free vector of the linear system.

After determining the unknowns at the boundary, the values of the electrical potential at the nodes in the center of the electrodes without prescribed values are collected in the vector $\mathbf{V}$. Such vector will be compared with the vector of measures $\bar{\mathbf{V}}$ during the process of solving the inverse problem.

The implementation of the Boundary Elements Method to solve Laplace's equation was written in Fortran language.

### 2.3 The inverse problem

As was said before, the aim of the EIT is to generate an image of the electrical resistivity from measures of electrical potential at the external boundary. This problem can be formulated as a minimization problem in which one wants to find the model of electrical resistivity that minimizes the distance between measured ($\bar{\mathbf{V}}$) and computed ($\mathbf{V}$) potentials. In this work, the objective is to recover the shape of the ventricular cavities under the circumstances explained before. Therefore, the resistivity model is obtained via the estimation of the vector $\mathbf{t}$ defined in Section 2.1.1. In this case, the vector contains 15 parameters $t_i$, with $i = 1, 2, ..., 15$ as described before. In other words, the goal is to estimate the parameter vector **t** that minimizes $f$:

$$f = \frac{1}{2}\mathbf{R}(\mathbf{t})^T\mathbf{R}(\mathbf{t}) \tag{19}$$

with

$$\mathbf{R}(\mathbf{t}) = \bar{\mathbf{V}} - \mathbf{V}(\mathbf{t}) \tag{20}$$

where $f$ is the objective function ($f : \mathbb{R}^n \to \mathbb{R}$), $\mathbf{R}(\mathbf{t})$ is the residual function ($\mathbf{R} : \mathbb{R}^n \to \mathbb{R}^m$), $m$ is the number of measures and $n$ is the number of parameters. The number of measures depends on the adopted protocol to inject current and measure electrical potential.

Equation 19 shows that the problem leads to a non-linear least square problem. So, many techniques can be used to solve it. The so called global convergent methods, for example, Genetic Algorithms (Eiben & Smith, 2003; Michalewicz, 1996), has the advantage of avoid the convergence to local minimum. However, they demand a large number of evaluations of the objective function. On the other hand, the local minimization methods converge faster to the minimum because they use the derivatives of the objective function with respect to the parameters. They also demand a suitable initial approximation to converge to the global minimum. Hybrid strategies, that combine the advantages of local and global methods can be used with success (Hsiao et al., 2001; Peters et al., 2010). In this work, the features of the problem allows the use of a local strategy, the called Levenberg-Marquard Method, that will be briefly described as follows.

### 2.3.1 Levenberg-Marquardt method

The Levenberg-Marquardt Method was adopted to solve the non-linear least square problem represented by Equation 19. The detailed description about this method is vastly found in the literature (Dennis & Schnabel, 1996; Fletcher, 1980; Madsen et al., 2004). The Levenberg-Marquardt Method can be understood as the Gauss-Newton method modified by the model trust region approach. In this method, the minimizer of the non-linear least-square problem is obtained iteratively. Each update of **t** is given by the minimizer $\mathbf{t}_+$ of the following constrained linear least-square problem:

$$\text{minimizes } \|\mathbf{R}(\mathbf{t}_0) + \mathbf{J}(\mathbf{t}_0)(\mathbf{t}_+ - \mathbf{t}_0)\|_2 \tag{21}$$

$$\text{subject to } \|\mathbf{t}_+ - \mathbf{t}_0\|_2 \leq \delta_0 \, . \tag{22}$$

where $\mathbf{t}_0$ is the current value for the vector of minimization parameters and $\mathbf{t}_+$ is the updated vector. $\mathbf{R}$ is the same residual function mentioned before. $\mathbf{J} \in \mathbb{R}^{m\times n}$ is the Jacobian matrix, storing the derivatives of each element of the residual vector with respect to the optimization variables ($J_{ij} = \partial R_i / \partial t_j$). $\delta_0$ is the initial value of the radius of the trust region.

The solution of this constrained minimization problem is the updated vector of variables $\mathbf{t}_+$:

$$\mathbf{t}_+ = \mathbf{t}_0 - \left(\mathbf{J}\left(\mathbf{t}_0\right)^T \mathbf{J}\left(\mathbf{t}_0\right) + \mu \mathbf{I}\right)^{-1} \mathbf{J}\left(\mathbf{t}_0\right)^T \mathbf{R}\left(\mathbf{t}_0\right) \, , \tag{23}$$

where **I** is the identity matrix and $\mu$ is the parameter that modifies the Gauss-Newton method. If $\left\| \left(\mathbf{J}\left(\mathbf{t}_0\right)^T \mathbf{J}\left(\mathbf{t}_0\right)\right)^{-1} \mathbf{J}\left(\mathbf{t}_0\right)^T \mathbf{R}\left(\mathbf{t}_0\right) \right\|_2 \leq \delta_0$, $\mu = 0$, otherwise, $\mu \neq 0$.

There are some different implementations of this method with respect to the update of the parameter $\mu$. In this work, the implementation of the Levenberg-Marquardt Method is provided by MINPACK-1, a standard package of subroutines written in Fortran language to solve non-linear equations and non-linear least squares problems, that is available at the Netlib repository (*http://www.netlib.org/minpack*). More details about the adopted implementation can be found in Moré et al. (1980). In the numerical experiments presented in this work, the subroutine LMDIF of MINPACK-1 was used. Such subroutine demands only the computation of the residual function $\mathbf{R}(\mathbf{t})$. The jacobian matrix is approximated by finite differences. So, the element $J_{ij}$ of the Jacobian matrix is computed as follows:

$$J_{ij} = \frac{\partial R_i}{\partial t_j} \approx \frac{R_i(\mathbf{t} + h_j \mathbf{e}_j) - R_i(\mathbf{t})}{h_j} \tag{24}$$

where $h_j$ is a small finite perturbation at the $j$-th element of the original vector of optimization variables $\mathbf{t}$ and $\mathbf{e}_j$ is the $j$-th column of the identity matrix.

The value of the parameter $h_j$ is computed by the product $\sqrt{\varepsilon} t_j$, where $\varepsilon$ is a parameter provided by the user. If the machine precision is greater than the computed $h_j$, this value is substituted by the machine precision.

### 2.4 Numerical experiments

#### 2.4.1 Stimulation patterns

An important aspect of the EIT problem is the choice of the protocols of current injection and electrical potential measurements. Since the problem is ill-conditioned, the suitable choice can be determinant to the success of the image generation. However, a deep study of the influence of different protocols on the solution of the inverse problem is not the focus of this work. More information on this topic can be found in other works, for instance, Peters & Barra (2010). Here we are limited to compare two patterns of electrical current injection. The first is called diametrical and the second is called alternative. Furthermore, all the experiments were done considering 16 electrodes equally spaced on the external boundary of the torso.

The name of the first pattern, diametrical, comes from an analogy. If the domain were circular, the electrodes used to inject current are diametrically opposed. Although the torso is not circular, the name of the pattern remains. In this pattern, 8 different cases of current injection is taken and 13 measures of potential for each case. So, the diametrical pattern yields 104 measures.

The second pattern, here called alternative, is a tentative of illuminating the region of interest better than other regions. Therefore, in this pattern, the electrodes used to inject current, the driven electrodes, are taken near to the heart. So, 6 cases of current injection with 13 measures each one give a total of 78 measures. Each double arrow of Fig. 5 indicates the driven electrode pair in each case of current injection. In both patterns, measurements on driven electrodes are not considered.

It is important to note that, in this work, the "measured" electrical potential values ($\bar{\mathbf{V}}$) were also synthetically generated, i.e., also numerically obtained.

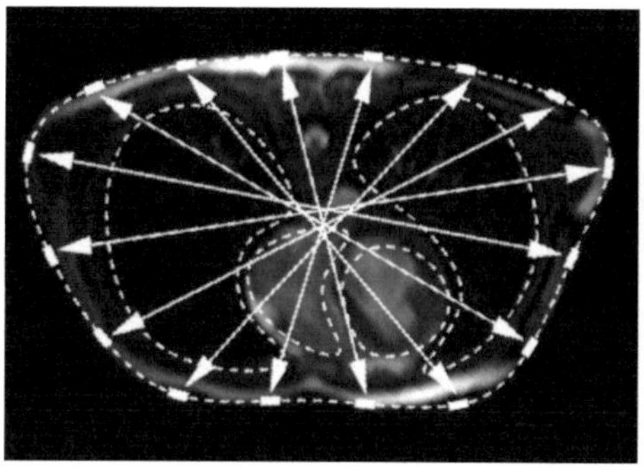

(a) Diametrical Pattern

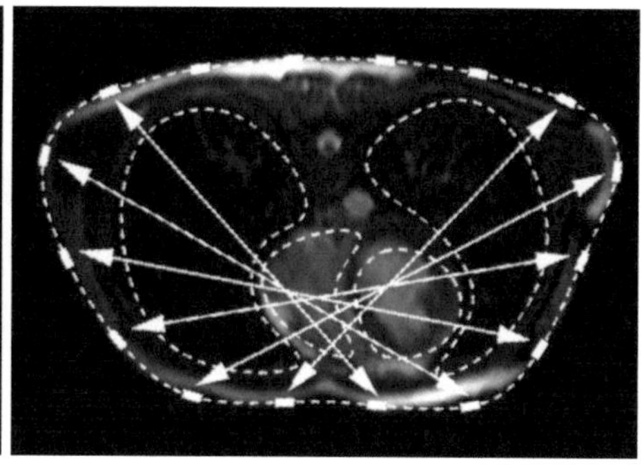

(b) Alternative Pattern

Fig. 5. Two stimulation patterns used in this work. Each double arrow indicates one pair of driven electrodes.

### 2.4.2 Problem

From MR images taken at the end of the systole and at the end of the diastole the cardiac ventricles were manually segmented. In this work we are considering an image of just one transversal section of the thorax. Therefore, the problem is treated as 2D and an approximation of the ejection fraction is needed.

Here, the section of the cavities were assumed to be proportional to their volumes, i.e. a cylindrical approximation. So that, in accordance to Equation 1, EF is approximated by:

$$EF = \frac{EDA - ESA}{EDA} \tag{25}$$

where $EDA$ is the end-diastolic area and $ESA$ is the end-systolic area.

Therefore, after segmentation, the EF is calculated in accordance to Equation 25. The EF of the left ventricle is 59.24% and the EF of the right ventricle is 29, 95%. These values characterize the initial situation of the heart cicle. From this moment, the EIT can be used to monitor the EF.

Later, a cardiac dysfunction was synthetically generated. In this simulated dysfunction model the end-diastolic volume is the same as in the normal cycle but the end-systolic volume is greater than the normal one. In this pathological situation new cardiac cycle, the EF of the left ventricle is 33.01% and the EF of the right ventricle is 16.19%. These dysfunction values are the target values to be estimated by the here proposed method.

As mentioned in Section 2.1, we have also tested the methods considering two different 2D models. Each with a different value for the resistivity of the lungs: 20000$\Omega cm$ (RLT = 20) and 50000$\Omega cm$ (RLT = 50).

As was said before, the solution depends on the initial guess provided for the local minimization method. So that, for each of 4 optimization problems (2 stimulus patterns times 2 RLT models) we have tested the optimization method with two different initial guesses. One guess corresponds to the shape of the ventricles at the end of the diastole of normal heart, i.e. $t_i = 1, \forall i$ and the other at the end of the systole for the normal tissue, i.e. $t_i = 0, \forall i$ . The initial guesses and the target can be compared in Fig. 6. Thus, the method was executed a total of 8 times (2 stimulus patterns times 2 RLT models times 2 initial guesses). Each execution computes the parameters **t** of the end of the systole. The areas inside the curves defined by **t** are the $ESA$. These values together with the known $EDA$ values, that is supposed to be the same as the initial condition of the heart cycle, are used with Equation 25 to compute the EF. Therefore, each execution yields 2 values: EF of the left and right ventricle.

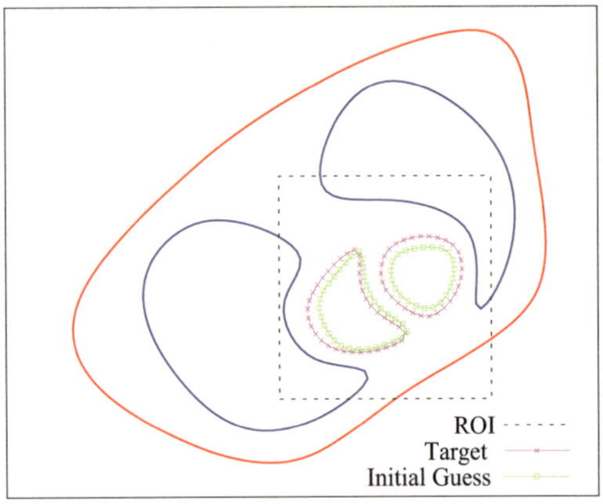


(a) $t_i = 0, \forall i$

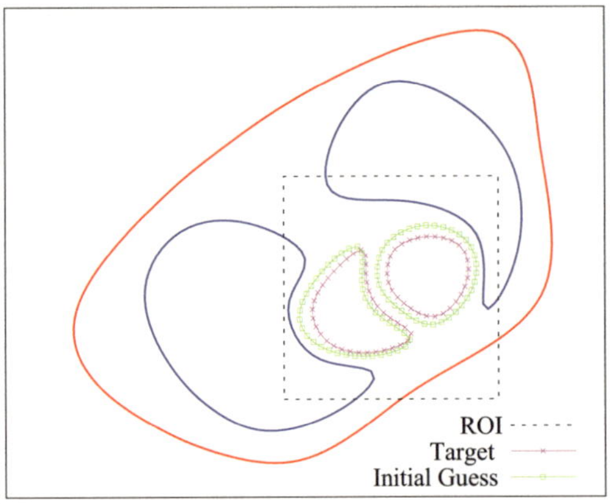


(b) $t_i = 1, \forall i$

Fig. 6. A typical target (pink) and the two initial guesses (green) given to the optimization procedure. The first one corresponds to the systole and the second one to the diastole. ROI denotes the region of interest.

## 3. Results

Table 2 presents the results of our numerical experiments that aim the EF estimation of the synthetically generated cardiac dysfunction. The columns present the results for the models with different values for the resistivity of the lungs: $20000\Omega cm$ (RLT = 20) and $50000\Omega cm$ (RLT = 50). Each couple of rows presents the comparison of the two stimulation patterns implemented: diametrical and alternative. In addition, for each pair (stimulus pattern, RLT) results are presented for two different initial guesses. The first one corresponds to the shape of the ventricles at the end of the systole for the normal heart, i.e. $t_i = 0, \forall i$ and the other at the end of the diastole of the normal heart, i.e. $t_i = 1, \forall i$. The last row of the table presents the target values for comparison: 16.19% the EF of right ventricle (RV) and 33.01% the EF of left ventricle (LV).

Table 3 shows the relative errors between the values of EF obtained in each execution and the target values for each ventricle. These values are computed as

$$\Delta\% = 100 \times \frac{|\tilde{EF} - EF|}{EF}, \tag{26}$$

where $\Delta\%$ is the error, $\tilde{EF}$ is the value achieved by the inverse problem solution for the ejection fraction and $EF$ is the target value. The relative errors are used to compute the mean relative errors used to compare patterns, initial guesses and models.

| Ejection Fraction (%) | | | | |
|---|---|---|---|---|
| Initial | RLT = 50 | | RLT = 20 | |
| Guess | RV | LV | RV | LV |
| Diametrical Pattern | | | | |
| $t_i = 0$ | 13.00 | 34.41 | 15.32 | 34.22 |
| $t_i = 1$ | 16.09 | 32.21 | 15.80 | 33.04 |
| Alternative Pattern | | | | |
| $t_i = 0$ | 12.97 | 35.86 | 20.54 | 29.94 |
| $t_i = 1$ | 18.72 | 32.84 | 20.89 | 29.40 |
| **Target** | **16.19** | **33.01** | **16.19** | **33.01** |

Table 2. Values of the ejection fraction estimated for the synthetic cardiac dysfunction for two resistivity models (RLT = 20 and RLT = 50), two different stimulation patterns (diametrical and alternative) and two initial guesses ($t_i = 0$ and $t_i = 1$). The last row shows the target values of the EF.

| Relative Errors (%) | | | | |
|---|---|---|---|---|
| Initial | RLT = 50 | | RLT = 20 | |
| Guess | RV | LV | RV | LV |
| Diametrical Pattern | | | | |
| $t_i = 0$ | 19.70 | 4.24 | 5.37 | 3.67 |
| $t_i = 1$ | 0.62 | 2.42 | 2.41 | 0.09 |
| Alternative Pattern | | | | |
| $t_i = 0$ | 19.89 | 8.63 | 26.87 | 9.30 |
| $t_i = 1$ | 15.63 | 0.51 | 29.03 | 10.94 |

Table 3. Relative errors of the obtained EF with respect to the target values.

Figure 7 allows a geometrical comparison between the final results and the actual (target) curves. In order to make the visualization easier, these figures show the region of interest defined in Fig. 6 without the curves of the lungs. It is important to emphasize that, to make the comparison fair, the results presented in these figures were obtained with the same initial guess, $t_i = 1, \forall i$.

The results show that, except in one case, the error of the ejection fraction of the left ventricle is smaller than the right ventricle value. The mean relative error of the eight results of the left ventricle results is 4.98% while the right ventricle is 14.94%.

Moreover, except in one case, the diametrical pattern provides results closer to the actual values than the alternative pattern. The diametrical pattern provides a mean relative value of 4.82% while the mean error of the alternative pattern is 15.10%.

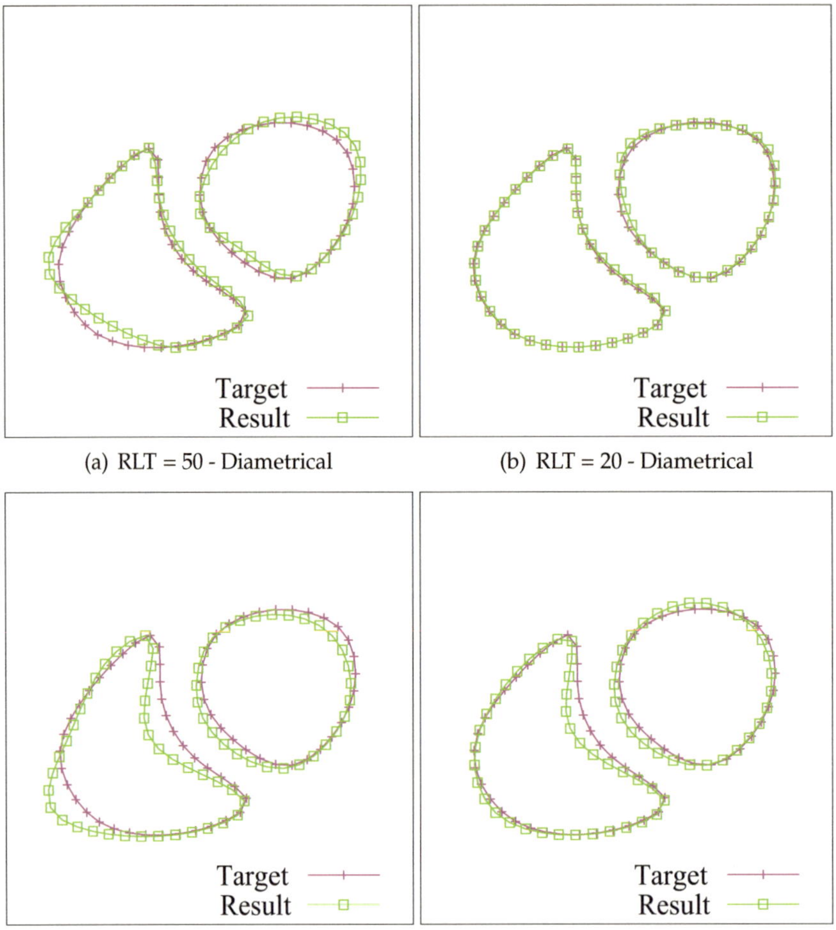


(a) RLT = 50 - Diametrical (b) RLT = 20 - Diametrical

(c) RLT = 50 - Alternative (d) RLT = 20 - Alternative

Fig. 7. Some results for the diametrical and the alternative pattern and the target.

About the initial guess, both of them provided good results. However, in this experiments, the best results were obtained with the guess of the original diastole curve, $t_i = 1$, with a mean relative error of 7.70% against an error of 12.21% for the other initial guess.

The geometrical results presented in Fig. 7, showing only the ventricular cavities, suggest that they become worse in the case the lung resistivity is greater. This behavior is expected because greater resistivities around the region of interest tend to block the electrical current to reach this area. For instance, for the best experimented pattern, the diametrical one, the mean relative error obtained with the greatest resistivity (RLT = 50) is 3.37% while the mean relative error obtained with the other lung resistivity (RLT = 20) is 1.44%.

The best result can be considered the one obtained for RLT = 20, diametrical pattern and $t_i = 1$. The relative error in the value of the ejection fraction is 0.09% for the left ventricle and 2.41% for the right ventricle. Figure 7(b) shows this result. In this case it is very difficult to see the difference between the result and the target.

## 4. Discussions and conclusions

The presented results suggest that the proposed methodology allows a suitable indication of the cardiac ejection fraction. We have observed that the error in the ejection fraction predictions for the right ventricle are greater than those found for the left ventricle and this is in agreement with other techniques, such as with echocardiography.

Concerning the different patterns for current injection tested in this work, the errors obtained with the diametrical pattern are smaller than those using the alternative pattern, in general. However this fact does not discard the use of the alternative pattern, as it presents good results and spends around 19 min. in a Pentium 4, 3.00 GHz, for a complete solution, 25% less then the diametrical.

Comparing the results obtained with different lung resistivities we may conclude that the inverse problem becomes more difficult to be solved as the RLT increases. Therefore, the results suggest the current injection should be triggered during the expiratory phase, when the air volume and the corresponding lung resistivity are smaller.

The preliminary results presented in this work suggest the proposed technique is a promising diagnostic tool that may offer continuous and non-invasive estimation of cardiac ejection fraction. However, the use of the EIT in real applications demands further improvements. The model could be improved, for instance, by the implementation of the complete electrode model (Cheney et al., 1999).

Another point is that, in this work, we assume the resistivities of the tissue known. Future works should include the resistivities of the tissue as parameters of the inverse problem, as well as deeper studies about the electrical properties of biological tissues. Furthermore, the behavior of the proposed method when subjected to real data should be evaluated.

## 5. Acknowledgements

This work was partially supported by FAPEMIG, UFJF, CAPES, CNPq and FINEP. In particular, the first author would like to thank CAPES for the Master's scholarship at Federal University of Juiz de Fora and CNPq for the Doctoral scholarship at Federal University of Rio de Janeiro.

## 6. References

Adler, A., Amyot, R., Guardo, R., Bates, J. H. T. & Berthiaume, Y. (1997). Monitoring changes in lung air and liquid volumes with electrical impedance tomography, *Journal of Applied Physiology* 83(5): 1762–1767.

Anderson, E., Bai, Z., Bischof, C., Blackford, L. S., Demmel, J., Dongarra, J. J., Du Croz, J., Hammarling, S., Greenbaum, A., McKenney, A. & Sorensen, D. (1999). *LAPACK Users' guide (third ed.)*, Society for Industrial and Applied Mathematics, Philadelphia, PA, USA.

Barber, D. C. & Brown, B. H. (1984). Applied potential tomography, *Journal of Physics E-Scientific Instruments* 17(9): 723–733.

Barra, L. P. S., Peters, F., Martins, C. P. & Barbosa, H. (2006). Computational experiments in electrical impedance tomography, *XXVII Iberian Latin American Congress on Computational Methods in Engineering*, Belém, Brasil.

Barra, L., Santos, R., Peters, F., Santos, E. & Barbosa, H. (2006). Parallel computational experiments in electrical impedance tomography, *18th Symposium on Computer Architecture and High Performance Computing*, Vol. 1, Sociedade Brasileira de Computação, High Perfomance Computing in the Life Sciences, Ouro Preto, Brasil, pp. 7–13.

Baysal, U. & Eyuboglu, B. M. (2000). Tissue resistivity estimation in the presence of positional and geometrical uncertainties, *Physics in Medicine and Biology* 45(8): 2373–2388.

Blanc, C. & Schlick, C. (1995). X-splines: A spline model designed for the end-user, *SIGGRAPH*, ACM - Association for Computing Machinery, Los Angeles, EUA, pp. 377–386.

Borsic, A., McLeod, C., Lionheart, W. & Kerrouche, N. (2001). Realistic 2d human thorax modelling for eit, *Physiological Measurement* 22(1): 77–83.

Brebbia, C., Telles, J. C. F. & Wrobel, L. C. (1984). *Boundary Elements Techniques: Theory and Applications in Engineering*, Springer-Verlag.

Brown, B. H., Barber, D. C. & Seagar, A. D. (1985). Applied potential tomography - possible clinical applications, *Clinical Physics and Physiological Measurement* 6(2): 109–121.

Bruder, H., Scholz, B. & Abrahamfuchs, K. (1994). The influence of inhomogeneous volume conductor models on the ecg and the mcg, *Physics in Medicine and Biology* 39(11): 1949–1968.

Cheney, M., Isaacson, D. & Newell, J. C. (1999). Electrical impedance tomography, *SIAM Review* 41(1): 85–101.

Choi, M. H., Kao, T. J., Isaacson, D., Saulnier, G. J. & Newell, J. C. (2007). A reconstruction algorithm for breast cancer imaging with electrical impedance tomography in mammography geometry, *IEEE Transactions on Biomedical Engineering* 54(4): 700–710.

Dennis, J. & Schnabel, R. B. (1996). *Numerical Methods for Unconstrained Optimization and Nonlinear Equations*, SIAM.

Eiben, A. E. & Smith, J. E. (2003). *Introduction to Evolutionary Computing*, Springer.

Fletcher, R. (1980). *Practical methods of optimization*, Wiley-Interscience, New York, NY, USA.

Gabriel, C. (1996). *The dielectric properties of biological tissue: I. literature survey*, Phys. Med. Biol.

Grimnes, S. (2008). *Bioimpedance and Bioelectricity Basics*, Academic Press.

Holder, D. (2005). Electrical Impedance Tomography: Methods, History and Applications, *Medical Physics* 32: 2731.

Hsiao, C. T., Chahine, G. & Gumerov, N. (2001). Application of a hybrid genetic/powell algorithm and a boundary element method to electrical impedance tomography, *Journal of Computational Physics* 173: 433–454.

Karhunen, K., Seppanen, A., Lehikoinen, A., Monteiro, P. J. M. & Kaipio, J. P. (2009). Electrical resistance tomography imaging of concrete, *Cement and Concrete Research* 40(1): 137–145.

Kim, M., Kim, K. & Kim, S. (2004). Phase boundary estimation in two-phase flows with electrical impedance tomography, *Int. Comm. Heat Transfer* 31(8): 1105–1114.

Lima, C. R., Mello, L. A. M., Lima, R. G. & Silva, E. C. N. (2007). Electrical impedance tomography through constrained sequential linear programming: a topology optimization approach, *Measurement Science and Technology* 18(9): 2847–2858.

Madsen, K., Nielsen, H. & Tingleff, O. (2004). Methods for non-linear least squares problems.

Mello, L. A. M., de Lima, C. R., Amato, M. B. P., Lima, R. G. & Silva, E. C. N. (2008). Three-dimensional electrical impedance tomography: A topology optimization approach, *Biomedical Engineering, IEEE Transactions on* 55(2): 531–540.

Michalewicz, Z. (1996). *Genetic Algorithms + Data Structures = Evolution Programs*, Springer Verlag.

Moré, J. J., Garbow, B. S. & Hillstrom, K. E. (1980). User guide for MINPACK-1, *Technical Report ANL-80-74*, Argonne National Laboratory, Argonne, IL, USA.

Park, B. G., Moon, J. H., Lee, B. S. & Kim, S. (2008). An electrical resistance tomography technique for the monitoring of a radioactive waste separation process, *International Communications in Heat and Mass Transfer* 35(10): 1307–1310.

Patterson, R. P. & Zhang, J. (2003). Evaluation of an eit reconstruction algorithm using finite difference human thorax models as phantoms, *Physiological Measurement* 24(2): 467–475.

Peters, F. & Barra, L. (2009). A strategy for parametrization refinement in the solution of a geometric inverse problem, *Computational Modeling (MCSUL), 2009 Third Southern Conference on*, pp. 136 –142.

Peters, F., Barra, L. & Santos, R. (2009). Determination of cardiac ejection fraction by electrical impedance tomography - numerical experiments and viability analysis, *Computational Science - ICCS 2009*, Vol. 5544/2009 of *Lecture Notes in Computer Science*, Springer Berlin / Heidelberg, pp. 819–828.

Peters, F. C. & Barra, L. P. S. (2010). Some numerical results on the influence of measurement strategies and load patterns in the eit inverse problem, *Journal of Physics: Conference Series* 224(1): 012145.

Peters, F. C., Barra, L. P. S. & Lemonge, A. C. C. (2010). Application of a hybrid optimization method for identification of steel reinforcement in concrete by electrical impedance tomography, *2nd International Conference on Engineering Optimization.*

Polydorides, N., Lionheart, W. & McCann, H. (2002). Krylov subspace iterative thechniques: On the brain activity with electrical impedance tomography, *IEEE Transactions on Medical Imaging* 21(6): 596–603.

Rush, S., McFee, R. & Abildskov, J. A. (1963). Resistivity of body tissues at low frequencies, *Circulation Research* 12(1): 40–50.

Schwan, H. P. & Kay, C. F. (1956). Specific resistance of body tissues, *Circulation Research* 4(6): 664–670.

Seo, J., Kwon, O., Ammari, H. & Woo, E. (2004). A mathematical model for breast cancer lesion estimation: Electrical impedance technique using ts2000 commercial system, *IEEE Transactions on Biomedical Engineering* 51(11): 1898–1906.

Trigo, F., Lima, R. & Amato, M. (2004). Electrical impedance tomography using extended kalman filter, *IEEE Transactions on Biomedical Engineering* 51(1): 72–81.

Yang, F. & Patterson, R. P. (2007). The contribution of the lungs to thoracic impedance measurements: a simulation study based on a high resolution finite difference model, *Physiological Measurement* 28(7): S153–S161.

Zlochiver, S., Freimark, D., Arad, M., Adunsky, A. & Abboud, S. (2006). Parametric eit for monitoring cardiac stroke volume, Vol. 27, Iop Publishing Ltd, pp. S139–S146.

13

# Assessment of Human Skin Microcirculation and Its Endothelial Function Using Laser Doppler Flowmetry

Helena Lenasi
*Institute of Physiology, Medical Faculty, University of Ljubljana*
*Slovenia*

## 1. Introduction

Human skin is the largest organ of the body: it accounts for approximately 5% of the total body weight, extends over about 1.8 $m^2$ and has an average thickness of 1-2 mm. Besides providing the mechanical barrier to protect the surface of the body and to prevent water loss it has other important functions. It is engaged in sensory perception and vitamin D metabolism, in inflammation, hemostasis and wound healing. Its role in human thermoregulation is essential (Roddie, 1983; Rowell, 1993).

The major role of blood flow to the skin is therefore concerned with temperature regulation. Accordingly, it is not surprisingly that blood flow to the skin goes far beyond its nutritive demands. The nutritive blood flow is estimated to comprise only 20% of the skin blood flow (SkBF), whereas the rest represents the functional blood flow. On the whole, the SkBF has been estimated to amount to 0.3 l/min at rest in thermoneutral conditions. During exposure to cold it can be reduced to almost zero, whereas it can increase up to 8 l/min during strenous exercise in a hot environment. It is thus obvious that it plays an important role in hemodynamics, since during strenous exercise and in severe heat stress it can comprise over 50% of the cardiac output, as compared to only 5% in resting thermoneutral conditions (Johnson, 1996; Rowell, 1993). The range of flows is therefore wide, and, in extreme conditions, high SkBF also represents a burden on the working heart. Indeed, many persons with borderline cardiac failure develop severe failure in a hot weather because of the extra load on the heart and then revert from failure in cool weather. As one of the major functions of the skin is to eliminate excessive heat, its temperature is generally under 37°C.

In recent years, the cutaneous microcirculation has gained increasing interest. Its easy and noninvasive accessibility renders skin microcirculation an ideal site for measuring. Moreover, as a dynamic structure it may serve as a model for generalized microvascular function as studies have shown a correlation of vascular reactivity between different vascular beds over the body (coronary arteries, brachial artery and skin microcirculation to list a few of them) in health and disease, at least with regard to endothelial function (Holowatz et al., 2008).

There is a constant competition between thermoregulatory and non-thermoregulatory challenges. Many different mechanisms, ranging from systemic to local factors, play in concert to balance these two demands and to eliminate redundant heat. This duality also explains the complex ultrastructure of the skin (Braverman, 1997). SkBF is regulated by centrally mediated neural mechanisms and by local humoral factors. Of local factors, the endothelium plays a pivotal role in the regulation of vascular tone. In spite of immense effort that was put in the investigation of endothelial function of skin microcirculation there are still many mysteries to be resolved. However, the term endothelial function is mostly used to refer to the ability of the endothelium to release substances that induce vasodilation by directly causing relaxation of the underlaying smooth muscle cells (SMC) (Crakowski et al., 2006).

Elucidating the role of endothelial vasodilators and their interactions as well as assessing endothelial function in human skin microcirculation is also important from the clinical point of view as early detectable endothelial dysfunction might precede clinical manifestation of the disease states.

One of the measures to improve endothelial dysfunction due to reduced nitric oxide (NO) bioavailability is regular physical activity. Nevertheless, the results on the impact of endurance training to the endothelium-dependent vasodilation, particularly in skin microcirculation of healthy persons, are controversial and the mechanisms induced by training remain to be elucidated.

Over the last years, new advanced techniques and strategies emerged in order to explain the function, the cell-to-cell communication and the complex interaction between pharmacological mediators in cutaneous microvasculature. Although different methods exist that tend to estimate skin blood flow none is optimal. A gold standard to evaluate skin microcirculation and its reactivity to various stimuli is laser Doppler flowmetry (LDF).

## 2. Skin microcirculation

### 2.1 Anatomy and physiology of skin microcirculation

The skin microcirculation is an anastomotic network of vessels with many crucial functions for the human as a whole. Namely, with its large capacity, it has to maintain nutrition of the epidermis and its adnexa, it is essential for human thermoregulation, in takes a major part in inflammation and wound healing, and, last but not least, it plays an important role in the determination of peripheral resistance. From all the above, it is obvious that the blood flow must be finely regulated and tuned in order to fulfill all the demands of the organism.

Because of its dimension, skin vasculature belongs to microcirculation only. It comprises arterioles, capillaries and venules (Braverman, 1997). The microvessels in the papillary dermis vary in diameter from 10 to 35 μm, but most range from 17 to 22 μm.

The cutaneous arteries arise from the subcutaneous tissue and enter the dermis to form the cutaneous arterial plexuses. The arterioles and venules of the cutaneous microcirculation form two important horizontal plexuses parallel to the skin surface: an upper horizontal plexus in the papillary dermis (subepidermal or subpapillary plexus) from which the nutritive capillary loops arise and a lower horizontal plexus at the dermal-subcutaneous border. These two plexuses communicate with each other with arterioles and venules and represent the physiologically important areas in the skin (Braverman, 1997).

Capillaries connect the arteriolar subpapillary plexus with the venous subpapillary plexus, and single capillary loops ascend to each papilla. They have a mean length of approximately 0.2 mm to 0.4 mm and each supplies on average 0.04 to 0.27 $mm^2$ of the skin surface.

Special feature of human skin microcirculation are arteriovenous anastomoses (AVAs). These are direct connections between arterioles and venules of the deep epidermal plexus and have thick muscular and richly innervated walls. They provide a low resistance short circuit for the passage of blood from arterioles to venules at high flow rates, as in response to body heating (Braverman, 1997; Roddie, 1983). They are found mainly in the apical regions of the skin (hands, feet, nose, lips and ears) and are most numerous in the nail beds, tips of digits, and palmar surfaces of digits, palms and soles, but they are almost absent from the dorsum of these areas.

The microvasculature of the skin varies significantly in different regions of the body, with respect to density and architecture of the vascular network as well as regarding blood flow. With respect to their structure and physiologic role, different skin parts could be divided into glabrous and nonglabrous areas: nonglabrous or hairy areas are areas over the skin of the trunk and extremities, whereas glabrous or nonhairy skin areas are found in palms, soles and lips. These regions differ with regard to the vascular control mechanisms. Nevertheless, there is not a discernible function that can be ascribed to one or another region.

### 2.2 Control of skin blood flow

As an important part of the cardiovascular system, SkBF undergoes periodic demands for increased and decreased blood flow in order to achieve cardiovascular adjustments during thermoregulatory challenges, during orthostasis and exercise.

Since SkBF takes part in the above-mentioned systemic reflexes its blood flow is mainly regulated by neural mechanisms rather than by local factors. However, local factors, in the first line factors released from the vascular endothelium and various substances co-transmitted from local nerve endings, can strongly modulate this general response to systemic challenges.

#### 2.2.1 Neural control mechanisms

With respect to the anatomical organisation of skin microcirculation, there are principally two types of neural control mechanisms (Johnson & Kellogg, 2010; Kellog, 2006).

I. All skin areas (glabrous and nonglabrous) throughout the body are supplied with sympathetic vasoconstrictor fibers that secrete norepinephrine at their nerve endings and, under resting conditions, exhibit a tonic vasoconstrictor influence on skin blood vessels. The resting tone is maintained by a continuous nerve discharge of 1-3 impulses per second and can be varied in both directions to produce vasoconstriction and, without need for any other specialised vasodilatory fibers, also vasodilation. Indeed, under exposure to cold, there is an increased discharge from this part of the sympathetic system, causing further vasoconstriction. On the other hand, under heat stress, the tonic outflow through sympathetic vasoconstrictor system is reduced. This constrictor system is extremely powerful in glabrous areas with abundant AVAs - areas that are most frequently exposed to severe cold. Thermoregulatory as well as other reflexes in these regions are mediated by changes in noradrenergic vasoconstrictor tone as well as direct effects of local temperatures on the skin (Johnson & Kellogg, 2010; Kellog, 2006).

II. In addition, nonglabrous skin areas also receive the so-called active (cholinergic) vasodilatory nerve fibers, most probably from the sympathetic origin too. Over the last years, many studies have been conducted to elucidate this cholinergic vasodilation mecanism, but the results are not conclusive. It is postulated that acetylcholine (ACh) is the most probable neurotrasmitter, possibly linked to sweating. The current hypothesis proposes a co-transmitter released by the nerve endings innervating either blood vessels directly or sweat glands and exerting its relaxant action on the vascular SMC. A putative co-transmitter has not been identified yet: the candidates include vasoactive intestinal peptide, substance P, histamine from mast cells acting on histamine $H_1$ receptors, prostanoids, and NO (Johnson & Kellogg, 2010; Kellog, 2006).

It should be mentioned that there are modulators of the neuraly mediated mechanisms involved in cutaneous vasoconstriction and vasodilation. In women, skin vascular reactivity depends on the phase of the menstrual cycle: progesteron resets the treshold for active cutaneous vasodilation (Charkoudian & Johnson, 2000). Furthermore, SkBF and the cutaneous microvascular reactivity are subject to diurnal rhytms (Aoki et al., 2003). Another modulator that resets the threshold for active cutaneous vasodilation is physical exercise (Johnson, 1996; Rowell, 1993) that is covered in more detail elsewhere in the chapter.

### 2.2.2 Local control mechanisms

Apart from neural mechanisms, local factors also impact SkBF. The standard meaning of the term applies to the mechanisms independent of nerves and hormones, by which organs and tissues alter their own arteriolar resistance. Included are classical vasodilators, such as decreased oxygen partial pressure, hydrogen ion, and locally released metabolites as adenosin, and increased concentrations of potassium. Their effect on the local vascular tone is more pronounced when inducing short-term hypoxia, such as a transient occlusion of the proximal artery. All things considered, little is know about these local mechanisms in controlling human skin microcirculation although their role seems to be of minor importance.

Much more important seems to be the role of vascular endothelium as a local regulator of vascular tone, also with respect to the skin microcirculation (Johnson, & Kellog, 2010; Kellog, 2006). The role of endothelium as a local regulator of vascular tone (in glabrous as well as in nonglabrous parts) has been assessed and confirmed by different independent studies.

Last but not least, local thermal factors, i.e. local heating and cooling of the skin, also play an important role in modulating vascular tone (Johnson, & Kellog, 2010; Kellog, 06).

Besides the above mentioned neural and local control mechanisms, skin microvessels also exhibit local and autonomous variations of blood diameter that cause corresponding flow variations and have been termed vasomotion. The contractions have a low frequency that can be obtained by transforming the signal of the laser Doppler flux (1-2 cycles/min) using spectral analysis. Vasomotion is suggested to facilitate blood flow through microvessels and can be amplified under conditions of circulatory and metabolic stress, as for examle by inducing a transient ischemia (Kvandal et al., 2006; Rossi et al., 2008). The origin of vasomotion remains to be fully elucidated: it has been proposed that the spontaneous muscular contractions are due to the intrinsic myogenic activity of vascular SMC.

### 2.3 Endothelium as a local regulator of vascular tone

In the last decades, a number of studies conducted in animals as well as in humans extensively expanded the knowledge about the pivotal role of endothelium in the regulation of vascular tone (Vanhoutte, 1989). In response to physical forces and neurohumoral mediators, endothelial cells secrete several vasoactive substances that affect vascular tone by inducing contraction and relaxation of the underlying smooth muscle. The most important endothelial vasodilators are NO, prostacyclin ($PGI_2$) and endothelium-derived hyperpolarizing factor (EDHF), whereas vasoconstrictors include endothelin (ET), platelet activating factor (PAF), etc. We will focus on the role of vasodilators.

Physical stimuli are shear stress exerted on the vascular wall by the flowing blood, and pulsatility of the vessel wall, whereas pharmacological stimuli include a variety of endothelial agonists, such as ACh, bradykinin, thrombin, serotonin, estrogens etc. In general, endothelial function *in vivo* can be estimated by applying pharmacological agonists to induce endothelium-dependent vasodilation. When estimating endothelial function, the terms NO-dependent and nonNO-dependent vasodilation (Higashi & Joshizumi, 2003) are often used to discern between different mediators involved.

NO is constitutively secreted by endothelial cells upon the action of endothelial nitric oxide synthase (eNOS) that is constitutively expressed in all endothelial cells. eNOS can further be activated by increases of calcium ions or by different agonists that induce changes in the phosphorylation of specific aminoacid residues of the enzyme (Fleming, 2010). Its action depends on the bioavailability of substrats (such as L-arginine) and cofactors, such as tetrahydrobiopterin ($BH_4$). NO induces vasodilation by activating soluble guanilat cyclase in SMC that further catalyses cGMP, causing vasorelaxation of SMC.

As for the role of $PGI_2$ and other prostanoids, their importance in skin microcirculation is unequivocal. They are synthesised by the family of cyclooxygenase (COX) enzymes. $PGI_2$ acts principally to modulate the function of vascular SMC and platelets; it is suggested to play only minor role in the regulation of vascular tone in health. On the contrary, it may play a compensatory role in the settings of decreased NO bioavailability (McCord et al., 2006; Szerafin et al., 2006).

The vasodilatation that remains after the combined eNOS and COX blockade has been ascribed to a yet unidentified mechanism. As it induces hyperpolarization of endothelial and vascular SMC by activating different families of $K^+$ channels, it has been termed EDHF (Feletou & Vanhoutte, 2009). The potential mechanisms leading to the hyperpolarization of endothelial cells and SMC include arachidonic acid metabolites derived from cyclooxygenases, lipooxygenases and cytochrome P450 (CYP) pathways, as well as $H_2O_2$, CO and $H_2S$. Another putative mechanism associated with the hyperpolarization of both endothelial and vascular SMC is suggested to be electrical coupling through myoendothelial gap junctions following small and intermediate conductance $Ca^{2+}$ activated $K^+$ channels ($IK_{Ca}$ and $SK_{Ca}$, respectively.).

The contributions of NO, EDHF and $PGI_2$ to the endothelium-dependent vasodilation are difficult to define, as their importance may vary depending on the vessel type and size as well as on the agonist used to stimulate the endothelium (Feletou & Vanhoutte, 2009; Schrage et al., 2005). There is a redundancy in endothelial vasodilator mechanisms and in the settings of compromised endothelial function, one vasodilator may overcome the deficiency of another one and in this way restore normal endothelial function. The same holds true when one or more pathways of vasodilator synthesis are inhibited, i.e. blocking eNOS and/or COX causes an increased production of the nonblocked substance(s). Also, a complex interaction and crosstalk between different mechanisms has been suggested (Feletou & Vanhoutte, 2009; Nishikawa et al., 2000; Osanai et al., 2000). It has been established that NO is involved predominantly in the control of vascular tone in larger conductance vessels, whereas in microcirculation, the role of EDHF seems to be more important (Pohl & deWit, 1999; Urakami-Harasawa et al., 1997). Most observations are based predominantly on animal studies and little is known about the impact of EDHF in humans *in vivo* (Yang et al., 2007). In spite of several investigations, the exact interaction of these mechanisms is still not well defined, specially not in human skin microcirculation.

## 3. Methods for assessing skin microcirculation

A number of methodologies have been used to provide indexes of SkBF. As SkBF is dynamically changing the technique employed must be able to detect these dynamic changes. Furthermore, the method has to be safe, easy to apply, accurate and reproducible, and should not affect SkBF. Usually it is not the basal flow that is of interest but rather vascular reactivity that can give insight into the vascular function. Thus, the measurement techniques are usually coupled to some provocation tests which can estimate vascular reactivity. The latter is usually tested to investigate the mechanisms involved in the regulation of SkBF, or to detect functional changes associated with the development of various diseases, and to evaluate the progression of a disease and efficiency of the disease treatment.

In general, there is no optimal method to assess SkBF; none of them is able to give accurate quantitative values of SkBF. Rather, the flow is presented in relative units. All of the methods have their advantages and disadvantages. Moreover, as they employ different principles, the direct comparison of the data obtained by different techniques is often not relevant, if at all possible.

Most frequently used methods to study the dynamics of the skin microcirculation include optical methods such as intravital dynamic capillaroscopy, photoplethysmography, venous occlusion plethysmography, laser Doppler flowmetry (LDF) and laser Doppler imaging (Serup et al., 2004). Alternative methods are based on thermographic assessment of blood flow or on measuring transcutaneous pO2 or on $^{133}$xenon clearance. The most recently developed methods include orthogonal polarization spectral imaging technique, sidestream dark field imaging technique (Treu et al., 2011), and laser speckle contrast imaging (Turner et al., 2008).

### 3.1 Laser Doppler flowmetry

LDF is a noninvasive method that has been developed and accomplished over the past 20 years. It enables a sensitive, continuous, noninvasive and real-time assessment of blood flow, being uninfluenced by the underlying skeletal muscle blood flow (Saumet et al., 1988).

In research, it has been used to study reflex control of cutaneous blood flow, and, in conjunction with other techniques (iontophoresis, microdialysis, and local warming and heating) to address the involvement of the endothelium in the local control of SkBF. Furthermore, the responses to drugs can be evaluated with respect to their local effect on skin microcirculation. Its use goes far beyond research purposes as it has currently also been used in clinical practice either as part of the diagnostic procedures or to follow the effectiveness of treatment.

### 3.1.1 Principles of laser Doppler flowmetry

The fundamental principles of LDF applied to the measurement of SkBF have been described in detail in several publications (Serup et al., 2006; Shepherd & Oberg, 1990).

The method is based on the Doppler shift of the emitted laser light when it travels through tissue and is reflected off the moving objects, such as the moving red blood cells. The Doppler effect is a physical phenomenon that occurs between two objects, a wave source and a wave receiver. The relative motion of the wave source and the wave detector causes a change in the wave frequency and wavelength. The difference between the frequencies of the emitted and received waves is called Doppler frequency shift.

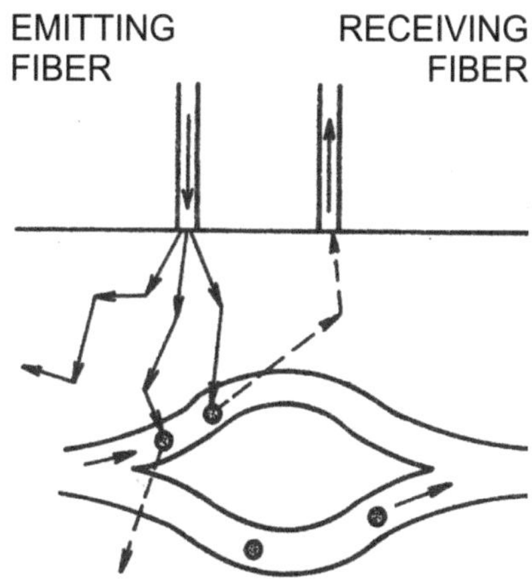


Fig. 1. A schematic diagram showing the detection of a red cell flux by laser Doppler flowmetry. Laser light is conducted to the skin via fiber optics. In the skin, a small fraction of the light is reflected by moving red cells with a shifting frequency (Doppler effect), whereas the rest is reflected by the same frequency. Both reflected beams are transmitted to the receiving optical fiber.

Prerequisites for LD technique are the characteristics of the laser beam, emitted to the tissue, such as monochromaticity and spatial and temporal coherence. The classical single-point probe consists of an emitting optical fiber with the source of laser light and usually, of two separate optical fibers that serve as receivers. The emitted light is guided through an optical fiber to the tissue where it is scattered, absorbed and only a small fraction is reflected (Fig.1). Stationary tissue reflects the light with the same frequency whereas moving cells reflect the light with a shifting frequency (optical Doppler effect). The frequency shift of the emitted light is proportional to the velocity of the moving erythrocytes. The reflected light is transmitted through one or more receiving optical fibers, and the nonshifted reference and Doppler-shifted beam are mixed on a photodetector and processed. The signal is then converted into electrical output that is fed through high-pass filters and amplifiers to finally obtain the signal as fluctuating voltage expressed in millivolts. The LDF signal is a stochastic representation of the number of erythrocytes in the sample volume multiplied by their velocity and is referred to as flux; rather than flowmetry, LDF is termed LD fluxmetry. Since the red blood cell flux is linearly correlated with SkBF it is taken as an estimation of blood flow. That is why the flux signal obtained by LDF is usually expressed in arbitrary perfusion units (PU). Due to the complex structure and the random orientation of the cutaneous microcirculation the obtained measurements are only semiquantitative and relative.

Due to the scattering of the emitted light in the tissue, only a small portion of the light incident on a tissue surface will penetrate very deeply and return to the surface. This is one of the reasons why LDF is ideally suited for measuring superficial tissues such as skin and mucosa.

The penetration depth of laser light depends on its wavelength (shorter wavelengths penetrate superficially, whereas longer penetrate more deeply) and on the distance between the transmitting and receiving fibers. It has been estimated that at small fiber separations, the signal is obtained from more superficial layers, such as capillary loops whereas at greater separations the contribution of deeper venous plexuses may dominate. In brief, different fiber separations or the use of lasers with lights of different wavelengths may enable the inspection of different depths of the cutaneous microcirculation.

The depth of measurement by LDF varies among tissues: for skin, it is estimated to be 0.5-1 mm. Considering the anatomical organisation of skin microvessels, the LD devices capture signals predominantly from the deeper subpapillary layer - the site of subpapillary arterial and venous plexuses. Thus, it records the thermoregulatory blood flow rather than the nutritive blood flow from papillary loops and superficial plexuses (Yvonne-Tee et al., 2006).

From the above, it is obvious that the variables which influence the measurement in one individual are the structure of skin surface and skin thickness as well as hematocrit.

Many commercial devices from different manufacturers are available today (Fig.2). Most of the current devices use a two- or five mW-powered helium-neon lasers with a wavelength of 632,8 nm and small probes. The surface area captured by such devices is estimated to be about 1 $mm^2$, whereas the penetration depth is 1 mm, resulting in a theoretical total measured tissue volume of 1 $mm^3$. Other available instruments nowadays use infrared light with a wavelength of 780 nm, applied by a diode laser. It is a challenge to develop devices using lasers with wavelengths below 600 nm, which will be able to record signals from the epidermis-dermis border. This would enable a more selective distinction between the deeper lying thermoregulatory component of blood flow and the more superficial nutritional component of the blood flow (Yvonne-Tee et al., 2006).

### 3.1.2 Application in humans: Calibration, validation and precautions

Before any measurement, the device has to be calibrated to instrumental zero (standard or instrumental calibration) and later on, the biological zero has to be determined. Instrumental zero calibration is obtained by placing the probe against a white surface. To test the sensitivity and to calibrate the device the probe tip is placed into a suspension of latex particles undergoing Brownian motion and the output of the flowmeter is tested.

The term biological zero applies to the LD flux that remains after an occlusion of a proximal artery. Before any measurement, biological zero can be assessed. The relative ratio between the normal resting flux and the biological zero value varies from region to region: biological zero LD flux can amount up to 20% of the resting flux (Tonneson, 2006, as cited in Serup et al., 2006). The sources of the biological zero seem to be blood cells that remained in the peripheral vessels during arterial occlusion and are still moving randomly and producing minor LD components recorded by the instrument as well as the Brownian movement of the interstitium (Kernick et al., 1999).

Before the measurement, the subject should rest for at least 20 minutes to acclimatize and calm down (Fig.2). Namely, a wide range of factors strongly influence the LDF signal and should be kept at minimum for a more relevant interpretation of the data. Such factors are subject-related: anatomical position of the probe, the subject's position, physical and mental activity, previous consumption of food, beverages containing caffeine or alcohol, smoking, taking drugs, menstrual cycle and temporal variations (circadian rhythms, inter-day variability, seasonal variations). Environment-related factors are first of all ambient temperature, air humidity and movement of the adjacent air. Factors that cannot be influenced and can have an impact on LDF are age, gender and, possibly, ethnic background. All these aspects must be taken into consideration and effort should be made to eliminate them or at least minimize to get the best possible results.

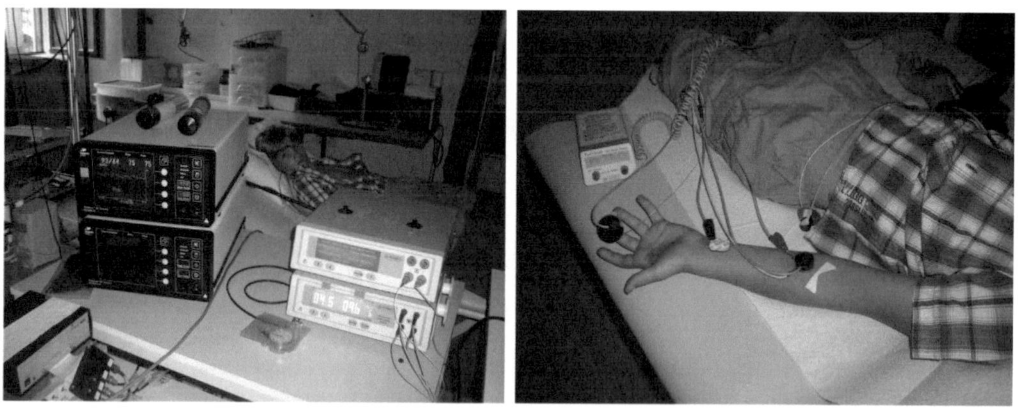

Fig. 2. A typical equipment for assessing skin microcirculation: Laser Doppler flowmeter (LDF, Perimed), the device to register blood pressure in the finger artery (Finapress, Ohmeda), and the transducer for a simultaneous transmission of the digital signals to the computer (left-hand). A typical position of the LDF probes: a standard LD probe (placed on the finger pulp, i.e. representative of glabrous site) and an iontophoretical delivery LD probe (placed on the volar forearm, i.e., representative of nonglabrous area) combined with the device for the application of iontophoresis (right-hand).

Debatable is also the temperature of the skin: while some authors recommend preheating the skin to a constant temperature and then performing a perturbation, others use the 'natural' skin without preheating.

Another problem are movement artifacts. To avoid it, person must lie completely still. Further, the probe must be in close contact with the measured skin; to do so, special two-sided adhesive tapes to fix the probe holder are available.

Due to the small measuring area and the anatomical architecture of the dermal microcirculation, there are considerable variations in blood flow (Braverman et al., 1990). To minimize the problem of spatial variability, several subsequent measurements have to be repeated and the data obtained averaged. Furthermore, newer devices include multiple point probes that have been designed to overcome the problem of immense spatial variability.

When performing LDF measurement, usually multi-channel devices are used that enable a continuous measurement of LDF in many sites simultaneously (Fig.2). Usually, the measurements are performed in the representative sites of glabrous and nonglabrous areas. Mostly measured glabrous sites in the upper extremity are palms, finger pulps and nailfolds, whereas nonglabrous sites include volar forearm and dorsal aspect of the hand and fingers.

### 3.1.3 Interpretation of the results

Many methodological issues must be taken into consideration when interpreting the results.

First, the strong site- and time-dependence of the obtained LDF signal and a great inter-individual variability must be taken into account. An accurate measurement should include the assessment of reproducibility in terms of the intraindividual variability coefficient that, based on some reports, could come up to 40%.

It is also important to realize that SkBF is very dynamic and apart from known factors that influence the variations (vasomotion, neural and humoral activity, heart beat and respiration related changes, respectively) there are also factors that cannot be ascribed to any known factor and thus explained. As a consequence, a wandering baseline is usually obtained. The seemingly random variation is much lesser when SkBF is perturbed, e.g. increased by heating or decreased by cooling. This is the basis for the provocation tests to be applied. Accordingly, more information is obtained in assessing vascular reactivity as a response to these perturbations. Rather than in absolute values, changes in LDF after such a perturbation are usually expressed as a percent of the baseline value.

Furthermore, it is advised to apply perturbation to induce maximal vasodilation (i.e. heating the skin to 44°C or applying an NO donor in excess) and thus achieve the highest (peak) flow and then express the quantity of the measured LDF relative to the peak flow. This would allow a comparison with the values assessed either by other devices or in other experimental conditions. Indeed, in many studies, the flow is expressed as a percent of the maximal flow (Crakowski et al., 2006; Turner et al., 2008).

Another recommendation is to express SkBF in terms of cutaneous vascular conductance (CVC) rather than in terms of flow. CVC is obtained by dividing the LD flux by mean arterial pressure. It is worth mentioning that all the measurements of LDF are usually performed with concomitant continual recordings of the blood pressure and the skin temperature.

The mostly exposed problem remains the standardization of the method as well as interpretation of the results that would enable a more accurate and relevant comparisons among studies using different devices and protocols. There is an urge to standardize the method as well as the protocols used (Crakowski et al., 2006; Turner et al., 2008; Yvonne-Tee et al., 2006).

### 3.1.4 Advantages and disadvantages

LDF enables a semiquantitative assessment of skin blood flow and is thus expressed in arbitrary PU. One of its disadvantages is thus inability to determine absolute blood flow.

Another disadvantage is great spatial and temporal variability. This must be taken into consideration when designing the measurements and interpreting the results. On the other hand, LDF has many advantages over some other methods: it is noninvasive, it can determine dynamic changes in skin microcirculation being uninfluenced by the underlying muscle blood flow (Saumet et al., 1988), it is easy applicable, reproducible, and, compared to many other methods, is relatively attractive regarding its price. As such, it remains the gold standard for assessing skin microcirculation and its reactivity in research purposes as well as in clinical practice.

### 3.2 How to study the endothelial function of the skin microcirculation

As with other techniques, there is no uniform technique that would separately evaluate only the endothelial function of skin microcirculation. Namely, the endothelium is not an entity per se but it is strongly associated with other structures, in terms of anatomy as well as physiology. There is a complex interaction between neural and other humoral mechanisms and the endothelium, so the methods used for evaluating separate mechanisms show considerable overlapping too. Therefore there is no single method that could give an insight into endothelial function but many different methods and tests have to be performed in order to get the clearest possible information.

Several methods to study endothelial function of the cutaneous microcirculation have been developed in recent years and are currently being used, each with their own advantages and disadvantages. By these methods, it is actually the vascular reactivity or vasodilator capacity that is being estimated: a part of this response also encompasses the endothelial component. So it is obvious that the results must be interpreted carefully when determining 'endothelial function'.

The usual approach to test endothelial function is to induce either a local or a systemic perturbation that will change the LDF. The stimuli used are pharmacological and physical ones. Of locally applied physical stimuli, flow mediated vasodilatation is important as well as locally induced changes in temperature, i.e. local heating and cooling (Johnson & Kellog, 2010; Kellogg, 2006). Flow mediated vasodilation is usually simulated by releasing a temporal occlusion of the proximal artery, and has thus been termed postocclusive reactive hyperemia (PRH).

The pharmacological stimuli are various agonists and antagonists that act directly on the endothelium or on the vascular SMC to induce changes in LDF. Often, they are coupled with the application of different blockers to inhibit the synthesis or release of the substance under investigation, as for example blockade of eNOS or COX or different adrenergic and cholinergic receptors as well as channels on the endothelial cells and SMC. There are various technique of application of these substances directly to the skin: their collective pitfall is that the exact concentration of the substance in the very tissue could not be determined accurately.

Let us briefly mention also commonly used systemic challenges that are often applied when studying skin microcirculation. These include systemic heating and cooling (more often the term whole body heating/cooling has been used), changing the oxygen partial pressure to induce hypo- or hyperoxia, and changes to perturb the baroreflexes: classic orthostatic test with a tilt-table or negative low body pressure and different mental tests. Namely, all the systemic changes also impact skin microcirculation and have been used to estimate the involvement of skin in reflexes associated with thermoregulation, exercise and other cardiovascular adjustments.

### 3.2.1 Pharmacological approach: Application of vasoactive substances

Endothelial function can be assessed by applying vasoactive substances locally and directly to the skin and recording the LDF response. In conjunction with LDF, this is performed most commonly by using iontophoresis and alternative methods, intradermal microinjection and microdialysis.

*Iontophoresis*

This is a method that enables application of soluble charged substances into the skin by means of an externaly applied direct electrical current (Kalia et al., 2004). Special iontophoretic drug-delivery electrodes have been designed that could be attached to the direct laser-Doppler probe (Figs.2,3). The quantity of the drug that penetrates into the skin is proportional to the magnitude of electrical current used. Usually, the quantity applied is expressed in milli Coulombs (mC), which are obtained as a product of the magnitude of electrical current (usually in order of μA) and the duration of the electrical current application. There are different modes of current application depending on the substance used and the protocol chosen: either protocol with a continuous application of current is used, or, more often, intermittent (interval) application of a constant or increasing current is accomplished. It must be taken into consideration that also curent alone causes vasodilation, referred to as 'galvanic response' (Abou-Elenin et al., 2002; Khan et al., 2004; Morris & Shore, 1996; Noon et al., 1998). The magnitude of the current-induced vasodilation depends on the vehicle used: a range of preparations have been used, including deionized water, tap water, sodium chloride and mannitol solutions, as well as different cellulose gels. The proposed mechanisms for the current-induced vasodilation are induction of an axon reflex (Noon et al., 1998), competition between ions of active substance and the vehicle (Khan et al., 2004), etc.

Another aspect that might influence drug delivery to the skin is skin resistance (Ramsay et al., 2002). It depends on the skin site, on the hydration status of the skin and also shows great inter-subject variability. To minimize the problem of skin resistance, skin should be cleaned with alcohol and gently rubbed mechanically to strip off the epidermis.

Nevertheless, iontophoresis has advantages over some other techniques. Compared to microinjection and microdialysis, it does not induce trauma affecting SkBF (Crakowski et al., 2007; Leslie et al., 2003). The quantity of drug is minimal and causes no systemic effects. Its disadvantage is the current-induced hyperemia, which can be minimalized by using an appropriate vehicle solution or by applying topical anesthesia (Crakowski et al., 2007; Morris & Shore, 1996); yet, the latter can impact the results in other way.

*Microinjection and microdialysis*

As alternatives to iontophoresis, microinjection or microdialysis have been used for the application of various pharmacological agents into the skin. By these techniques, either a solution containing a single substance or a mixture of different compounds can be applied. By microinjection, very small amounts (up to 10 μl) of agents of low concentrations are applied intradermally (Leslie et al., 2003). The advantage of microdialysis over microinjection is that the skin can be continuously perfused with the solution containing the active substance and in this way enables a constant stimulus or blockade of a certain compound (Crakowski et al., 2007; Turner et al., 2008). Moreover, using microdialysis, it is also possible to remove effluent fluid from the tissue and to determine certain substances of interest in the dialysate. The major disadvantage of microdialysis is its invasiveness (Crakowski et al., 2007).

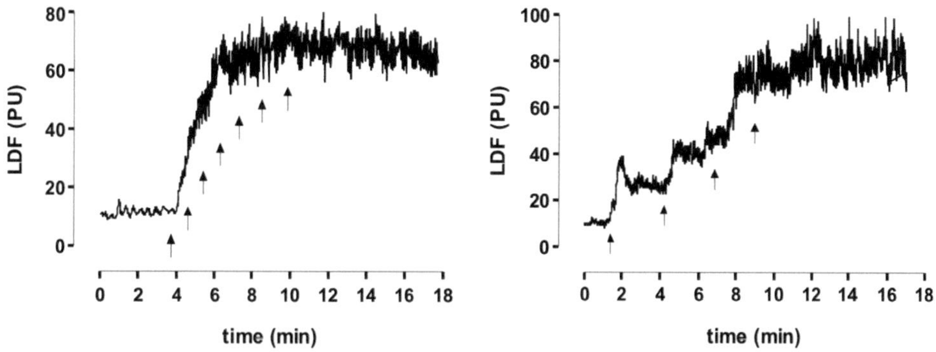


Fig. 3. A representative laser Doppler flux (LDF) response to pulsed iontophoretical application of acetylcholine, an endothelium-dependent agonist (left-hand) and sodium nitroprusside, an endothelium-independent agonist (right-hand) in the volar forearm of one subject. Arrows denote electrical pulses. PU, perfusion units.

Conventionally, ACh has been used as a standard drug to assess endothelial function (Fig.3, left-hand). It has been established, though, that apart from acting on muscarinic receptors expressed in endothelial cells it also affects other parts of the vessel wall: its potential action on the local nerve endings has also been proposed (Berghoff et al., 2002; Morris & Shore, 1996). In light of such observations, the data must be interpreted cautiously. Further, its action on the endothelium is debatable; multiple mechanisms have been proposed, including the involvement of NO, prostaglandins and EDHF (Holowatz et al., 2005; Kellogg et al., 2005; Khan et al., 1997; Morris & Shore, 1996; Noon et al., 1998; Turner et al., 2008).

Other commonly used drugs are metacholine, bradykinin, histamine, and substance P (Kalia et al., 2004). To test the reactivity of vascular SMC, sodium nitroprusside has been most commonly applied, usually by iontophoresis (Fig.3, right-hand).

### 3.2.2 Postocclusive reactive hyperemia

PRH refers to an increase in SkBF over the baseline following the release of a temporal occlusion of a proximal artery and has been used as an index of endothelial function (Fig.4), for research purposes as well as in clinical practice. It is characterised by an initial peak flux reached in a few seconds after the release that depends on the duration of the occlusion (Yvonne-Tee et al., 2008), and a subsequent return of the LDF to the baseline. However, PRH is a complex phenomenon that comprises metabolic and endothelial vasodilators, as well as a myogenic response and a sensory component (Lorenzo et al., 2007; Yvonne-Tee et al., 2008).

The endothelial component of the PRH response is believed to result from vasodilators (NO, $PGI_2$ and EDHF) released from the endothelium in response to augmented shear stress due to an increase in blood flow following the release of an occlusion. Yet, the results on the contribution of different endotehlial vasodilators are unequivocal (Bingelli et al., 2003; Dalle-Ave et al., 2004; Durand et al., 2004; ; Medow et al., 2007; Wong et al., 2003).

In the upper extremity, PRH has been performed by a compression of either brachial artery or diferent finger arteries, respectively to suprasystolic blood pressure. The most commonly used occlusion time is 3 or 5 min, but it can range from 1 and up to 15 minutes. Many parameters can be deduced from PRH; unfortunately, they are not standardised (Crakowski et al., 2006; Yvonne-Tee et al., 2008). Indices that are assessed most commonly are: the maximal (peak) LDF response after occlusion release ($LDF_{peak}$), the time to reach the peak response ($t_{peak}$), the half time in which the LDF returns to 50% of the baseline, the duration of hyperemia (time to recovery, $t_{rec}$) and the area under the curve (AUC) (Fig.4). The response of the microvasculature strongly dependes on the occlusion time (Wong et al., 2003; Yvonne-Tee et al., 2008).

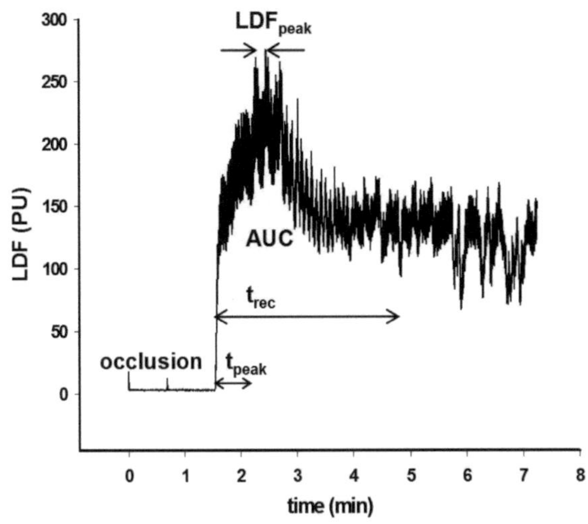


Fig. 4. A representative laser Doppler flux (LDF) response of postocclusive reactive hyperemia (PRH) obtained in the finger pulp after the release of a 3-min occlusion of the brachial artery. Typical indices of the PRH are indicated. PU, perfusion units.

PRH has also been used to induce or amplify the vasomotion in skin microcirculation (Rossi et al., 2008). It is proposed that amplified LDF oscillations are due to the local synchronicity of oscillatory blood flow in a group of cutaneous capillaries during ischemia. It is conceivable that these oscillations represent the local myogenic component of the PRH (Rossi et al., 2008).

### 3.2.3 Locally induced thermal changes: Heating and cooling

They are used to investigate the mechanisms involved in the local cooling and heating (Johnson & Kellog, 2010; Minson, 2010), as well as in clinical practice to determine microvascular (dys)function in different diseases.

Local heating is usually achieved by applying LD probes with a built-in heater; maximal vasodilation is obtained at a temperature between 42-44°C. As noted previously, maximal vasodilation is sometimes assessed to obtain the maximal vasodilating capacity; all other measurements are referred to this maximal vasodilation.

As for the cooling either LD probes with a built-in cooler or cold water of different degrees is used or flexible cold-gel packages are applied over the skin (Fig.5). Cooling by cold water or flexible packs also evoke a systemic response that can be tracked in other parts of the skin, as for example in the contralateral arm (Fig.5).

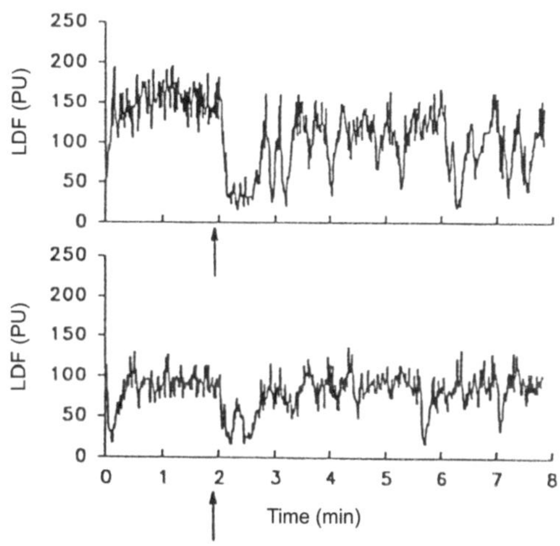


Fig. 5. A representative laser Doppler flux (LDF) response to local cooling obtained in the finger pulp of the ipsilateral hand (direct response, upper panel) and the contralateral hand (indirect response, lower panel), respectively. PU, perfusion units.

Both, heating and cooling, show typical patterns: an immediate response to the thermal stimulus as well as a later, sustained response. Part of the response is mediated by axon reflex, whereas there is also impact of NO and the endothelium. Cooling probably acts to inhibit NOS whereas heating causes activation of NOS (Johnson & Kellogg, 2010). Apart from eNOS, also involvement of neuronal NOS is proposed (Kellogg et al., 2009), which renders the interpretation of the results difficult. Additional studies are needed to clarify the exact contribution of different NOS isoforms (Kellogg et al., 2009).

### 3.2.4 Spectral analysis of the LDF signal

By means of spectral analysis, the LDF signal can be decomposed into components with different frequencies. It has been postulated that low frequencies around 0.01 Hz might reflect endothelial function, the frequencies at arround 0.04 Hz might reflect the neurogenic influence on the vessel wall, the ones around 0.1 Hz myogenic activity, whereas oscillations of higher frequencies at around 0.3 Hz and 1 Hz reffer to respiratory and heart beat activity, respectively (Kvandal et al., 2006). This is one of the tools used to assess endothelial function in physiologic (Kvernmo et al., 2003) and pathologic (Rossi et al., 2011) conditions. The most widely used spectral methods are fast Fourier transform, autoregressive modeling and wavelet analysis.

## 4. Human skin microcirculation and the endothelium: Impact of NO, prostaglandins and EDHF

The role of endothelium as a local regulator of vascular tone in skin microcirculation has been investigated in many studies. Furthermore, many studies have established an impairment of endothelium-dependent vasodilation in human skin microcirculation with aging (Black et al., 2008; Holowatz et al., 2007) and in disease (Colberg et al., 2005; Rossi et al., 2011; Taddei et al., 2006). Nevertheless, the exact contribution of various endothelial vasodilators to endothelium-mediated vasodilation has to be elucidated as the results are discrepant. The discrepancy may partly be due to different methods and agonists used to test endothelial function. It might be due to the use of different inhibitors of endothelial vasodilators or different mode of their application (oral, iontophoretical application, perfusion of the brachial artery). A mechanistic explanation would propose that inhibiting one pathway may lead to an upregulation of another one and thus blur the actual effect of the substance under investigation (Feletou & Vanhoutte, 2009; Nishikawa et al., 2000; Osanai et al., 2000). Furthermore, different endothelial vasodilators show a strong site-dependency (Schrage et al., 2005). All above must be taken into account when interpreting the results. It has not been extensively studied to what extent the endothelium contributes to the regulation of vascular tone and vasodilation in glabrous and nonglabrous skin area.

Although it is generally accepted that ACh mediates a NO-dependent response of endothelium (Kellogg et al., 2005; Turner et al., 2008), there are studies that did not confirm an involvement of NO (Hollowatz et al., 2005; Khan et al., 1997; Noon et al,1998). It has also been claimed that the contribution of NO to the ACh-induced vasodilation may be site-dependent: Noon et al (Noon et al.,1996) suggested that NO may be more important in the regions rich in AVAs (glabrous areas) than in areas with predominantly nutritive blood flow (dorsum of the hand). Even more debatable remains the role of prostaglandins in the ACh-mediated response in human skin microcirculation. While some studies have confirmed their role (Durand et al., 2004; Holowatz et al., 2005, Kellogg et al., 2005; Khan, 1997; Noon et al., 1998), others failed to do so (Abou-Elenin et al., 2002; Dalle-Ave et al., 2004; Morris& Shore, 1996).

A compelling study was performed by Hendry & Marshall: contrary to most other studies they showed that the inhibition of COX actually augmented the ACh- mediated increase in LDF (Hendry & Marshall, 2004). They speculate that in this setting, the vasoconstrictor products released by the endothelium (such as thromboxane $A_2$ and prostaglandin $H_2$) may limit the response to ACh, and not until the COX is blocked, could the maximal response to ACh be detected. In fact, it has been shown by other authors that thromboxane $A_2$ exerts its inhibitory effects on bioavailable NO by increasing oxidative stress (Tang et al., 2005) and inhibiting NOS (Yamada et al., 2003). Furthermore, Higashi et al. (2003) have shown that apart from NO, potassium-ATP channels, and cytochrome P-450, but not prostaglandins, may play a role in the ACh-induced vasodilation. Yet, their study was performed using a strain-gauge plethysmography (Higashi et al., 2003). In other studies, a portion of the ACh-mediated response, however, was attributed to an axon reflex (Berghoff et al., 2002;).

As for the role of NO and prostaglandins in the PRH, the results are controversial too (Dalle-Ave et al., 2004; Medow et al., 2007; Wong et al., 2003,). The role of NO seems less important than it was predicted. Namely, Wong et al. showed no effect of NOS inhibition on the PRH in the forearm skin (Wong et al., 2003). The results were substantiated by the study of Zhao et al., who assessed the concentration of NO in the microdyalisate using a NO selective amperometric electrode (Zhao et al., 2004). Other studies have confirmed an involvement of NO in the PRH response (Bingelli et al., 2003; Medow et al., 2007), yet it seems only of minor importance compared to other mechanisms. A conceivable speculation has been made by Medow et al: they propose that the COX inhibition unmasks the NO dependence of PRH in human skin (Medow et al., 2007). The results could strengthen the hypothesis on the crosstalks between various endothelial vasodilators in human skin. The role of the cross-talk between angiotensin II and NO has also been proposed (Loot et al., 2009).

As part of the ACh- and PRH –induced vasodilation in human skin microcirulation persists after simultaneous eNOS and COX blockade, it is speculated that other endothelial mediators might also be involved. There are also cross-talks between endothelial and neural mechanisms: NO has been shown to attenuate cutaneous responsiveness to norepinephrine via postsynaptic mechanisms (Shibasaki et al., 2008); furthermore, it is the $\alpha_2$-adrenergic receptor on the endothelium to mediate the NO-induced as well as prostaglandin-mediated vasodilation (Hermann et al., 2005). NO released from neuronal nNOS might be even more important than the one from eNOS (Kellogg et al., 2009). From above observations it is clear that different mechanisms contribute to the local regulation of vascular tone but their exact role has yet to be elucidated.

In the light of the aforementioned studies, we aimed at addressing the role of the nonNO-nonPGI$_2$-dependent mechanism in human skin in different measuring sites as well as using different provocation tests to stimulate the endothelium. We simultaneously applied eNOS and COX inhibitors to the volar forearm using intradermal micro-injection and performed iontophoresis of ACh. Our results have shown no effect of the combined inhibition on the baseline LDF. Furthermore, about 80% of the ACh-induced vasodilation persisted after combined NOS and COX blockade. We may only speculate about the mechanisms involved but according to other observations, it may be attributable to an endothelial mechanism other than NO and PGI$_2$, such as a putative EDHF. Other mechanisms, such as axon reflex, might also be involved; by applying an anesthetic cream to the measuring site we would be able to eliminate the potential axon reflex. This is one of the pitfalls of our study. Another pitfall is the microinjection tehnique; as mentioned previously, the quantity of a substance applied could not be determined. It might be that we were not able to achieve an adequate concentrations of the drugs *in situ*. In this regard, microdialysis would seem to be more suitable. In another set of experiments, we induced PRH after blockade of eNOS and COX to assess the role of nonNO-nonPGI$_2$-dependent mechanisms involved. After having obtained indices of PRH, the results have shown no differences in the L-NMMA and diclofenac treated sites as compared to the control sites, but there were differences in the AUC. Namely, AUC was slightly smaller in the treated sites (unpublished observation) which again points to only a minor role of NO and PGI$_2$ in the LDF response induced by PRH.

With respect to the role of EDHF in human skin *in vivo*, the studies are scarce. The existence of endothelium-dependent, NO/PGI$_2$-independent relaxations, potentially attributable to an EDHF, has been confirmed in humans *in vivo*. Based on studies in patients who exhibited a NO/PGI$_2$-independent response to an endothelial challenge, it has been suggested that EDHF might serve as a backup vasodilator in the settings of compromised endothelial function (Fichtlscherrer et al., 2004; Fischer et al., 2007; Taddei et al., 2006; Yang, 2007). Different putative mechanisms are proposed to mediate the EDHF-mediated vasodilation:

in humans, the most probable candidate is a CYP derived metabolite (Feletou & Vanhoutte, 2009). Indeed, a mechanism sensitive to CYP epoxygenase inhibition was confirmed (Bellien et al., 2005; Fischer et al., 2007; Fischtlscherer et al., 2004; Hillig et al., 2003; Taddei et al., 2006). Moreover, the CYP2C9 isoform was already confirmed on the endothelium of some human arteries where also a functional role of a CYP-derived EDHF was shown (Hillig et al., 2003; Larsen et al., 2006).

Based on the results from previous *in vivo* studies in humans our aim was to further characterize the nonNO-non$PGI_2$-dependent vasodilation in the skin microcirculation in the forearm. Therefore, we assessed the LDF response to ACh and PRH in the presence and absence of the selective CYP 2C9 inhibitor, sulfaphenazole, respectively. Contrary to most other studies that mainly applied the CYP inhibitors by perfusion of the brachial artery, we applied it by an intradermal microinjection. Sulfaphenazole had no effect either on the baseline LDF or on the vasodilation induced by ACh (Lenasi, 2009) or PRH (unpublished results). This is in agreement with some studies using venous plethysmography performed in healthy humans (Passauer et al., 2003, 2005), whereas at odds with most studies performed in patients (Fischer et al., 2007; Fischtlscherer et al., 2003; Taddei et al., 2006). We may explain the discrepancy with the studies performed in patients by the fact that the expression of CYP might be upregulated in patients due to a decrased bioavailability of NO. Again, methodological limitations must be taken into consideration, such as microinjection and the selection of a proper CYP inhibitor. Also, to evaluate the impact of EDHF in the control of skin microcirculation, it would be suitable to apply another endothelial agonist besides ACh. Namely, it has been proposed that the nonNO-nonPGI-dependent vasodilation might be more sensitive to bradykinin than to ACh (Schrage et al., 2005). Furthermore, the assumption that the NO/$PGI_2$-independent relaxation is indeed due to an EDHF would be strengthened had we applied an inhibitor of $Ca^{2+}$-activated K-channels or a depolarizing agent to at least indirectly prove an endothelium-dependent hyperpolarization (Feletou and Vanhoutte, 2009).

Taken together, different endothelial vasodilators are involved in the control of vascular reactivity of the skin microcirculation. The exact mechanisms involved and the role of a putative EDHF remain to be established.

## 5. Exercise augments the endothelium dependent vasodilation in skin microcirculation

Beneficial effects of exercise on the vascular reactivity of human skin microcirculation have been reported in many studies (Hodges et al., 2010). In general, the collective finding is that regular physical exercise enhances endothelium-dependent vasodilation. Moreover, it has been shown that exercise also improves the decline of endothelium-dependent vasodilation of cutaneous microcirculation in age (Black et al., 2008) and disease (Colberg et al., 2005; Rossi et al., 2011; Taddei et al., 2006).

The exact mechanisms of exercise-induced adaptations in human skin microcircultion remain unresolved. Various mechanisms have been proposed, the most likely one seems to be an increased production of NO by increased eNOS activity, probably due to repetitively increased shear stress on the endothelium (Green et al., 2004). Apart from endothelial adaptations, changes in the sensitivity of vascular SMC to endothelial vasodilators or alterations in neural vascular control may play a role. By inducing local heating as a vasodilating stimulus, the study of Tew et al. has shown that aerobic fitness affects the contribution of noradrenergic sympathetic fibers to the heating-induced LDF response (Tew et al., 2011). Indeed, it has been shown that endurance trained athletes have a diminished temperature threshold for active vasodilation in skin compared to matched sedentary controls (Fritzsche & Coyle, 2000). It is thus obvious that apart from local, possibly endothelial mechanisms, neural mechanisms also are subject to adaptations.

We aimed at assessing vascular reactivity in highly endurance-trained athletes with a high maximal aerobic capacity ($V_{O2max}$ 65 ml/min/kg) and comparing it with age-matched, sedentary controls ($V_{O2max}$ 41 ml/min/kg). Vascular reactivity was assessed at two representative sites with different control mechanisms: glabrous and nonglabrous area, respectively. Namely, it has been shown that the hemodynamic changes associated with acute exercise differ between these two sites (Yamazaki & Sone, 2006). The amplitude of changes, expressed as CVC as well as the time in which the changes occur during exercise differ between these two sites which might point to different control mechanisms. We hypothesised that similar differences might also be observed regarding adaptation to chronic exercise. We determined vascular reactivity by an iontophoretical application of ACh and SNP as well as by inducing PRH. Unfortunately, we were able to aplly ACh and SNP only to nonglabrous skin sites. As for the glabrous areas, we assessed the response to a 4 min brachial artery occlusion on the finger pulp and compared it with the response in the volar forearm. As expected, we found an increased responsiveness, as assessed by peak response to ACh and the indices of PRH, respectively, in the trained. Yet, the differences in indices of PRH were observed only in the glabrous sites and not in the nonglabrous, respectively (Lenasi & Štrucl, 2010). This may prove that glabrous parts with abundant AVAs are indeed more strongly involved in thermoregulatory adaptations to exercise. The adaptation of skin microcirculation to exercise might be explained by a direct effect of exercise-induced shear stress on the vessels, as well as by adaptive changes attending thermoregulatory challenges. The discrimination between these two mechanisms is not possible as they overlap each other. Nevertheless, Lorenzo & Minson have shown that skin microcirculation also undergoes thermoadaptative changes as a part of acclimation to heat without eliciting reflexes engaged in exercise (Lorenzo & Minson, 2010). To do so, they trained subjects only at 50% of their $V_{O2max}$, intensity that assumingly does not induce changes in the reflexes affecting exercise. Another interesting approach was by Rossi et al.: by performing spectral analysis of the LDF signal, they showed an augmented amplitude of the low frequency band presumably reflecting endothelial function in the trained (Rossi et al., 2006). Similar observations were found in the study performed by Kvernmo et al. (Kvernmo et al., 2003).

Exercise training probably induces adaptations in all age groups. Namely, a recent study performed in adolescents showed an enhanced endothelium-dependent vasodilation in nonglabroous skin in the group of trained subjects (Roche et al., 2010). Also, in the group of postmenopausal women who underwent a 48-week regime of aerobic exercise training the endothelium-dependent and –independent vasodilation was enhanced as well as the response to local heating (Hodges et al., 2010). Black et al. have shown that age-related decline in endothelial function can be improved already after 24 weeks aerobic training (Black et al., 2008). Contrary to the observation by Hodges et al (Hodges et al., 2010) on an increased endothelium-independent vasodilation (induced by an application of SNP) we found a decreased response to SNP in the trained. The result is at odds with most other studies that either showed no differences in the SNP-induced vasodilation between the sedentary and the trained or an increased response in the trained. Our observation is difficult to interpret; we suggested a decreased sensitivity of vascular SMC to a NO donor (Gori & Parker, 2002) which seems in certain respect illogical. The data on the vasodilator response to heating show that the LDF increase to the application of ACh occurs prior to the increase induced by SNP (Kellog et al., 2005). This might suggest that the endothelium is modified by exercise sooner then the vascular SMC. The observation would support the results of the studies that found no differences in endothelium-independent vasodilation between the trained and the sedentary.

Interestingly, most studies found no differences in the baseline LDF between the trained and the sedentary. The same holds true also for longitudinal studies that were performed in a cohort of subjects who underwent training and thus are more reliable (Black et al., 2008; Hodges et al., 2010). This seems logical as under resting conditions the nutritional needs of skin microcirculation are similar for the trained and the sedentary. When performing exercise, the trained exhibit a greater vasodilator capacity, probably of endothelial origin that may fulfil the increased demands for heat elimination in the trained.

It has been accepted that augmented endothelium vasodilator capacity induced by training are due to increased bioavailability of NO (Green et al., 2004). The speculative functional studies were confirmed by Wang, who has shown an increased response to ACh as well as an increased level of plasma NO metabolites after 8 weeks of training in healthy subjects. (Wang, 2005). Also, Vassalle et al. have shown an enhanced release of NO in the trained combined to an increased LDF response induced by PRH (Vassalle et al., 2003). Increased NO might be due to an upregulation of eNOS or its enhanced activity. Other mechanisms are proposed, such as an increase in plasma antioxidant activity (Franzoni et al., 2004) that prevent the scavenging of NO by free radicals and increase the bioavailability of its precursors (Doutreleau et al., 2010) and cofactors and thus increase its bioavailability. Apart from changes in the bioavailability of NO, an increase of other vasodilators, such as prostanoids (McCord et al., 2006) and EDHF (Taddei et al., 2006), may also be involved. It has been shown that prostanoids contribute to endothelium-mediated vasodilation in response to acute exercise (Duffy et al., 1999). Studies performed in animals have shown an increase in EDHF-mediated vasodilation induced by training (Minami et al., 2002). The same mechanisms are speculated to also play a role in humans. Additional studies in humans are needed to clarify this issue.

## 6. Conclusion

Skin microcirculation and the mechanisms controlling it remain an interesting area of research. As a dynamic structure, it is engaged in various thermoregulatory and non-thermoregulatory reflexes. Apart from neural control, the endothelium has been suggested to play an important role in the regulation of vascular tone and reactivity in skin microcirculation. However, glabrous and nonglabrous skin areas differ with respect to the control of vascular tone, also regarding the endothelium.

Laser Doppler flowmetry (LDF) represents an easy-to-apply, noninvasive and reproducible method to investigate skin microcirculation, yet with some disadvantages, such as great spatial and temporal variability. Coupled to LDF, many methods have been developed over the last 20 years in order to assess the endothelial function of human skin. Most frequently used are iontophoresis of ACh, postocclusive reactive hyperemia, and locally induced thermal changes. Apart from research purposes, they are often applied in clinical practice to assess the endothelial (dys)function and its response to therapy. They are suggested to be applicable indices of global microvascular function. Nevertheless, none of them is able to detect specifically endothelial function: rather, they provide integrated indices of vascular reactivity. This must be taken into consideration when interpreting the results obtained.

As skin microcirculation is often compromised in disease, also due to endothelial dysfunction, strategies on how to improve it are being sought. One of the measures to improve endothelial function seems to be participation in regular aerobic exercise, as it has been shown to be associated with enhanced mirovascular reactivity, in particular endothelium-dependen vasodilation, in glabrous and nonglabrous areas over the body.

The mechanisms involved in adaptations to exercise training as well as the exact contribution of various endothelial vasodilators (NO, $PGI_2$ and EDHF) to the regulation of vascular tone in human skin microcirculation, remain to be resolved. Nevertheless, they represent putative therapeutical targets and are thus important also from the clinical point of view.

## 7. Acknowledgement

The author wish to thank Olga Shrestha for language editing.

## 8. References

Abou-Elenin, K., Xydakis, A., Hamdy, O., Economides, P.A., Horton, E.S., & Veves, A. (2002). The effect of aspirin and various iontophoresis solution vehicles on skin microvascular reactivity. *Microvasc Res*, 63, 1, 91-5.

Aoki, K., Stephens, D.P., Saad, A.R., & Johnson, J.M. (2003). Cutaneous vasoconstrictor response to whole body skin cooling is altered by time of day. *J Appl Physiol*, 94, 930-934.

Bellien, J., Joannides, R., Iacob, M., Arnaud, P., & Thuillez, C. (2005). Evidence for a basal release of a cytochrome-related endothelium-derived hyperpolarizing factor in the radial artery in humans. *Am J Physiol Heart Circ Physiol*, 290, 4, H1347-52.

Berghoff, M., Kathpal, M., Kilo, S., Hilz, M.J., & Freeman, R. (2002) Vascular and neural mechanisms of ACh-mediated vasodilation in the forearm cutaneous microcirculation. *J Appl Physiol*, 92, 780-788.

Binggeli, C., Spieker, L.E., Corti, R., Sudano, I., Stojanovic, V., Hayoz, D., Lüscher, T.F., & Noll, G. (2003). Statins enhance postischemic hyperemia in the skin circulation of hypercholesterolemic patients: a monitoring test of endothelial dysfunction for clinical practice? *J Am Coll Cardiol*, 42, 1, 71-7.

Black, M.A., Green, D.J., & Cable, N.T. (2008). Exercise prevents age-related decline in nitric-oxide-mediated vasodilator function in cutaneous microvessels. *J Physiol*, 586, 14, 3511-24.

Braverman, I., Keh, A., & Goldminz, D. (1990). Correlation of laser Doppler wave patterns with underlying microvascular anatomy. *J Invest Dermatol*, 95, 283-286.

Braverman, I.M. (1997). The cutaneous microcirculation: Ultrastructure and Microanatomical Organization. *Microcirc*, 4, 3, 329-340.

Charkoudian, N., & Johnson, J.M. (2000). Female reproductive hormones and thermoregulatory control of skin blood flow. *Exerc Sport Sci Rev*, 28, 108-112.

Colberg, S.R., Parson, H.K., Nunnold, T., Holton, D.R., Swain, D.P., & Vinik, A.I. (2005). Change in cutaneous perfusion following 10 weeks of aerobic training in type 2 diabetes. *J Diabetes Complications*, 19, 276-283.

Crakowski, J-L., Minson, C.T., Salvat-Melis, M., & Halliwill, J.R. (2006). Methodological issues in the assessment of skin microvascular endothelial function in humans. *TRENDS Pharmacol Sci*, 27, 9, 503-508.

Crakowski J.-L., Lorenzo, S., & Minson, C.T. (2007). Effects of local anaesthesia on subdermal needle insertion pain and subsequent tests of microvascular function in human. *Eur J Pharmacol*, 559, 150-154.

Dalle-Ave, A., Kubli, S., Golay, S., Delachaux, A., Liaudet, L., Waeber, B., & Feihl, F. (2004). Acetylcholine-induced vasodilation and reactive hyperemia are not affected by acute cyclo-oxygenase inhibition in human skin. *Microcirculation*, 11, 4, 327-36.

Doutreleau, S., Rouyer, O., Di Marco, P., Lonsdorfer, E., Richard, R., Piquard, F., & Geny, B. (2010). L-arginine supplementation improves exercise capacity after a heart transplant. *Am J Clin Nutr*, 91, 5, 1261-7.

Duffy, S.J., New, G., Tran, B.T., Harper, R.W., & Meredith, I. (1999). Relative contribution of vasodilator prostanoids and NO to metabolic vasodilation in the human forearm. *Am J Physiol*, 276, H663-H670.

Durand, S., Tartas, M., Bouye, P., Koitka, A., Saumet, J.L., & Abraham, P. (2004). Prostaglandins participate in the late phase of the vascular response to acetylcholine iontophoresis in human. *J Physiol*, 561, 3, 811-819.

Feletou, M., & Vanhoutte, P.M. (2009). EDHF: an update, *Clin Sci*, 117, 139-155.

Fichtlscherer, S., Dimmeler, S., Breuer, S., Busse, R., Zeiher, A.M., & Fleming, I. (2004). Inhibition of cytochrome P450 2C9 improves endothelium-dependent, nitric oxide-mediated vasodilatation in patients with coronary artery disease. *Circulation*, 109, 2, 178-83.

Fischer, D., Landmesser, U., Spiekermann, S., Hilfiker-Kleiner, D., Hospely, M., Müller, M., Busse, R., Fleming, I., & Drexler, H. (2007). Cytochrome P450 2C9 is involved in flow-dependent vasodilation of peripheral conduit arteries in healthy subjects and in patients with chronic heart failure. *Eur J Heart Fail*, 9, 8, 770-5.

Fleming, I. (2010). Molecular mechanisms underlying the activation of eNOS. *Pflugers Arch – Eur J Physiol*, 459, 6, 793-806.

Franzoni, F., Plantinga, Y., Femia, F.R., Bartolomucci, F., Gudio, C., Regoli, F., Carpi, A., Santoro, G., & Galetta, F. (2004). Plasma antioxidant activity and cutaneneous microvascular endothelila function in athletes and sedentary controls. *Biomed Pharmacotherap*, 58, 432-436.

Fritzsche, R.G., & Coyle, E.F. (2000). Cutaneous blood flow during exercise is higher in endurance-trained humans. *J Appl Physiol*, 88, 2, 738-44.

Gori, T., Parker, J.D. (2002). Nitrate Tolerance A Unifying Hypothesis. *Circulation*, 106: 2510-2513.

Green, D.J., Maiorana, A., O'Driscoll, G., & Taylor, R. (2004). Effect of exercise training on endothelium-derived nitric oxide function in humans. *J Physiol*, 561, 1, 1-25

Hendry, R,G,, & Marshall, J.M. (2004). Vasoconstrictor products of cyclo-oxygenase activity limit acetylcholine-induced cutaneous vasodilatation in young men. *Clin Sci (Lond)*, 107, 3, 323-30.

Hermann, D., Schlereth, T., Vogt, T., & Birklein, F. (2005). Clonidine induces nitric oxide- and prostaglandin-mediated vasodilation in healthy human skin. *J Appl Physiol*, 99, 6, 2266-70.

Higashi, Y., & Yoshizumi, M. (2003). New methods to evaluate endothelial function: Method for Assessing Endothelial Function in Humans Using a Strain-Gauge Plethysmography: Nitric oxide-dependent and –Independent Vasodilation. *J Pharmacol Sci*, 93, 399-404.

Hillig, T., Krustrup, P., Fleming, I., Osada, T., Saltin, B., & Hellsten, Y. (2003). Cytochrome P450 2C9 plays an important role in the regulation of exercise-induced skeletal muscle blood flow and oxygen uptake in humans. *J Physiol*, 546(Pt 1), 307-14.

Hodges, G.J., Sharp, L., Stephenson, C., Patwala, A.Y. George, K.P., Goldspink, D.F., & Cable, N.T. (2010). The effect of 48 weeks of aerobic exercise training on cutaneous vasodilator function in pst-menopausal females, *Eur J Appl Physiol*. 108, 1259-1267.

Holowatz, L.A., Thompson, C.S., Minson, C.T., & Kenney, W.L. (2005) Mechanisms of acetylcholine-mediated vasodilatation in young and aged human skin. *J Physiol*, 563, 965-973.

Holowatz, L.A., Thompson-Torgerson, C.S., & Kenney, W.L. (2007). Altered Mechanisms of Vasodilation in Aged Human Skin. *Exerc Sport Sci Rev*, 35, 3, 119-25.

Holowatz, L.A., Thompson-Torgerson, C.S., & Kenney, W.L. (2008). The human cutaneous circulation as a model of generalized microvascular function. *J Appl Physiol*, 105, 1, 370-2.

Johnson, J.M., & Proppe, D.W. (1996). Cardiovascular adjustments to heat stress. In: *Handbook of Physiology*. Environmental Physiology, 215-243, Am. Physiol. Soc., Bethesda.

Johnson, J.M., & Kellogg, D.L.Jr. (2010). Thermoregulatory and thermal control in the human cutaneous circulation. *Front Biosci*, S2: 825-853.

Kalia, Y.N., Naik, A., Garrison, J., & Guy, R.H. (2004). Iontophoretic drug delivery. *Adv Drug Deliv Rev*, 56, 619-658.

Kellogg, D.L.Jr., Zhao, J.L., Coey, U, & Green, J.V. (2005). Acetylcholine-induced vasodilation is mediated by nitric oxide and prostaglandins in human skin. *J Appl Physiol*. 98, 629-632.

Kellogg, D.L.Jr. (2006). In vivo mechanisms of cutaneous vasodilation and vasoconstriction in humans during thermoregulatory challenges. *J Appl Physiol*. 100, 1709-1718.

Kellogg, D.L.Jr., Zhao, J.L., & Wu, Y. (2009). Roles of nitric oxide synthase isoforms in cutaneous vasodilation induced by local warming of the skin and whole body heat stress in humans. *J Appl Physiol*, 107, 5, 1438-44.

Kernick, D.P., Tooke, J.E., & Shore, A.C. (1999). The biological zero signal in laser Doppler fluximetry - origins and practical implications. *Pflugers arch Eur J Physiol*, 437, 624-631.

Khan, F., Davidson, N.C. , Littleford, R.C., Litchfield, S.J., Struthers, A.D., & Belch., J.J. (1997). Cutaneous vascular responses to acetylcholine are mediated by a prostanoid-dependent mechanism in man. *Vasc Med*, 2, 82-6.

Khan, F., Newton, D.J., Smyth, E.C., & Belch, J.J. (2004). Influence of vehicle resistance on transdermal iontophoretic delivery of acetylcholine and sodium nitroprusside in humans. *J Appl Physiol*, 97, 883-887.

Kvandal, P., Landsverk, S.A., Bernjak, A., Stefanovska, A., Kvernmo, H.D., & Kirkebøen, K.A. (2006). Low-frequency oscillations of the laser Doppler perfusion signal in human skin. *Microvasc Res*, 72, 120-127.

Kvernmo, H.D., Stefanowska, A., & Kirkeboen, K.A. (2003). Enhanced endothelial activity reflected in cutaneous blood flow oscillations of athletes. *Eur J Appl Physiol*, 90, 16-22.

Larsen, B.T., Miura, H., Hatoum, O.A., Campbell, W.B., Hammock, B.D., Zeldin, D.C., Falck, J.R., & Gutterman, D.D. (2006). Epoxyeicosatrienoic and dihydroxyeicosatrienoic acids dilate human coronary arterioles via BK(Ca) channels: implications for soluble epoxide hydrolase inhibition. *Am J Physiol Heart Circ Physiol*, 290, 2, H491-9.

Lenasi, H. (2010). The role of nitric oxide- and prostacyclin-independent vasodilatation in the human cutaneous microcirculation: effect of cytochrome P450 2C9 inhibition. *Clin Physiol Funct Imaging*, 29, 4, 263-70.

Lenasi, H., & Štrucl, M. (2010). Regular physical activity alters the postocclusive reactive hyperemia of the cutaneous microcirculation. *Clin Hemorheol Microcirc*, 45, 365-374.

Leslie, S.J., Affolter, J., Denvir, M.A., & Webb, D.J. (2003). Validation of laser Doppler flowmetry coupled with intra-dermal injection for investigating effects of vasoactive agents on the skin microcirculation in man. *Eur J Clin Pharmacol*, 59, 99-102.

Loot, A.E., Schreiber, J.G., Fisslthaler, B., & Fleming, I. (2009). Angiotensin II impairs endothelial function via tyrosine phosphorylation of the endothelial nitric oxide synthase. *J Exp Med*, 206, 13, 2889-2896.

Lorenzo, S., & Minson, C.T. (2007). Human cutaneous reactive hyperaemia: role of $BK_{Ca}$ channels and sensory nerves. *J Physiol*, 585, 1, 295-303.

Lorenzo, S., & Minson, C.T. (2010). Heat acclimation improves cutaneous vascular function and sweating in trained cyclists. *J Appl Physiol*, 109, 6, 1736-43.

McCord, G.R., Cracowski, J-L. & Minson, C.T. (2006). Prostanoids contribute to cutaneus active vasodilation in humans. *Am J Physiol Regul Integr Comp Physiol*, 291, R596-R602.

Medow, M.S., Taneja, I., & Stewart, J.M. (2007). Cyclooxygenase and nitric oxide synthase dependence of cutaneous reactive hyperemia in humans. *Am J Physiol Heart Circ Physiol*, 293, H425-H432.

Minami, A., Ishimura, N., Harada, N., Sakamoto, S., Niwa, Y., & Nakaya, Y. (2002). Exercise training improves acetylcholine-induced endothelium-dependent hyperpolarization in type 2 diabetic rats, Otsuka Long-Evans Tokushima fatty rats. *Atherosclerosis*, 162, 1, 85-92.

Minson, C.T. (2010). Thermal provocation to evaluate microvascular reactivity in human skin. *J Appl Physiol*, 109: 1239-1246.

Morris, S.J., & Shore, A.C. (1996). Skin blood flow responses to the iontophoresis of acetylcholine and sodium nitroprusside in man: Possible mechanisms. *J Physiol*, 496, 531-542.

Nishikawa, Y., Stepp, D.W., & Chilian, W.M. (2000). Nitric oxide exerts feedback inhibition on EDHF-induced coronary arteriolar dilation in vivo. *Am J Physiol Heart Circ Physiol*, 279, H459–H465.

Noon, J.P., Haynes, W.G., Webb, D., & Shore, A.C. (1996). Local inhibition of nitric oxide generation in man reduces blood flow in finger pulp but not in hand dorsum skin. *J Physiol*, 490, 501-8.

Noon, J.P., Walker, B.R., Hand, M.F., & Webb, D.J. (1998). Studies with iontophoretic administration of drugs to human dermal vessels in vivo: cholinergic vasodilatation is mediated by dilator prostanoids rather than nitric oxide. *Br J Clin Pharmacol*, 45, 545-550.

Osanai, T., Fujita, N., Fujiwara, N., Nakano, T., Takahashi, K., Guan, W., & Okomura, K. (2000). Cross talk of shear-induced production of prostacyclin and nitric oxide in endothelial cells. *Am J Physiol Heart Circ Physiol*, 278, H233–H238.

Passauer, J., Pistrosch, F., Lässig, G., Herbrig, K., Büssemaker, E., Gross, P., & Fleming, I. (2005). Nitric oxide- and EDHF-mediated arteriolar tone in uremia is unaffected by selective inhibition of vascular cytochrome P450 2C9. *Kidney Int*, 67, 5, 1907-12.

Passauer, J., Bussemaker, E., Lassig, G., Pistrosch, F., Fauler, J., Gross, P., & Fleming, I. (2003). Baseline blood flow and bradykinin-induced vasodilator responses in the human forearm are insensitive to the cytochrome P450 2C9 (CYP2C9) inhibitor sulphaphenazole. *Clin Sci (Lond)*, 105(4), 513-8.

Pohl, U., & deWit, C. (1999). A Unique Role of NO in the Control of Blood Flow. *News Physiol Sci*, 14, 74-80.

Ramsay, J.E., Ferrell, W.R., Greer, I.A., & Sattar, N. (2002). Factors critical to iontophoretic assessment of vascular reactivity: implications for clinical studies of endothelial dysfunction. *J Cardiovasc Pharmacol*, 39, 9-17.

Roche, D.M., Rowland, T.W., Garrard, M., Marwood, S., & Unnithan, V.B. (2010). Skin microvascular reactivity in trained adolescents. *Eur J Appl Physiol*, 108, 1201-1208.

Roddie, I.C. Circulation to skin and adipose tissue. In: *Handbook of Physiology*. J. T. Shepherd, and S. R. Geiger (Eds.). Bethesda: American Physiology Society, 1983, pp: 285-309.

Rossi, M., Santoro, G., Maurizio, S., & Carpi, A. (2006). Spectral analysis of skin blood flowmotion before and after exercise in healthy trained subjects. *Int J Sports Med*, 27: 540-545.

Rossi, M., Carpi, A., Galetta, F., Franzoni, F., & Santoro, G., (2008). Skin vasomotion investigation: A useful tool for clinical evaluation of microvascular endothelial function? *Biomed Pharmacother*, 62: 541-545.

Rossi, M., Bradbury, A., Magagna, A., Pesce, M., Taddei, S., & Stefanovska A. (2011). Investigation of skin vasoreactivity and blood flow oscillations in hypertensive patients: effect of short-term antihypertensive treatment. *J Hypertens*, 29, 8, 1569-76.

Rowell, LB. (1993). *Human cardiovascular control*. Oxford University Press, New York, Oxford.

Saumet, J.L., Kellogg, D.L.Jr., Taylor, W.F., & Johnson, J.M. (1988). Cutaneous laser-Doppler flowmetry: influence of underlying muscle blod flow. *J Appl Physiol*, 65, 478-481.

Schrage, W.G., Dietz, N.M., Eisenach, J.H., & Joyner, M.J. (2005). Agonist-dependent variablity of contributions of nitric oxide and prostaglandins in human skeletal muscle. *J Appl Physiol*, 98, 4, 1251-7.

Serup, J., Jemec, G.B.E., & Grove, G.L. (eds.) (2006). *Handbook of Noninvasive Methods and the Skin*, CRC Taylor & Francis Group, ISBN 0-8493-1437-2, Boca Raton, London, New York.

Shepherd, A.P., & Oberg, P.A. (Eds.) (1990). *Laser-Doppler blood flowmetry*, Kluwer Academic Publishers, ISBN 0-7923-0508-6, Boston Dordrecht London.

Shibasaki, M., Low, D.A., Davis, S.L., & Crandall, C.G. (2008). Nitric oxide inhibits cutaneous vasoconstriction to exogenous norepinephrine. *J Appl Physiol*, 105, 5, 1504-8.

Szerafin, T., Erdei, N., Fulop, T., Pasztor, E.T., Edes, I., Koller, A., & Bagi, Z. (2006). Indcreased cyclo-oxygenase-2 expression and prostaglandin-mediated dilation in coronary arteries of patients with diabetes mellitus. *Circ Res*, 99, 112-117.

Taddei, S., Versari, D., Cipriano, A., Ghiadoni, L., Galetta, F., Franzoni, F., Magagna, A., Virdis, A., & Salvetti, A. (2006). Identification of a cytochrome P450 2C9-derived endothelium-derived hyperpolarizing factor in essential hypertensive patients. *J Am Coll Cardiol*, 48, 508-15.

Tang, M., Cyrus, T., Yao, Y., Vocun, L., & Pratico, D. (2005). Involvement of thromboxane receptor in the proatherogenic effect of isoprostane F2alphaIII: evidence from apolipoprotein E- and LDL receptor-deficient mice. *Circulation,* 112: 2867-2874.

Tew, G.A., Saxton, J.M., Klonizakis, M., Moss, J., Ruddock, A.D., & Hodges, G.J. (2011). Aging and aerobic fitness affect the contribution of noradrenergic sympathetic nerves to the rapid cutaneous vasodilator response to local heating. *J Appl Physiol,* 110, 1264-1270.

Treu, C.M., Lupi, O., Bottino, D.A., & Bouskela, E. (2011). Sidestream dark field imaging: the evolution of real-time visualization of cutaneous microcirculation and its potential application in dermatology. *Arch Dermatol Res,* 303, 69-78.

Turner, J., Belch, J.J.F., & Khan, F. (2008). Current Concepts in Assessment of Microvascular Endotehlial Function Using Laser Doppler Imaging and Iontophoresis. *Trends Cardiovasc Med,* 18, 109-116.

Urakami-Harasawa, L., Shimokawa, H., Nakashima, M., Egashira K, & Takeshita A. (1997). Importance of endothelium-derived hyperpolarizing factor in human arteries. *J Clin Invest,* 100, 2793-2799.

Vanhoutte, P.M. (1989). Endothelium and control of vascular function. *Hypertension,* 13, 658-667.

Vassalle, C., Lubrano, V., Domenici, C., & L'Abbate, A. (2003). Influence of chronic aerobic exercise on microcirculatory flow and nitric oxide in humans. *Int J Sports Med,* 24, 1, 30-5.

Wang, J.S. (2005). Effects of exercise training and detraining on cutaneous microvascular function in man: the regulatory role of endothelium-dependent dilation in skin vasculature. *Eur J Appl Physiol,* 93, 429-34.

Wong, B.J., Wilkins, B.W., Holowatz, L.A., & Minson, C.T. (2003). Nitric oxide inhibitions does not alter the reactive hyperemic response in the cutaneous circulation. *J Appl Physiol,* 95, 504-510.

Yamada, T., Fujino, T., Yuhki, K., Hara, A., Karibe, H., Takahata, O., Okada, Y., Xiao, C.Y., Takayama, K., Taniguchi, T., Shiokoshi, T., Ohsaki, Y., Kikuchi, K., Narumyia, S., & Ushikubi, F. (2003). Thromboxane $A_2$ regulates vascular tone via its inhibitory effect on the expression of inducible nitric oxide synthase. *Circulation,* 108, 2381-2386.

Yamazaki, F., & Sone, R. (2006). Different vascular responses in glabrous and nonglabrous skin with increasing core temperature during exercise. *Eur J Appl Physiol,* 97, 5, 582-90.

Yang, Q., Yim, A.P.C., & He, G.-W. (2007). The Significance of Endothelium-Derived Hyperpolarizing Human Circulation. *Curr Vasc Pharmacol,* 5, 85-92.

Yvonne-Tee, G.B., Rasool, A.H.G., Halim, A.S., & Rahman, A.R.A. (2006). Noninvasive assessment of cutaneous vascular function in vivo using capillaroscopy, plethysmography and laser-Doppler instruments: Its strengths and weaknesses. *Clin Hemorheol Microcirc,* 34, 457-473.

Yvonne-Tee, G.B., Rasool, A.H.G., Halim, A.S., Wong, A.R., & Rahman, A.R.A. (2008). Method optimization on the use of postoclussive hyperemia model to assess microvascular function. *Clin Hemorheol Microcirc,* 38, 119-133.

Zhao, J.L., Pergola, P.E., Roman, L.J., & Kellogg, D.L.Jr. (2004). Bioactive nitric oxide concentration does not increase during reactive hyperemia in human skin. *J Appl Physiol,* 96, 628-632.

# 14

# Determination of Limb Hemodynamics During Rhythmical Muscle Contractions Assessed by Doppler Ultrasound

Takuya Osada[1,2] and Göran Rådegran[2,3]
[1]*Department of Sports Medicine for Health Promotion, Tokyo Medical University, Tokyo*
[2]*The Copenhagen Muscle Research Centre, Rigshospitalet University of Copenhagen, Copenhagen*
[3]*The Clinic for Heart Failure and Valvular disease, Skåne University hospital and Department of Cardiology, IKVL, Lund University, Lund*
[1]*Japan*
[2]*Denmark*
[3]*Sweden*

## 1. Introduction

Ultrasound Doppler instruments may provide valuable measurements of hemodynamic changes with high temporal resolution. In the clinical setting, Doppler velocity profiles may be useful for the evaluation of cardiac function, valvular disease and major conduit vascular disease. Furthermore, arterial stiffness and limb conduit arterial vessel dilatation following cuff-ischemia as measured by 2-dimentional echo imaging and Doppler ultrasound method are useful as surrogate parameters in atherosclerosis and hypertension.

Lifestyle related diseases such as obesity, hypertension, hyperlipidemia, and diabetes mellitus may be prevented by physical activity. Furthermore, a decreased amount of physical fitness or long term bed rest may lead to reduction of exercise tolerance (maximum oxygen consumption) due to cardiovascular-, respiratory- and muscle-dysfunction.

Circulatory changes following physical activity may also be used for studying cardiovascular regulation. For instance, cardiac output increases with increasing exercise intensity along with enhanced skeletal muscle vasodilatation and muscle pumping in the exercising muscle. Perfusion in the active muscle is furthermore one indicator of oxygen delivery to the muscles. Therefore, non-invasive Doppler measurements of blood velocity and flow in the feeding conduit arteries to working skeletal muscle may give us valuable information of the hemodynamic response in peripheral upper or lower limbs.

## 2. Exercise model

Determinations of blood flow to contractile muscles are the most important focus of the present chapter. Precise and stable measurements in conduit arteries assessed by Doppler ultrasound may be performed during exercise. Whole body exercise methods such as walking and running on a treadmill would be even better for the investigation of exercising leg blood flow. However, methods do not easily allow measurement of upper- and lower-limb blood flow using Doppler ultrasound in these models as motion artifacts are present. There is also difficulty in fixing the ultrasound Doppler probe. Local lower limb muscle blood flow may be measured using the one-legged, dynamic knee-extensor exercise model described by Andersen and Saltin (1985). This exercise model allows stable measurements of femoral arterial blood velocity using Doppler ultrasound (Figure 1). Therefore, all hemodynamic data described in this chapter are from dynamic knee-extension exercise.

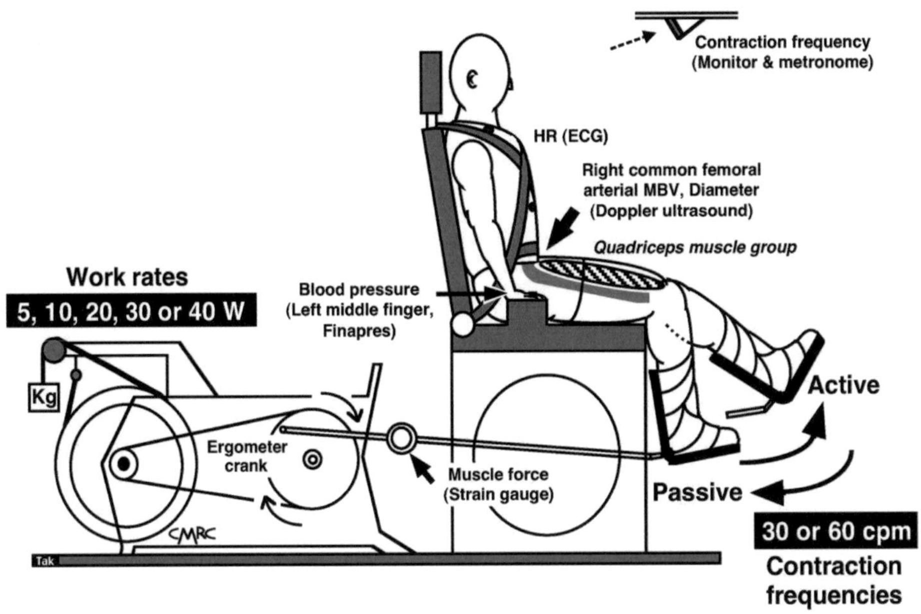


Fig. 1. Rhythmic thigh muscle contractions (one-legged dynamic knee extensor) model. Modified figure, reprinted with permission from Osada, T. & Rådegran, G. (2005). *Japanese Journal of Physiology,* Vol. 55, No. 1, pp. 19-28. by The Physiological Society of Japan.

## 3. Participants

All healthy male volunteers were familiarized with the above mentioned one-legged, dynamic knee-extensor exercise model before starting the experiments (Andersen et al., 1985; Andersen & Saltin, 1985). They trained at 30 and 60 contractions per minute at external target work rates of 10, 20, 30 and 40 W. Their hamstring muscles were allowed to fully relax, so that only the knee extensor musles performed the work. The subject's thigh was positioned horizontally with the knee joint bent. The lower leg moved up to ~ $60^{o}$ angle from the bent knee joint. All subjects provided written informed consent to participate in the study, which was approved by the Ethical Committees of Copenhagen and Frederiksberg (KF-01-013/96). The study adhered to the principles of the Helsinki Declaration.

## 4. Hemodynamic measurements

### 4.1 Doppler instrumentation

The measurements were performed using a Doppler ultrasound instrument (Model CFM 800, Vingmed Sound, Horten, Norway) equipped with an annular phased array transducer (Vingmed Sound) probe (11.5-mm diameter). The imaging frequency was 7.5 MHz and the Doppler frequencies varied between 4.0 and 6.0 MHz (high-pulsed repetition frequency mode, 4 - 36 kHz). Blood velocity was measured with the probe at the lowest possible insonation angle and always < 60° (Gill, 1985). The mean value of the insonation angle was ~ 50°, which remained constant throughout the experiments for each individual. The probe position was stable and the sample volume was precisely positioned in the center of the vessel and adjusted to cover the diameter width of the vessel.

### 4.2 Measurement of blood velocity, vessel diameter and blood flow in femoral artery

The measurements of blood velocity and blood flow in the femoral artery using Doppler ultrasound has previously been validated and shown to produce accurate absolute values both at rest and during leg exercise such as rhythmical thigh muscle contractions (Hughson et al., 1997; Osada, 2004; Rådegran, 1997; Shoemaker et al., 1994; Walløe & Wesche, 1988). Compared with thermodilution, the high temporal resolution of Doppler ultrasound additionally enables continuous measurement of blood velocity throughout the kicking cycle during exercise (Osada & Rådegran, 2002; Rådegran, 1997; Rådegran & Saltin, 1998; Roberg et al., 1997; Shoemaker et al., 1994; Walløe & Wesche, 1988).

The angle-corrected, time and space-averaged, and amplitude-weighted mean ($V_{mean}$) and maximum ($V_{max}$; outer envelope) blood velocities, respectively, were measured. $V_{mean}$ was defined by averaging the mean blood velocity trace (Osada & Rådegran, 2002; Rådegran, 1997). $V_{max}$ was defined as the maximum outer envelope (Leyk et al., 1992; Osada et al., 1999; Osada et al., 2003). The $V_{max}$ obtained in the present study was expressed as the blood velocity measured at the center of the vessel. Each blood velocity parameter was measured in relation to the blood pressure curve. The site of blood velocity and vessel diameter measurements in the femoral artery was distal to the inguinal ligament but above the bifurcation into the branch of the superficial and deep femoral artery. This location minimizes turbulence from the femoral bifurcation and the influence of blood flow from the inguinal region. In addition, the arterial diameter is not affected by the contractions and relaxations at this site located proximal to the muscle.

The blood velocity measurements were performed for approximately 2 to 3 min, when steady-state had been reached after 3 min of one-legged, dynamic knee extensor (Osada, 2004; Rådegran & Saltin, 1998), as previously described (Rådegran, 1997). The systolic and diastolic diameters of the femoral artery were measured on a monitor relative to the ECG at rest. The mean vessel diameter was calculated in relation to the temporal duration of the blood pressure curve as; [(systolic vessel diameter value × 1/3) + (diastolic vessel diameter value × 2/3)] (Rådegran, 1997). The diameters were measured under perpendicular insonation at rest before exercise. The value of the vessel diameter at rest (pre-exercise) was used to calculate femoral arterial blood flow during rest and during one-legged, dynamic knee extensor, since the diameter does not significantly vary between rest and steady-state exercise (Hughson et al., 1997; Isnard et al., 1996; Leyk et al.,

1992; MacDonald et al., 1998; Osada et al., 1999; Rådegran, 1997). Steady-state leg blood flow was calculated by multiplying the cross-sectional area [Area = $\pi \times$ (vessel diameter/2)$^2$] of the femoral artery, with the angle corrected, time and space-averaged, and amplitude (signal intensity) weighted mean-blood velocity, where blood flow = mean-blood velocity × cross sectional area.

## 5. Validation of blood flow during incremental one-legged, dynamic knee-extensor as measured by Doppler ultrasound

In previous reports, central and peripheral hemodynamic measurements have been demonstrated using the thermodilution technique for cardiac output and limb blood flow during incremental cycling ergometer exercise. However, this invasive technique has the limitation of poor time resolution of blood flow. Several techniques have previously been developed that enable estimates to be made of arterial inflow, venous outflow, and local blood flow within a muscle. Whereas many of the techniques are impaired by different methodological limitations, the indicator methods and the ultrasound Doppler method have both been found to give repeatable measurements of the same magnitude during both rest and dynamic knee extensor exercise (Rådegran, 1997).

The Doppler ultrasound is unique as it allows continuous blood flow measurements non-invasively with a high temporal resolution. With continuous measurements, transitional changes in blood flow can be characterized (Walløe & Wesche, 1988; Wesche, 1986). The technique's precision and accuracy have furthermore been improved by sampling of the blood velocity continuously during dynamic knee extensor exercise (Rådegran, 1997). Doppler ultrasound may therefore be suitable for the investigation of transitional changes of limb hemodynamics in the conduit brachial, femoral and poplitial artery during rest and upper forearm or lower limb exercise.

Temporal blood flow changes due to muscle contractions during dynamic knee extensor exercise have been well described (Osada, 2004). Doppler ultrasound has furthermore been used to examine the hyperaemic response at the onset of exercise (Hughson et al., 1993; Rådegran & Saltin, 1998), steady-state (Osada & Rådegran, 2002) and recovery after exercise (Osada et al., 2003). At the onset of exercise as well as recovery after exercise, variations in blood flow may be influenced by changes in blood pressure, heart rate or strength of muscle contractions.

Furthermore, femoral arterial blood velocity and blood flow increases linearly with incremental target exercise intensities of work rate (workload) during steady-state rhythmic thigh muscle contractions. This implies that an enhanced vasodilatation is elicited, in relation to the increased average muscle force exerted at higher workloads, to meet the elevated metabolic activity.

Figure 2 shows the relationship between limb femoral arterial blood flow and target workload (10, 20, 30 and 40 W) in relation to rhythmic thigh muscle contractions at 60 contractions per minute. In addition, thermodilution blood flow measurements obtained under similar experimental conditions by Andersen and Saltin (1985) are closely related to those obtained by Doppler ultrasound. Thus, blood flow measured by Doppler ultrasound is valid not only at rest but also during incremental one-legged dynamic knee extensor exercise.

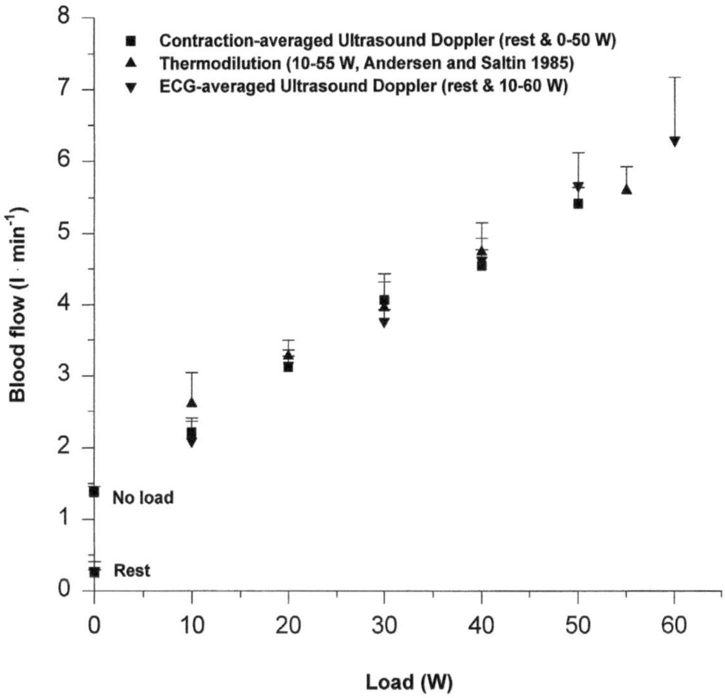


Fig. 2. Blood flow during incremental one-legged dynamic knee extensor exercise, estimated from mean blood velocity and averaged on a beat-by-beat basis or continuously measured and analyzed in relation to muscle contraction cycle. Reprinted with permission from Rådegran, G. (1997), *Journal of Applied Physiology*, Vol. 83, No. 4, pp. 1383-1388, by The American Physiological Society.

## 6. Variation of blood velocity and blood flow modified by muscle contraction-relaxation cycles

It is well known that conduit arterial blood velocity and blood flow is markedly influenced by intramuscular pressure, as well as the superimposed influence of the arterial blood pressure. The high intramuscular pressure during muscle contractions may consequently temporarily reduce or even reverse the blood velocity, depending on the relationship between the intramuscular- and arterial blood pressure. The major extent of the blood velocity and flow consequently occurs during the muscle relaxation phase. Figure 3 shows that mean blood velocity increased to its highest value at the systolic blood pressure phase during muscle relaxation, and significantly decreased to its lowest value at the diastolic blood pressure phase during muscle contraction. Mean blood velocity showed an intermediate value at the systolic blood pressure phase during muscle contraction and at the diastolic blood pressure phase during muscle relaxation, respectively. The blood velocity curve was furthermore retrograde in the diastolic blood pressure phase during muscle contraction. The figure below shows the contribution to the magnitude of the physiological variability in blood velocity and flow by the contraction-relaxation-induced variations in muscle force, and consequently the intramuscular pressure variations, along with the superimposed influence of the blood pressure as well as the tonic influence of the state of vasodilatation. Moreover, the exercise blood velocity and blood flow fluctuations due to muscle contractions and relaxations, with the superimposed influence of the cardiac cycle, are described in Figure 4.

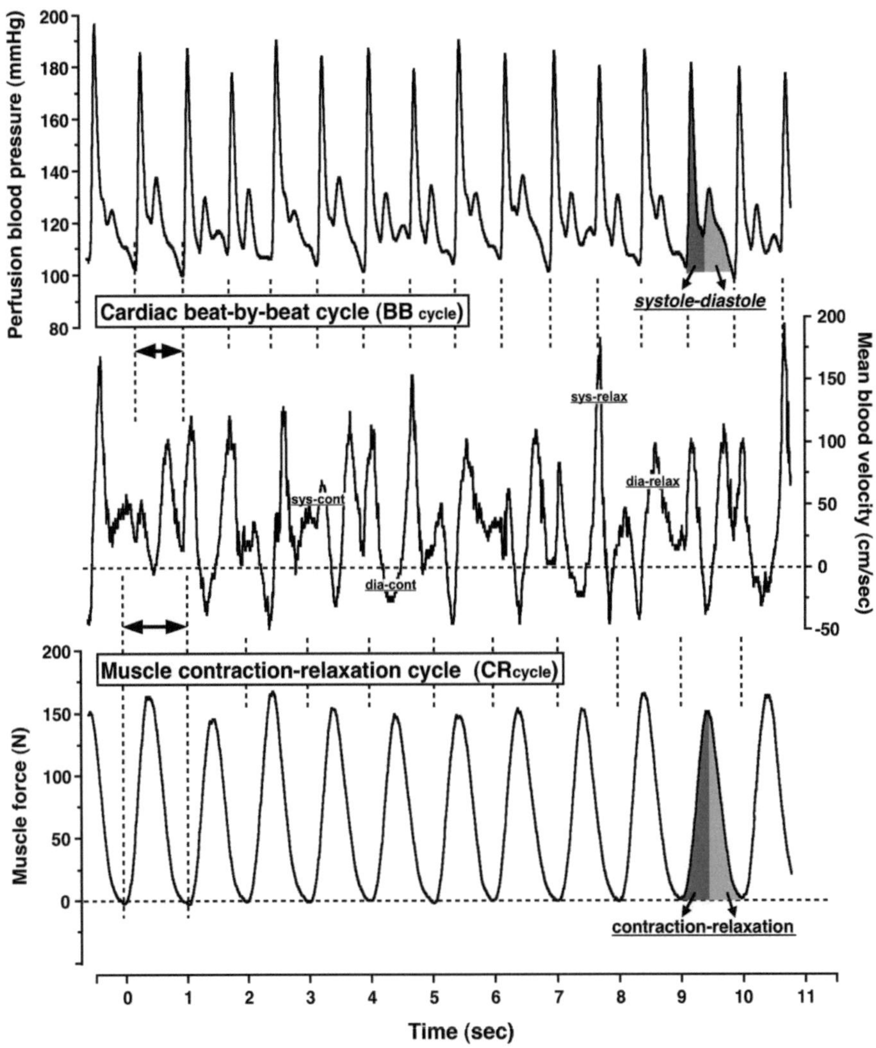


Fig. 3. Continuous recording of mean blood velocity, blood pressure and muscle force during steady-state one-legged dynamic knee extensor at 20 W and 60 contractions per minute in one subject: sys, systole; dia, diastole; cont, muscle contraction; relax, muscle relaxation. Modified figure, reprinted with permission from Osada, T. & Rådegran, G. (2006). *Journal of Sports Medicine and Physical Fitness*, Vol. 46 No. 4, pp. 590-597, by Edizioni Minerva Medica.

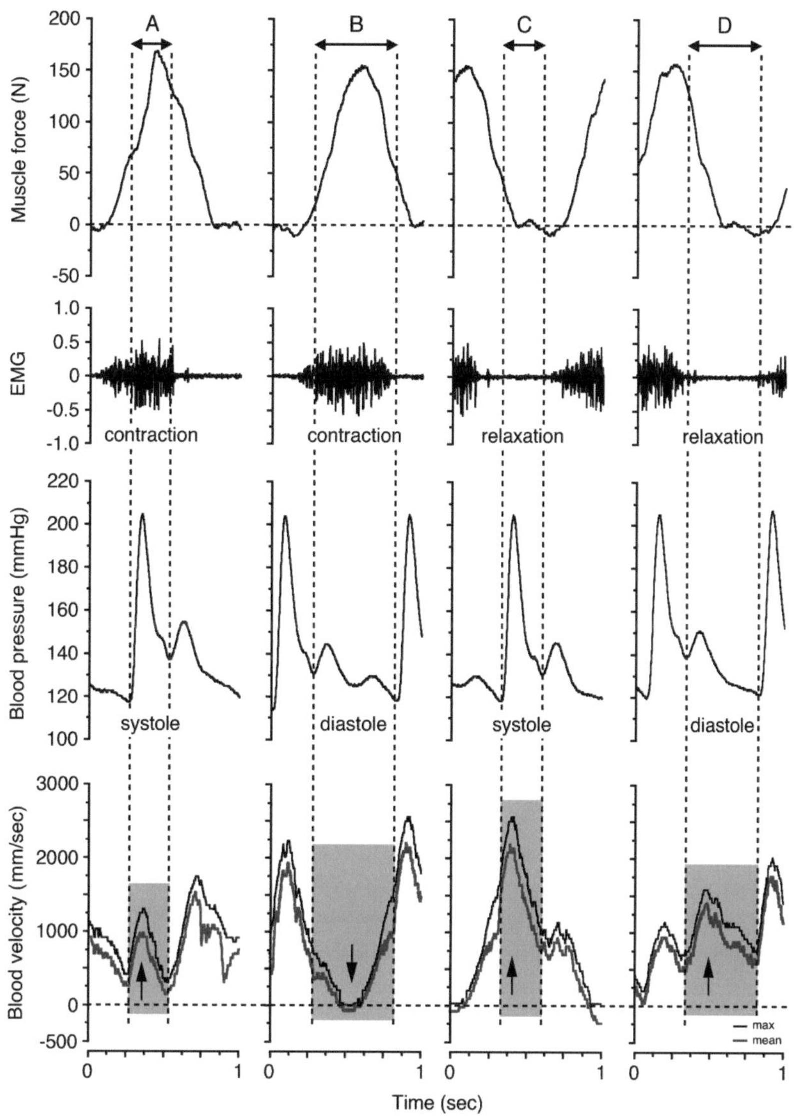


Fig. 4. Flow profile in the blood velocity ($V_{max}$ and $V_{mean}$) in the limb femoral artery for the cardiosystolic and cardiodiastolic phases during the muscle contraction and muscle relaxation phases of one-legged dynamic knee-extensor exercise at 20 W and 60 contractions per minute. Reprinted with permission from Osada, T. & Rådegran, G. (2006), *Journal of Physiological Science*, Vol. 56, No. 3, pp. 195-203, by The Physiological Society of Japan.

As seen in Figure 4, blood velocities ($V_{\max}$ and $V_{\text{mean}}$) during the cardiosystolic and cardiodiastolic phases were measured continuously in parallel with the blood pressure curve during the muscle contraction and muscle relaxation phases determined from the electromyography (EMG) and the muscle force curve. Blood velocity fluctuated in relation to the state of vasodilatation and the muscle contraction-relaxation duty cycles, indicated by the oscillations in muscle force.

Four variations (A–D) in the coupling between the blood pressure curve and the state of contraction and relaxation were indicated; (A) the cardiosystolic phase during muscle contraction, (B) the cardiodiastolic phase during muscle contraction, (C) the cardiosystolic phase during muscle relaxation, and (D) the cardiodiastolic phase during muscle relaxation. $V_{max}$ and $V_{mean}$ were determined as the "average" transient maximum (outer envelope) and mean (amplitude-weighted, time-and-spatial averaged) angle-corrected blood velocity values, respectively, for the cardiosystolic and cardiodiastolic phases. The formation of the blood velocity profile and flow was modified by the intramuscular pressure, as indicated by the muscle force curve, and the superimposed influence of the blood pressure in relation to the cardiosystolic and cardiodiastolic phases. The arrow down (↓) and up (↑) indicates the influence on the blood velocity and flow, depending on the magnitude of, and temporal relation between, the intramuscular pressure and the arterial blood pressure, respectively.

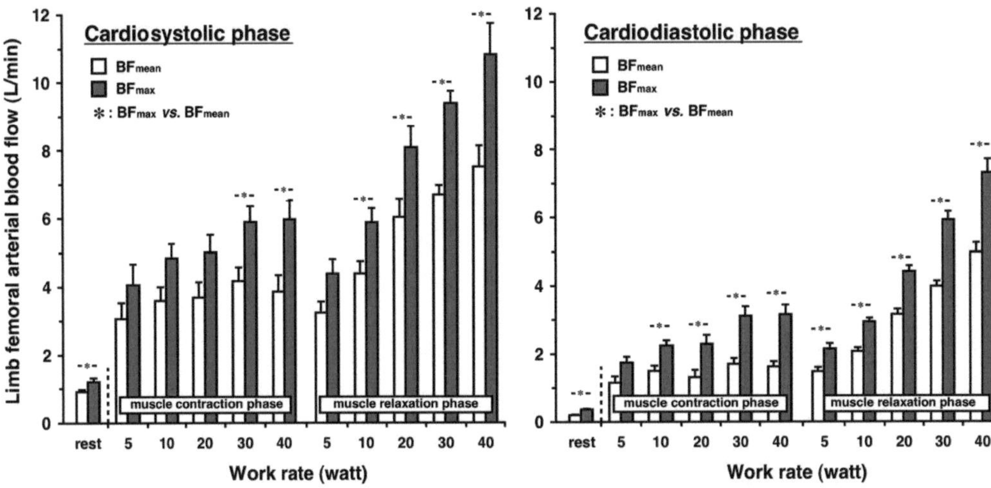


Fig. 5. Blood flow for the cardiosystolic and cardiodiastolic phases during the muscle contraction and muscle relaxation phases of one-legged dynamic knee-extensor exercise at 60 contractions per minute, *$P < 0.05$. Reprinted with permission from Osada, T. & Rådegran, G. (2006), *Journal of Physiological Science*, Vol. 56, No. 3, pp. 195-203, by The Physiological Society of Japan.

There is furthermore information available regarding differences in blood flow variations induced by muscle contractions and muscle relaxations at incremental exercise intensities at 5, 10, 20, 30 and 40 W (Fig. 5). These data clearly demonstrated that blood flow in the femoral artery increases during muscle relaxation, rather than muscle contraction. Also, there is a large difference in blood flow magnitude between cardiosystole and cardiodiastole at incremental exercise intensities. In consequence, the average exercise blood flow value may be over- or under-estimated if the time for measurement is restricted to only a single phase among the muscle contraction and muscle relaxation phases and the cardiosystolic and cardiodiastolic phases. This evidence of blood flow response due to muscle mechanical factor and cardiac pumping cycle is a clear physiological phenomenon, but the blood flow response in relation to the variations in the force of muscle contractions (≈ intramuscular pressure, workload) should be further clarified.

Of further interest is whether sudden changes in workload and rhythm may exert influence upon the magnitude of blood flow. Such information may be useful for the temporal evaluation of exercising blood flow during consecutive rhythmic muscle contractions with large variation due to poor exercise performance.

## 7. Changes in blood flow due to spontaneous changes of workload

Limb femoral arterial blood flow during steady-state rhythmic thigh muscle contractions increases linearly with incremental target workloads (work rates) (Hughson et al., 1996; 1997; Osada & Rådegran, 2002; Rådegran, 1997; Shoemaker et al., 1994; Tschakovsky et al., 2006). This implies that enhanced vasodilatation is elicited in relation to the increased average muscle force, exerted at higher workloads, to meet the elevated metabolic activity (Fig. 2). However, these blood flow values are a mean of steady-state exercising blood flow measurements, and temporary muscle contraction-induced blood flow variations may therefore be conveyed in the mean average blood flow value (Fig. 2, 4 and 5). For human voluntary exercise, it is of value to consider how variations in repeated muscle contractions at target muscle strength (muscle force) directly influence exercise blood flow in conduit arteries. Therefore, we've investigated whether sudden physiological and spontaneous changes in exercise rhythm, and consequently workload, temporarily alter blood flow to the working muscle.

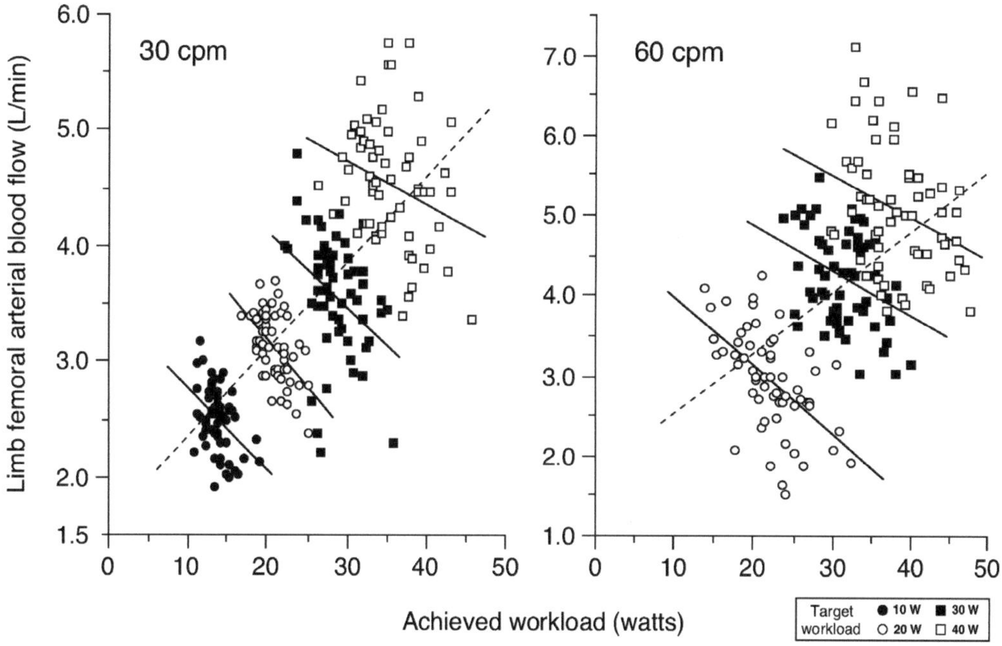


Fig. 6. Relationship between steady-state limb femoral arterial blood flow and the achieved workload during incremental one-legged dynamic knee-extensor exercise at 30 or 60 contractions per minute during a minute measurement in one subject (60 samplings at each workload). Modified figure, reprinted with permission from Osada, T. & Rådegran, G. (2009), *Clinical Physiology and Functional Imaging*, Vol. 29, No. 4, pp. 277-292, by John Wiley & Sons Ltd.

The results showed that limb femoral arterial blood flow increased positively and linearly (dotted line) with increasing target workload. However, limb blood flow was inversely and linearly related (solid line) to the actually achieved workload, when measured over 60 consecutive contraction-relaxation cycle bouts for each target intensity at 30 and 60 contractions per minute, respectively (Figure 6).

Thus any sudden spontaneous increase or decrease in the achieved workload transiently altered the relationship between limb femoral arterial blood flow and the achieved workload. The influence upon the magnitude of limb femoral arterial blood flow, due to fluctuations in the achieved workload from the target workload was similar at target workload sessions of 30 and 60 contractions per minute, respectively. These findings indicate that a transient sudden increase in the workload during rhythmic muscle contractions more rapidly impedes limb femoral arterial blood flow, than that vasodilatation may be elicited to restore the intensity related steady-state limb blood flow response, in relation to the average metabolic activity. This evidence in human applied science may contribute to the evaluation of exercise hemodynamics for rhythmic, dynamic-isotonic exercise training, leading to exercise prescriptions (muscle contraction frequency or muscle contraction intensity) for healthy participants as well as for patients, requiring additional physical activity in the rehabilitation or clinical setting.

## 8. Conclusion

Measuring exercise blood velocity and blood flow in working skeletal muscle assessed by Doppler ultrasound can be performed, however there are still limitations with regards to the exercise model, target vessel, muscle contraction-intensity and -frequencies, in upper or lower limbs.

## 9. Acknowledgment

The authors would like to acknowledge the support given by Professor Bengt Saltin, the staff of The Copenhagen Muscle Research Centre, as well as the volunteers who participated in this study. This study was supported by the Danish National Research Foundation Grant 504-14 (CMRC), in part by "a Grant-in-Aid for Young Scientists (B) (No. 16700471) in 2004-2005" as well as by the "Excellent Young Researchers Overseas Visit Program (No. 21-8285) in 2010" in Scientific Research from the Ministry of Education, Culture, Sports, Science and Technology (MEXT) of Japan and the Japan Society for the Promotion of Science (JSPS) (T. Osada).

## 10. References

Andersen, P., Adams, R.P., Sjøgaard, G., Thorboe, A. & Saltin, B. (1985). Dynamic knee extension as model for study of isolated exercising muscle in humans. *Journal of Applied Physiology*, Vol. 59, No. 5, pp. 1647-1653, ISSN 8750-7587

Andersen, P. & Saltin, B. (1985). Maximal perfusion of skeletal muscle in man. *Journal of Physiology (London)*, Vol. 366, pp. 233-249, ISSN 0022-3751

Gill, R.W. (1985). Measurement of blood flow by ultrasound: Accuracy and sources of error. *Ultrasound in Medicine and Biology*, Vol. 11, No. 4, (July-August) pp. 625-641, ISSN 0301-5629

Hughson, R.L., Cochrane, J.E. & Butler G.C. (1993). Faster O2 uptake kinetics at onset of supine exercise with than without lower body negative pressure. *Journal of Applied Physiology*, Vol. 75, No. 5, pp. 1962-1967, ISSN 8750-7587

Hughson, R.L., MacDonald, M.J., Shoemaker, J.K. & Borkhoff, C. (1997). Alveolar oxygen uptake and blood flow dynamics in knee extension ergometry. *Methods of Information in Medicine*, Vol. 36, No. 4-5, pp. 364-367, ISSN 0026-1270

Hughson, R.L., Shoemaker, J.K., Tschakovsky, M.E. & Kowalchuk, J.M. (1996). Dependence of muscle $VO_2$ on blood flow dynamics at onset of forearm exercise. *Journal of Applied Physiology*, Vol. 81, No. 4, pp. 1619-1626, ISSN 8750-7587

Isnard, R., Lechat, P., Kalotka, H., Chikr, H., Fitoussi, S., Salloum, J., Golmard, J .L., Thomas, D. & Komajda, M. (1996). Muscular blood flow response to submaximal leg exercise in normal subjects and in patients with heart failure. *Journal of Applied Physiology*, Vol. 81, No. 6, pp. 2571-2579, ISSN 8750-7587

Leyk, D., Eßfeld, D., Baum, K. & Stegemann, J. (1992). Influence of calf muscle contractions on blood flow parameters measured in the arteria femoralis. *International Journal of Sports Medicine*, Vol. 13, No. 8, pp. 588-593, ISSN 0172-4622

MacDonald, M.J., Shoemaker, J.K., Tschakovsky, M.E., & Hughson R.L. (1998). Alveolar oxygen uptake and femoral artery blood flow dynamics in upright and supine leg exercise in humans. *Journal of Applied Physiology*, Vol. 85 No. 5, pp. 1622-1628, ISSN 8750-7587

Osada, T., Katsumura, T., Hamaoka, T., Inoue, S., Esaki, K., Sakamoto, A., Murase, N., Kajiyama, J., Shimomitsu, T. & Iwane, H. (1999). Reduced blood flow in abdominal viscera measured by Doppler ultrasound during one-legged knee extension. *Journal of Applied Physiology*, Vol. 86, No. 2, pp. 709-719, ISSN 8750-7587

Osada, T., Katsumura, T., Murase, N., Sako, T., Higuchi, H., Kime, R., Hamaoka, T. & Shimomitsu, T. (2003). Post-exercise hyperemia after ischemic and non-ischemic isometric handgrip exercise. *Journal of Physiological Anthropology and Applied Human Science*, Vol. 22, No. 6, pp. 299-309, ISSN 1345-3475

Osada, T. (2004). Muscle contraction-induced limb blood flow variability during dynamic knee extensor. *Medicine and Science in Sports and Exercise*, Vol. 36, No. 7, 1149-1158, ISSN 0195-9131

Osada, T. & Rådegran, G. (2002). Femoral artery inflow in relation to external and total work rate at different knee extensor contraction rates. *Journal of Applied Physiology*, Vol. 92, No. 3, pp. 1325-1330, ISSN 8750-7587

Osada, T. & Rådegran, G. (2006). Alterations in the blood velocity profile influence the blood flow response during muscle contractions and relaxations. *Journal of Physiological Science*, Vol. 56, No. 3, pp. 195-203, ISSN 1880-6546

Osada, T. & Rådegran, G. (2006). Differences in exercising limb blood flow variability between cardiac and muscle contraction cycle related analysis during dynamic knee extensor. *Journal of Sports Medicine and Physical Fitness*, Vol. 46, No. 4, pp. 590-597, ISSN 0022-4707

Osada, T. & Rådegran, G. (2009). Femoral artery blood flow and its relationship to spontaneous fluctuations in rhythmic thigh muscle workload. *Clinical Physiology and Functional Imaging*, Vol. 29, No. 4, pp. 277-292, ISSN 1475-0961

Rådegran, G. (1997). Ultrasound Doppler estimates of femoral artery blood flow during dynamic knee extensor exercise in humans. *Journal of Applied Physiology*, Vol. 83, No. 4, pp. 1383-1388, ISSN 8750-7587

Rådegran, G. & Saltin, B. (1998). Muscle blood flow at onset of dynamic exercise in humans. *American Journal of Physiology Heart and Circulatory Physiology*, Vol. 274, No. 1, pp. H314-H322, ISSN 0002-9513

Robergs, R.A., Icenogle, M.V., Hudson, T.L. & Greene, E.R. (1997). Temporal inhomogeneity in brachial artery blood flow during forearm exercise. *Medicine and Science in Sports and Exercise*, Vol. 29, No. 8, pp. 1021-1027, ISSN 0195-9131

Shoemaker, J.K., Hodge, L. & Hughson, R.L. (1994). Cardiorespiratory kinetics and femoral artery blood velocity during dynamic knee extension exercise. *Journal of Applied Physiology*, Vol. 77, No. 6, pp. 2625-2632, ISSN 8750-7587

Tschakovsky, M.E., Saunders, N.R., Webb, K.A., & O'Donnell, D.E. (2006). Muscle blood-flow dynamics at exercise onset: Do the limbs differ? *Medicine and Science in Sports and Exercise*, Vol. 38, No. 10, pp. 1811-1818, ISSN 0195-9131

Walløe, L. & Wesche, J. (1988). Time course and magnitude of blood flow changes in the human quadriceps muscles during and following rhythmic exercise. *Journal of Physiology (London)*, Vol. 405, pp. 257-273, ISSN 0022-3751

# Part 4

## Advances in Medical Imaging Techniques

# 15

# Current State of the PET/CT Hybrid Technique and Clinical Indications

Patricia Carreño-Morán and María de las Nieves Gómez León
*Clinical University Hospital of Salamanca and Princesa Hospital of Madrid*
*Spain*

## 1. Introduction

In the year 2000, Townsend developed a prototype that integrates FDG-PET and CT, thus creating the possibility of performing both tests sequentially, in order to obtain an image that is the result of the fusion of hardware of anatomical (CT) and metabolic information (PET) of the section under study (Townsend & Beyer, 2002). Since then, PET/CT imaging has been a revolution in the diagnosis of tumours, staging, restaging and detection of local and distant recurrence and assessment of therapy response.

Applications have been developed in very different areas such as oncology, cardiology (cardiac viability), neurology (Alzheimer disease and epilepsy before surgery), etc.

## 2. Techniques

### 2.1 Hybrid technique

Therefore, the CT, which was the anatomical imaging technique of choice in the staging and monitoring of the treatment of oncological patients as well as in the planning of radiotherapy, joined the FDG-PET, which is a more functional technique that allows for an early detection of the disease and with which the residual lesions after treatment can be characterized as scar tissue or neoplastic lesions. PET/CT might improve the precision of the initial staging and the detection of residual diseases and recurrences in these patients. This would then optimize the treatment schemes for each patient and prevent the complications of other, more aggressive diagnostic techniques, as well as the toxicity of unnecessary chemotherapy and/or radiotherapy (Beyer, 2011).

### 2.2 PET/CT imaging protocol

The patients must not eat anything for 4-6 hours prior to the test. Immediately after the administration of a 370 MBq dose of intravenous 18FDG, the patient rests for 45-60 minutes. During this time, each patient receives 1500 ml of oral contrast (Gastrographin 3%), except for the studies on lung cancer, in which water is administered as an oral contrast. Nowadays the data are obtained with a hybrid system PET/CT which combines 4-64 slice multi-detector CT with a PET scanner of 18 bismuth germinate (BGO), lutetium oxyorthosilicate (LSO), or gadolinium silicate(GSO) crystal detector rings. At first, a CT scan is performed at low doses and without intravenous iodated contrast.

The images are taken 45-60 minutes after an injection at rest, starting at the base of the skull, down to the upper area of the thigh. Initially, in Spain, in 2003 (Gómez-León et al., 2007), low dose CT images were obtained at 140 mV, 80 mA, gantry rotation time of 0.5 seconds, 2x5 cm collimation, section thickness of 5 mm and reconstruction interval of 3 mm. Immediately after that, the PET scan acquired 4-6 contiguous volumes. Finally, the diagnostic CT could be studied after an injection of intravenous contrast (Iobitridol 300 mg iodine/ml), with a 50-70 seconds delay for the acquisition of the images (depending on the pathology under study). The parameters used were the same that those for low dose CT, except for the intensity of the current, which varied according to an automatic intensity modulation system that depends on the weight of the patient, with a maximum of 300 mA. A few minutes after the end of the test, PET images went through attenuation correction with the CT data and then reconstructed, like the CT images and the combined PET/CT images (Gómez-León et al., 2007).

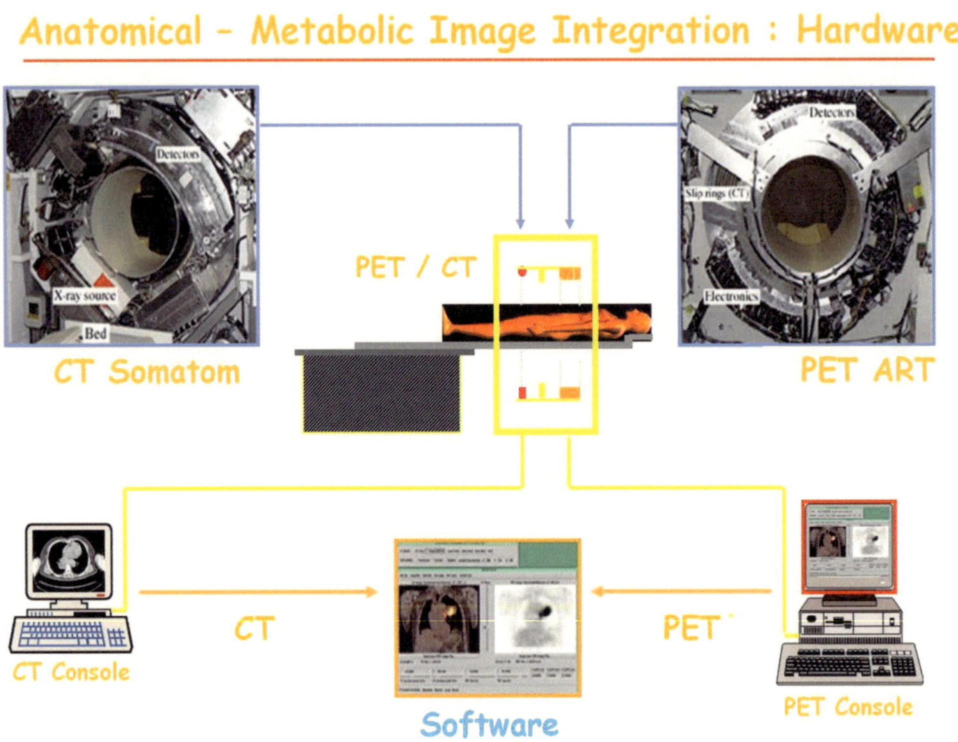


Fig. 1. PET/CT (modified from Townsend, 2002)

Nowadays, PET/CT images can be studied without a prior low-dose CT, using the data obtained in the diagnostic CT with intravenous contrast. There are no differences between PET attenuation with low-dose CT and diagnostic CT with intravenous contrast (Pinilla et al., 2010).

### 2.3 Assessment of the PET image or CT image

The main limitations of these techniques separately are the inability to distinguish, in many cases, benign lesions from malignant lesions, especially in the lymph nodes, the inability to establish the response to the treatment and the impossibility to distinguish, in some cases, between the changes in recurrences after therapy (chemotherapy, radiotherapy, surgery).

### 2.4 Advantages of combined PET/CT over PET and CT

- Improvement in locating the lesions thanks to a quasi-perfect anatomical and functional co-register.
- Different physiological and pathological uptake in PET.
- Functional changes precede anatomical alterations.
- Planning of RT.
- CT data can be used for the correction of data attenuation in PET (shorter times).
- PET/CT shows a higher sensitivity and specificity than each of its components individually, and probably higher than the combined retrospective reading of both separated components.
- The most relevant effect is the fact that CT provides more specificity to PET, which allows for a precise anatomical location of PET uptakes and a higher degree of certainty in the interpretation of the tests (Czernin et al., 2010).
- PET, on the other hand, provides some valuable functional information.
- Tumour cells present an increased glucose transport rate and an increased rate of glucose metabolism.

### 2.5 Implications of CT-based attenuation correction

- Artifacts due to respiratory and deglutition movements.
- Artifacts due to beam hardening (upper limbs) and obesity.
- Artifacts due to the use of contrasts and high-density objects.
- Other artifacts due to the patient's weight, the patient's BMI, the patient's lean weight, the administered dose of FDG, the level of basal glycemia, crystal PET detectors (BGO vs. LSO), etc.
- Asymmetrical uptake of FDG in the muscles, previous record of traumatisms or inflammation.

### 2.6 PET/CT: Physiological uptake

- 18FDG uptake is more intense in the brain, in which metabolism depends on glycolysis, and in the myocardium, which uses glycol tic metabolism in basal situations.

- 18FDG is excreted through urine, and intense activity can be found in the urinary system, the ureters and the bladder.
- It is present in the liver, the spleen, the bone marrow and the renal cortex.

### 2.6.1 Physiological uptakes

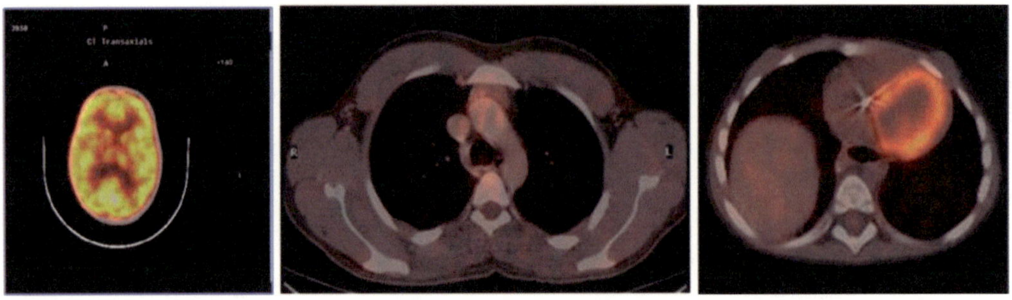

Fig. 2, 3 & 4. Physiological uptake of the brain, thymus and myocardium.

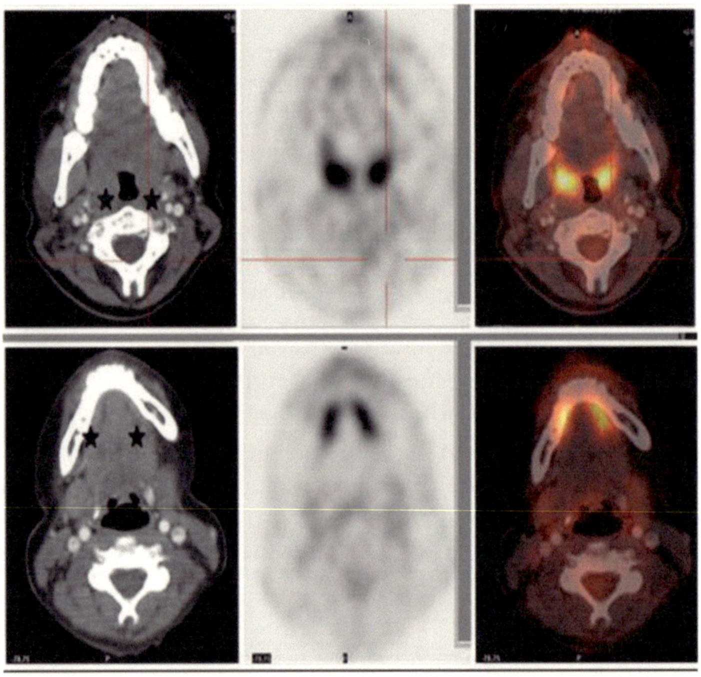

Fig. 5a & b. Physiological uptake of lymph tissue (asterisks) and tongue (asterisks).

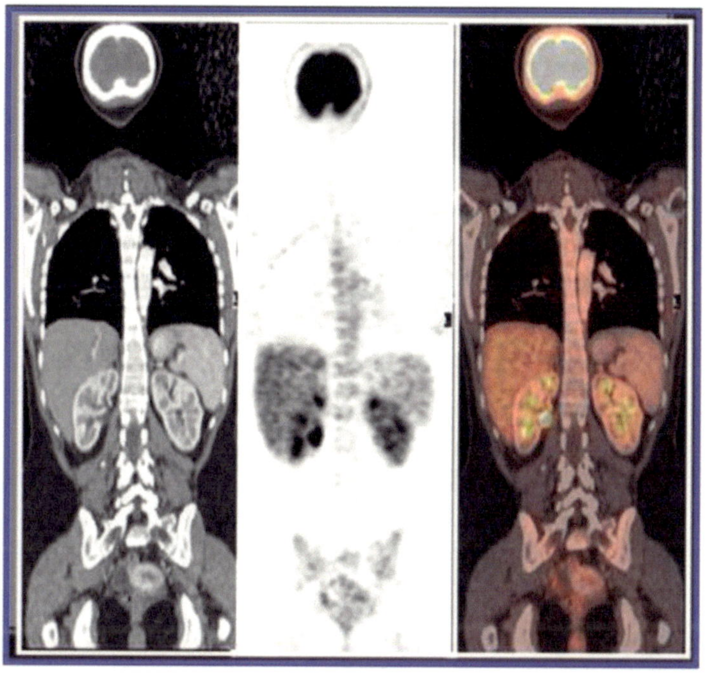

Fig. 6. Physiological uptake of the kidneys and bladder.

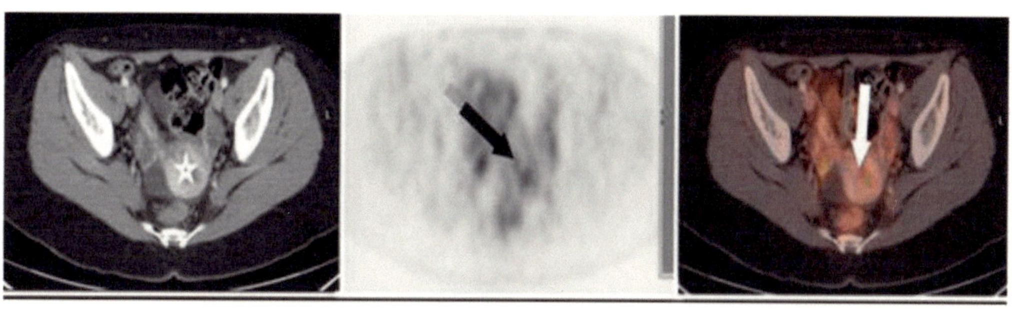

Fig. 7. Uptake of the endometrium (arrow) and bowel loops filled with oral contrast.

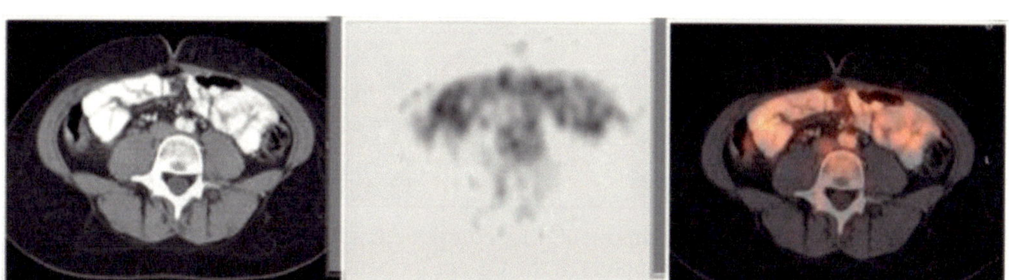

Fig. 8. Uptake of the endometrium and bowel loops filled with oral contrast.

### 2.6.2 Physiological uptakes after treatment

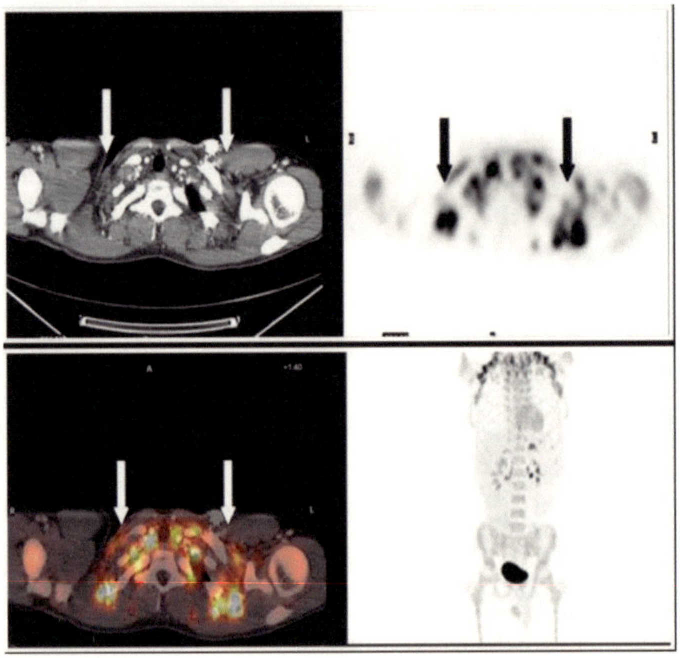

Fig. 9. Axial CT section with intravenous contrast, axial section of the PET component, combination of both techniques and coronal section of the entire PET study. Brown fat (arrows on the different sections).

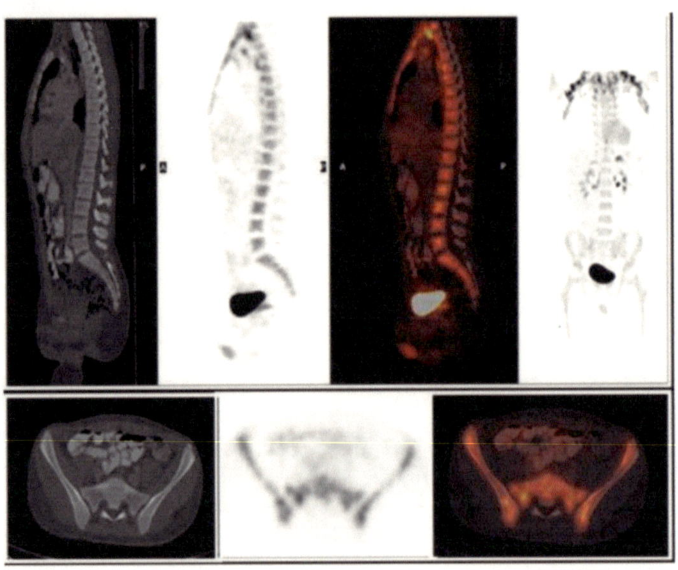

Fig. 10. Sagittal sections of CT component, PET component and combined image. Coronal PET section. Axial sections of the pelvis of the CT component, PET component and combined image. The patient received a bone marrow transplant, with uptake in the entire axial and peripheral skeleton due to granulocyte colony-stimulating factor.

### 2.7 FDG PET/CT: Limitations

This is a list of tumours with low uptake of FDG: Well-differentiated tumours, hypocellular tumours, mucine-producing tumours, HCC (hepatocell carcinoma), BAC and intraductal mucinous papillary tumours.

On the other hand, there are some difficulties in the detection of the pathological collection:

- High physiological uptake: brain, tonsils
- Physiological elimination: Urothelial carcinoma of the renal pelvis, bladder cancer

### 2.8 Applications of PET/CT in oncology

PET/CT is used in the staging and re-assessment of specific neoplasias, and it is especially useful in non-small cell lung cancer, lymphomas, colorectal cancer, sarcomas and melanomas.

PET/CT is particularly useful in patients under suspicion of clinical recurrence with conventional imaging techniques, as well as in the characterization of residual masses after chemotherapy and radiotherapy.

We want to highlight an article that was published in Euroradiology in 2011, which analyzed the increase in the use of PET/CT in Europe (Høilund-Carlsen et al., 2011). The most notable results dealt with the fact that the diagnosis, staging and treatment may change in up to 36% of the cases, according to some studies published in the USA: Initial results of The National Oncologic PET registry.

Danish experience: A 3-year clinical experience in a large new Danish PET/CT centre in relation to national and European developments. The use of PET/CT in cancer was registered from early 2006 to 2009, in order to judge the impact on patient management and to compare it with national and European trends.

- Referrals came primarily from the departments of oncology (23.0%), hematology (21.6%), surgery (12.6%), internal medicine (12.7%) and gynecology (5.5%).
- Referral indications were diagnosis (31.3%), staging (22.3%), recurrence detection (21.2%), response evaluation (17.0%) and other causes (8.2%). Response from nearly 60% of users showed that PET/CT caused a change in diagnosis and/or staging and/or treatment plan in 36.0% of cases.
- The working diagnosis was confirmed in 53.7% of the cases, the staging in 42.7% of the cases and the treatment plan in 49.9% of the cases, and changes took place in diagnosis (14.3% of the cases), in staging (22.1%), and in treatment plan (28.3%).
- According to the EANM, during the study period, there was a steep increase in the national use of FDG and in the European use of PET/CT from 166 cases (in 27 countries) to 463 cases (in 46 countries), which represents an increase of 179%, and an increase of the number of studies of 69%.

## 3. Indications for the monitored use of FDG: High-level research NLCAHR contextualized health research synthesis: PET/CT programs

1. Solitary pulmonary nodule
2. Non-small cell lung cancer
3. Recurrent colorectal cancer
4. Staging and re-staging of lymphoma

5. Recurrent malignant melanoma.
6. Identification of cancer of unknown primary origin
7. Malignant tumours in head and neck
8. Breast cancer.
9. PET-CT and it´s applications in radiation therapy.
10. The future: Neuroradiology and cardiovascular diseases (Demeter et al., 2009).

### 3.1 Solitary pulmonary nodule

- The role of PET-CT in clinical assessment in indeterminate pulmonary nodules shows two options: biopsy or resection and monitoring over 2 to 5 years. The use of PET-CT in the management of pulmonary nodules helps to stratify patients better according to the risk of malignancy.
- Accuracy depends on: Nodule size ≥ 1cm and FDG-Avidity SUV 2.5: overlapping
- Improvements in the increase of the uptake compared with background activity
- S: 83-100% E: 63-90%, NPV: 95% and change the management in 26% of patients.

#### 3.1.1 Limitations of PET/CT

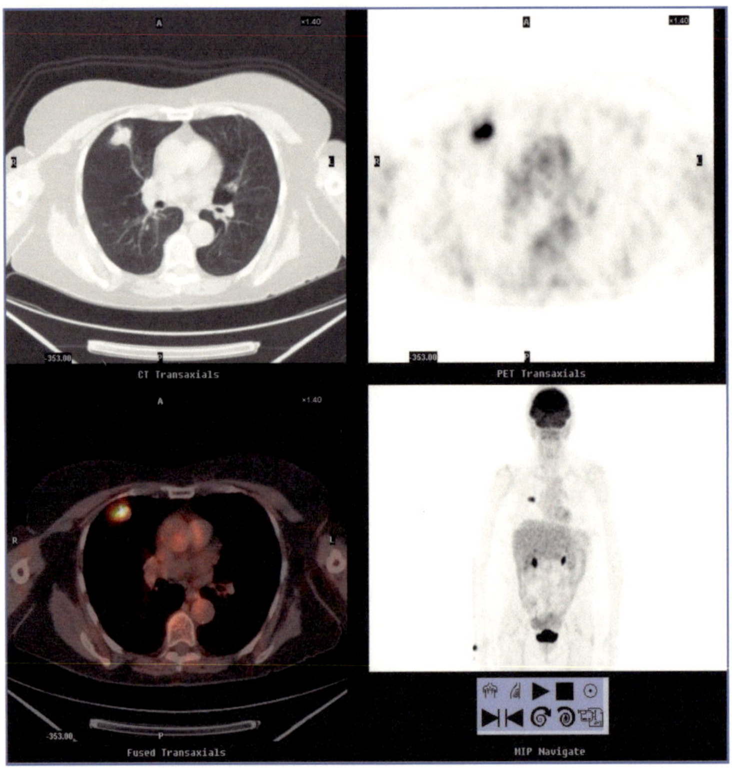


Fig. 11. False positive: Axial section of CT, PET and combined images and coronal section of the PET study. The pulmonary nodule of the right upper lobe shows an intense uptake of 18FDG in the PET and combined image. The anatomopathological analysis revealed a tuberculoma in a patient with colon carcinoma.

Benign uptakes:

- Physiological uptakes. Brown fat
- Inflammation: sarcoidosis, vasculitis, etc.
- Inflammation after surgery (1-2 months) or after radiation therapy (2-3 months)
- Active infections
- Benign tumours

False positive: Tuberculosis, granuloma, sarcoidosis, abscess and fungal infection (aspergillosis, coccidioidomycosis), necrotizing pneumonia, benign tumours: sclerosing hemangioma, myofibroblastic tumour and leiomyoma.

False negative: Well-differentiated adenocarcinoma, BAC (bronchioalveolar carcinoma), carcinoid and nodules of less than 1 cm.

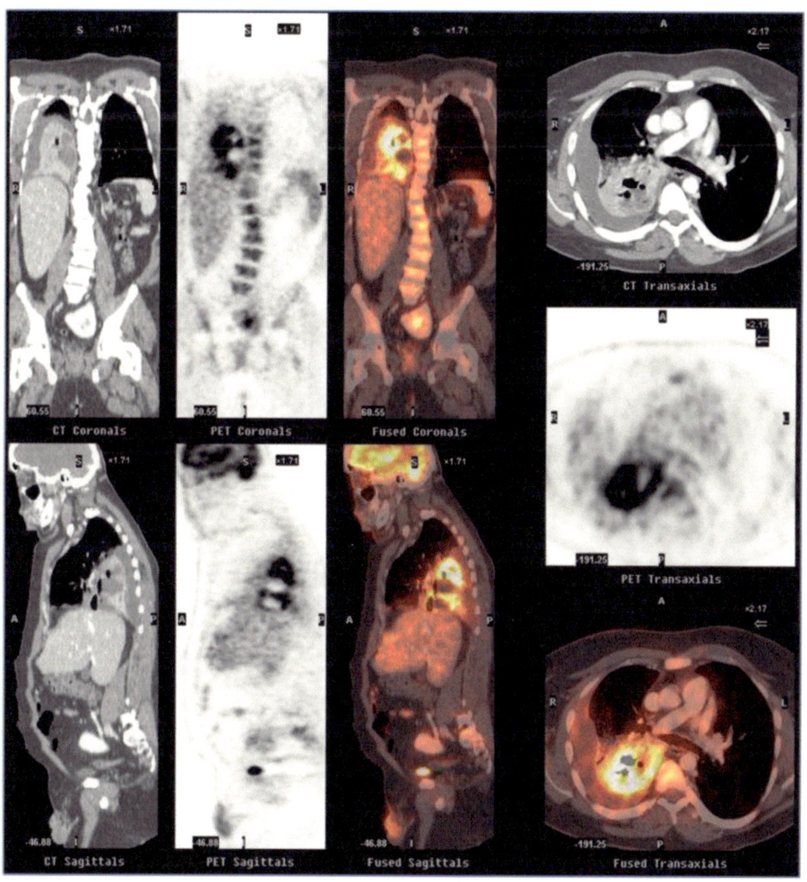


Fig. 12. Coronal and sagittal sections of the entire body with CT, PET and combined images. Axial sections. False positive: Necrotizing pneumonia of middle lobe and lower right lobe with effusion.

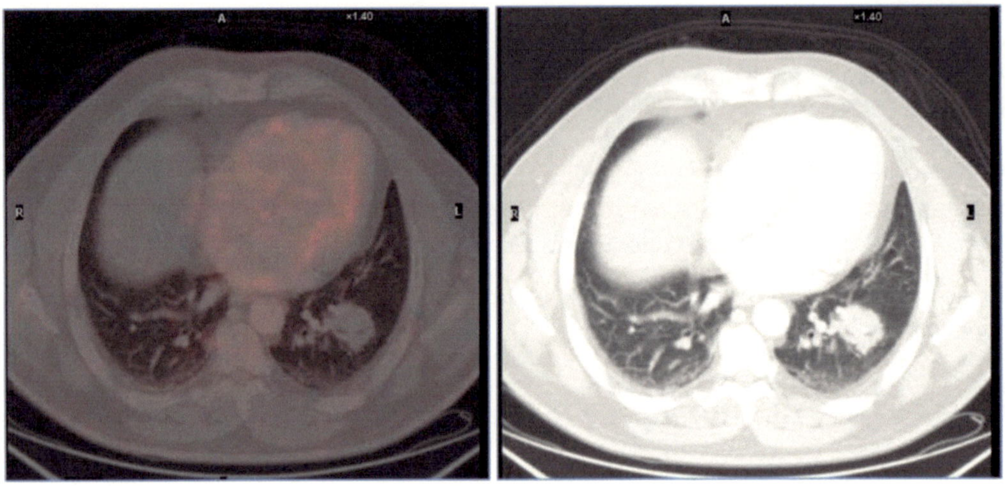

Fig. 13a & b. Axial sections of CT and PET/CT combined image. Lesion on the lower right lobe with air bronchogram, without 18FDG uptake. False negative: Bronchioalveolar carcinoma.

### 3.2 Non-small-cell lung carcinoma

PET/CT improves the identification and location of the lesions as well as the detection of the involvement of small nodes and neoplastic lesions with low FDG avidity. Diagnostic accuracy of PET/CT: T 70-97%; N: 78-93%; TNM: 83-96%. Global staging is significantly better. It leads to a change of stage in approximately 26% of the patients, and it changes the management approach in 9-19% of the cases.

Advantages of PET/CT:

- Techniques: Better quality than PET study. The PET element is shorter (examination time decreases by 40%), and it provides a more effective use of PET radiotracers.
- For the patient: A single preparation session and study session, and a better clinical management of complementary examinations
- At diagnosis: More sensitivity and specificity than isolated CT and PET.
    - CT adds specificity: Better location, safer reading.
    - PET adds sensitivity: it detects infiltrations without morphological alterations.

#### 3.2.1 Limitations of PET/CT

- Tumours with a decrease in the 18F-FDG uptake: Well-differentiated tumours, hypocellular tumours or mucin-producing tumours.
- Difficult detection of pathological deposits:
    - High physiological uptake: brain, tonsils.
    - Physiological elimination: Urothelial carcinoma of the renal pelvis, bladder cancer

### 3.2.2 T staging

PET/CT is a better choice because it provides an accurate correlation between the extension of the FDG deposit and the anatomy of the area.

- Improvement of the CT component: Focal chest wall infiltration, invasion of the mediastinum and vascular invasion.
- PET Component: It distinguishes between tumours and atelectasis; malignant pleural effusion (T4) with an accuracy of 92%; metabolic activity with prognostic value.

### 3.2.3 N staging

PET increases sensitivity and NPV. PET/CT adds specificity and improves accuracy: Improvement of the exact location of the uptake in patients with atelectasis, mediastinal deviation and anatomical variants and proper identification of the node stage.

The problems derived from false positives in granulomatous disease and inflammatory changes caused by a coexistent lung disease leads to a lower PPV. For this reason, a mediastinoscopy is advised if the tumour can be operated, as well as an histological confirmation.

PET/CT is a good guide for an invasive biopsy, if the glands show positive results for the aortopulmonary window, the anterior mediastinum or the posterior subcarinal region. It is useful for a mediastinotomy, a transbronchial biopsy, ultrasound-guided fine-needle aspiration or transbronchial ultrasound-guided endoscopy.

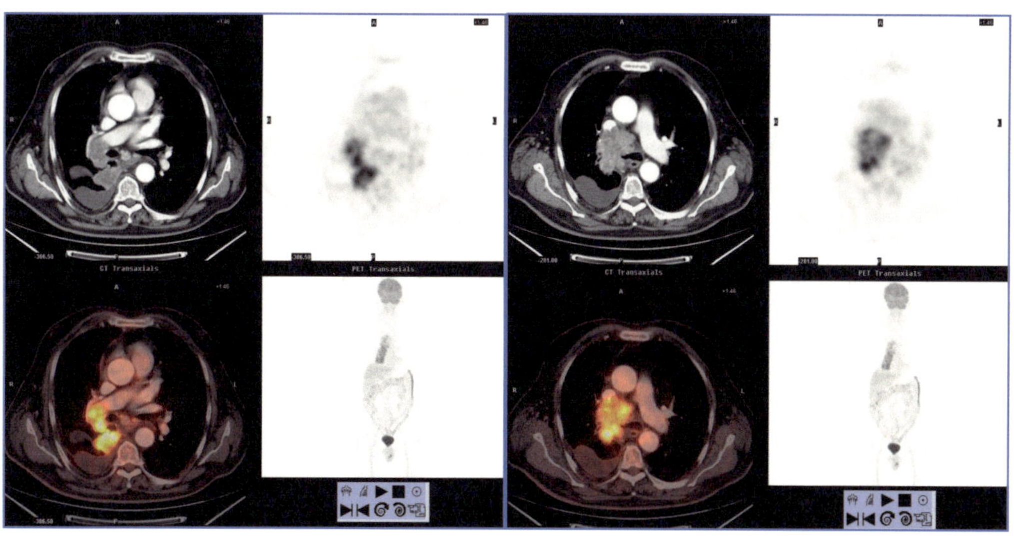

Fig. 14. PET/CT: Staging of NSCLC with mediastinal adenopathies, with an important 18FDG uptake. The invasion of the right main pulmonary artery can be seen thanks to the intravenous contrast. The pleural effusion does not show an 18FDG uptake.

### 3.2.4 M staging

PET provides an excellent detection of thoracic metastases, detection of unsuspected distant metastases 28% and change of treatment in 53% of the cases. PET/CT allows a more accurate location in adrenal metastases, with diagnostic accuracy in 92 % of the cases. It reduces the number of unnecessary thoracotomies by 25%.

- Hepatic metastases: The specificity and sensitivity of PET/CT is similar to those of other diagnostic techniques. It offers additional information for unspecific lesions.
- Adrenal metastases: Up to 10% of all NSCLC include a metastatic adrenal nodule at diagnosis. The accuracy of PET/CT is 92%, and its specificity ranges between 80 and 100% of all cases. An undetermined nodule in the CT with negative results in the PET scan generally means that it will be benign. False negatives have been described in adrenal metastases for very small lesions or when there is hemorrhage or necrosis.
- Bone metastases: Sensitivity goes up to 90% (similar to scintigraphy with Tc99m), although its specificity is better than scintigraphy with Tc99 (61%). The main limitation can be seen in blastic bone metastases, in which scintigraphy with Tc99m shows higher accuracy, or peripheral bone metastases. However, most bone metastases of NSCLC are central and lithic, which means that PET/CT might replace scintigraphy with Tc99m.
- Limitations of PET/CT in brain metastases are explained by the difficulty of finding small lesions due to cerebral physiological FDG activity. For this reason, brain NMR is recommended in these uncertain cases.

### 3.2.5 Re-staging

Post-therapy changes are known to make CT assessment more difficult. PET/CT improves the post-therapy accuracy, because 18F-FDG accumulates in the viable tumour cells instead of being captured by post-therapy necrosis and fibrosis.

Recurrence diagnosis in NSCLC with PET/CT improves sensitivity (77-100%) and specificity (62-92%), although this last factor can be reduced due to inflammation after radiation therapy or chemotherapy. For this reason, the diagnosis should be carried out 1-2 months after chemotherapy and 2-3 months after radiation therapy.

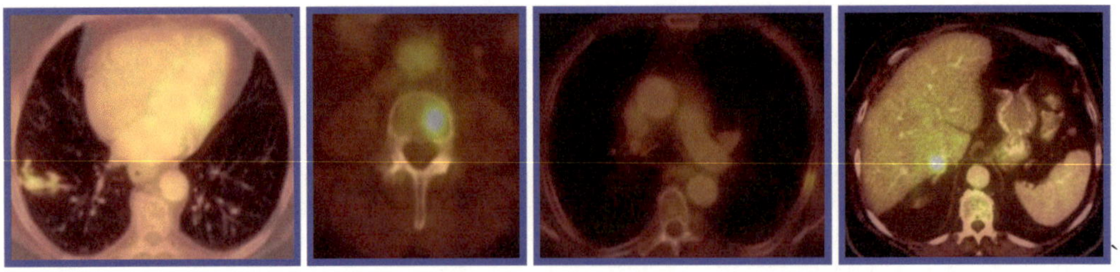

Fig. 15. NSCLC staging on upper left lobe with metastases on the liver, bones (sternum and vertebras) and peripheral pancreas (arrow). The patient is a 61-year-old male with NSCLC (initial stage: N1, according to a recent CT scan), and with several unsuspected metastatic lesions on the spine, liver and ribs.

### 3.3 Colorectal cancer

At diagnosis, colorectal cancer is found only in 36% of the patients. 39% of them showed lymph node metastases, and 19% of them presented distant metastases. Up to 15-20% of the patients presented liver metastases when their primary tumour was surgically resected. Surgery (of the primary tumour and the liver metastases) is the only known curative treatment.

- Resection of liver metastases is only indicated for patients with 1-4 lesions located on a single lobe (whenever there is no other evidence of more adenopathies or distant metastases)
- Up to 5% of the patients present synchronous colon carcinomas, and 30% of all patients present adenomatous polyps. Moreover, another 5% will develop a metachronic carcinoma of the colon in the future.

PET/CT is very useful in:

- Detection of recurrences in the following cases: high CEA with conventional imaging techniques, non specific or erroneous findings with conventional techniques or presacral masses after treatment.
- Monitoring of treatment with chemotherapy and radiotherapy.

PET/CT is not to be used in: Screening, initial diagnosis and patients with a known disseminated disease

Recurrence of colorectal cancer takes place in 37-44% of the patients within the first two years after the resection of the tumour with curative purposes. An early detection of potentially resectable metastases or local recurrences leads to an increase in survival rates. Serum CEA levels can be used to monitor the presence of recurrences (S: 59%; E: 84%), but they cannot locate the place of the recurrence. PET showed more than 90% sensitivity and more than 95% specificity, compared with CT levels, which were 60-85% sensitivity and 60-90% specificity. PET modifies the therapeutic management in up to 25-35% of the patients, and it detects up to 33% more metastases, compared with conventional methods.

Diagnostic accuracy of PET ranges between 90 and 100%, compared with 50-65% for CT.

Between 15 and 20% of patients with local recurrences are candidates for curative resection. However, long-term survival in these cases is only 35% (due to the presence of hidden metastases).

Correct differentiation between a viable tumour and a post-therapy fibrosis (due to surgery and/or radiation therapy) on the pelvis is vital for a proper management of the patients with suspicion of local recurrence. PET is very useful for a correct classification of these patients, and it can also find additional unsuspected metastatic sources. FDG accumulation 6 months after radiation therapy or later are a sign of a residual tumour or a recurrence.

Importance in liver metastases: The use of PET in the assessment of patients before a curative liver resection probably leads to the selection of a subgroup of "ideal" patients-candidates who can benefit greatly from this technique. 3-year survival rate improves up to 77% (compared with 40-45% with CT), and 3-year disease-free survival rates also improve up to 40% (compared with 15-28% with CT).

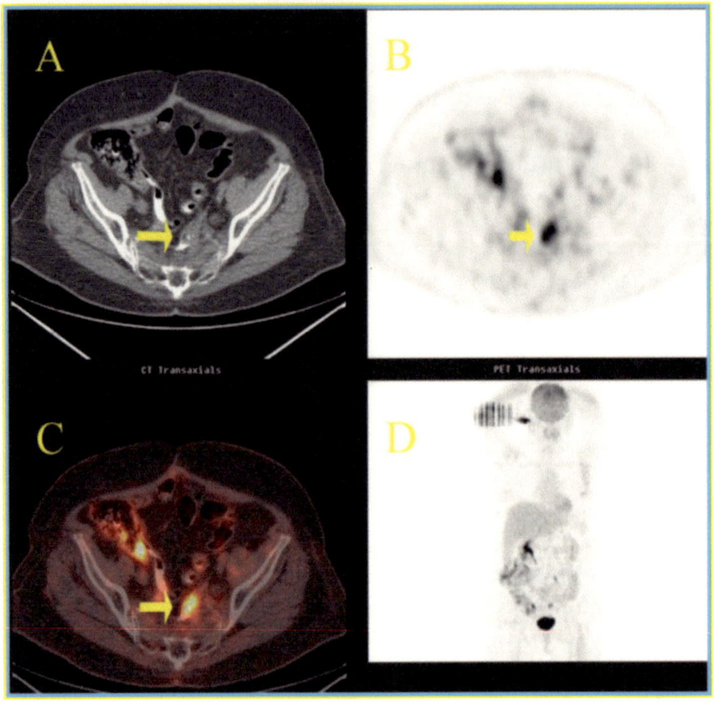


Fig. 16. I. Axial section of CT (A). 64-year-old woman with adenocarcinoma, treated with surgery, chemotherapy and radiation therapy, with clinical suspicion of recurrence. Axial section of PET (B) and combined image (C). PET study in a coronal section (D). A small mass can be seen on the surgical site, showing an intense 18FDG uptake. The recurrence was confirmed with surgery.

### 3.4 Lymphomas

- In most HL and NHL there is an increase in avidity: HL, DLC-NHL, follicular lymphoma
- Staging and re-staging: higher sensitivity and specificity than CT and PET: sensitivity: 91-94%, specificity: 88-100%.
- PET/CT detects normal-sized node diseases, characterization of residual masses; it detects partial or slow responses and less false positives than PET
- It identifies small lesions and specific locations: Base of lungs, skin and non-distant metastasis
- Residual mass: Early detection of remains/recurrence, more effective treatment.
- Disease exclusion prevents invasive diagnostic procedures and unnecessary treatments and guided biopsy towards uptake regions in the mass.

Non-Hodgkin lymphomas (NHL) can be roughly classified into 3 groups: low grade, intermediate grade and high grade. Low-grade NHL represents 40% of all NHL, and they are usually indolent. Most of the patients are treated with a monochemotherapy regime (or even with a wait-and-see approach). PET can represent an important role in the assessment of patients in which the low-grade NHL is suspected to have turned into a high-grade NHL (this happens in 10-20% of the cases).

Intermediate-grade NHL represents 40% of all NHL, and high-grade NHL represent 5-10% of all cases. Both are treated with chemotherapy and radiation therapy. PET plays several roles in the management of these patients. It determines the extension of the disease (staging) and the response to treatment (therefore, chemotherapy treatments can be modified if they are not being effective).

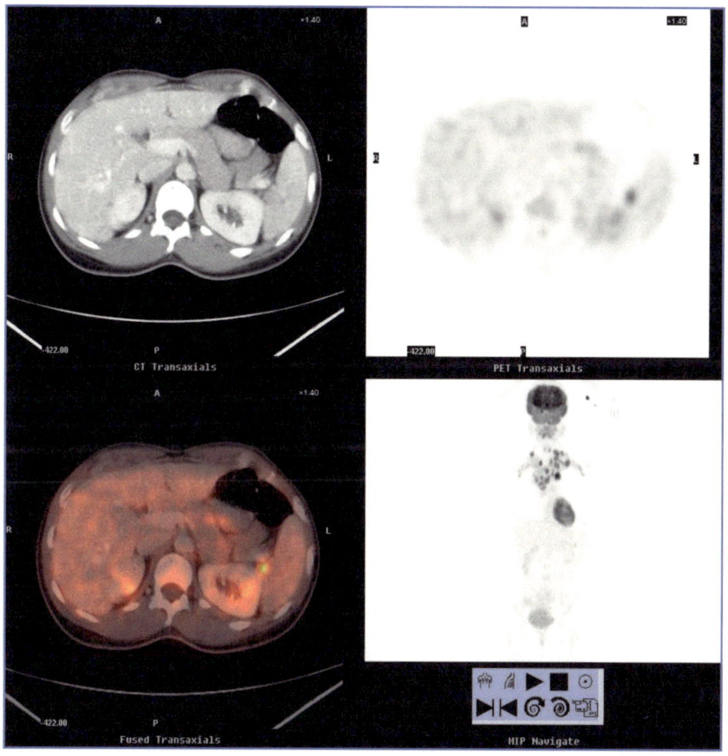


Fig. 17. Axial section of CT with normal intravenous contrast. Axial section of PET. PET/CT detected a pathological FDG uptake in a small adenopathy in the splenic hilium. Therefore, the stage was increased from II to III.

Hodgkin's lymphoma (HL): The extension of the disease is, when taken by itself, the most important prognostic factor for a proper management with regard to global survival and recurrence-free survival in HL patients. Conventional methods are often incapable of revealing the real extension of the tumour (for example, between 20% and 30% of all patients with a HL that is allegedly located over the diaphragm also present infradiaphragmatic involvement when an exploratory laparotomy is performed).

PET provides an excellent contrast for the lesions and a relatively good anatomical location thanks to the tomographic nature of the images, greatly improved with the new PET/CT.

It makes it possible to study, in a single exploration, all the affected organs.

The detection of the lesions depends on their biochemical signal instead of on anatomical criteria. A certain correlation between the FDG uptake degree and the histological degree of the lymphoma has been observed.

However, low-degree lymphomas may not accumulate enough FDG to be detected. PET fulfills two important aspects that are being more and more taken into account in health services: on the one hand, it reduces the number of invasive diagnostic procedures, and on the other hand, it is a technique with a good cost-effectiveness ratio (a study which included PET into the diagnostic algorithm of lymphoma patients showed that expenses were reduced by 50%). Some studies have shown that PET modifies the management of lymphoma patients in up to 62% of the cases (Pinilla et al., 2010).

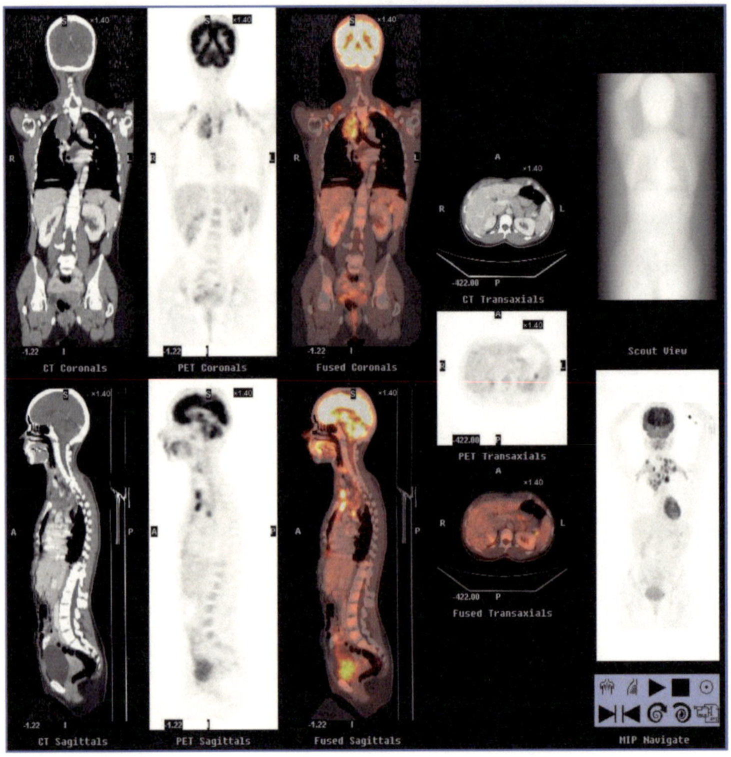


Fig. 18. PET/CT can change the stage of the disease in approximately 10% of all lymphoma patients. Study of PET/CT in initial staging of a patient with nodular sclerosis Hodgkin's lymphoma with laterocervical, supraclavicular and mediastinal involvement.

### 3.4.1 Lymph node involvement

PET shows high sensitivity for the detection of lymph nodes and staging the patients. Published sensitivities vary between 62% and 100%. In spite of this variability, PET seems to be more sensitive than CT for the staging of lymphoma patients, because it can detect more lesions inside and outside the nodes, than conventional methods. It alters the stage of patients, in any of both directions, in up to 44% of the cases, according to some studies.

### 3.4.2 Extranodal involvement

Extranodal involvement is associated with a worse prognosis of patients. PET can detect up to 57% more extranodal lesions than CT. Diffuse infiltration in the spleen, bone marrow and liver cannot be detected with CT. Up to 30% of lymphoma patients with splenomegaly do not present tumour infiltration of the spleen and a significant number of patients presents tumour involvement of the spleen without splenomegaly. FDG uptake by the bone marrow represents a tumour infiltration, although an increased uptake of the bone marrow can also be expected if the patient has undergone chemotherapy or has received colony-stimulating factors recently (post-therapy medullary hyperplasia).

Bone marrow involvement (stage IV) means a worse prognosis in lymphoma patients, and it is more frequent in NHL patients. In order to be detected by CT, the bone involvement must be focused and accompanied by bone destruction. Unfortunately, a diffuse infiltration of the bone marrow does not show bone destruction, and it is usually asymptomatic. PET can detect both the focal involvement and the diffuse infiltration of the bone marrow. According to several studies, it is more sensitive than bone scintigraphy with Tc99m.

### 3.4.3 Monitoring of response to treatment

Conventional methods (CT, NMR) only show a reduction of the size of the lesions, and they are not very reliable as predictors of the clinical success of the lymphoma treatment. Some studies with CT showed that less than 50% with positive findings in CT developed a recurrence of the disease in the long term. Unlike conventional techniques, PET determines the metabolic activity of a lesion, which reflects the mass of viable cells inside a tumour. After the beginning of chemotherapy or radiation therapy, there is a series of metabolic changes in the tumour before any changes on the size of the mass. Several recent studies suggest that, after successful chemotherapy, the metabolic activity of the tumour rapidly decreases (SUV decrease by 75-90% 7 days after the beginning of treatment). An intense and persistent FDG uptake after the end of chemotherapy cycles shows an absence of therapeutic response.

Patients who show persistently positive PET studies after the first chemotherapy cycle present a much higher risk of recurrence (a recurrence rate of 90%, according to one study) than patients with a positive response (decrease in FDG uptake). Likewise, some studies observed that 85% of all patients with a negative PET study after the first chemotherapy cycle remain in remission (minimum monitoring time of 18 months). A PET study after the first chemotherapy cycle also has been proven to be a better predictor for response to treatment than a PET study at the end of the treatment (diagnostic accuracy of 87% versus 70%).

An early assessment of response to treatment would not only avoid the toxicity of an ineffective treatment, but also reduce the costs of that therapy. In these cases, patients could benefit from second-line therapies. A variation of SUV over 25% must be considered as a real finding.

Differentiation of fibrotic tissue versus viable in a post-therapy residual mass: The presence of a residual mass after the end of lymphoma therapy is a challenge for the clinical diagnosis, because it can represent either a viable tumour or a residual diagnosis. Conventional diagnostic techniques do not offer reliable enough signs that can tell the difference between a viable tumour and a fibrosis, but with PET, FDG accumulates in the viable tumour, whereas fibrosis do not reveal any accumulation. In patients with mediastinal lymphoma, up to 64% of them show some anatomical alteration after the end of the treatment. However, only 18% of them will show a recurrence. FDG uptake in a residual mass is associated to a higher rate of recurrence and worse global survival rates, compared with patients without FDG uptake. The presence of persistent metabolic activity in a residual mass may motivate a change in the treatment or the addition of new chemotherapeutic agents. In spite of the fact that 25% of all patients with negative PET results and a residual mass will have a recurrence, it will take place in a different location from the residual mass in 80% of the cases (Cronin, 2010).

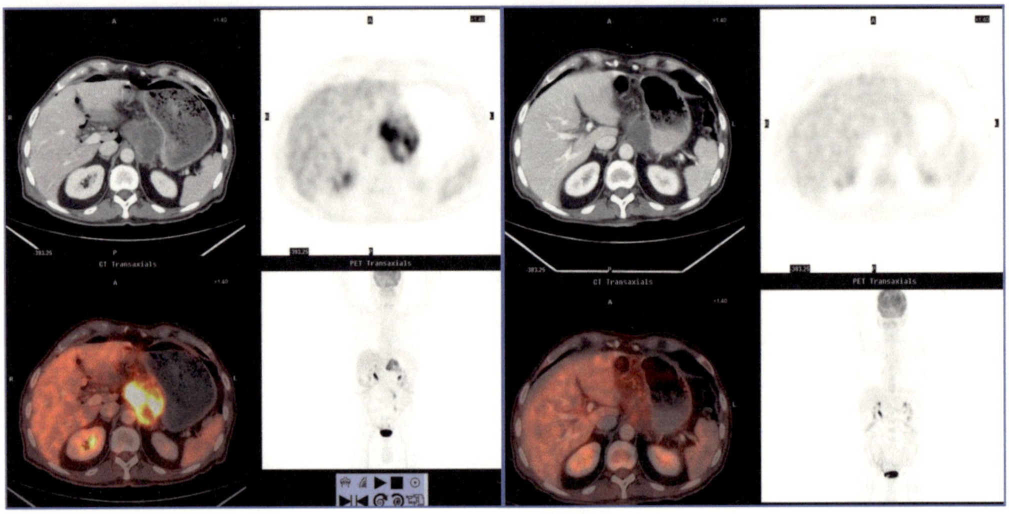

Fig. 19a & b. 45-year old patient with Diffuse large B-cell NHL with a mass that shows an intense FDG avidity at diagnosis (a). The mass persists after the end of the treatment, without FDG uptake. The recurrence was confirmed with monitoring, without additional treatment (b).

### 3.5 Melanoma

It is one of the tumours with the highest FDG avidity, and it has the potential to metastasize in any part of the body. Therefore, it benefits from a PET/CT assessment, which shows a great sensitivity for the detection of metastases, with the exception of the brain.

PET is useful in the detection of adenopathies and distant metastases (particularly with melanomas thicker than 1.5 mm - Clark level 4). The sensitivity and specificity of PET in the detection of distant metastases is 80% and 87%, respectively (higher than in conventional methods).

PET's sensitivity for the detection of adenopathies in patients with melanoma depends on the size of the metastases (sensitivity is almost 100% for adenopathies >1 cm, and only 23% for adenopathies <5 mm). All data accumulated until now suggest that the diagnostic accuracy of PET is higher for systemic staging than for local staging of regional lymph nodes (especially in Stage I or II patients). Therefore, PET cannot replace sentinel node biopsy in the clinical management of the patients.

### 3.6 Cancer of unknown primary origin

- Guided biopsy identifies primary tumours in more than 33% of the cases (Wartski et al 2006) and diagnosis of distance metastasis
- Controversial cost-effectiveness analysis in first test for epidermoid carcinoma
- Useful in cervical metastases of adenocarcinoma.

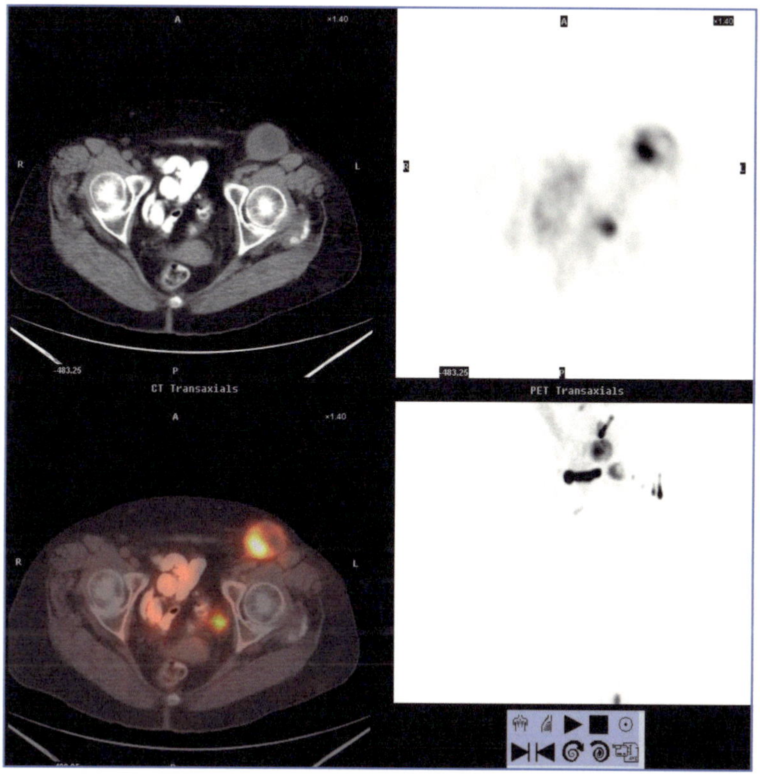


Fig. 20. Patient with melanoma on the leg and inguinal and iliac node involvement.

### 3.7 Head and neck tumours

They are useful to distinguish, in some cases, between the changes in recurrences after therapy (chemotherapy, radiotherapy, surgery).

#### 3.7.1 Applications of PET/CT in the assessment of head and neck tumours

- Unknown primary tumour: detection of the primary lesion in up to 33% of the cases.
- Staging.
- Re-staging: post-therapy changes versus recurrence.
- Thyroid cancer: especially when the I-131 scintigraphy is negative.
- Metachronic/synchronic tumours: respiratory and digestive tract (up to 30% of the patients).

#### 3.7.2 Possible interpretation errors

- Asymmetrical uptake of FDG in the muscles.
- Submaxillary glands
- Treatment with surgery and radiation therapy.
- Uptake in supraclavicular area fat.
- Hashimoto's thyroiditis.

### 3.7.3 Esophageal cancer

- USA's Medicare currently includes two indications for PET in esophageal cancer:
  - Preoperative staging and post-therapy re-staging.
  - Monitoring of the treatment (when there is evidence of a potential recurrence).
- Primary tumour: PET is not useful in the assessment of primary esophageal cancer or in the detection of a local invasion of the tumour. A PET/CT combination improves staging.
- Lymph node metastases: The presence of adenopathies on the neck, the supraclavicular areas or the celiac trunk is a sign of M1 metastasis (which means that its detection represents a great impact on the management of the patient).
- Distant metastases: The main advantage of PET with regard to conventional imaging techniques is its capability to detect distant metastasis (diagnostic accuracy of 84% versus 63% for CT). The presence of distant metastases has a great impact on the management of the patient because they are not resectable. PET detects metastatic diseases that are not identified by conventional studies in up to 20% of the patients.
- Recurrent esophageal cancer: The sensitivity of PET for the detection of distant metastases is 95% (specificity of CT is 79%). Moreover, PET provides additional diagnostic information in 27% of the patients with suspicion of tumour recurrence.

### 3.7.4 Thyroid cancer

- Diagnosis: PET is not indicated in the diagnosis of thyroid cancer (not all carcinomas attract FDG, and some benign lesions can accumulate FDG).
- Staging: Although there are no data in this regard, PET probably does not play an important role in the initial staging of patients with thyroid cancer.
- Patients with suspicion of recurrent cancer and a negative I-131 scintigraphy: The published sensitivity of PET for the detection of recurrent thyroid cancer in patients with negative I-131 scintigraphies ranges between 60% and 94% (specificity between 42-95%). One advantage of PET is the fact that it can detect tumour sites in nodes smaller than 1 cm. However, PET cannot detect small lung metastases.
- Prognosis: 3-year survival rates are significantly reduced in patients with postive PET results (survival of 60%), with regard to patients with a negative result (survival of 98%), which means that PET has an important prognostic value.

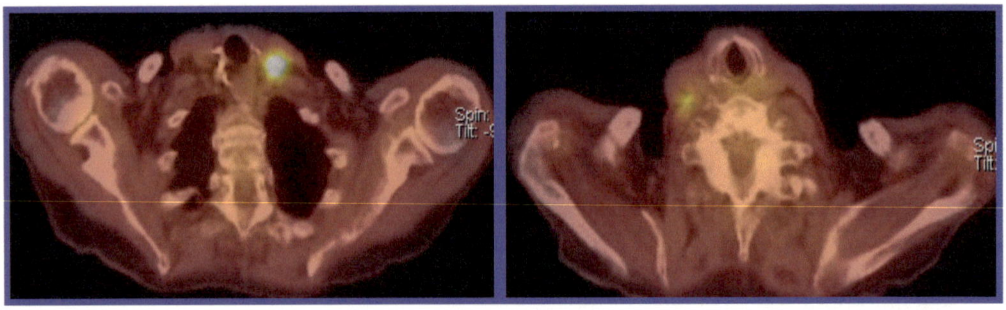

Fig. 21a & b. Recurrent thyroid cancer. The patient is a 73-year-old woman with a record of papillary thyroid cancer. She showed a recent increase of serum thyroglobulin with negative results for I-131 scintigraphy. PET/CT: Tumour remains on the surgical site and right laterocervical adenopathy.

### 3.7.5 Head and neck tumours

Most head and neck tumours are epidermoid carcinomas. Up to 60% of the patients present an advanced stage of the lesion at diagnosis. The involvement of lymph nodes is the most important prognostic factor with regard to survival. Conventional studies with CT and/or NMR have certain limitations in the assessment of lymph node involvement, because they are mainly based on the size of the nodes (> 1 cm) in order to classify them as pathological nodes. However, up to 40% of all lymph node metastases take place in nodes smaller than 1 cm. PET is particularly useful in the assessment of patients with a clinical stage N0. In this clinical context, between 16% and 60% of all patients reveal hidden lymph node metastases after a PET study.

- Proper preoperative staging (TNM) is essential when planning the type of lymph node dissection and when assessing the need of postoperative radiation therapy or chemotherapy.
- A relatively common presentation of head and neck tumours is the appearance of cervical adenopathies. A careful ENT examination, together with CT/NMR can identify the primary tumour in most cases. However, in up to 32-40% of the patients, the primary lesion will not be identified. PET, particularly combined with CT, is especially useful in these cases.
- Assessment of response to treatment: PET (PET/CT) can be used to monitor the response to treatment in head and neck tumours. Tumours that respond to treatment show a reduced metabolic activity, and those that present a persistent uptake one month after radiation therapy usually contain viable or residual tumour cells. In more than 80% of the cases, PET can establish the difference between a residual tumour and post-radiation therapy fibrosis.

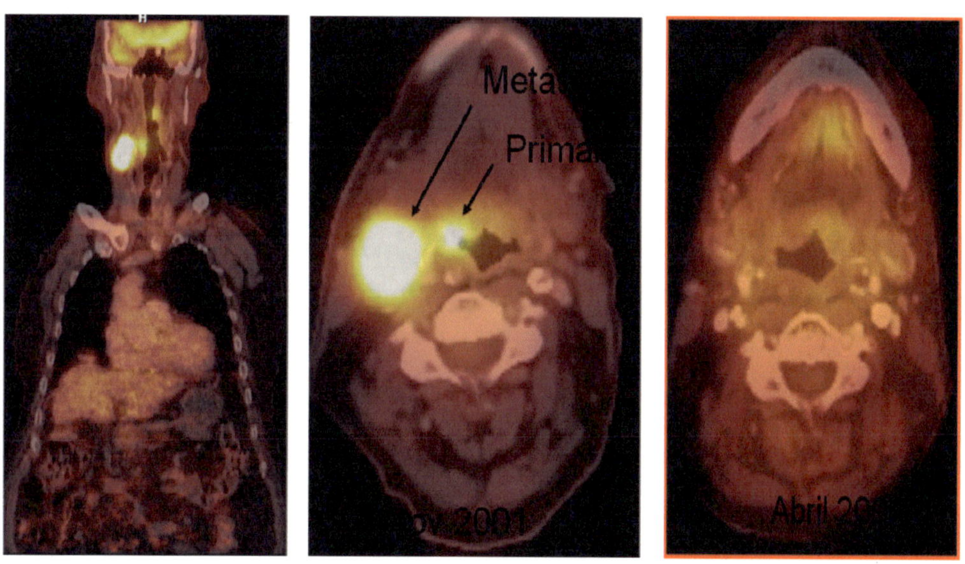

Fig. 22a, b & c. Head and neck tumour: unknown primary tumour. The patient is a 70-year-old male with a recent biopsy of a right cervical mass that was positive for epidermoid carcinoma (unknown primary mucosal lesion). PET/CT shows a favorable response after treatment with surgery and radiation therapy.

- The quantification of FDG uptake by the tumour (through SUV) correlates with the biological behavior of the tumour, and it has been proved that an intense FDG uptake (SUV>5.5) identifies a group of patients who can benefit from a more aggressive treatment.

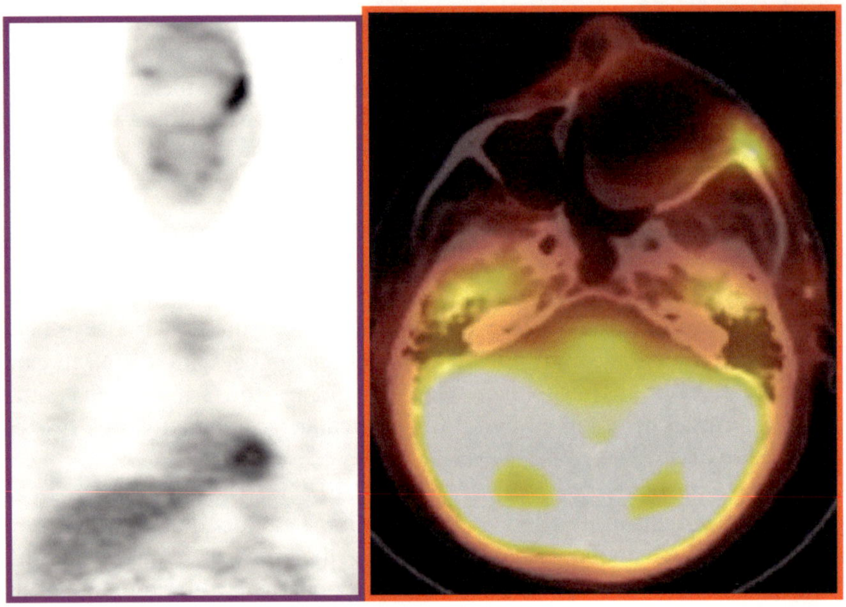

Fig. 23a & b. Re-staging of head and neck tumour. The patient is a 72-year-old male with adenopathy in an adenocarcinoma of the left nasal cavity with extension into the orbitary region that was surgically operated. 6 weeks later, the tests reveal a FDG-uptake area on the anterior region of the left zygomatic arch, compatible with persistence of viable tumour.

### 3.8 Breast cancer

Assessment of systemic metastases, identification of recurrence locations and possible role in the radiotherapy planning.

- CT Component: extended towards chest wall and skin.
- PET provides a more accurate detection of metastases in the internal mammary gland.

PET studies can have a very significant impact on the management of patients, especially in those with suspicion of advanced disease. PET can modify the clinical stage in up to 36% of the cases (it increases the clinical stage in 28% of the cases and reduces it in 8% of the cases). In 20% of the cases, unsuspected metastases are discovered, and the clinical management of patients is modified in up to 58% of the cases, once that the PET results are taken into account.

#### 3.8.1 Local disease

Breast cancer presents a significantly variable FDG uptake. Generally speaking, a higher proliferation rate of the tumour and a higher degree of undifferentiation mean a higher rate of metabolic activity of the tumour and higher FDG avidity. Invasive ductal carcinoma shows a FDG uptake significantly higher than invasive lobular carcinoma. Focal node lesions also present high levels of FDG uptake, compared with infiltrative/diffuse lesions. PET/CT has an advantage in the fact that it is not altered by the density of the mammary tissue, and the quality of the image is not altered in case of previous surgery (radiation therapy or mammary prosthesis). Its sensitivity ranges between 64% and 96%, and its specificity is around 75-100%. The main limitation of PET is the fact that it cannot detect lesions smaller than 1 cm, due to the partial volume effect and the physiological accumulation of FDG in the mammary tissue.

### 3.8.2 Lymph node metastases

The sensitivity that has been published in the literature for PET detection of locoregional adenoapthies ranges between 50% and 100%, and its specificity is around 86-92%. If nodes of less than 1 cm and micrometastases are taken into account, the sensitivity of PET studies significantly decreases. For these reasons, PET cannot replace axillary node dissection. PET is particularly useful in the detection of adenopathies in the mediastinum and the internal mammary chain (PET sensitivity: 85%; CT sensitivity: 54%). The identification of these adenopathies has a very significant impact on the management of the patients (either increasing the radiation field or applying a more aggressive chemotherapy regime) and in their prognosis (Escalona et al., 2010).

### 3.8.3 Metastatic disease

PET is more accurate in the detection of unsuspected distant metastases, both at initial diagnosis and during the monitoring stage.

### 3.8.4 Monitoring of response to treatment

The assessment of response to treatment can be established with PET before any other diagnostic method (before there is a noticeable or measurable reduction in the size of the tumour). A PET study after a single chemotherapy cycle can predict the response (or lack of response) of the tumour to the treatment, with a sensitivity of 90-100% and a specificity of 74-85%).

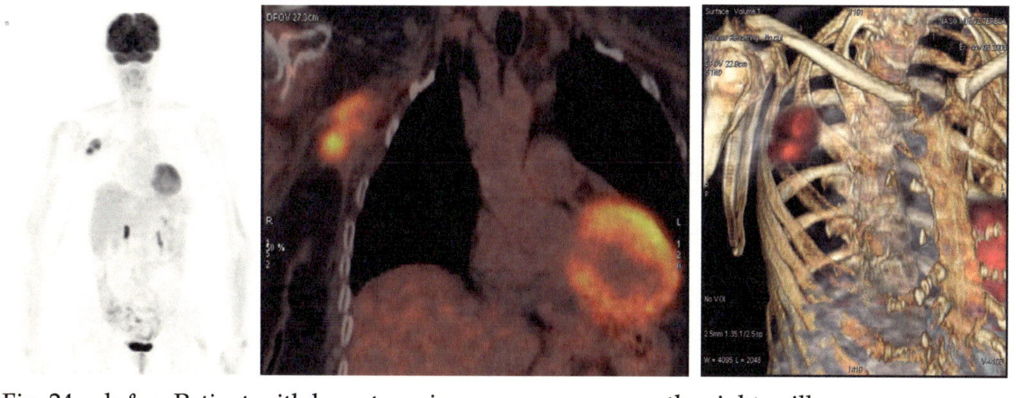

Fig. 24 a, b & c. Patient with breast carcinoma, recurrence on the right axilla.

### 3.8.5 Assessment of tumour recurrence

Previous surgery and/or radiation therapy can produce fibrosis/scar tissue that will complicate the assessment of potential locoregional recurrences (particularly on the axillary region), although potential distant metastatic areas can be detected.

### 3.8.6 Other applications of PET in breast cancer patients

The presence or absence of estrogen receptors has a great influence on the choice of a systemic treatment. Between 30% and 40% of the patients with advanced breast cancer and positive result for estrogen receptors (ER) will respond to treatment with antiestrogens (tamoxifen). Another important percentage of patients will have a stable condition for a clinically significant period of time. The presence of ER can be assessed with the use of an estrogen tracer (FES). If a tumour shows SUV>1 in a PET study with FES, it is considered to be a positive result for ER. When the tamoxifen treatment has started, ER are blocked, which means that any tumour that responds to antiestrogen therapy will show a fast decrease of SUV in PET studies with FES.

## 3.9 PET/CT and its applications in radiation therapy

Ideally speaking, the radiation therapy should administer a dose of ablative radiation to the tumor, leaving the peritumoral healthy tissue intact. With 3D conformational radiation therapy, the doses for the tumor and the other tissues can be calculated more accurately, the therapeutic effect increases, and toxic complications are reduced. In order to apply this therapy, the tumor needs to be accurately located. CT provides anatomical information, as well as the dosimetric bases for the calculation of radiation absorption. However, it also has

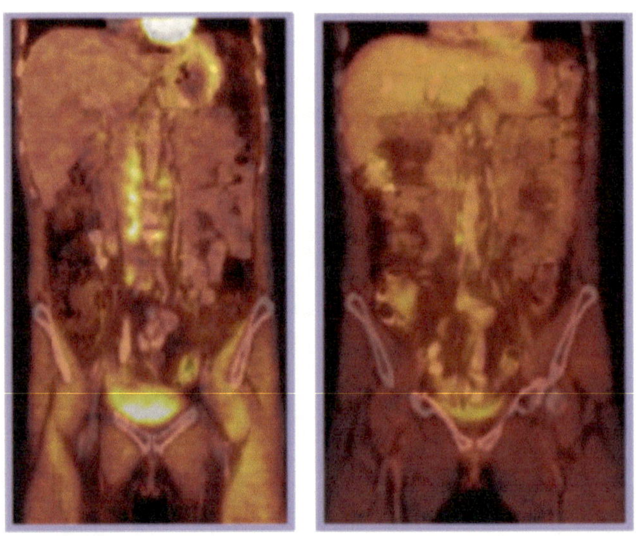

Fig. 25a & b. Intensity-modulated radiation therapy in a patient with cervical cancer (pre- and post-treatment)

important limitations, such as the delimitation of tumor margins, unnecessarily large radiation areas or infiltrated areas that remain untreated. PET/TC integrates structural and molecular information. Therefore, it provides a more accurate estimation of the tumor size and it identifies better areas with tumor viability. The use of this new "anatomobiological outline" in the planning of radiation therapy represents a clinically significant change with regard to the volume of radiation therapy that the patients receive. It can change the treatment approach, avoid unnecessary radical radiation therapy and adjust the volume of treatment, with the possibility of increasing the doses in specific locations.

- PET/CT before treatment: Cervical cancer with inguinal and paraaortic adenopathies. Definition of target volume.
- Planning of radiation therapy. The axial section of the radiation field is extended 14 mm in order to include paraaortic adenopathies, and additional radiation is applied to the pelvic adenopathy.
- Intensity modulated radiation therapy is administered in order to achieve higher effectiveness in the treatment with less side-effects.
- The response to treatment is assessed after the end of the therapy.

### 3.10 The future: Neuroradiology and cardiac viability

#### 3.10.1 Drug-resistant epilepsy

MRI and PET co-registration in pediatric epilepsy FDG-PET represents a useful tool for presurgical evaluation of epilepsy, particularly when MRI is nonlesional. Previous studies have shown FDG-PET to have 63–100% sensitivity in lateralizing temporal lobe epilepsy (TLE) and to provide complementary information to MRI. For extratemporal lobe epilepsy (ETLE), studies have shown FDG-PET to have slightly lower sensitivity at 36–83%. In addition to increasing detection postsurgical prognostic information independent of information provided by MRI, FDG-PET might thus provide complementary as well as supplementary functional information in regard to the etiology of seizure activity. Given the parallel roles of MRI and FDG-PET in presurgical evaluation for epilepsy patients, co-registration of MRI and FDG-PET might enhance presurgical management of intractable epilepsy. This has not been unequivocally established, but it is already recommended that FDG-PET images be interpreted in light of all structural imaging information. In the recent UCLA cohort, FDG-PET and MRI co-registration demonstrated favorable postsurgical outcomes (Engel class I–II) in 80% of the patients with intractable epilepsy with the application of co-registered imaging to maximally resect the functional abnormal area. This technique uses anatomic imaging to help define the limits of resection, despite previous MRI findings that had been considered to be nonlesional.

#### 3.10.2 PET and brain development in pediatrics

Functional development of the pediatric brain has been evaluated by FDG-PET. Chugani et al. demonstrated that the metabolic pattern of a developing brain follows the order of anatomical, evolutional and behavioral development. Increased glucose metabolism is shown in the visual, sensorimotor cortex and the cerebellum, and this is correlated with early visuospatial and sensorimotor function and primitive reflexes. Hypermetabolism in the basal ganglia is known to be associated with developing movement and sensorimotor function.

The quantitative analysis of brain FDG-PET has demonstrated that the degree of glucose metabolism of infants is significantly lower than that of adults. The degree of metabolic activity of neonates is about 30% that of adults and it continues to increase with age. It is hypothesized that increased metabolism is associated with increased metabolic demands from neuronal plasticity development. By a child's third year, the metabolic level exceeds that of adults, and it reaches its plateau between ages 4 and 9 with a value 1.3 times higher than that of normal adults. After this period, the value decreases to adult level by the end of the second decade.

Future applications include combined PET-MRI imaging and neuroreceptor imaging.

### 3.10.3 Dementia

Conventional anatomic imaging (e.g., MRI and CT) play a minimal role in the early detection of dementia, especially for Alzheimer's Dementia AD. There is evolving literature that supports that FDG PET may be more sensitive and specific than conventional nuclear medicine imaging (i.e., ECD and HMPAO imaging) in the diagnosis of dementia, especially in early detection. A more recent multicentre study (Mosconi et al., 2008) enrolled 548 patients (110 normal, 114 with mild cognitive impairment, 199 with AD, and 125 with other forms of dementia). Based on clinical endpoints they found that FDG PET correctly classified 94% of normal variants, 95% of AD, and between 92% and 94% of other types of dementia. There was significant heterogeneity in FDG patterns for patients with mild cognitive impairment. They developed standardized automated methods to analyze FDG brain scans and thought this automated consistent approach resulted in more homogeneous results than previously reported in the literature.

### 3.10.4 Cardiac viability

A stress PET examination can reliably demonstrate myocardial blood flow using 82Rb or 13Nammonia. PET radiopharmaceuticals can be used to assess both cardiac perfusion (i.e., 13N-ammonia, 15O-water, 82Rb) and heart muscle viability (FDG) (Machac et al., 2006). This section will only address evidence related to FDG viability assessment. Cardiac imaging tests can be roughly stratified into those which assess coronary blood flow/cardiac muscle perfusion, systolic function (i.e., how well the heart is pumping), heart muscle viability (i.e., living, but potentially at risk, heart muscle versus dead/scarred tissue) and other less common studies which assess very specific metabolic processes (e.g., fatty acid metabolism) or neuromuscular function (e.g., MIBG studies). PET can be used to assess all of these areas the CT component, can also assess coronary artery anatomy (e.g., CT angiogram) and coronary calcium scoring. These parameters can also be assessed through conventional CT or with SPECT/CT (Hesse et al., 2005).

## 4. Conclusion

PET/CT is a multidisciplinary technique which involves nuclear, radiology, radio physics, radio pharmacology and oncology and combines the advantages of the functional information by PET and the special and contrast resolution of CT. This improves the diagnosis, staging and follow-up of some types of cancer and other pathologies, and new indications could appear in the future.

## 5. References

Beyer, T.; Townsend, D.W.; Czernin, J. & Freudenberg, L.S. (2011) The future of hybrid imaging - part 2: PET/CT Insights Imaging REVIEW. *Insights into imaging*, Vol. 2, No. 3, pp. 225-234.

Cronin, C.G.; Swords, R.; Truong, M.T.; Visswanathan, C.; Rohren, E.; Giles, F.J.; O'Dwyer, M. & Bruzzi, J.F. (2010) Clinical utility of PET/CT in lymphoma. *American Journal of Roentgenology*, Vol. 194, No. 1, pp. W91-W103, ISSN 0361-803X.

Czernin, J.; Benz, M.R. & Allen-Auerbach, M.S. (2010) PET/CT imaging. The incremental value of assessing the glucose metabolic phenotype and the structure of cancers in a single examination. *European journal of radiology*, Vol. 73, No. 3, pp. 470-480, ISSN 0720-048X.

Demeter, S.; Bornstein, S.; Butler, J.; Cramer, B.; Hollett, P. & Jones, L. (2009). *The Development of a PET/CT Program in Newfoundland and Labrador*, Newfoundland and Labrador Centre for Applied Health Research, Memorial University, St. John's, NL.

Escalona, S.; Blasco, J.A.; Reza, M.M.; Andradas, E. & Gómez, N. (2010). A systematic review of FDG-PET in breast cancer. *Medical Oncology*, Vol. 27, No. 1, pp. 114-129, ISSN 1357-0560.

Gómez-León, N.; Pinilla, I.; Rodríguez-Vigil Junco, B.; Coya, J.; Herández, D.; Andradas, E.; Reza, M. & Madero, R. (2007). Uso del sistema híbrido PET/TC: experiencia inicial del Hospital Universitario La Paz. *Radiología*, No. 49, pp. 29-36, ISSN 0033-8338.

Hesse, B.; Tägil, K.; Cuocolo, A.; Anagnostopoulos, C.; Bardies, M.; Bax, J. et al. (2005) EANM/ESC procedural guidelines for myocardial perfusion imaging in nuclear cardiology. *Eur J Nucl Med Mol Imaging*, No. 32, pp. 855-897, ISSN 1619-7070.

Høilund-Carlsen, P.F.; Gerke, O.; Vilstrup, M.H.; Lerberg Nielsen, A.; Thomassen, A.; Hess, S.; Høilund-Carlsen, M.; Vach, W. & Petersen, H. (2011) PET/CT without capacity limitations: a Danish experience from a European perspective. *European Radiology*, Vol. 21, No. 6, pp. 1277-1285, ISSN 0938-7994.

Machac, J.; Bacharach, S.L.; Bateman, T.M.; Bax, J.J.; Beanlands, R.; Bengel, F. et al. (2006) Positron emission Tomography myocardial perfusion and glucose metabolic imaging. *Journal of Nuclear Cardiology*, No. 13, pp. 121-151, ISSN 1071-3581.

Pawaroo, D.; Cummings, N.M.; Musonda, P.; Rintoul, R.C.; Rassl, D. & Beadsmoore, C. (2011) Non-small cell lung carcinoma: accuracy of PET/CT in determining the size of T1 and T2 primary tumours. *American Journal of Roentgenology*, Vol. 196, No. 5, pp. 1176-1181, ISSN 0361-803X.

Pinilla, I.; Gómez-León, N.; Del Campo-Del Val, L.; Hernandez-Maraver, D.; Rodríguez-Givil, B.; Jover-Díaz, R. & J. Coya, J. (2010) Diagnostic value of CT, PET and combined PET/CT performed with low-dose unenhanced CT and full-dose enhanced CT in the initial staging of lymphoma. *Q J Nucl Med Mol Imaging*, EPUB ahead of print, ISSN 1827-1936.

Townsend D. W, Beyer T. (2002) A combined PET/CT scanners: a hardware approach to image fusion. *British J Radiol*; No. 75, pp. 24-30.

# 16

# Advances in Medical Imaging Applied to Bone Metastases

Àngel González-Sistal[1], Alicia Baltasar Sánchez[1], Michel Herranz Carnero[2] and Álvaro Ruibal Morell[2]
[1]*Medical Imaging Research Laboratory, Dpt. Physiological Sciences II Faculty of Medicine, University of Barcelona*
[2]*Nuclear Medicine Service, Complexo Hosp. Universitario Santiago de Compostela Molecular Imaging Group, IDIS*
*Spain*

## 1. Introduction

Bone metastases are the result of a primary cancer invasion which spreads into the bone marrow through the lymphogenous or hematogenous pathways. Bone metastases are a common complication of cancer.The primary cancers that most frequently metastasize to bone are breast and prostate cancer (65 - 75 %) amongst many others (thyroid 42 %, lung 36 % or kidney 35 %) (Suva et al., 2011). Although the exact incidence of bone metastases is unknown given its dependence on the type of primary cancer, it is estimated that 350,000 people die of bone metastases annually in the United States.

### 1.1 Bone structure and microenvironment

Bone is the third most common site of hematogenous tumor metastases after liver and lungs. The imbalance in bone turnover results in a favorable environment for the growth of metastatic tumors, a process known as the vicious cycle of bone metastases (Fili et al., 2009).

Bone consists of cortical, trabecular and marrow components. Cortical bone, is compact and has canals containing vessels. A layer of compact bone surrounds trabecular bone, which contains the bone marrow. Most of the red marrow (hematopoietic) is located in axial bones (spine, ribs, pelvis, proximal femora), whereas fat marrow is found in appendicular bones (long bones). Bone tissue contain the cells types: osteoblasts, osteoclasts, osteocytes and bone-lining cells.

Breast and prostate carcinomas have a great avidity for bone because the molecular interactions between these cancer cells and host cells favor the establishment of osseous lesions. Thyroid, lung, kidney, gastric, colon and skin cancers also metastasize usually to bone but, to a lesser degree, because these cell types do not possess the properties needed for invasion and residence in the bone microenvironment (Weilbaecher et al., 2011).

A number of factors contribute to the high incidence of bone metastases (Eriksen, 2010): high blood flow in the red marrow; adhesive molecules on tumor cells that bind them to marrow stromal cells and bone matrix (tumor cells increase the production of angiogenic and bone-resorbing factors that further enhance tumor growth in bone); growth factors (transforming growth factor *b* (TGF *b*), insulin-like growth factors I and II (IL-I and IL-II), fibroblast growth factors (FBG), platelet-derived growth factors and bone morphogenetic proteins (BMPs)) that are released and activated during bone resorption, providing fertile ground in which tumor cells can grow (Suva et al., 2009).

The adult skeleton continually turns over and remodels itself. There is a balanced remodeling sequence: osteoclasts resorb bone on trabecular surfaces and then osteoblasts form bone at the same site (Hadjidakis et al., 2006).

### 1.2 Types and localization of bone metastases

Most tumor implants occur through the hematogenous pathway. The preference for axial involvement is also due to the greater vascularity of the red marrow found in the axial skeleton as opposed to the yellow marrow (high-fat) found in the appendicular bone. Bone metastases are characterized as "lytic"(bone destructive), "blastic / sclerotic" (bone forming) or "mixed" according to the radiographic and/or pathologic appearance of the lesion. This classification represents the dysregulation of the normal bone remodeling process mediated by osteoblasts, osteoclasts and tumor cells.

Patients with breast cancer have predominantly osteolytic lesions (Trinkaus et al., 2009), although 15 to 20 percent of them have osteoblastic lesions. Bone metastases from kidney, lung or thyroid cancers more often are osteolytic. In addition, secondary formation of bone occurs in response to bone destruction. Only in multiple myeloma do purely lytic bone lesions develop. In contrast, the lesions in prostate cancer are predominantly osteoblastic. (Logothetis & Lin, 2005; Ye et al., 2007).

### 1.3 Clinical features

Bone metastases represent a major cause of morbidity and mortality, once tumors metastasize to bone they are usually incurable (Coleman et al., 2011). Bone metastases are rarely silent. They can give rise to a number of life-threatening complications (Coleman et al., 2006). Osteolytic metastases can cause severe pain, pathologic fractures, decreased mobility, hypercalcemia, anemia, spinal cord compression and other nerve-compression syndromes. Patients with osteoblastic metastases have bone pain and pathologic fractures because of the poor quality of the bone produced by the osteoblasts. Patients with fewer metastases or solitary lesions appear to have a better prognosis than those with multiple metastatic deposits.

### 1.4 Biomarkers of bone turnover

Biochemical markers of bone turnover have been used to assess the response to therapy or for the detection of bone metastases. Levels of bone-specific alkaline phosphatase, osteocalcin and type I procollagen C-propeptide are serum markers of osteoblast activity. Whereas, serum levels of C-terminal telopeptide of type I collagen or tartrate-resistant acid phosphatase and urinay levels of type I collagen cross-linked N-telopeptides are indicators of osteoclast activity (Roodman, 2004).

There are limitations to the clinical utility of many of these bone markers. Recently, some new markers have been described as potentially important role: CXXL16/CXCR6 (Ha et al., 2011), OPG/RANKL (Mercatali et al., 2011) or CCN3 (Ouellet et al., 2011).

## 2. Pre-clinical cancer research optical imaging modalities

Optical imaging is based on the detection of photons emitted from living cells, tissues or animals. It can be divided into bioluminescence imaging (BLI) and fluorescence imaging (FLI). The role of molecular imaging in pre-clinical research is evolving. In small animal models optical imaging technologies are used to visualize normal as well as aberrant cellular processes at a molecular-genetic or cellular level of function (Chaudhari et al., 2005; Kwon et al., 2010; Snoeks et al., 2011).

The mechanism for creating luminescent light is that luciferase, which acts as a catalyst in the presence of oxygen and ATP, converts chemical luciferin into oxyluciferin, releasing light in the process. The substrate D-luciferin is injected, distributes rapidly throughout the body of the animal and is taken up by the cells. The emitted light is detected by a cooled charged coupled device camera (CCD) and has a wavelength from 500 to 620 nm which is sufficient to penetrate small animal tissue (Ntziachristos et al., 2005).

As regards FLI, fluorescence occurs when the excited state is caused by external stimulation by light (Leblond et al., 2010). As for BLI, luminescence is caused by a chemical reaction (either a natural, biological one- bioluminescence, or a purely chemistry based once chemiluminescence) (Kim et al., 2010). Despite its distinctive features each modality revealed differences in sensitivity, signal-to-noise-ratio (SNR) and background emission from tissues. Autofluorescence of tissue reduces the signal-to-noise ratio, so in fluorescence imaging the SNR is expected to be greater than in bioluminescence imaging.

In vivo expression of reporter genes encoding bioluminescent or fluorescent proteins can be detected externally by sensitive detection systems. BLI could easily image in vivo a bone metastatic lesion that in the end-point histological analysis results in a tumor of $\approx 0.5$ mm$^3$ volume, corresponding to $\approx 1.7 \times 10^4$ cells.

Optical imaging only provides semi-quantitative data because of tissue-dependent signal attenuation and poor positional information due to photon scattering. However, new advances have made it possible to extend BLI and FLI to 3D imaging by optical tomography, ensuring better quantification of photon emission. As a result of the development of fluorescence molecular tomography (FMT) and other 3D fluorescence and bioluminescence data capturing methods, it is now possible to acquire 3D optical data and use different modalities (radiography, μCT, PET, SPECT or MRI) to ensure spatial resolution and anatomical detail (Nahrendorf et al., 2010).

The main advantage of optical imaging is by a noninvasive study its ability to visualize biological processes, such as angiogenesis, inflammation or matrix degradation in the development and growth of bone metastases (Snoeks et al., 2011).

## 3. Diagnosis imaging modalities: Algorithm choice

Imaging plays a major role given that early identification of skeletal metastases could lead to changes in patient management and quality of life. Imaging modalities are based on either direct anatomic visualization of the bone or tumor or indirect measurements of bone tumor metabolism (figure 1). Clinical evaluation demands multimodal diagnostic imaging owing to the limitations of the diagnostic techniques. Four main modalities are currently used in clinical practice: radiography, computed tomography (CT), scintigraphy and magnetic resonance imaging (MRI). At present, positron emission tomography (PET) and single photon emission computed tomography (SPECT) have a potential for evaluation (Rybak et al., 2001; Costelloe et al., 2009).

These techniques differ in performance in terms of sensitivity and specificity, but none of the modalities alone seem to be able to yield a reliable diagnostic outcome. There is currently no consensus about the best modality for diagnosing the bone metastases and for assessing their response to treatment. In clinical practice, most oncologists do not even use the same criteria, which results in disparate assessments of bone metastases (González-Sistal, 2007; Welch & Black, 2010).

Although bone metastases can be treated, their response to treatment is considered "unmeasurable", which excludes patients with cancer and bone metastatic disease from participating in clinical trials of new treatments (Hamaoka et al, 2010).

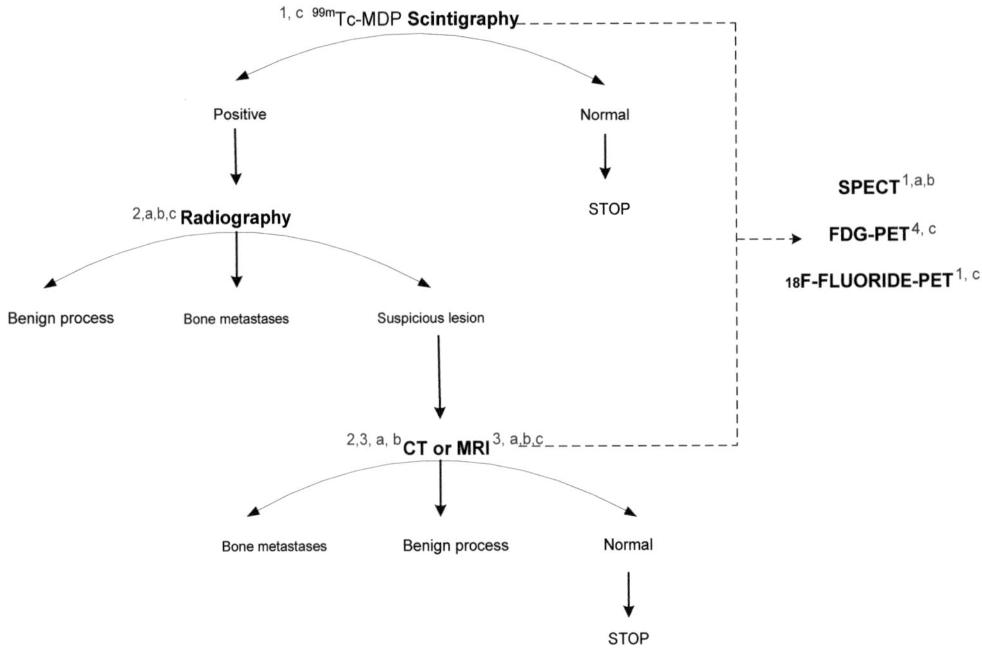


Fig. 1. Protocol for detection of bone metastases. Each imaging modalities visualize different aspects of bone tissue or tumor. (**Visualization**: 1 bone metabolism, 2 cortical/trabecular bone, 3 bone marrow / tumor, 4 tumor metabolism; **Extension**: a local, b regional, c whole body)

The algorithm of figure 1 shows a classical protocol for detection of bone metastases. The proposed algorithm is based in:

- Scintigraphy remains the technique of choice in asymptomatic patients in whom skeletal metastases are suspected (whole-body screening). This technique, albeit very sensitive, is poorly specific, and thus a bone scan finding is double-checked with an additional examination (radiography, CT or MRI).
- Radiography is used to evaluate symptomatic sites (bone pain) or confirm findings of other imaging modalities

- CT and MRI can depict anatomic changes in more detail. CT is preferable for assessing axial bone metastases, regardless of whether the main tumor involves the bone marrow or cortex. MRI, on the other hand, is better for detecting bone marrow disease or spinal cord compression.
- If MRI and CT cannot detect the disease and clinical suspicion of bone metastases remains, a PET/CT is made
- SPECT is not typically used for the initial detection of metastatic disease. SPECT-CT is useful for the assessment of lesions that are not determined in scintigraphy

## 4. Gamma-ray techniques

### 4.1 $^{99m}$Tc-MDP bone scintigraphy

Bone scintigraphy is a nuclear medicine tomographic imaging technique using gamma rays. Technetium-99m bound to methylene diphosphonate ($^{99m}$Tc-MDP) is the most frequent radionuclide used in scintigraphy. The patient is injected this radiopharmaceutical and then he is scanned with a gamma camera (a device sensitive to the radiation emitted by the patient) which it produces a 2D picture.

$^{99m}$Tc-MDP bone scintigraphy is the method used to screen the whole body for bone metastases. It detects increases in osteoblastic activity and the flow of the blood level. It is a marker of bone turn-over or bone metabolism (Moore et al., 2007).

Scintigraphy is indicated for the following procedures: screening or staging in asymptomatic patients, evaluation of persistent bone pain with a negative radiography, determination of the extent of bone metastases in patients with positive radiography, differentiation of metastatic from traumatic fractures and determination of the therapeutic response to bone metastases (Hamaoka et al., 2004).

A classic pattern is the presence of randomly distributed focal lesions throughout the skeleton (figure 2) which appear as areas of increased tracer uptake ("hot spots"). Other typical patterns in scintigraphy are superscan (diffuse metastatic disease), cold lesions (due to complete absence of reactive bone, they are associated with aggressive carcinomas), normal scintiscan, flare phenomenon (osteoblastic activity that reflects bone healing after chemotherapy but not advancing disease) and hypercaptation in soft-tissue lesions.

As regards the degree of confidence, scintiscans are non specific for determining the cause of increased uptake (lower specificity) since the findings of scintigraphy reflect the metabolic reaction of bone. Bone scintiscans have a poor spatial and contrast resolution. Many benign processes can produce an isotope uptake that mimics metastases (false-positive finding) and approximately one third of patients show a solitary area associated with a benign process. Thus, biopsy confirmation may also be needed for the final diagnosis of suspicious lesions. The differential diagnosis includes metabolic illness, osteomalacia, trauma, arthritis, osteomyelitis, infarctions and Paget's disease. Therefore, suspicious lesions or a single "hot spot" should be verified by other imaging modalities such as radiography, CT, or MRI.

Scintigraphy does not detect pure lytic metastases when bone turnover is slow or when the site is avascular. The main advantages of scintigraphy are widely available and can screen rapid whole-body images at a reasonable cost.

When assessing the therapeutic response, scintigraphy should be supplemented by images obtained with other modalities to provide a valid baseline for the assessment of bone tumor. In addition, it can take six months or longer to detect a response in the scintigraphy because of the confounding effect of the flare phenomenon.

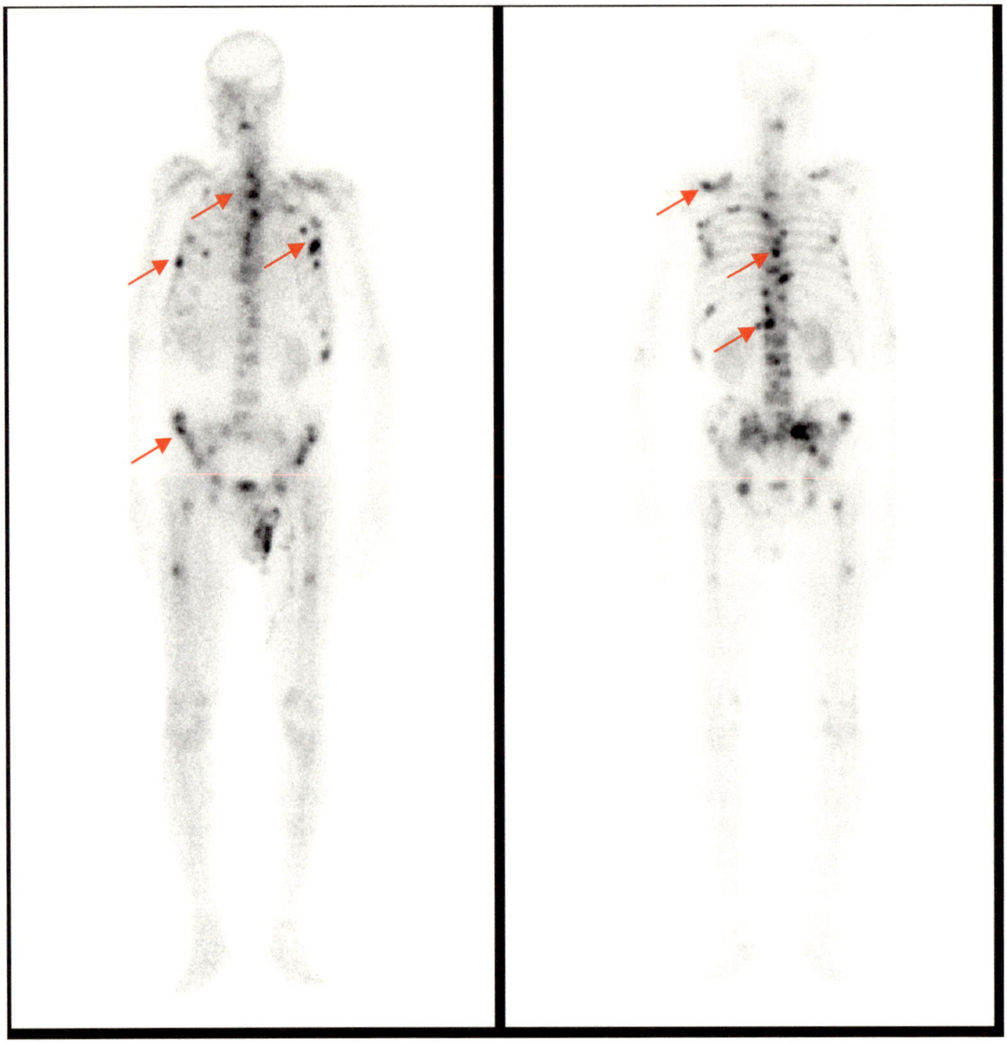

Fig. 2. $^{99m}$Tc bone scintigraphy images of a patient with prostatic carcinoma. This is a classical pattern with the presence of randomly distributed focal lesions throughout the skeleton. Bone metastases appear as areas of increased tracer uptake ("hot spots") (red arrows).

### 4.2 Single-photon-emission computed tomography (SPECT)

SPECT is a nuclear medicine tomographic imaging technique using gamma rays. $^{99m}$Tc-MDP, the same radionuclide used in conventional skeletal scintigraphy is the most frequent radionuclide used. It is very similar to conventional nuclear medicine planar imaging using a gamma camera. However, images are acquired in a cross-sectional rather than a planar fashion. It is able to provide 3D information. Compared with a conventional scintigraphy, the precise anatomic localisation provided by SPECT ensures a better differentiation between benign and malignant diseases. SPECT has greater sensitivity and specificity than scintigraphy for detecting vertebral and pelvis metastases (sensitivity 87-92% and specificity 73-100%). Like scintigraphy, it is possible that SPECT does not detect lytic lesions (Beheshti et al., 2009).

Because of limited availability and poor diagnostic imaging quality, SPECT is not typically used for the initial detection of metastatic disease (Chua, 2009). SPECT-CT is useful for the assessment of lesions that are not determined in scintigraphy. When scintigraphy are reviewed immediately, SPECT or SPECT-CT imaging can be performed in the same session without administering a second dose of radionuclide.

### 4.3 Positron emission tomography (PET)

PET is a nuclear medicine imaging technique that produces tomographic images through the detection of high-energy photon pairs emitted during positron decay of a radioisotope. PET visualizes the uptake of positron-emitting radioisotope by tissues, but, for skeletal metastases, two radiopharmaceuticals are typically used: $^{18}$F-Fluoride, a bone turnover tracer, and $^{18}$FDG a tumor tracer. PET can be used for whole-body scanning to detect metastases in either soft tissue or bone. PET provides a 3D image of tracer concentration within the body that is then constructed by computer analysis. In modern scanners, 3D imaging is often accomplished with the CT or MRI on the patient in the same machine. PET has a limited spatial resolution and complementary CT scanning or MRI is required to localize the specific area (Costelloe et al., 2009; Cook ,2010).

Its main advantages are: high sensitivity (84-100%), biochemical and molecular information (does not always coincide with morphological explorations). PET is an effective technique that is used in the evaluation of skeletal metastatic disease, particularly when combined with CT, because of its high resolution and coverage of the whole body (Ben-Haim, 2009 & Israel, 2009). PET has the advantage of permitting quantification of therapeutic response using the maximum standard uptake (mSUV) value. PET can be a sensitive modality for diagnosing and monitoring osteolytic response (Beheshti et. al, 2009; Wahl et al., 2009). However, the disadvantages may include PET cyclotron or the generator method, its high radiation, its high cost, its limited availability, and the additional time required for scanning with respect to other imaging modalities.

### 4.4 $^{18}$FDG-PET

$^{18}$FDG (2-deoxy-2-[18F]-fluoro-D-glucose or fluorodeoxyglucose) has been used to measure glucose metabolism in many types of primary cancer and can be useful for distinguishing benign from malignant bone lesions. It is an analog of glucose and represents the most widely used PET radiotracer in daily practice. The mechanism of uptake in tumor cells consist in the diffusion facilitated by glucose transporters (GLUTs), phosphorylation by hexokinase and subsequent metabolic trapping within the cell. It is a reflection of glucose metabolism consumption or tissue level.

Although it is a very sensitive marker, it is not very specific, since increases in tissue uptake of $^{18}$FDG is not always synonymous with cancer. The main clinical application of this technique consists in diagnosing, staging and restaging of various cancer types (figure 3). It is very effective in detecting metastases of breast, lung, esophagus, colon, thyroid, head, neck, melanoma and lymphoma.

From the dosimetric point of view, it should be noted that an administration of 350 MBq of $^{18}$FDG results in a radiation exposure of approximately 6,3-7 mSV and PET/CT examination may result in a radiation exposure of more than 22-23 mSv, near the upper range of the dose given for regular diagnostic abdomen CT (3,5-25 mSv).

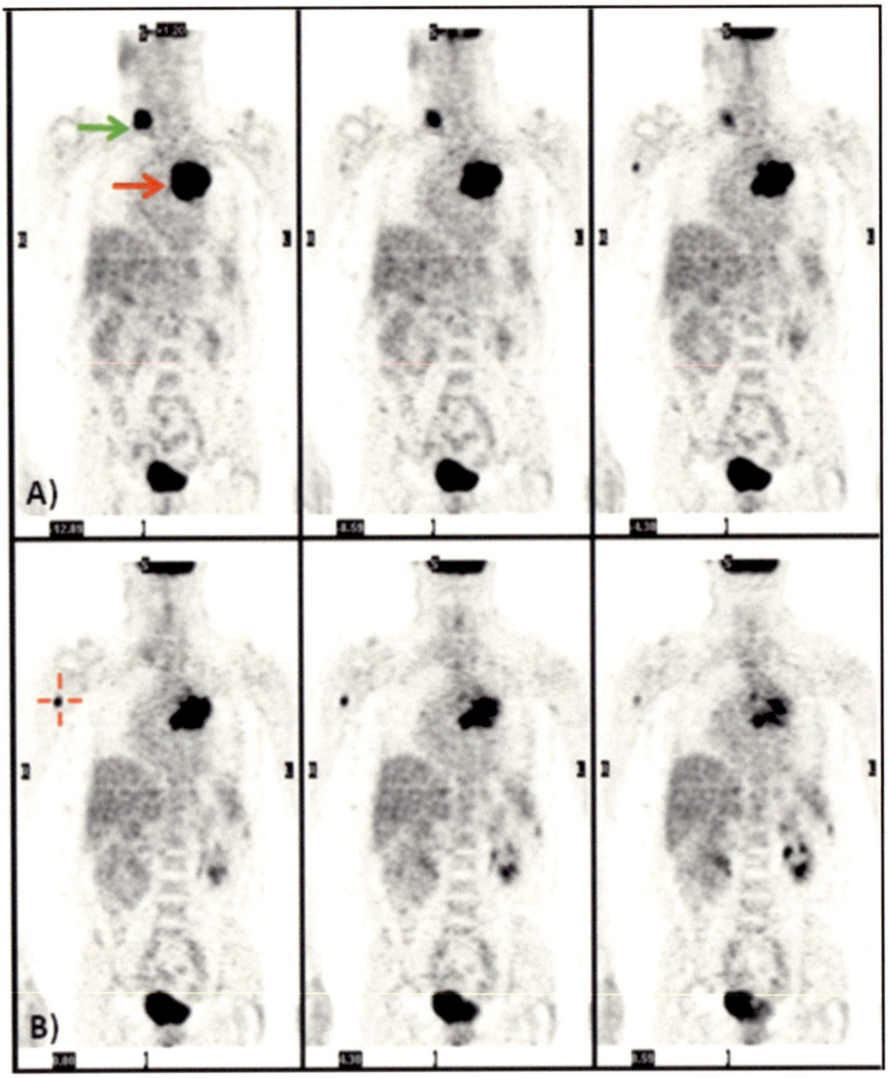


Fig. 3. PET images in a patient with lung carcinoma. **(A)** $^{18}$FDG PET shows the primary tumor (red arrow, 4x4.3cm, mSUV=27) with contralateral clavicle nodal metastases (green arrow, 2.7x2.5 cm, mSUV=19.2). **(B)** Incidental right humerus focal uptake is noted (red cross) which is suspicious for bone metastases modifying the initial disease staging from the patient to stage IV.

### 4.5 $^{18}$F-fluoride-PET

The mechanism of $^{18}$F-Fluoride uptake is similar to that of $^{99m}$Tc-MDP, the tracer used in scintigraphy: its accumulation depends on osteoblastic activity and local blood flow. It is an indicator of bone turnover, but not of a specific tracer of bone metastases. At present, it is the second most commonly used technique in oncology, playing an important role in the detection of bone involvement. A number of studies have shown that the diagnostic accuracy of $^{18}$F-fluoride–PET is better than scintigraphy (95,7% vs 75,4%) for detecting bone metastases in lung, prostate, thyroid and breast cancer, especially when using PET/CT (Withofs et al., 2011). Moreover, it appears to be more sensitive than SPECT.

The specificity of $^{18}$F-Fluoride when used with PET alone is 62% (Groves et al., 2007), which demands a CT, mainly pelvic and lumbar injury, and may also detect extra-osseous metastases. An advantage is that it can detect early osteoblastic changes in slow growing tumors, where $^{18}$FDG has a limited value. $^{18}$F-fluoride appears to be equally sensitive to osteoblastic and osteolytic metastases and can identify extremely early osteoblastic changes in response to metastatic deposits. It also seems to be superior in the detection the low avidity of bone tumor metastases for $^{18}$FDG as in some thyroid cancers.

Moreover, quantitative $^{18}$F-Fluoride PET can determine kinetics of fluoride incorporation into bone as a measure of fluoride transport, bone formation and turnover. Kinetic analysis (fluoride transport and flux) may be useful in assessing changes in bone turnover in response to therapy, and in bone metastases with values exceeding those of normal bone (Doot et al., 2010).

## 5. X-ray techniques

### 5.1 Radiography

Radiography is an x-ray imaging technique that produces a 2D picture of human body structures superimposed on each other, whose insides absord different amounts of radiation depending on the densities of its components. Bone metastases can appear on radiography as areas of absent density (osteolytic), as disrupted bone structure or as high density (osteoblastic). Radiography is a good method for characterizing bone metastases: osteolytic, osteoblastic or mixed. The ocurrence of bone metastases suggests a primary tumor, eg. osteolytic metastases are typical in breast and lung carcinomas whereas osteoblastic metastases are more common in prostatic carcinoma (Hamaoka et al., 2004). Radiography is used to evaluate symptomatic sites (bone pain) or confirm findings of other imaging modalities (especially for evaluating suspicious lesions on scintigraphy). Radiography may be used to assess the risk of a pathological fracture. False positive diagnosis may result because osteolytic metastases can mimic osteoarthritis. Osteoblastic metastases may be difficult to distinguish from other sclerotic bone lesions such as tuberous sclerosis.

The disadvantage is that between 30 and 50% of normal bone mineral content must be lost before lytic lesions become apparent on radiography (Wahl et al., 2009). Moreover, lesions in trabecular bone are more difficult to detect by radiography than cortical. The main advantages of radiography are that it is cost effective and widely available. However, it is not recommended for screening because of its limited sensitivity, which depends partly on location (Rybal & Rosenthal, 2001).

Radiography can detect the response of osteolytic lesions by depicting active bone formation (blastic change) or the reappearance and normalization of bone structure. But, it may be difficult to differentiate bone metastases from healing or previously unidentified sclerotic lesions. In several studies, indicators of response to treatment on radiography are correlated with clinical symptoms or other changes better than scintigraphy. Nevertheless, changes in radiography are not apparent until three to six months after the initiation of treatment (Even-Sapir, 2005).

### 5.2 Computed tomography (CT)

CT consists of a large series of 2D x-ray images taken around a single axis of rotation. The computer assisted reconstruction is used to generate 3D pictures. The radiologic appearance in the CT bone window setting offers skeletal detail because it can distinguish between materials of different densities. It is more sensitive than radiography in the detection of bone metastases. CT is useful for evaluating radiography negative areas in symptomatic patients or where metastases are suggested clinically. CT is important in the evaluation of focal abnormalities observed in bone scintigraphy that cannot be confirmed using radiographs.

Osteolytic, osteoblastic and mixed bone metastases are well despicted on CT. It can detect metastases in the marrow. Bone metastases appear more attenuated than the marrow. But the usefulness of CT in detecting early deposits in bone marrow is limited. Although CT is superior to radiography some advanced destructive lesions on trabecular bone may not be visible in the absence of cortical bone involvement, so CT is less apparent than the marrow changes visualized on MRI (Hamaoka et al., 2004). CT is also better than radiography and scintigraphy for depicting lesions in the spine and calvarium. CT is useful in guiding needle biopsy in bones such as vertebrae or ilia.

The disadvantage of CT is that its high radiation dose makes CT unsuitable as a screening tool. Thus, limited anatomic areas can be scanned simultaneously (Rybal & Rosenthal, 2001).

When assessing the therapeutic response, sclerosis of a lytic component on CT suggests a response to treatment. Notwithstanding, lysis or the appearance of new lysis or an increase in the size of blastic lesion represents a disease progression (Hamaoka et al., 2009; Wahl et al., 2009).

### 5.3 Dual-energy X-ray absorptiometry (DXA)

DXA is a method for the evaluation of bone mineral density (BMD) and monitoring patients with osteopenia or osteoporosis, entailing minimal exposure to radiation (x-ray). Two x-ray beams with differing energy levels are aimed at the patient's bones. When soft tissue absorption is subtracted out, the BMD can be determined from the absorption of each beam by bone.

BMD reflects the balance between bone formation and resorption. This method has also been applied in several clinical trials to assess the therapeutic outcome of patients with bone metastases receiving systemic treatments (Vassiliou et al., 2011). The BMD of skeletal metastases increases in patients responding to treatment and was significantly correlated with the changes imaged on skeletal x-rays and CT.

## 6. Magnetic resonance imaging (MRI)

MRI produces high quality images of the inside of the human body. It uses a powerful magnetic field to align the magnetization of some atoms in the body (hydrogen nuclei or protons of the water molecules) and a radiofrequency fields to systematically alter the alignment of this magnetization. When a patient is subjected to the powerful magnetic field of the scanner, the magnetic moments of some of these protons change and align with the direction of the field. An image can be constructed because the protons in different tissues return to their state of equilibrium at different rates (tissue variables: spin density, T1 and T2 relaxation times, flow and spectral shifts) (Wu, 2011). Unlike the other techniques, MRI does not use ionizing radiation.

MRI diagnosis of bone metastases is characterized by long T1 relaxation times, whereas T2 relaxation times are variable, depending on tumor morphology. Metastases are seen as focal or diffuse areas of hypointensity on T1-weighted images which contrasts with the surrounding high signal marrow fat. Metastases can often be distinguished from focal deposits of red marrow because the latter are more focal and may have centrally located fat (bull's eye sign). In the case of T2-weighted images, bone metastases are seen as areas of intermediate or high signal intensity which contrast with normal marrow because of their high water content, and they are commonly, surrounded by a rim of bright signal (halo sign) (Schmidt, 2007).

MRI can identify bone metastases at an early stage. CT can also visualize bone marrow lesions, but the resolution is poor. The advantages of MRI include distinguishing benign (osteoporotic) from malignant causes of vertebral compression fracture, detecting spinal cord compression and the capability to obtain sagittal views of the entire spine to be assessed in one imaging session. Nevertheless, MRI is less advisable than radiography or CT for detecting the destruction of cortical bone structure because, cortical appears black on T1 and T2-weighted sequences.

Difussion-weighted imaging (DWI) is a MRI technique based on the imaging of molecular mobility of water (i.e. diffusion). Recently, DWI has been proposed as a time-and cost-effective detection to image tumor deposits throughout the whole body. DWI is considered a highly sensitive method for the detection of bone metastases (Luboldt, 2008; Takenaka, 2009).

With whole-body MRI, technical problems arise from the relatively long examination times (45–60 min) and the limited depiction of metastases in small bones. However, the development of ultrafast pulse sequences (Turbo STIR (short tau inversion recovery)) for whole-body MRI may substantially decrease imaging time. MRI scanning has contraindications, these include: pacemakers, metallic implants or ferromagnetic foreign bodies (e. g. shell fragments). Many benign process can produce the appearance of bone metastases on MRI ( e.g in vertebral column: degenerative disk disease, osteomyelitis, benign compression fracture, infarcts or Schmorl's nodes).

When assessing the therapeutic response, MRI is optimal for showing spinal cord status and changes in the bone marrow but not suited to showing lytic or blastic change in bone structure.

## 7. Imaging modalities in major cancer entities

### 7.1 Breast cancer

The skeleton is the most common site of distant metastases in breast cancer (30%–85%). The vertebral column is the most common site of spread followed by the ribs. Bone metastases of breast cancer are lytic, blastic or mixed. Scintigraphy is indicated in patients with advanced disease or when bone involvement is clinically suspected. The use of $^{18}$F-FDG PET it is not a routine staging procedure. $^{18}$F-FDG PET allows for the detection of both soft-tissue and skeletal sites of disease. The superiority of $^{18}$F-FDG PET was reflected mainly in the detection of bone metastases, which were predominately lytic. By using PET/CT, sclerotic lesions overlooked by the PET part of the study can be identified on the CT part. In this setting, the high sensitivity of $^{18}$F-FDG PET for detecting marrow and lytic lesions and the high sensitivity of CT for detecting sclerotic lesions are complementary. Notwithstanding, some types of breast cancer, primarily well-differentiated histologic subtypes including some of the tubular and lobular ones, are less $^{18}$F-FDG avid and so are their metastases. A recognized scintigraphy effect of antiestrogen therapy commonly applied in patients with breast cancer is the "flare reaction". Clinically, it may be difficult to differentiate the flare reaction from disease progression. The initial agonist effect to therapy is also associated with increased tumor $^{18}$F-FDG uptake. A change in $^{18}$F-FDG uptake can be detected as early as 10 days after initiation of treatment compared with several weeks that are often required to make this assessment on the basis of clinical symptoms (Niikuraet al., 2011).

### 7.2 Prostate cancer

Prostate cancer frequently metastatizes to bone (35-85%). Bone metastases of prostate cancer are predominantly blastic. The vertebral column (lumbar), pelvis, sternum, ribs and femur are the most common sites of spread. Staging of newly diagnosed prostate cancer is essential for guiding treatment. Patients with low-risk prostate cancer are unlikely to have metastatic disease on scintigraphy. Patients are referred for scintigraphy mainly if they are considered to be at high risk for bone metastases, with high PSA levels, a locally advanced disease, or a high Gleason score. Scintigraphy is the most widely used method for evaluating skeletal metastases of prostate carcinoma. The role of $^{18}$F-FDG PET seemed to be limited in this type of cancer as both the soft-tissue sites of disease and bone metastases were reported to be $^{18}$F-FDG negative or to show only a low-intensity uptake in many patients. PET/CT was suggested to overcome the problem of pelvic tumor sites being obscured by the radioactive urine. Using $^{18}$F-FDG PET for monitoring the response to treatment, a decline in tumor glucose uptake measured as early as 48 h after androgen withdrawal, preceding any change in tumor volume or in PSA levels. Other PET tracers suggested for assessment of prostate cancer include $^{11}$C- or $^{18}$F-labeled choline and acetate, $^{11}$C-methionine, $^{18}$F-fluorodihydrotestosterone, and $^{18}$F-fluoride. The latter may be highly sensitive for detecting bone metastases in patients with prostate cancer (Even-Sapir, 2007).

### 7.3 Lung cancer

Bone metastases are diagnosed at initial presentation in 4%–60% of patients with non-small-cell lung cancer (NSC). Bone pain is usually considered an indicator of skeletal metastases, but up to 40% of lung cancer patients with proven bone metastases are asymptomatic.

Surgical resection offers the highest probability of a favorable outcome in patients with NSC lung carcinoma. However, the survival of patients who undergo surgery remains low, probably because of presurgical understaging. Clinical staging at presentation has been performed by means of CT of the thorax through the liver and adrenals, CT or MRI of the brain, and scintgraphy for assessment of bone involvement. This staging algorithm remains the most commonly used in places where $^{18}$F-FDG PET is not a routine staging modality of lung cancer. Including SPECT in the acquisition protocol of scintigraphy could improve the diagnostic accuracy scintigraphy in detecting bone metastases in patients with lung cancer. If necessary, scintigraphy can be complemented by CT or regional MRI for further assessment of unclear lesions. $^{18}$F-FDG PET and PET/CT were recently reported to be of value in assessing the presence of soft-tissue and bone spread in patients with NSC lung cancer. They reported that $^{18}$F-FDG PET had a high positive predictive value and a lower false-positive rate compared with scintigraphy (Even-Sapir, 2007).

The utility of PET in the detection of bone metastases is demonstrated in the following case (figures 4 and 5). A patient with lung carcinoma where the scintigraphy did not detect pure lytic metastases caused by slow bone turnover or an avascular site. The PET scan revealed a focus of increase FDG uptake suspicious for osteolytic metastases in the spine. MRI was requested for confirmation of diagnosis.

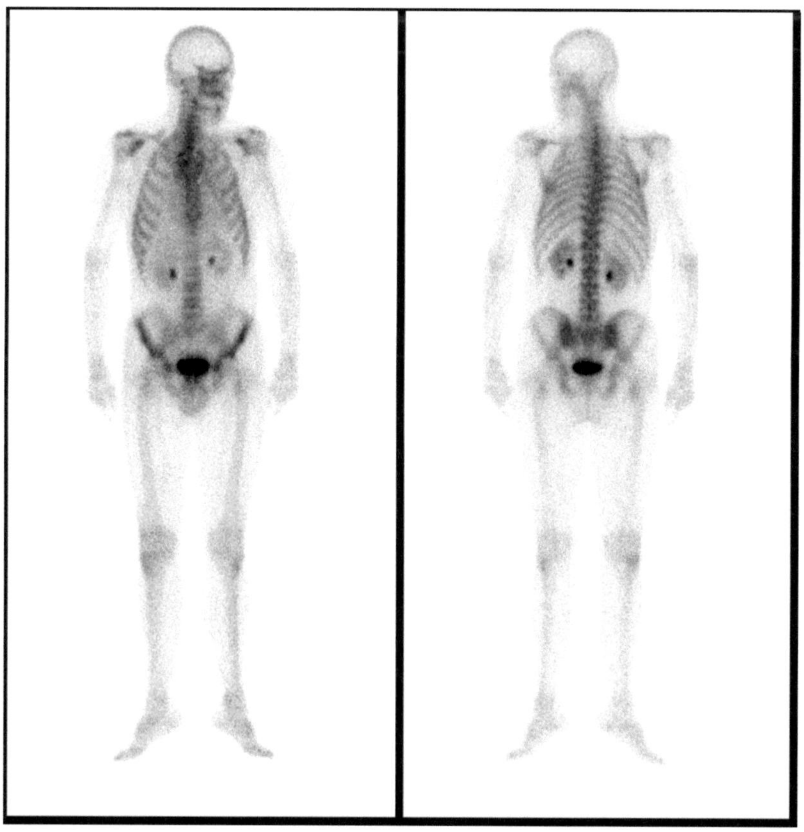

Fig. 4. $^{99m}$Tc-MDP bone scintigraphy images of a patient with lung carcinoma. It is a normal scintiscan. The bone scan does not revealed suspicious foci of uptake

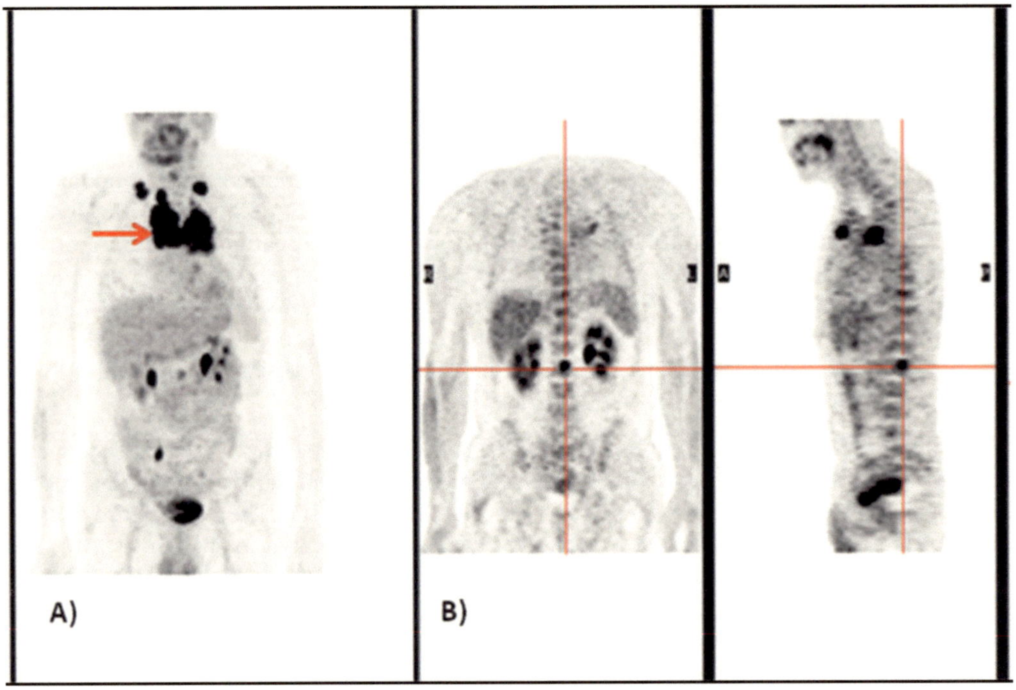


**(A)** PET show the primary tumor (red arrow). **(B)** A subsequent PET scan revealed a focus of increased FDG uptake in the spine (L2 vertebral body, red cross) which is suspicious for a osteolytic metastases.

Fig. 5. PET images in a patient with lung carcinoma. The utility of PET in the detection of bone metastases is demonstrated in this case. The bone scan, of the same patient, is showed in figure 4: a normal scintiscan (false negative case).

## 8. References

Beheshti M, Langsteger W, Fogelman I. (2009). Prostate cancer: role of SPECT and PET in imaging bone metastases. *Semin Nucl Med* 39: 396-407

Ben-Haim S, Israel O. (2009). Breast cancer: role of SPECT and PET in imaging bone metastases. *Semin Nucl Med* 39(6):408-15

Chaudhari AJ, Darvas F, Bading JR, Moats RA, Conti PS, Smith DJ et al 2005. Hyperspectral and multispectral bioluminescence optical tomography for small animal imaging. *Phys Med Biol* 50:5421–5441

Chua S, Gnanasegaran G, Cook GJR. (2009). Miscellaneous cancers (lung, yhyroid, renal cancer, myeloma, and neuroendocrine tumors): Role of SPECT and PET in imaging bone metastases. *Semin Nucl Med* 39: 416-430

Coleman RE. (2006). Clinical features of metastatic bone disease and risk of skeletal morbidity. *Clin Cancer Res* 15;12(20 Pt 2):6243s-6249s

Coleman RE & McCloskey EV. (2011). Bisphosphonates in oncology. *Bone* 49(1):71-6

Costelloe CM, Rohren EM, Madewell JE, Hamaoka T, Theriault RL, Yu TK, Lewis VO, Ma J, Stafford RJ, Tari AM, Hortobagyi GN, Ueno NT. (2009). Imaging bone metastases in breast cancer: techniques and recommendations for diagnosis. *Lancet Oncol* 10(6):606-14

Cook GJ. (2010) PET and PET/CT imaging of skeletal metastases. *Cancer Imaging* 10: 1-8

Doot RK, Muzi M, Peterson LM, Shubert EK, Gralow JR, Specht JM et al.(2010). Kinetic analysis of 18F-fluoride PET images of breast cancer bone metastases. *J Nucl Med* 51: 521-7

Eriksen EF. (2010). Cellular mechanisms of bone remodeling. *Rev Endocr Metab Disord* 11(4):219-27

Even-Sapir E. (2005). Imaging of malignant bone involvement by morphologic, scintigraphic, and hybrid modalities. *J Nucl Med* 46(8):1356-67

Even-Sapir E. (2007). PET/CT in malignant bone disease. *Semin Musculoskelet Radiol* 11(4):312_321

Fili S, Karalaki M, Schaller B. (2009). Mechanism of bone metastasis: the role of osteoprotegerin and of the host-tissue microenvironment-related survival factors. *Cancer Lett* 28;283(1):10-9.

González-Sistal, A. Baltasar Sánchez, A (2006). A complementary method for the detection of osteoblastic metastases on digitized radiographs. *J Digit Imaging* 19(3):270-5

González-Sistal A. (2007) Diagnostic Imaging Modalities of Osteoblastic Metastases *Hospital Imaging & Radiology Europe* 2 (1): 16-17

Groves AM, Win T, Haim SB, Ell PJ. (2007). Non-[18F]FDG PET in clinical oncology. *Lancet Oncol* 8(9):822-30

Ha HK, Lee W, Park HJ, Lee SD, Lee JZ, Chung MK. (2011). Clinical significance of CXCL16/CXCR6 expression in patients with prostate cáncer. *Mol Med Report* 4(3):419-24

Hadjidakis DJ, Androulakis II. (2006). Bone remodeling. *Ann N Y Acad Sci* 1092:385-96

Hamaoka T, Madewell JE, Podoloff DA, Hortobagyi GN, Ueno NT. (2004) Bone imaging in metastatic breast cáncer. *J Clin Oncol* 15;22(14):2942-53

Hamaoka T, Costelloe CM, Madewell JE, Liu P, Berry DA, Islam R, Theriault RL, Hortobagyi GN, Ueno NT. (2010). Tumour response interpretation with new tumour response criteria vs the World Health Organisation criteria in patients with bone-only metastatic breast cancer. *Br J Cancer* 16;102(4):651-7

Kim JB, Urban K, Cochran E, Lee S, Ang A, Rice B, Bata A, Campbell K, Coffee R, Gorodinsky A, Lu Z, Zhou H, Kishimoto TK, Lassota P. (2010). Non-invasive detection of a small number of bioluminescent cancer cells in vivo. *PLoS One* 23;5(2):e9364

Kwon H, Enomoto T, Shimogawara M, Yasuda K, Nakajima Y, Ohmiya Y. (2010). Bioluminescence imaging of dual gene expression at the single-cell level. *Biotechniques* 48(6):460-2

Leblond F, Davis SC, Valdés PA, Pogue BW. (2010). Pre-clinical whole-body fluorescence imaging: Review of instruments, methods and applications. *J Photochem Photobiol B* 21;98(1):77-94

Logothetis CJ, Lin SH. (2005). Osteoblasts in prostate cancer metastasis to bone. *Nat Rev Cancer* 5(1):21-8

Luboldt W, Kufer R, Blumstein N, Toussaint TL, Kluge A, Seemann MD, Luboldt HJ. (2008). Prostate carcinoma: diffusion weighted imaging as potential alternative to conventional MR and 11C-choline PET/CT for detection of bone metastases. *Radiology* 249: 1017- 1025

Mercatali L, Ibrahim T, Sacanna E, Flamini E, Scarpi E, Calistri D, Ricci M, Serra P, Ricci R, Zoli W, Kang Y, Amadori D. (2011). Bone metastases detection by circulating biomarkers: OPG and RANK-L. *Int J Oncol* 39(1):255-61

Moore AE, Blake GM, Fogelman I. (2007). A study to determine the dependence of 99mTc-MDP protein binding on plasma clearance and serum albumin concentration. *Nucl Med Commun* 28(3):187-92

Nahrendorf M, Keliher E, Marinelli B, Waterman P, Feruglio PF, Fexon L, Pivovarov M, Swirski FK, Pittet MJ, Vinegoni C, Weissleder R.(2010). Hybrid PET-optical imaging using targeted probes. *Proc Natl Acad Sci USA* 27;107(17):7910-5

Niikura N, Costelloe CM, Madewell JE, Hayashi N, Yu TK, Liu J, et al (2011). FDG-PET/CT Compared with conventional imaging in the detection of distant metastases of primary breast cáncer. *Oncologist*; 16 (8):1111-9

Ntziachristos V, Ripoll J, Wang LV, Weissleder R. 2005 Looking and listening to light: the evolution of whole-body photonic imaging. *Nat Biotechnol* 23:313–320

Ouellet V, Tiedemann K, Mourskaia A, Fong JE, Tran-Thanh D, Amir E, Clemons M, Perbal B, Komarova SV, Siegel PM. (2011). CCN3 impairs osteoblast and stimulates osteoclast differentiation to favor breast cancer metastasis to bone. *Am J Pathol* 178(5):2377-88

Roodman GD. (2004). Mechanisms of bone metastasis. *N Engl J Med* 15;350 (16):1655-64.

Rybak LD, Rosenthal DI. (2001). Radiological imaging for the diagnosis of bone metastases. *Q J Nucle Med* 45(1):53-64

Schmidt GP, Schoenberg SO, Schmid R, Stahl R, Tiling R, Becker CR, Reiser MF, Baur-Melnyk A. (2007). Screening for bone metastases: whole-body MRI using a 32-channel system versus dual-modality PET-CT. *Eur Radiol* 17(4):939-49

Snoeks TJ, Khmelinskii A, Lelieveldt BP, Kaijzel EL, Löwik CW (2011). Optical advances in skeletal imaging applied to bone metastases. *Bone* 48(1):106-14

Suva LJ, Washam C, Nicholas RW, Griffin RJ.(2011). Bone metastasis: mechanisms and therapeutic opportunities. *Nat Rev Endocrinol* 7(4):208-18

Takenaka D, Ohno Y, Matsumoto K, Aoyama N, Onishi Y, Koyama H, Nogami M, Yoshikawa T, Matsumoto S, Sugimura K. (2009). Detection of bone metastases in non-small cell lung cancer patients: comparison of whole-body diffusion-weighted imaging (DWI), whole-body MR imaging without and with DWI, whole-body FDG-PET/CT, and bone scintigraphy. *J Magn Reson Imaging* 30(2):298-308

Trinkaus M, Ooi WS, Amir E, Popovic S, Kalina M, Kahn H, Singh G, Gainford MC, Clemons M. (2009). Examination of the mechanisms of osteolysis in patients with metastatic breast cancer. *Oncol Rep* 21(5):1153-9

Vassiliou V, Andreopoulos D, Frangos S, Tselis N, Giannopoulou E, Lutz S. (2011). Bone Metastases: Assessment of Therapeutic Response through Radiological and Nuclear Medicine Imaging Modalities. Clin *Oncol (R Coll Radiol)* [Epub ahead of print]

Wahl RL, Jacene H, Kasamon Y, Lodge MA. (2009). From RECIST to PERCIST: Evolving Considerations for PET response criteria in solid tumors. *J Nucl Med* 50 Suppl 1:122S-50S

Welch HG, Black WC. (2010). Overdiagnosis in cáncer. *J Natl Cancer Inst*. 5;102(9):605-13

Weilbaecher KN, Guise TA, McCauley LK. (2011). Cancer to bone: a fatal attraction. *Nat Rev Cancer* 2011 Jun;11(6):411-25

Withofs N, Grayet B, Tancredi T, Rorive A, Mella C, Giacomelli F, et al. (2011). 18F-fluridePET/CT for assessing bone involvement in prostate and breast cancers. *Nucl Med Commun* 32: 168-76

Wu LM, Gu HY, Zheng J, Xu X, Lin LH, Deng X, Zhang W, Xu JR. (2011). Diagnostic value of whole-body magnetic resonance imaging for bone metastases: a systematic review and meta-analysis. *J Magn Reson Imaging* 34(1):128-35

Ye XC, Choueiri M, Tu SM, Lin SH.(2007). Biology and clinical management of prostate cancer bone metástasis. *Front Biosci* 1;12:3273-86

# 17

# A Hierarchical Framework for Mitosis Detection in Time-Lapse Phase Contrast Microscopy Image Sequences of Stem Cell Populations

Anan Liu[1]*, Kang Li[2] and Tong Hao[3]
[1]*School of Electronic Information Engineering, Tianjin University*
[2]*Microsoft Corporation*
[3]*School of Chemical Engineering and Technology, Tianjin University*
[1,3]*China*
[2]*USA*

## 1. Introduction

Measurement of the proliferative behaviors of cells in vitro is important to many biomedical applications ranging from basic biological research to advanced applications, such as drug discovery, stem cell manufacturing, and tissue engineering. Critical to such measurement is accurate identification and localization of mitosis, which is the process whereby a eukaryotic cell separates the chromosomes in its cell nucleus into two identical sets in two daughter nuclei. In the early years, it is possible to manually identify incidents of mitosis because mitotic cells in culture tend to retract, round up, and exhibit intensified surrounding halos under phase contrast illumination (Fig.1) for short-period, small-scale studies. Recently, many cell proliferation assays have been developed for high throughput cell imaging and analysis. Especially, phase contrast microscopy is a superior imaging modality because it enables continuous monitoring of live cells without requiring destructive methods of cell manipulation, such as cell lysis and staining. Consequently, the need for extended-time observation and the proliferation of high-throughput imaging have made automated image analysis mandatory.

The state-of-the-art mitosis detection methods can be categorized into three classes, tracking-based, tracking-free, and hybrid approaches. Tracking-based approaches rely on cell tracking to determine individual cell trajectories, and then identify mitosis based on the temporal progression of cell features along their trajectories (Al-Kofahi et al., 2006; Bise et al., 2009; Debeir et al., 2005). The dependency on cell tracking is a severe burden because tracking *per se* is a challenging task. Tracking-free approaches alleviate this burden and can detect mitosis directly in an image sequence. One representative technique was proposed by Li et al (Li, Kanade, Chen, Miller & Campbell, 2008), which applies a cascade classifier to classify volumetric sliding windows of an image sequence with 3D Haar-like features. Major drawbacks of this approach include the requirement of a large amount of training

---

*Corresponding Author

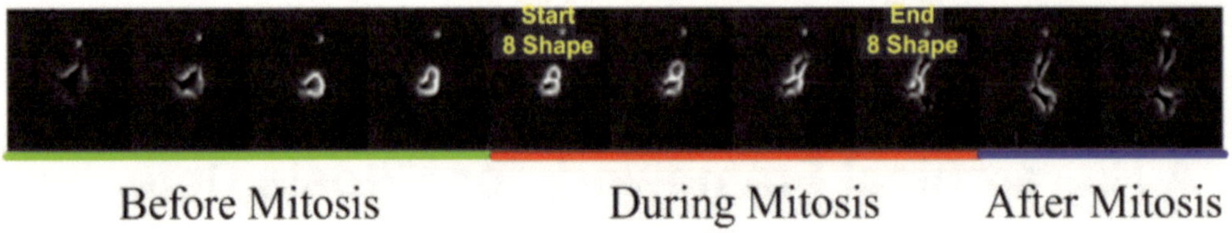


Fig. 1. Mitosis Sample. All the frames in one mitosis sequence are concatenated into one figure to show the visual pattern transition. One mitosis sequence can be visually divided into three stages, before mitosis, during mitosis, and after mitosis. Especially, all mitotic regions within the stage of during mitosis appear like 8 shape.

data and the lack of location specificity of detection. Hybrid approaches aim to construct a self-contained solution by leveraging the advantages of the previous two methods. These approaches typically consist of candidate sequence detection, sequence feature extraction, and classification as consecutive steps. To detect mitosis candidates, earlier methods (Eccles & Klevecz, 1986) apply thresholding and morphological filtering to extract bright halos surrounding potentially mitotic cells in each image, and then group the extracted regions in successive images based on their spatial relationship. Subsequently, to identify mitosis, Eccles et al (Eccles & Klevecz, 1986) employed a ring shape detector to locate the mother and two daughter cells; Gallardo et al (Gallardo et al., 2004) adopted a hidden Markov model to classify candidates based on temporal patterns of cell shape and appearance features; Liang et al (Liang et al., 2007) utilized conditional random field model to identify mitosis with shape and texture features in the mitotic regions. However, these methods can only recognize mitosis event without precise spatial and temporal localization during cell proliferation because of the lack of the ability to analyze the latent structure of mitosis progression.

Different from previous work simultaneously identifying and localizing mitosis event, we divided the problem of mitosis event detection into two sub-tasks: 1) mitosis identification: identifying the visual pattern transition from 0 shape mother cell to 8 shape mother cell and finally to two separate daughter cells in Fig.1; 2) mitosis localization: localizing the starting point, the first 8 shape pattern, and ending point, the last 8 shape pattern, during mitosis progression in Fig. 1. The proposed framework follows the spirit of the hybrid approach. It takes a phase contrast microscopy image sequence as input, and automatically pinpoints the time point at which mitosis occurs. First, model-based microscopy image preconditioning (Li & Kanade, 2009) and volumetric segmentation are utilized to extract spatiotemporal sub-regions in the input image sequence where mitosis potentially occurred. Then, a hidden conditional random field classifier (Quattoni et al., 2007) is applied for mitosis identification. By making significant extension on our previous work on mitosis sequence identification (Liu et al., 2010a;b), a conditional random field model (Lafferty et al., 2001) is implemented for mitosis localization. The first two stages jointly optimize the recall and precision for mitosis identification while the third stage pinpoints the time point at which mitosis occurs, minimizing the mean error and standard deviation of mitosis location. The superiority lies in three aspects: 1) nonnegative mixed-norm preconditioning method can avoid over segmentation and *ad hoc* image processing; 2) volumetric region grow method can avoid the explicit cell tracking; 3) latent contextual information can be discovered by hidden conditional random field and conditional random field classifiers for both sub-tasks. Consequently the proposed framework has high generalization ability and can be straightforwardly adapted to different cell types.

The rest of the paper is structured as follows. In Section 2, we introduce the hierarchical framework for mitosis event detection. Then, the experimental methods and results are respectively detailed in Section 3 and 4. At last, the conclusion and future work are presented.

## 2. Mitosis detection framework

As shown in Fig.2, the proposed hierarchical framework for mitosis event detection consists of three steps: *Mitosis Candidate Extraction*, *Mitosis Identification*, and *Mitosis Localization*. We will present the technical details of each step in the subsequent sections.

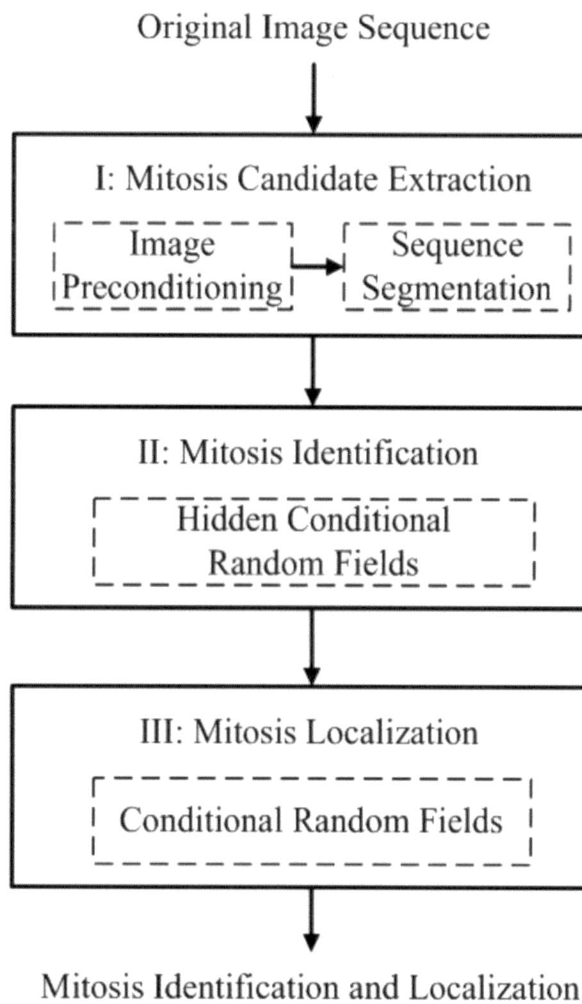


Fig. 2. Mitosis detection framework

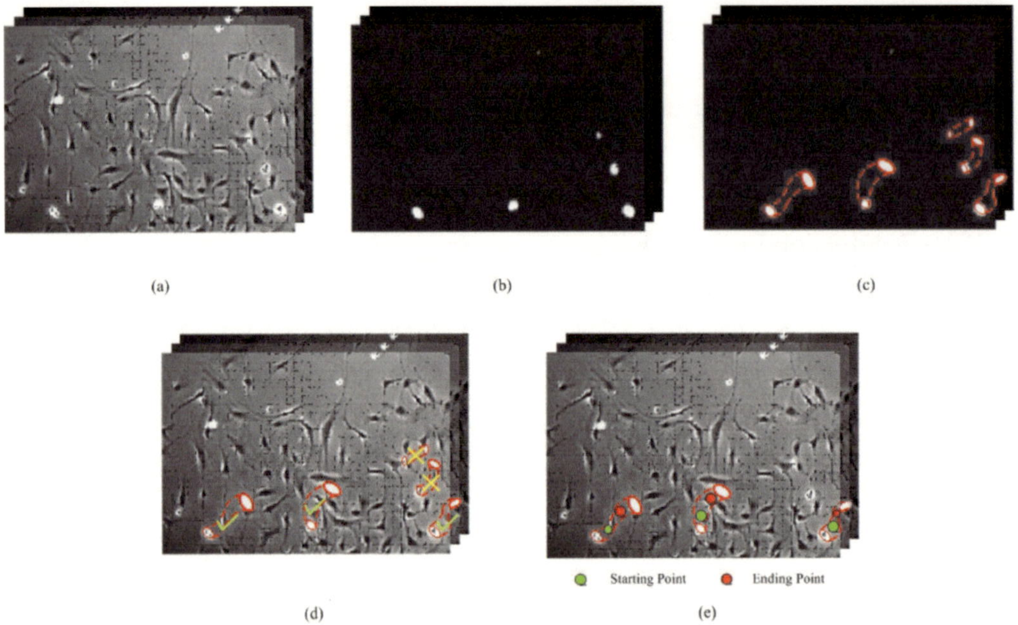


Fig. 3. Outputs by the key steps of the proposed framework. (a) Original image sequence; (b) Outputs of image preconditioning; (c) Outputs of mitosis candidate extraction; (d) Outputs of mitosis identification; (e) Outputs of mitosis localization.

### 2.1 Mitosis candidate extraction

This step serves the purposes of eliminating "easily" negative regions in the image sequence where mitosis is unlikely to occur and extracting temporally continuous sub-sequences with potential mitosis to facilitate subsequent sequence classification. The algorithm consists of two sub-steps, image preconditioning and sequence segmentation.

#### 2.1.1 Image preconditioning

Image segmentation in microscopy, especially in non-fluorescence optical microscopy modalities, is notoriously challenging due to inherent optical artifacts. Rather than treating phase contrast microscopy images as general natural images and rushing into the image processing warehouse for solutions, we study the properties of phase contrast optics to model its image formation process. Li et al's research revealed that the phase contrast imaging system can be relatively well explained by a linear imaging model (Li, 2009; Li & Kanade, 2009; Yin et al., 2010). With this model, a quadratic optimization function with sparseness and smoothness regularizations can be formulated to enhance cell regions and transforms the original image into an ideal image with zero background and nonzero foreground regions that correspond to potential mitotic cells as shown in Fig.3.(b). The detailed method contains following two steps.

***(a) Algebraic image model***

The generic model for microscopy images consists of three components: 1) an imaging model $h(\cdot)$ that represents the image formation process of the microscope; 2) an additive bias $b(x,y)$

that compensates for a nonzero background level, nonuniform illumination, and spatial sensitivity variations of the detector; and 3) a noise model $n(\cdot)$ that accounts for imaging and detection noise. The model can be written as:

$$g(x,y) = n(h(f(x,y)) + b(x,y)), \tag{1}$$

with $g(x,y)$ being the observed image, and $f(x,y)$ being the ideal object image that we want to retrieve, which could represent the optical path length distribution in the object, fluorescence intensities, or an phenomenological image that simply facilitates object segmentation. Under the assumption of additive noise, the model above can be expressed succinctly in a linear algebraic framework, given by

$$g = Hf + b + n \approx Hf + constant, \tag{2}$$

where $g$ denotes a vectoried representation of the observed image, which is formed by concatenating the image pixels in raster order. The vectors $f, b, n$ are defined likewise for the object, bias, and noise, respectively. The imaging model is expressed as a matrix-vector multiplication between the $N \times N$ transfer matrix $H$ and $f$, which is adequate for representing a wide range of microscopy image formation processes. Depending on the physics of phase contrast microscopy, we choose the image formation model, $H$, defined by an effective point spread function (or EPSF) in (Li, 2009):

$$EPSF(x,y) \propto \delta(x,y) - (\alpha e^{-(x^2+y^2)/\sigma_1^2} - \beta e^{-(x^2+y^2)/\sigma_2^2}) \tag{3}$$

where $\delta(\cdot)$ is a Dirac delta function, and $\alpha, \beta$ are scaling factors. The EPSF approximates the imaging function of phase contrast optics, which accounts for the formation of halo effects around imaged cells.

***(b) Nonnegative mixed-norm preconditioning***

With the image model specified in Eq.2 and the assumption of additive noise, we need to compute the ideal object image $f$ given an observed image $g$. This inverse problem can be tackled through a two-step process. Then an observed image which is unfriendly for computer analysis can be transformed into the one that facilitates automated object segmentation and measurement.

*a.Bias Elimination*:As the first step of preconditioning, a bias-corrected image can be obtained by estimating the bias field from an image. Under the assumption that the bias field is smooth and spatially slowly varying, it can be modeled as a $K$-th order polynomial surface:

$$b = Xp \tag{4}$$

where $p = (p_0, p_1, p_2, \ldots)^\top$ is the coefficient vector, and $X$ is a matrix of $N$ rows and $(K+1)(K+2)/2$ columns with the $i$-th row being $(1, x_i, y_i, x_i^2, x_i y_i, y_i^2, \ldots)$. To eliminate the bias, the optimal coefficients can be computed firstly by solving the over-determined linear system $Xp = g$. This amounts to solving the least-squares problem $p^* = \arg\min_p ||Xp - g||_2^2$, which has a closed-form solution $p^* = (X^\top X)^{-1} X^\top g$. The bias-corrected image is then computed as $g^* = g - Xp^*$.

*b.Object Reconstruction via Convex Optimization*: The second step of preconditioning reconstructs the object from the bias-corrected image. It is achieved by minimizing:

$$O(f) = ||g^* - Hf||_2^2 + \gamma Smoothness(f) + \beta Sparsity(f), \quad s.t. f \geq 0 \tag{5}$$

where $||\cdot||_2$ denotes a L2 norm; the positive coefficients $\gamma$ and $\beta$ control the importance; the first term promotes data fidelity; the second and third terms encourage the spatial smoothness and sparseness of the reconstructed image, respectively.

By employing an L2 (Tikhonov) smoothness term (Tikhonov, 1977) and a weighted L1 sparseness term (Donoho, 2004), Eq.5 can be transformed into:

$$O_1(f) = ||g^* - Hf||_2^2 + \gamma||Rf||_2^2 + \beta||Wf||_1, \quad s.t. f \geq 0 \tag{6}$$

The smoothness term penalizes the L2 norm of the Laplacian of $f$, where the $N \times N$ matrix $R$ represents an algebraic Laplacian operator with symmetric boundary condition. The sparseness term penalizes the weighted L1 norm of $f$, where $W$ is a diagonal matrix with positive weights $w_1 \dots w_N$ on the diagonal and zeros elsewhere.

By rewriting $O_1(f)$ in terms of the symmetric positive definite matrix $Q = H^\top H + \gamma R^\top R$ and the vector $l = -H^\top g^*$, and letting $w$ denote the weight vector $(w_1 \dots w_N)$, the minimization problem can be expressed as the following nonnegative-constrained quadratic program:

$$f^* = \arg\min_f \frac{1}{2} f^\top Q f + (l + \beta w)^\top f, \quad s.t. f \geq 0 \tag{7}$$

We utilized the simple and efficient iterative algorithm, the sparseness-enhanced multiplicative update (SEMU) algorithm (Li & Kanade, 2009), to solve the object function above.

### 2.1.2 Sequence segmentation

After preconditioning, 3D seeded region growing (Silvela & Portillo, 2001) is applied to the transformed image sequences to extract spatiotemporal sub-regions that correspond to candidate mitosis sequences (Fig.3(c)). The algorithm relies on two automatically-determined thresholds: a seeding threshold computed by Otsu's optimal thresholding algorithm (Otsu, 1979)is used to detect seeds; and a lower threshold determined by Rosin's unimodal thresholding algorithm (Rosin, 2001) is used as the stopping criterion of region growing.

## 2.2 Mitosis identification

With the extracted candidate mitosis sequences, the goal of mitosis identification is to classify the candidate mitosis sequences detected in the previous step as mitosis or not as shown in Fig.3(d). To take advantages of the spatiotemporal context and the flexible constellation of latent structure during mitosis progression, the hidden conditional random field (HCRF) classifier is utilized to model the visual pattern transition shown in Fig.1.

HCRF is a powerful discriminative model for temporal inference (Quattoni et al., 2007). Comparing to generative models, like Hidden Markov Models (HMMs) (Rabiner, 1989), HCRF does not assume observations are independent of each other and therefore can incorporate long range dependencies for inference. On the other hand, different from other discriminative models, like Conditional Random Fields(CRFs) (Lafferty et al., 2001), HCRF use intermediate hidden variables to model the latent structure of the input domain and can infer a single label for the entire input sequence with the training data not explicitly labeled. Therefore, several literatures show that HCRF always outperforms HMMs and CRFs (Gunawardana et al., 2005; Quattoni et al., 2007; Wang et al., 2006).

Mitosis identification can be formulated as the problem of predicting a label $y$ given an observation sequence $\boldsymbol{X} \equiv \{\boldsymbol{x}_t\}_{t=1}^T$, where $\boldsymbol{x}_t$ denotes the feature descriptor of the $t$-th frame in the observation sequence and $y$ is a member of a sequence-wise label set $Y \equiv (Mitosis, Non - mitosis)$. HCRF model also consists of a vector of hidden variables $\boldsymbol{h} \equiv \{h_t\}_{t=1}^T$ where $h_t \in \mathcal{H}$ captures the latent structure of the input domain and $\mathcal{H}$ is the set of potential hidden states. A graphical representation of the HCRF model $G = (V, E)$ where $V$ denotes the vertex set and $E$ denotes the edge set, is shown in Fig.4 (a).

Given the definitions of the sequence-wise label $y$, the observation sequence $\boldsymbol{X}$, the hidden variables $\boldsymbol{h}$ and the model parameters $\theta$, the HCRF model can be defined by:

$$p(y|\boldsymbol{X},\theta) = \sum_{\boldsymbol{h}} p(y,\boldsymbol{h}|\boldsymbol{X},\theta) = \frac{1}{Z}\sum_{\boldsymbol{h}} exp(\psi(y,\boldsymbol{h},\boldsymbol{X};\theta)) \tag{8}$$

where $Z = \sum_{y' \in Y, \boldsymbol{h} \in \mathcal{H}} exp(\psi(y',\boldsymbol{h},\boldsymbol{X};\theta))$ is a partition function; $\psi(y,\boldsymbol{h},\boldsymbol{X};\theta) \in \mathcal{R}$ is a potential function parameterized by $\theta$ as:

$$\psi(y,\boldsymbol{h},\boldsymbol{X};\theta) = \sum_{j \in V}\sum_{p \in P_1} f_{1,p}(j,y,h_j,\boldsymbol{X})\theta_{1,p} + \sum_{(j,k) \in E}\sum_{p \in P_2} f_{2,p}(j,k,y,h_j,h_k,\boldsymbol{X})\theta_{2,p} \tag{9}$$

where $f_{1,p}$ and $f_{2,p}$ denote the $P_1$ node feature functions and $P_2$ edge feature functions respectively; $\theta_{1,p}, \theta_{2,p}$ are the components of $\theta$, corresponding to node and edge parameters.

For mitosis identification, we define the two kinds of node feature functions, $f_{1,1}$ and $f_{1,2}$, as follows:

$$f_{1,1}(j,h_j,\boldsymbol{X}) = \phi(\boldsymbol{x_j}), \quad f_{1,2}(j,h_j,y) = \begin{cases} 1, \text{ if } h_j \in \mathcal{H} \text{ and } y \text{ is } Mitosis, \\ 0, \text{ otherwise.} \end{cases} \tag{10}$$

where $\phi(\boldsymbol{x_j})$ is the feature descriptor of frame $\boldsymbol{x}_j$. Correspondingly, $\theta_{1,p}$ consists of two parts, $\theta_{1,1}$ for $f_{1,1}$ measuring the compatibility between observation $\boldsymbol{x_j}$ and hidden state $h_j$, and $\theta_{1,2}$ for $f_{1,2}$ measuring the compatibility between latent variable $h_j$ and segment-wise label $y$. We also define the edge feature function as follows:

$$f_{2,1}(j,k,y,h_j,h_k,\boldsymbol{X}) = \begin{cases} 1, \text{ if } (h_j,h_k) \in \mathcal{T} \text{ and } y \text{ is } Mitosis, \\ 0, \text{ otherwise.} \end{cases} \tag{11}$$

where $\mathcal{T}$ denotes all possible hidden state transitions from $h_j$ to $h_k$ within a mitosis sequence. Correspondingly, $\theta_{2,1}$ for $f_{2,1}$ measures the compatibility between an edge with hidden state $h_i$ and $h_j$ and the segment-wise label $y$.

Given $Tr = \{(\boldsymbol{X_1}, y_1), (\boldsymbol{X_2}, y_2), \ldots, (\boldsymbol{X_N}, y_N)\}$ be a set of training examples, the model parameters can be learned by optimizing the objective function (Lafferty et al., 2001):

$$L(\theta) = \sum_{i=1}^{N} \log p(y_i|\boldsymbol{X}_i, \theta) - \frac{1}{2\sigma^2}||\theta||^2 \tag{12}$$

where $N$ is the total number of training sequences. The first term in Eq.12 is the log-likelihood of the data; the second term is the log of a Gaussion prior with variance $\sigma^2$, i.e., $p(\theta) \sim exp(\frac{1}{2\sigma^2}||\theta||^2)$. The optimal model parameter $\theta^* = \arg\max_\theta L(\theta)$ can be obtained with gradient ascent algorithm, such as BFGS (Avriel, 2003). Given an unseen test sequence $\boldsymbol{X}$, the best corresponding label $y^*$ can be computed by

$$y^* = \arg\max_y p(y|\boldsymbol{X}, \theta^*) \tag{13}$$

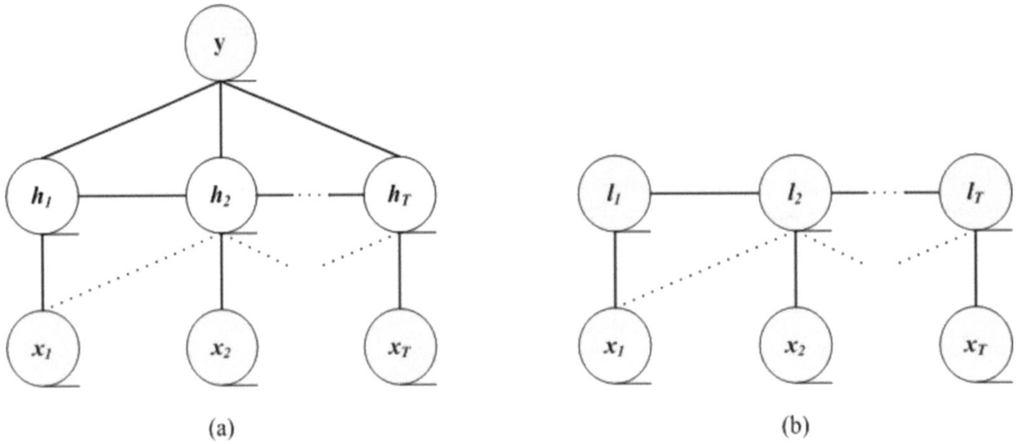


Fig. 4. A comparison of graphical structure. (a)HCRF; (b)CRF

### 2.3 Mitosis localization

Comparing to previous work only focusing on coarse level mitosis localization (Gallardo et al., 2004; Liang et al., 2007), it is more important to localize the start and end of mitosis event in spatio-temporal domain which will benefit real-time quantitative analysis of mitotic rate and the correlation between the mother cell and the daughter cells during cell division (Li, Miller, Chen, Kanade, Weiss & Campbell, 2008). Different from our previous work only considering the start and end of mitosis as a spatial visual pattern like 8 shape (Liu et al., 2010b), we regard mitosis progression as the spatio-temporal visual pattern changes from 0 shape mother cell to 8 shape cell and finally to two separate daughter cells. Consequently we propose to model the visual pattern transition between adjacent frames with Conditional Random Model (CRF), the most notably discriminative model proposed by Lafferty et al(Lafferty et al., 2001), to localize the start and end of one mitosis event as shown in Fig.3(e). Comparing to Support Vector Machine (Liu et al., 2010b) using only spatial information for mitotic cell modeling, CRF can take good advantages of spatio-temporal context to refine the frame-wise annotation for accurate mitosis localization. Furthermore, CRF can incorporate long range dependencies between observations and their labels without the assumption of generative dynamic Bayesian network models that the observations are independent given the values of hidden variables.

The task of mitosis localization can be considered as the problem of predicting a sequence of labels $\boldsymbol{L} = \{l_t\}_{t=1}^{T}$ given an observation sequence $\boldsymbol{X} = \{\boldsymbol{x}_t\}_{t=1}^{T}$ , where $l_t$ is a member of a frame-wise label set $\mathcal{L}$ of all possible labels. For one mitosis event, we designate $\mathcal{L}$ contains three members, before mitosis (BM), during mitosis (DM), after mitosis (AM). Therefore, the first and the last frames of a segment with label DM within one mitosis sequence respectively correspond to the start and end of mitosis event. CRF is an undirected probabilistic graphical model ($G' = (V', E')$) as shown in Fig.4 (b).

Given the definitions of the frame-wise label sequence $\boldsymbol{L}$, the observation sequence $\boldsymbol{X}$, and the model parameters $\gamma$, the CRF model can be mathematically formulated by:

$$p(\boldsymbol{L}|\boldsymbol{X}, \gamma) = \frac{1}{Z'} exp(\varphi(\boldsymbol{L}, \boldsymbol{X}; \gamma)) \tag{14}$$

where $Z' = \sum_{\boldsymbol{L}'} exp(\varphi(\boldsymbol{L}', \boldsymbol{X}; \gamma))$ is a partition function; $\varphi(\boldsymbol{L}, \boldsymbol{X}; \gamma) \in \mathcal{R}$ is a potential function parameterized by $\gamma$ as:

$$\varphi(\boldsymbol{L}, \boldsymbol{X}; \gamma) = \sum_{j \in V'} \sum_{q \in Q_1} f'_{1,q}(j, l_j, \boldsymbol{X})\gamma_{1,q} + \sum_{(j,k) \in E'} \sum_{q \in Q_2} f'_{2,q}(j, k, l_j, l_k, \boldsymbol{X})\gamma_{2,q} \tag{15}$$

where $f'_{1,q}$ and $f'_{2,q}$ denote the $Q_1$ node feature functions and $Q_2$ edge feature functions respectively; $\gamma_{1,q}$ and $\gamma_{2,q}$ are the components of $\gamma$, corresponding to node and edge parameters. We define the node feature function as follows:

$$f'_{1,1}(j, l_j, \boldsymbol{X}) = \phi(\boldsymbol{x_j}) \tag{16}$$

where $\phi(\boldsymbol{x_j})$ is the feature descriptor of frame $x_j$ and $\gamma_{1,1}$ for $f'_{1,1}$ measures the compatibility between observation $x_j$ and frame-wise label $l_j$. We also define the edge feature function as follows:

$$f'_{2,1}(j, k, l_j, l_k, \boldsymbol{X}) = \begin{cases} 1, \text{ if } (l_j, l_k) \in \mathcal{T}', \\ 0, \text{ otherwise.} \end{cases} \tag{17}$$

where $\mathcal{T}'$ denotes all possible state transitions from $l_j$ to $l_k$ within a mitosis sequence and $\gamma_{2,1}$ measures the compatibility between an edge linking label $l_j$ and $l_k$ and the frame $x_j$ and $x_k$.

Given $Tr' = \{(\boldsymbol{X_1}, \boldsymbol{L_1}), (\boldsymbol{X_2}, \boldsymbol{L_2}), \ldots, (\boldsymbol{X_M}, \boldsymbol{L_M})\}$ be a set of training examples, the model parameters can be learned by optimizing the objective function:

$$L(\gamma) = \sum_{i=1}^{M} \log p(\boldsymbol{L_i}|\boldsymbol{X_i}, \gamma) - \frac{1}{2\sigma^2}||\gamma||^2 \tag{18}$$

where $M$ is the total number of training sequences. The first term in the objective function is the log-likelihood. The second term denotes the Gaussian prior with variance $\sigma^2$. Learning the parameters of a CRF model is a convex problem so that the global optimality $\gamma^* = \arg\max_{\gamma} L(\gamma)$ can be guaranteed and obtained with gradient ascent algorithm, such as BFGS

(Avriel, 2003). Given a testing sequence $\boldsymbol{X}$, with the optimal model parameters $\gamma^*$, the label $\boldsymbol{L}^*$ of the input sequence is

$$\boldsymbol{L}^* = \arg\max_{\boldsymbol{L}} p(\boldsymbol{L}|\boldsymbol{X},\gamma^*) \tag{19}$$

## 3. Experimental method

### 3.1 Data

Five phase contrast image sequences of C3H10T1/2 mouse mesenchymal stem cell populations (American Type Culture Collection, Manassas, VA) were acquired, each containing 1000 images. The multipotent C3H10T1/2 stem cells serve as a model for the adult human mesenchymal stem cells that can differentiate into a variety of cell types. The growing environment consists of Dulbecco's Modified Eagle's Media (DMEM; Invitrogen, Carlsbad, CA), 10% fetal bovine serum (Invitrogen, Carlsbad, CA) and 1% penicillin streptomycin (PS; Invitrogen, Carlsbad, CA). The cells were observed during growth under a Zeiss Axiovert 135TV inverted microscope with a 5×, 0.15 N.A. objective and phase contrast optics. Time-lapse image acquisition was performed every 5 minutes using a 12-bit Qimaging Retiga EXi Fast 1394 CCD camera at 500ms exposure with a gain of 1.01. Each image consists of 1392×1040 pixels with a resolution of 19 $\mu$m/pixel.

### 3.2 Feature representation

From Fig.1, it is obvious that mitotic regions typically do not have rich features, and their shapes and appearances are highly irregular and flexible. To represent the feature of each frame within one mitosis sequence, we computed the GIST descriptor for each frame to formulate $\phi(\boldsymbol{x_i})$. GIST is a well-known visual feature for image classification and can represent all levels of processing, from low-level features (e.g., color, spatial frequencies) to intermediate image properties (e.g., surface, volume) and high-level information (e.g., objects, activation of semantic knowledge) (Oliva & Torralba, 2001). The superiorities of GIST for mitotic region description lie in three aspects: 1) GIST representation can bypass the segmentation of individual objects. Precise cell region segmentation in phase contrast microscopy is a notoriously difficult problem due to the phenomena of halo or shade-off. Consequently, shape features, like Histogram of Oriented Gradients (Dalal & Triggs, 2005) and Shape Context (Belongie et al., 2002), are usually not satisfactory descriptors for this task. Comparatively, the computation of GIST only uses spectral and coarsely localized information and therefore formulates a holistic representation of entire image without requirement to precisely extract edge or boundary in the image; 2) GIST is invariant to scale and rotation. Mitotic regions usually experience drastic changes in both size and orientation during mitosis progression. GIST physically represents the dominant spatial structure of an image including a set of perceptual dimensions, naturalness, openness, roughness, expansion, and ruggedness. Therefore GIST is a robust descriptor for mitotic regions; 3) GIST is a compact descriptor. GIST can be formulated from localized energy spectrum (spectrogram) with both intensity and local structure information. Due to the high dimension and redundancy of spectrogram, dimensionality reduction of Karhunen-Loeve Transform (KLT) is implemented on it to formulate a compact representation.

### 3.3 Experiments

***(a)Mitosis Identification***: The proposed model-based microscopy image preconditioning and sequence segmentation methods are implemented on the original image sequences to extract mitotic candidate sequences. Then, an HCRF classifier is learned with manually labeled mitotic and non-mitotic candidate sequences by the previous step for mitosis identification. In HCRF model, we can incorporate long range dependencies controlled by a sequence window length $w$ which defines the amount of past and future observations to be used when predicting the state at time t ($w = 0$ indicates only the current observation is used). To select the best window size $w$, we tuned this parameter and trained the corresponding HCRF classifiers to compare their performances with Area Under Curve (AUC) of ROC curve. After obtaining the best window size, we randomly selected one image sequence as training set and tested on the other four image sequences. Four different outcomes of the mitosis identification algorithm are examined: 1) true positive (TP): the identified sequence contains one mitosis event; 2) false positive (FP): the identified sequence does not contain any mitosis event; 3) true negative (TN): the discarded sequence does not contain any mitosis event; 4) false negative (FN): the discarded sequence contains mitosis events. Then, Precision (the ratio of TP to TP+FP) and recall (the ratio of TP to TP+FN), and the F1 score (a harmonic mean of precision and recall) are used as quantitative metrics for measuring the accuracy of mitosis identification. To evaluate the performance of the proposed method, it is quantitatively compared with two different methods: 1) to show the superiority of HCRF for sequence classification, it is compare to CRF model (Liang et al., 2007) which can not discover the latent structure of the entire sequence for classification; 2) to validate the advantage of integrating temporal information, it is also compared to a frame-by-frame classification approach using a support vector machine (SVM) classifier as we did previously (Liu et al., 2010b).

***(b)Mitosis Localization***: With the identified mitosis sequences, we manually annotate the three states, before mitosis, during mitosis, and after mitosis, with label 1, 2, and 3 correspondingly. Then, a CRF classifier is trained for mitosis localization. In CRF model, we can also incorporate long range dependencies with a sequence window length $w'$ which defines the amount of past and future observations to be used when predicting the state at time t. To select the best window size $w'$, we tuned this parameter and trained the corresponding CRF classifiers to compare their performances with Area Under Curve of ROC curve. After getting the best window size, we selected the same training set for model learning and tested on the other four image sequences. To evaluate the accuracy of mitosis localization, we calculated the mean and standard deviation (SD) of the timing error of the start and end of the state of during mitosis. The timing error is defined as the absolute difference of the first/last frame with label 2 by the proposed method against the manually-labeled ground truth.

## 4. Experimental results

### 4.1 Mitosis identification

With preconditioning and volumetric region growing, we extracted candidate mitosis sequences in each input sequence. This step achieved 100% recall with relatively low precision around 42%. To improve precision, we trained HCRF models with GIST features to refine the identification results. To optimize the performance of HCRF model, 4 HCRF classifiers were learned by varying window size from 0 to 3. From Fig.5, the optimal window size can be set with 2 (AUC=0.929) by plotting the ROC curve of each model and comparing the AUC values.

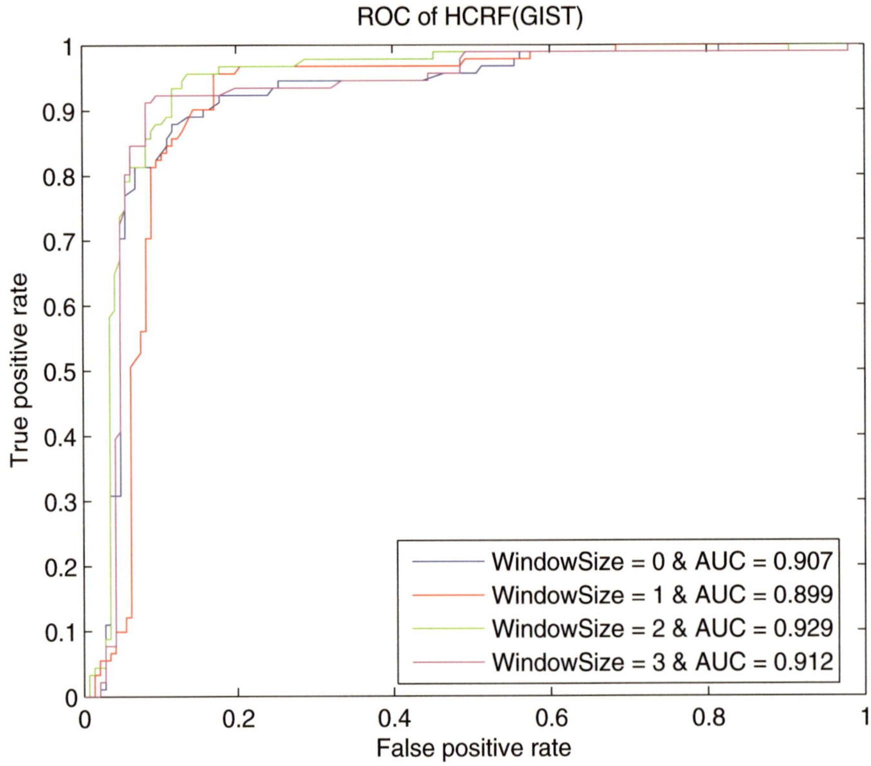


Fig. 5. ROC curves of HCRF models with different sequence window sizes from 0 to 3.

Thereafter, the HCRF classifier was trained with GIST feature and window size 2 on the training set. The ROC curves of the test results on the four test sequences are shown in Fig.6. By choosing the threshold corresponding to the maximum F score, we identify the mitosis events in each input sequence. Fig.7 shows the four kinds of samples decided by our method. From Table 1, we can achieve an average precision of 0.83 and an average recall of o.92 with a corresponding maximum F score of 0.88.

| Sequence No. | Precision (%) | Recall (%) | *MaximumF* (%) |
|---|---|---|---|
| 1 | 85 | 95 | 90 |
| 2 | 83 | 90 | 87 |
| 3 | 79 | 94 | 86 |
| 4 | 84 | 90 | 87 |
| Average | 83 | 92 | 88 |

Table 1. Precision and recall of mitosis identification by HCRF

To demonstrate the superiority of HCRF for sequence classification, we compared its performance to the CRF model trained with fully-labeled sequences. To utilize CRF for

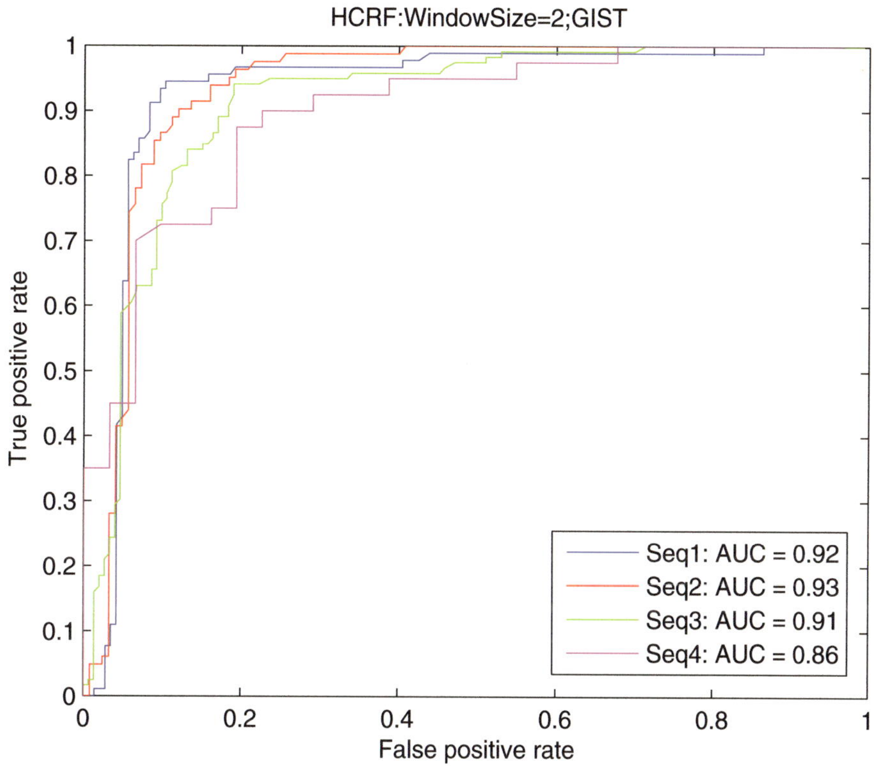


Fig. 6. ROC of HCRF with GIST feature and window size = 2

mitosis identification, it is first applied to label the full sequence. Then, a candidate sequence is classified as mitosis if the number of frames assigned with labels 2 (during mitosis) is greater than a certain threshold. By varying the threshold, we plot the ROC curves to evaluate the performance of CRF models and obtained the optimal AUC of 0.78. Moreover, to show the advantage of integrating temporal information, we compare its performance to a frame-by-frame classification approach using a support vector machine (SVM) classifier. We implemented a mitotic cell detector using SVM with a radial basis function (RBF) kernel. The best parameters for the SVM models were selected by cross validation. The detector was applied independently to each frame of a candidate sequence. Different from the training strategy of CRF, we labeled the frames during mitosis as positive samples, and the other frames as negative samples. A candidate sequence is classified as mitosis if the number of frames assigned to be mitotic exceeds a certain threshold. By varying the threshold, we plot the ROC curves to evaluate the performance of SVM models and obtained the optimal AUC of 0.77.

To compare the overall classification performances of HCRF, CRF and SVM trained with GIST features, we utilize the balanced F score as a complementary metric to AUC. We separately computed the AUC and the best achievable F score of each sequence with each classifier. From Table.2, the results indicate that the HCRF classifier consistently outperformed both CRF and

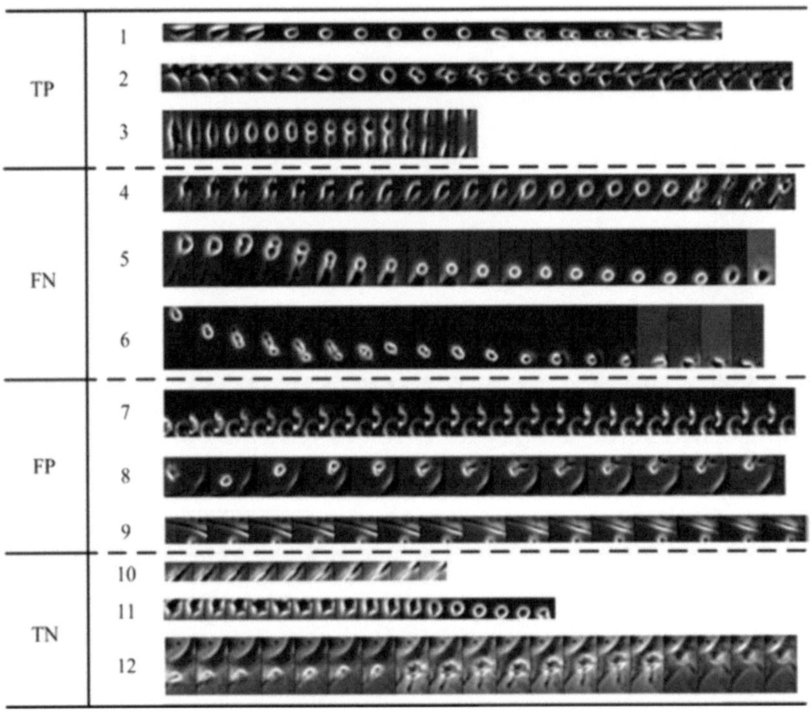


Fig. 7. Mitosis identification results by HCRF.

SVM, with a best-case performance of 92% AUC and 90% maximum F score when precision and recall are 85% and 95% respectively.

| Sequence No. | AUC (%) | | | Maximum F (%) | | |
|---|---|---|---|---|---|---|
| | HCRF | CRF | SVM | HCRF | CRF | SVM |
| 1 | 92 | 78 | 77 | 90 | 84 | 80 |
| 2 | 93 | 73 | 71 | 87 | 83 | 77 |
| 3 | 91 | 73 | 70 | 86 | 84 | 81 |
| 4 | 86 | 62 | 55 | 87 | 75 | 80 |

Table 2. Comparison between HCRF, CRF and SVM

#### 4.2 Mitosis localization

To localize the starting and ending points of mitosis events, we used CRF to label each frame of the identified mitosis candidates by HCRF. To optimize the performance of CRF model, 4 CRF classifiers were learned by varying window size from 0 to 3. From Fig.8, the results showed that the model trained with GIST features and window size 1 outperformed the others with the best AUC value of 0.933.

The CRF classifier was trained with GIST feature and window size 1 on the training set. The ROC curves of the test results on the four test sequences are shown in Fig.9. By choosing the

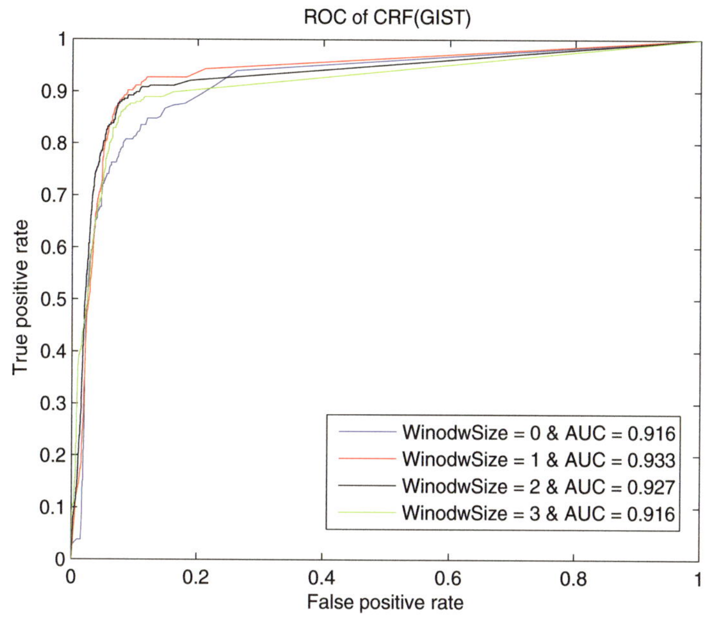


Fig. 8. ROC curve of CRF models with different sequence window lengths from 0 to 3.

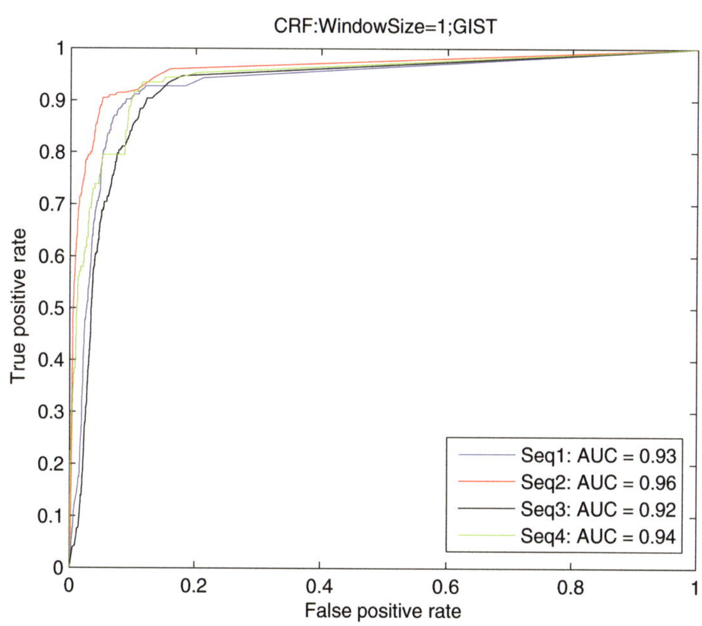


Fig. 9. ROC of CRF with GIST feature and window size = 1.

threshold corresponding to the maximum F score, we located the starting and ending points in each input sequence as shown in Fig.10. The experimental result shows that the proposed method can achieve an average localization error of $1.35 \pm 1.46$ frames for the start of mitosis

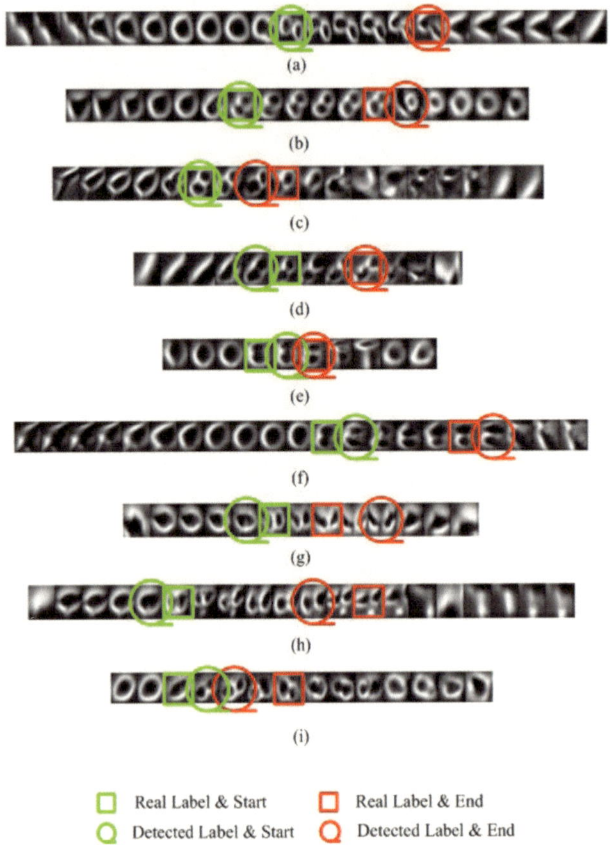


Fig. 10. Mitosis localization results by CRF. (a) Both starting and ending points are labeled correctly; (b-c) The starting point is labeled correctly while the ending point is labeled wrongly; (d-e) The starting point is labeled wrongly while the ending point is labeled correctly; (f-i) Four cases of locating both starting and ending points wrongly.

event and $1.68 \pm 1.73$ frames for the end of mitosis event. From Fig.10, it is understandable that the start point can usually be localized more precisely than the end point because the appearances and shapes of mitotic cells always change drastically when two daughter cells separate with each other physically.

## 5. Conclusion

We propose a hierarchical framework of mitosis event detection for cell populations imaged with time-lapse phase contrast microscopy. The method consists of three stages: mitosis candidate extraction, mitosis identification, and mitosis localization, which jointly optimize recall and precision for mitosis identification and minimize the mean error and standard deviation of mitosis location. The proposed detection method achieved two kinds of excellent results in very challenging image sequences of multipolar-shaped C3H10T1/2 mesenchymal stem cells. For mitosis identification, we can achieve an average precision of 0.83 and a recall of o.92 with a corresponding maximum F score of 0.88. For mitosis location, the proposed method can achieve an average localization error of $1.35 \pm 1.46$ frames for the start of mitosis event and $1.68 \pm 1.73$ frames for the end of mitosis event. Moreover, the proposed method does not depend on empirical parameters, *ad hoc* image processing, or cell tracking and consequently can be straightforwardly adapted to different cell types.

## 6. Acknowledgement

We would like to thank Prof. Takeo Kanade, Dr. Phil G. Campbell, Dr. Lee E. Weiss, Dr. Mei Chen, Dr. Eric D. Miller, Dai Fei Elmer Ker, Dr. Sung Eun Eom, Dr. Zhaozheng Yin, Jiyan Pan, and Ryoma Bise for their helpful discussions. This work was supported in part by the National Natural Science Foundation of China (61100124, 21106095), Tianjin Research Program of Application Foundation and Advanced Technology (10JCYBJC25500), China Postdoctoral Science Foundation (2011M500512), 2010/2011 Innovation Foundation of Tianjin University.

## 7. References

Al-Kofahi, O., Radke, R., Goderie, S., Shen, Q., Temple, S. & Roysam, B. (2006). Automated cell lineage construction: A rapid method to analyze clonal development established with murine neural progenitor cells, *Cell Cycle* 5(3): 327–335.

Avriel, M. (2003). *Nonlinear Programming: Analysis and Methods*, Dover Publishing.

Belongie, S., Malik, J. & Puzicha, J. (2002). Shape matching and object recognition using shape contexts, *IEEE Trans. Pattern Anal. Mach. Intell.* pp. 509–522.

Bise, R., Li, K., Eom, S. & Kanade, T. (2009). Reliably tracking partially overlapping neural stem cells in dic microscopy image sequences, *MICCAI Workshop on Optical Tissue Image Analysis in Microscopy Histopathology and Endoscopy*, Vol. 12, pp. 67–77.

Dalal, N. & Triggs, B. (2005). Histograms of oriented gradients for human detection, *Proc. 2005 IEEE Int. Conf. Computer Vision and Pattern Recognition (CVPR05)*, pp. 886–893.

Debeir, O., Ham, P. V., Kiss, R. & Decaestecker, C. (2005). Tracking of migrating cells under phase-contrast video microscopy with combined mean-shift processes, *IEEE Trans. Med. Imag.* 24: 697–711.

Donoho, D. L. (2004). For most large underdetermined systems of linear equations the minimal l1-norm solution is also the sparsest solution, *Comm. Pure Appl. Math* 59: 1848–1853.

Eccles, B. A. & Klevecz, R. R. (1986). Automatic digital image analysis for identification of mitotic cells in synchronous mammalian cell cultures, *Anal. Quant. Cytol. Histol.* 8: 138–147.

Gallardo, G., Yang, F., Ianzini, F., Mackey, M. & Sonka, M. (2004). Mitotic cell recognition with hidden Markov models, *Proc. SPIE: Medical Imaging*, Vol. 5367, pp. 661–668.

Gunawardana, A., Mahajan, M., Acero, A. & Platt, J. C. (2005). Hidden conditional random fields for phone classification, *Proc. Int. Conf. Speech Communication and Technology*, pp. 1117–1120.

Lafferty, J. D., McCallum, A. & Pereira, F. C. N. (2001). Conditional random fields: Probabilistic models for segmenting and labeling sequence data., *ICML'01*, pp. 282–289.

Li, K. (2009). *Large-Scale Stem Cell Population Tracking in Phase Contrast and DIC Microscopy Image Sequences*, PhD thesis, Carnegie Mellon University, 5000 Forbes Avenue, Pittsburgh, PA.

Li, K. & Kanade, T. (2009). Nonnegative mixed-norm preconditioning for microscopy image segmentation, *Proc. Int. Conf. Information Processing in Med. Imaging*, pp. 362–373.

Li, K., Kanade, T., Chen, M., Miller, E. D.and Weiss, L. E. & Campbell, P. G. (2008). Computer vision tracking of stemness, *Proc. IEEE Int. Symp. Biomed. Imaging*, pp. 847 – 850.

Li, K., Miller, E., Chen, M., Kanade, T., Weiss, L. & Campbell, P. (2008). Cell population tracking and lineage construction with spatiotemporal context, *Med. Image Anal.* 12(5): 546–566.

Liang, L., Zhou, X., Li, F., Wong, S., Huckins, J. & King, R. (2007). Mitosis cell identification with conditional random fields, *Proc. Life Sci. Sys. App. Workshop*, pp. 9–12.

Liu, A., Li, K. & Kanade, T. (2010a). Mitosis sequence detection using hidden conditional random fields, *Proc. 7th IEEE International Symposium on Biomedical Imaging: From Nano to Macro*, pp. 580–583.

Liu, A., Li, K. & Kanade, T. (2010b). Spatiotemporal mitosis event detection in time-lapse phase contrast microscopy image sequences, *2010 IEEE International Conference on Multimedia and Expo (ICME10)*, pp. 161–166.

Oliva, A. & Torralba, A. (2001). Modeling the shape of the scene: A holistic representation of the spatial envelope, *Int. J. Comput. Vision.* pp. 145–175.

Otsu, N. (1979). A threshold selection method from gray level histograms, *IEEE Trans. Syst., Man, Cybern.* 9: 62–66.

Quattoni, A., Wang, S., Morency, L.-P., Collins, M. & Darrell, T. (2007). Hidden conditional random fields, *IEEE Trans. Pat. Anal. Mach. Intel.* 29(10): 1848–1852.

Rabiner, L. R. (1989). A tutorial on hidden markov models and selected applications in speech recognition, *Proceedings of the IEEE*, Vol. 77, pp. 257–286.

Rosin, P. L. (2001). Unimodal thresholding, *Patt. Recog.* 34(11): 2083–2096.

Silvela, J. & Portillo, J. (2001). Breadth-first search and its application to image processing problems, *IEEE. T. Image. Process.* 10(8): 1194–1199.

Tikhonov, A.-I. N. (1977). *Solutions of Ill Posed Problems (Scripta Series in Mathematics)*, Vh Winston.

Wang, S. B., Quattoni, A., Demirdjian, M. D. & Darrell, T. (2006). Hidden conditional random fields for gesture recognition, *Proc. 2006 IEEE Int. Conf. Computer Vision and Pattern Recognition*, pp. 1521–1527.

Yin, Z., Li, K., Kanade, T. & Chen, M. (2010). Understanding the optics to aid microscopy image segmentation., *Proc. International Conference on Medical Image Computing and Computer Assisted Intervention (MICCAI10)*, pp. 209–217.

18

# Safety of Interactive Image-Guided Surgery

Alain Beaulieu
*Royal Military College of Canada*
*Canada*

## 1. Introduction

In this chapter, we discuss Interactive Image-Guided Surgery (IIGS) and present the current state of the art in the analysis and evaluation of this kind of computer-supported medical procedure. We also present the results of our research to evaluate the safety of IIGS. During our discussion of the current state of the art, we review the various approaches that have been proposed to analyze and evaluate IIGS systems including their strengths and weaknesses.

The original hypothesis that initiated our research was that: "it is possible to improve the safety analysis of computer-guided surgery if we model this kind of system as a process control model." The hypothesis was first elaborated in an initial research planning meeting while we were investigating a better way of developing a Verification and Validation method for IIGS. During the evolution of this research, this hypothesis has evolved significantly from a basic idea into a modelling language and a protocol that have been evaluated using a particular set of IIGS systems used for orthopedic surgery.

## 2. Using medical imaging for surgery

For many decades, medical imaging has been rapidly evolving as one of the most useful applications of scientific and engineering knowledge to improve the quality of health care. Medical imaging provides technology that enables physicians to see subcutaneous structures and tissues without the use of more invasive procedures[1].

The use of medical imaging increases the observability of areas of interest inside the patient. Increased observability allows for more complete diagnosis and better planning of surgical procedures leading to potential improvements in surgical outcome. The first use of medical imaging with clinical intent can be traced back to January 1896 in Birmingham, United Kingdom where an x-ray was used to plan the removal of a needle from a woman's hand Viergever (1998). Medical imaging for clinical procedures has therefore been around for over 100 years. The first use of medical images was static, but it demonstrated the usefulness of medical imaging in planning surgeries. Medical imaging progressed over the next 100 years with improvements in the quality of existing modalities and image processing, as

[1] The debate on the degree of invasiveness of ionizing and non-ionizing radiation is ongoing. Although it is clear that their side effects cannot be overlooked *Assessment and Management of Cancer Risks from Radiological and Chemical Hazards* (1998); on Radiological Protection (1960-Present); Profio (1979); Tenforde (1979), medical imaging is far less invasive and risky than open exploratory surgery Hindus (2001).

well as the addition of new imaging modalities. In today's medical imaging, there are numerous modalities that can be used in complementary fashion to improve diagnosis. Some of these modalities include: X-Ray, CAT[2], Magnetic Resonance Imagery (MRI), Single Photon Emission Computed Tomography (SPECT)[3], Positron Emission Tomography (PET), ultrasound and several other specialized forms of imaging Mösges & Lavallée (1996).

In recent years, it has been possible to acquire intraoperative volumetric data with the use of mobile medical imaging (CT, MRI and ultrasound). Mobility of 3-Dimensional medical imaging in the operating room has allowed surgeons to track surgical instruments through tissues in real-time during the surgery, leading to less invasive procedures or Minimally Invasive Surgery (MIS) Patel et al. (1998); van der Weide et al. (1998); Viergever (1998).

The benefits of MIS are significant. Although no single reference could be found that provided a comprehensive list of the potential benefits of MIS, several authors refer to such benefits to highlight the relevance of their work Choi et al. (2000); Gary et al. (2006); Hindus (2001); Mösges & Lavallée (1996); Patel et al. (1998); Peters (2001); Pieper et al. (1994); Robb (1996); van der Weide et al. (1998); Viergever (1998); Zamorano et al. (1994).

During the last decade, increased ability to process computer graphics and images in real-time has made possible the intraoperative use of 3-D computer models obtained from segmentation and volume rendering of preoperative imaging from CAT, MRI and ultrasound Viergever (1998). Without volumetric data, the surgeon would have to form his/her own mental model from imaging slices.

## 3. Interactive image-guided surgery

### 3.1 General

This section covers the general principles of orthopedic IIGS. We present the processes and methods involved in IIGS; the intent is to provide an overview and to illustrate the complexity of such systems. IIGS can be represented as a pipeline of operations which can be separated into six distinct phases as displayed in Figure 1. The parts of the process are defined as follows:

1. *Image Capture* - Preoperative images of the region of interest in the patient are acquired. The images of interest are represented by a set of CAT slices or a scene[4].
2. *Visualization* - Various complex operations are applied to images to extract information. Visualization has also been called rendering or more loosely refered to as image processing.
3. *Surgery Planning* - Preoperative planning of the surgery is conducted using the scenes from visualization that have been generated by the IIGS system. The planning phase can also include rehearsal of operations on some guidance systems. Training can also be included as a requirement.
4. *Registration* - In the operating theatre, the visualized images are registered to the patient to align the reference systems.

[2] Also known as Computed Axial Tomography or CT
[3] AKA tomoscintigraph
[4] A scene is a constructed 3-D image from a region of interest in the patient.

5. *Intraoperative Guidance* - During surgery, the position of surgical instruments is tracked and displayed superimposed on the preoperative visualized images, allowing the surgeon to accurately navigate through the area of interest in the patient.
6. *Postoperative Followup* - After surgery, the surgeon may want to confirm surgical outcome using the surgery planning information.

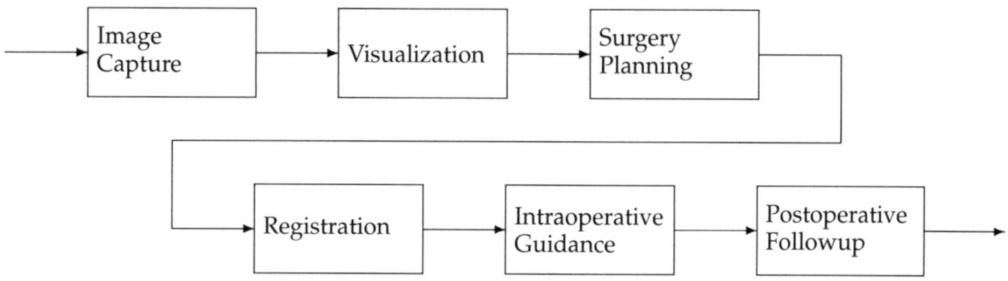


Fig. 1. The IIGS Pipeline

The above phases have also been presented in the literature as models containing three or four phases Breeuwer et al. (1998); Gauldie (2002). A three phase model could be composed of preoperative (phases 1-3 above), intraoperative (phases 4-5) and postoperative (phase 6). Regardless of the separation of phases or actual requirement of the system, the system follows this linear progression of operations. Below, we address the six phases of IIGS. Planning and post operative followup phases can be represented as single processes and depend in large measure on information generated during the other four phases. These two phases are highly dependent on competent human intervention derived from medical knowledge.

### 3.2 Image capture

The imaging modality depends on the procedure to be performed and the target area to be imaged. Apart from the physics of the modality, it is important to note that for a given modality, various health facilities will have different machines each with its own pixel resolution, slice thickness and storage format. The increased need to communicate medical images over networks and between machines has pushed the adoption of medical imaging standards such as Digital Imaging and Communication in Medicine-3 (DICOM-3). This standard only supports sets of 2-D slices and not volume models Starreveld et al. (2001). Further processing of the images as described in the following section depend on the ability of the algorithms to adapt to the parameters of various CAT scan machines and format of images that come from other systems.

Image capture can be preceded by the surgical implantation of fiducial markers if fiducial registration is to be performed. Physical markers such as these are made visible on medical images by selecting appropriate material for the markers.

### 3.3 Visualization

Prior to intraoperative mobile 3-D medical imaging and IIGS, the surgeon had a series of 2-D slices that he/she used to form a mental 3-D model. Visualization (sometimes referred to as rendering[5]) deals with the display of 3-D information on a 2-D matrix of pixels (computer screen). Using computer graphics methods and today's technology, this 3-D visualization can be built from the 2-D slices obtained from medical imaging modalities. Constructing a 3-D model is a complex process that is best viewed as a pipe-and-filter architecture for image transformations. This view is useful since the selection and ordering of various operations will determine the characteristics and quality of the visualization.

Several image processing operations can be applied to medical images including: filtering, segmentation, classification, interpolation, quantification and image rendering. There is a great number of algorithms and techniques described in the literature for each of these operations. Most techniques require interactive or manual assistance from an expert in 3-D image processing, but recently, automated algorithms are starting to appear in the literature Radau et al. (2000); Udupi et al. (2001); Zoroofi et al. (2001). One of the most helpful references in the domain of visualization is a survey paper on 3-D rendering in medicine by Jayaram K. Udupa Udupa (2001). In trying to create a concise survey of the operations used in visualization, we found that there is no consensus on terminology or clean interfaces between various operations. For example filtering and classification are often included as part of segmentation. We consider each operation as a step in visualization. The operations are presented in the following subsections.

Images on computer screens are represented by a set of pixels. Likewise, medical images produced from modalities like CAT are formed from matrices of pixels of various intensities identifying different tissues. Pixels and voxels are sometimes used synonymously in the literature. In 3-D visualization, it makes more sense to talk about voxels, the 3-D equivalent of a 2-D pixel Hindus (2001); Udupa (2001). This mixup in terminology can be explained when we consider that a 2-D slice has a thickness that is determined by the beam width of the CAT machine.

### 3.3.1 Filtering

Filtering is an operation that takes a scene and changes the intensity[6] of its voxels to reduce noise, distortion and other artifacts that have not been eliminated by the imaging machine. Filtering smoothes the edges of structures to provide clearer and crisper images. Filtering can either be linear or optimal Ayache et al. (1996).

There are two approaches to linear filtering: gradient or Laplacian. Both approaches assume a white Gaussian noise. If the noise does not have zero mean or there are a lot of irregularities in structures, linear filtering may require large convolution masks as well as complex algorithms. Because medical images are very large, the computational requirements of complex algorithms are very high.

Another less computation intensive approach for noisy images is optimal filtering. Canny, Deriche and Shen have proposed such filters Ayache et al. (1996).

[5] Visualization and rendering are often used interchangeably in the literature, but they are not synonymous. Visualization represents the entire process of image transforms where rendering is its last step of displaying the image.

[6] Depending on the modality of imaging, and the author, intensity is sometimes replaced by density. This is especially true for scenes that have vector-valued voxel intensity such as obtained with MRI.

### 3.3.2 Segmentation

Segmentation is crucial for the identification and extraction of information and structures from a given scene. For orthopaedic surgery the structures consist of bones, ligaments, cartilage and tendons. The ability to accurately locate structures in the body for planning and intraoperative tracking is directly linked to surgical outcome Ayache et al. (1996); Dean et al. (1998); Udupa (2001).

There are two main classes of approaches for segmentation: region-based segmentation which includes a set of voxels describing a sub-scene and boundary-based segmentation that outputs a set of voxels or geometric information from voxels (polygons) about the boundary of the object Udupa (2001).

Another way to characterize segmentation algorithms is in the way set membership is decided for voxels. In a hard segmentation, also called binary segmentation, set membership is either 0 or 1. Gray or fuzzy segmentation uses voxel intensity to decide the degree of belonging to the set with real values ranging between 0 and 1. Some methods, such as thresholding and clustering, use either binary or gray segmentation Udupa & Gonçalves (1996).

Region-based methods can be divided in two different groups: clustering and region-growing. Clustering uses voxel features to define each set in a scene. The simplest clustering method is thresholding. Region-growing, as the name indicates, grows sets of voxels based on homogeneity properties. These methods grow regions of interest from seed points by considering neighboring voxels for inclusion.

There is a great number of boundary-based (edge detection) methods described in the literature. Only a few are mentioned here. Filtering is often used as a first step in the process of edge detection. The following are examples of boundary based methods:

1. Simple thresholding and hysteresis-thresholding can be used to find contours. The problem with these simple methods is that there are many discontinuities between edges in the contour Ayache et al. (1996). These contours can be closed by domain experts who have knowledge of anatomy.
2. Active contours also called snakes, have been successfully used to solve the 2-D contour problem. In order to use these algorithms in a 3-D environment, one must find a 3-D generalization of the energy defining the border of an object. The user defines an initial contour and the algorithm optimizes this contour based on a balance between inside and outside energies.
3. Isosurface methods track the surfaces of structures through the assumption that the boundary of an object in a scene has a constant density. One such algorithm is Lorensen's marching cubes Lorensen & Cline (1987), which has been adapted for one of Queen's University IIGS systems. The marching cubes method constructs the surface of each structure by finding, for each voxel, the local direction of an isosurface through it.

From a validation perspective, it is important to note that not only are the results from boundary-based methods highly dependent on the algorithm but also on the skills of the user.

### 3.3.3 Classification

Classification is basically a problem of creating an opacity scene from a density scene Udupa & Gonçalves (1996). Classification deals with connecting like-pixels with the use of a luminescence histogram Ayache et al. (1996). Objects are defined by their belonging to a range of luminescence. Classification and segmentation are two different operations but gray segmentation is synonymous with classification Udupa & Gonçalves (1996).

### 3.3.4 Interpolation

In order to facilitate the processing of information and to complete the 3-D representation from slices, it may be necessary to combine or split voxels through interpolation. The preferred shape for a voxel in most algorithms is a cube. Because slice spacing (z-dimension) is 2-8 times greater than the voxel size in the x or y dimension, we want to fill the gap with fictitious voxels based on interpolated density information from neighboring voxels. If the slices overlap, some voxels may need to be split, again requiring interpolation. The result will provide an isotropic 3-D representation.

### 3.3.5 Rendering

Rendering is the last process in the visualization pipeline. As such the image that is rendered depends on several operations, as well as the sequencing of these operations. There are two kinds of rendering: surface and volume.

Surface rendering for which density has either value [0,1] portrays the boundary surface of a structure. Surface rendering can be displayed as a set of polygons obtained from segmentation. Each polygon has its own intensity level that is calculated based on the orientation of the surface with respect to the screen. This gives the impression of depth to the structures. Surface rendering can also be portrayed through volume rendering techniques but the opacity of the surface voxels will hide the elements behind them.

Volume rendering for which density has a real value in the interval [0..1] portrays a translucent structure through two distinct operations: projection and pixel intensity calculations. The projection can be done with either direct projection of object polygons or with ray casting. Pixel intensity calculations can be done in several ways, depending on the determination of normal vectors to the object surface. The quality of the rendition is highly dependant on the estimation of the normal vectors Udupa & Gonçalves (1996).

### 3.3.6 Safety implications of visualization

As we can observe by the number of transformations described above, visualization, can be the source of some significant accuracy errors in IIGS. Each of the transformations is a single point of failure and has cumulative effects on the next set of transformations. The results from visualization are fed to the subsequent phases. Hazards created by failures in the transformations will propagate to these phases.

As we have found during our research, tests with phantoms and computer code inspections of algorithms represent the two main mitigation strategies.

### 3.4 Surgery planning

As indicated above, surgery planning can be reduced to a single process that is highly dependent on information provided by the previous phases of IIGS. During this phase, the surgeon uses a part of the IIGS system to perform a simulated surgery where s/he can make changes to the virtual or visualized skeletal structure of the patient. The planning tool can provide the surgeon with a variety of options to visualize corrections. Depending on the tool, the surgeon can change the amount of correction applied to the bone structure, choose and change prosthesis size, view post simulated surgery results. More complex planning tools may allow the surgeon to obtain technical measurements and even view dynamic models after a correction.

### 3.5 Registration

Registration is the process of aligning coordinate systems so that we can match geometric data. Registration is also called co-registration, matching and fusion Taylor et al. (1996). Registration is done between coordinate systems of various modalities such as the registration of CAT and MRI 3-D models, and/or between imaging data and patient. Registration is critical to IIGS because it is directly linked to the execution of a preoperative plan through intraoperative navigation.

There are several approaches to registration. We describe three of them here, namely: fiducial markers, anatomical landmarks and surface based methods. Other methods are described in Gauldie (2002); Lavallé (1996). In the selection of a registration technique, there is a tradeoff between accuracy and invasiveness.

Fiducial markers are small posts that are surgically secured to bone tissue prior to imaging. Markers are chosen to be visible for the particular medical imaging modality. Immediately prior to surgery, registration is performed by touching each marker with a tracked probe. This procedure is the gold standard for registration because it minimizes errors in transformation. This procedure is, however more invasive than other methods Birkfellner et al. (1998); Starreveld et al. (2001).

Anatomical landmarks are an option for registration when it is desired to eliminate the extra surgical procedure needed by fiducial methods. The problem is to find a set of distinctive and unambiguous points that can be registered reliably. Depending on the procedure, the surgeon may only expose surfaces that are devoid of such features rendering this method difficult to use.

Surface-based registration is accomplished by acquiring points from the surface to be registered. These points form a description of the surface that must be matched to the 3-D model. The most prevalent method for acquiring these points is by touching the exposed surface of the bone at several locations with a tracked probe. The problem with this type of point collection is that the surgeon will expose as little bone as possible. Recently, A-Mode ultrasound has been used to perform transcutaneous surface registration at Queen's University Gauldie (2002). A-Mode ultrasound has also been used to perform anatomy-based registration for the spine Lavallé et al. (1996), but the point gathering method and the matching technique used by the authors resemble that of surface-based registration.

After the points are matched, the registration algorithm tries to find the best transformation that will best align the coordinate systems. For bones, a rigid-body transformation ($\overrightarrow{F}(x)$) consisting of a 3 by 1 translation vector $\overrightarrow{T}$ and a 3 by 3 rotation matrix $\overrightarrow{R}$ is sufficient because the deformations of images are negligible Lavallé (1996). The transformation therefore has the form:

$$\overrightarrow{F}(x) = \overrightarrow{R}x + \overrightarrow{T} \tag{1}$$

Registration must be accurate in order to maximize surgical outcome. From the many papers on the topic, it is generally accepted that registration accuracy of less than 1 mm and 0.5 degrees is surgically acceptable. No paper could be found in the literature that provided empirical justification for the acceptability of these limits on surgical accuracy. Some papers also talk about sub-pixel accuracy for localization. This provides a vague requirement, since pixels vary in size and geometry depending on the imaging machine and the settings.

### 3.6 Intraoperative guidance

After the scenes are registered to the patient, it is possible to display digitized models of the tools as part of the visualization, to provide these scenes in real-time and provide guidance information to the surgeon. Other technical data such as numerical values of location, angles and forces can also be displayed. As an example, during a High Tibial Osteotomy (HTO) which involves the removal of a wedge of bone tissue, the position and angle of a drill used to insert guide wires into the leg can be tracked and errors displayed on the preoperative plan in real-time. Force monitoring of the drill can be ascertained by measuring the current to determine torque Mösges & Lavallée (1996).

The accurate display of surgical instrument models depends on the tracking system used. There are two basic categories of instrument tracking: articulated arms and triangulated emitters Galloway et al. (1994).

#### 3.6.1 Articulated arms

Articulated arms can resolve positions though the use of instrumented joints (potentiometers, optical encoders, or resolvers) and simple kinematics. The surgeon manipulates a surgical instrument that is attached to the end of the arm. The arm can also have other useful characteristics such as limiters that are set to respect the preoperative plan or brakes that keep the position of the instrument fixed for long periods.

Articulated arms have good accuracy but this accuracy is limited by uncertainties related to deformations, backlashes, alignment errors and the like. Articulated arm signals cannot be obscured. However, arms have other limitations: accuracy is inversely proportional to the size of the operating envelope, only one instrument can be attached to a single arm, and sterility is a problem Galloway et al. (1994).

#### 3.6.2 Triangulated emitters

Three types of triangulated emitters are discussed in the literature, each having multiple implementations.

Ultrasound time-of-flight was one of the first methods used to triangulate instruments. This technology is simple and cheap to implement. A piezoelectric emitter on the instrument is synchronized with several receivers whose locations are known precisely. Time-of-flight of an ultrasound pulse provides distances between each receiver and the transmitter. Intersection of the spheres in space at the known radii provides the location of the instrument. The two main problems with ultrasound are that the speed of sound changes depending on the temperature and the signals can be obscured by the presence of surgical staff.

Electromagnetic systems can also be used. Three emitters generate magnetic fields in orthogonal planes and the signals are captured by receivers. The main advantages of this technology are that the signals do not suffer from line-of-sight obscuration and they are not sensitive to temperature changes. It is also possible to attach such a device to an endoscope and locate the end position of these instruments inside the body. The main problems with this technology are the susceptibility to metallic objects in the operating theater as well as electromagnetic interference from other electrical equipment Galloway et al. (1994).

Passive and active optical tracking can also be used for triangulation. Queen's University uses an active system composed of Charge-Coupled Detector (CCD) cameras in a linear arrangement and a series of Infrared Light Emitting Diode (IRED) mounted on surgical instruments. The IRED's on each instruments are mounted at specific locations and are sequentially pulsed at time-specific intervals. The position of an IRED can be located in less than 300 microseconds. This technology does however suffer from line-of-sight obscuration which can be limited by careful placement of the cameras.

In terms of accuracy, the active optical tracking system is the most accurate, capable of locating instruments within +/- 0.2 mm in a volume of $(500mm)^3$ Galloway et al. (1994); Mösges & Lavallée (1996).

### 3.7 Postoperative followup

After the surgery the patient will be evaluated to determine surgical outcome and general well-being. Some of the postoperative assessments will be done without the use of the IIGS systems, using physician evaluations and/or patient questionnaires. Some evaluations will make use of a subset of the IIGS system such as the Medical Imaging and Visualization to compare preoperative and postoperative results. It can also be useful to compare the plan to the actual result. Such postoperative followups should be undertaken with care considering the additional radiation that the patient has to be subjected to.

### 3.8 Failures in IIGS systems

It is important to identify what is meant by a failure within the scope of Integrated Image-Guided Surgery. Apart from the obvious hardware and software failures that can cause a system to crash or malfunction, we must consider errors that may affect surgical outcome. A concept that is advanced by Schneider and Hines, is that of *patient vulnerability from data*[7] provided by medical software Schneider & Hines (1990). In their paper Schneider and Hines define patient safety as *"freedom from harm by a medical device"*, while patient vulnerability

[7] Data as discussed here includes medical imaging and models derived from volume rendering, registration and tracking information.

is defined as *"potential harm due to erroneous system output"*. During orthopaedic surgery involving IIGS, the decisions made by the surgeon depend in large measure on the IIGS system[8]. Vulnerabilities in IIGS therefore come from the data that is provided in the form of rendered images, real-time display of surgical instruments within the model and numerical information. As indicated by Fitzpatrick, the knowledge of accuracy is as important as the accuracy itself Fitzpatrick et al. (1998) both of which are crucial to managing patient vulnerability. Since geometric accuracy is linked with surgical outcome and the skeletal structure of the body is modified from this information, any errors in accuracy that can have an impact on patient vulnerability are potential hazards. Failures must be identified based on the severity and likelihood of hazards. Another problem of introducing complex medical devices is that the surgeon does not know the level of confidence he can have Fitzpatrick et al. (1998).

### 3.9 IIGS conclusion

Interactive Image-Guided Surgery includes a complex set of process and interfaces which have traditionally been represented as a pipeline of operations. The image processing portion of the system can be represented with a pipe-and-filter software architecture. We argue that although this representation is excellent to illustrate an introductory discussion to IIGS, it is not sufficient to perform a safety analysis on IIGS. Throughout the discussion of the various phases of IIGS, there are many interfaces, equipment and interactions that are not visible in the pipeline architecture of the system. For example, the quality of the visualization depends on the selection of the operations applied to the medical images, the algorithm used to implement each operation, the ordering of the operations in the pipe-and-filter architecture and the skills of the operator performing the image transformations.

The potential sources of errors from devices, processes and interfaces vary widely in range, which can affect the quality of visualization, planning, registration, guidance and ultimately the surgical outcome. As well, we must identify unwanted disturbances and noise that interfere with the ideal operation of the IIGS system. In order to increase the completeness of the safety analysis, we must first identify and expose all system interfaces.

## 4. State of the art in the analysis and evaluation of IIGS systems

Before we describe our approach to safety analysis of IIGS systems, we present work that has been done in the area analysis and evaluation of these systems. The intent is to show through various approaches taken, the complexity of studying these systems from a safety perspective.

Little in the published research is directly relevant to the topic of analysis, evaluation or validation and verification of IIGS systems. The literature, however, contains many papers on spatial fidelity and accuracy of visualization, segmentation and registration algorithms. The words verification and validation are often used by these papers, but they mainly refer to mathematical and procedural accuracy verification. Accuracy and spatial fidelity are crucial to IIGS systems and it is generally accepted that they can significantly affect surgical outcome. Although necessary to the conduct of safe IIGS procedures, accuracy and spatial fidelity are, however, not synonymous with system safety. Saying that software is correct and the

[8] The surgeon also has his/her experience and coarse visual and tactile feedback to rely on.

calculations are accurate says nothing about possible omissions of safeguard requirements that could have made the system safer Gowen & Yap (1993).

Several papers have also been published on validation of user interfaces and clinical trials but none of the proposed methods or protocols are applicable or extendable to general clinical practice. We define general clinical practice as a hospital with no integral research and development department that would have knowledge of the internal design of the systems and could be called upon to operate IIGS technology.

In the following subsections we present several methods that have been used to perform some form of analysis, evaluation or validation activities for IIGS systems. At the end of each section, an evaluation of the scope, focus and aim of each method is given. The scope refers to the phase(s) that the method concentrates on: preoperative, intraoperative or postoperative. The focus localizes the area of interest or where the method is applied and can be one or more of: software, hardware, system, interfaces, patient, or surgeon. The aim identifies the goal of the method; the quality factor that is sought after: safety, reliability, usability, or effectiveness.

### 4.1 Clinical relevance

Two papers that closely address the validation of IIGS systems are from Verbeeck et al. (1995) and from Breeuwer et al. (1998). Both papers approach the validation of IIGS systems from the *clinical evaluation* perspective. Also, both papers recognize the necessity for verification of accuracy using phantoms. Breeuwer et al. also look at CAT and MRI image distortion and the impact of registration errors as part of their validation efforts.

In their paper, Verbeeck et al. establish some strong arguments for setting up a Clinical Relevance validation that in effect justifies or rejects the requirement for the system. The basic idea of Clinical Relevance validation is to use a set of questionnaires that ask the surgeon to evaluate the system based on a number of criteria which are rated on a three point scale. In their paper, they compare the results of an existing manual[9] method of performing stereotactic brain surgery and a new system for planning and guidance. The evaluation of the new IIGS system is done in two distinct phases, each phase including its own questionnaires.

The Functional Specification Phase uses prototyping and a functional specification questionnaire containing twelve questions to refine the system. Each question in this questionnaire has a weight factor, assigned by the surgeon, that depends on the patient's need for the new system, but does not depend on the technology. A second questionnaire that does not involve the patient and deals specifically with the surgeon's interaction with the new IIGS system contains ten questions without weight factors. This questionnaire deals mainly with the usability, usefulness and robustness of the new system from the surgeon's perspective.

The Clinical Acceptability Phase includes two questionnaires. The first questionnaire contains seven questions and compares the old and new IIGS systems as well as their defined medical protocols[10]. The questions deal with the clinical information that can be obtained from each system. The questions also evaluate the degree by which any additional information requirement from the new system outweighs the necessary activities to get this information.

[9] The method is said to be manual even though a computer is used to assist in the static planning phase.

[10] Because the two systems, manual and IIGS, differ in scope and information requirements, each must have its own medical protocol for use by the surgical team.

Because the protocols differ and the information requirements are not the same for both systems, a "not available" score can be assigned to a question. Because the information needs within a protocol may vary in importance, weight factors are assigned to each question by the surgeon. The second questionnaire for this phase contains six questions and addresses the beneficial aspects of the new technology for the patient. Here the surgeon answers questions that deal with overall benefits, risk, comfort, time, and perceived accuracy of the systems.

Breeuwer et al. also use a questionnaire for assessment by the surgeons. The eight questions posed to the surgeon are on a visual analog scale scored from -5 to +5. This is similar to a Likert scale Likert (1932).

Both validations ask a question about the perceived safety from the surgeon's point of view following a procedure. Breeuwer also asks a question about the effect upon the confidence of the surgeon during the procedure.

The questionnaire method used by both research groups is an efficient instrument to evaluate a quality factor such as Clinical Relevance or to measure the confidence of the surgeon in the new technology. This, however, is not the appropriate kind of instrument to use to validate or verify system safety. Another weakness of questionnaires is that they explore known issues at the time the questionnaire was developed; safety critical systems require instruments that bring to light issues we did not think about "*a priori*". Also because of the small samples used in both studies, the issue of statistical significance is questionable. Finally, as seen from both papers, the questionnaires are quite short and contain no validating questions to ensure that answers are consistent.

Clinical relevance and effectiveness remain important aspects of introducing new technology in the operating theater and should be evaluated as part of a validation protocol. On the other hand, the use of system designers to operate the new IIGS system in the operating rooms is not the norm in clinical practice. System designers have a complete understanding of the underlying technology of the IIGS system compared to general clinical technical staff so the results obtained from clinical evaluation in a research setting may not be transferable to a general clinical setting. Clinical relevance covers the intraoperative phase and is surgeon centric. The study aims at relevance from a usability analysis perspective. Safety is mentioned but as a single indivisible global quality factor.

### 4.2 Human error analysis

A paper that describes another aspect of the state of the art in the analysis of IIGS systems is by Jiang et al. (1998). This paper is most closely related to our research. In their research, the authors perform a tailored Failure Mode Effect Analysis (FMEA) technique to study human errors in IIGS. Their research takes an approach similar to that of conventional safety analysis of safety critical systems Chudleigh et al. (1995); Fries et al. (1996); Gowen (1994); Herrmann (1995); Jones et al. (2002); Leveson (1995); Loesh et al. (1999); Mojdehbakhsh et al. (1994); Murthy (1995) but explicitly examines only the software modules.

While the technique used by Jiang et al. has a lot of merit, their approach also has significant limitations. The aim of their research is to identify surgical errors by focussing on human factors and human errors that can occur in using software. Their analysis is limited to software component failure modes and human errors that could cause each software component to fail. The authors concentrate on errors caused by the operation of the software not on systematic faults. Because the computer human interactions are part of the study, errors in interface design may be uncovered by this approach. In order to study this human interaction errors from design the study should include the design of the human machine interfaces.

There are several reasons why FMEA alone is not sufficient for this kind of analysis:

1. The underlying assumption made by the authors in only using FMEA, is that there are only single points of failure in the system. FMEA is a stovepipe analysis that does not look at module interfaces or error propagation between modules. For example, if two human errors are made, one during segmentation and one during registration, the effect of one of the errors may not be significant enough to activate a protection measure, but the accrued errors could be surgically significant and not be discovered.
2. Because the analysis only studies the failures of the software modules that are in the current system architecture, and does not look at global system safety, there is a high probability of missing a safety requirement that could be solved by adding a new module or function such as a watchdog or built-in test.
3. Errors caused by hardware malfunctions may be overlooked if not anticipated as part of the failure modes of the software modules.
4. Because the technique used by the authors focuses on mistakes and failures, they do not analyze the effects of the new medical protocol as part of the safety analysis. There is no mention of modifying surgical gestures, system interfaces, human-machine interfaces, noise, or disturbances. This is important because some procedures change with the introduction of IIGS[11].
5. System failures that are not caused by software failures or human errors may be overlooked by this approach. For example the effects of motion artifacts, deformation of tissue due to changes in patient position between the imaging and the operating room, and system latency during tracking, may be overlooked.

The analysis would be more complete if complemented with other safety analysis techniques. The authors however, look at methods of prevention and protection against software failures and human errors by applying the concepts of FMEA to software. It is the only work of its kind that could be found in the open literature for the analysis of IIGS systems. Human-error analysis is software centric and includes preoperative and intraoperative phases, an improvement on other methods presented. The method aims at increasing safety by reducing failures induced by interaction with the software.

### 4.3 Component-based trusted architecture pattern

A recent paper suggests a drastically different approach to ensure safety of IIGS. The researchers claim that by using encapsulated Moore state machines and a "*trusted architectural pattern of components*" they can guarantee safety and reliability in the system Gary et al. (2006). They base this claim on the hypothesis that "*state machines ensure that component behavior is deterministic and that all components are in a known and error-free state at any given moment.*"

[11] For example for wrist alignment surgery the old protocol was to cut, distract, drill holes; the IIGS procedure changes this order to drill holes, cut and distract.

The paper also claims that the approach can predictably integrate third-party software by bounding these untrusted components' behavior using state machine wrappers.

The approach gives little consideration to the fact that the IIGS software interacts with a physical environment. The techniques they suggest do not consider safety hazards that are not related to the software and for which software design could provide mitigation and/or removal. This does not follow sound safety design principles elaborated in countless references Chudleigh et al. (1995); Elliott et al. (1994); Fei et al. (2001); Gowen (1995); Gowen & Collofello (1994); Halang et al. (1998); Jiang et al. (1998); Jones et al. (2002); Knight (1990); Leffingwell & Norman (1993); Leveson (1995). Leveson states that "*...the quality of a safety program is measured by its ability to influence design*" Leveson (1995); this ability comes in the form of safeguard requirements that comes from a safety analysis. These safeguards would be missed if we only use the trusted architecture paradigm as proposed by the authors.

By their own admission, communication with subject matter experts such as surgeons, to confirm requirements is difficult. In their research, the authors used Unified Modeling Language (UML) activity diagrams to show the process of state transitions and the safe behavior of the software.

The approach is entirely software centric and specifically addresses only the intraoperative phase of IIGS. The Component-Based Trusted Architecture Pattern is a sound design approach that may produce reliable[12] software, not safe systems.

### 4.4 Conclusion on state-of-the-art

The analysis and evaluation of IIGS systems discussed above focuses on narrow concerns and isolated parts of larger systems. This aspect of IIGS research is indeed in its infancy. There are several reasons for this lack of maturity. The complexity of the systems makes verification and validation activities difficult to identify and perform. Due to the nature of these interactive systems, with person in the loop, validation efforts are complex and difficult to express. Our research aims to increase the expressiveness of models in the conduct of safety analysis for these systems. By increasing expressiveness of the models we will better communicate with domain experts. Our aim is also to develop a system centric focus including pre, intra and post operative phases in our modeling and safety analysis. This allows to have a more complete analysis at the system level.

## 5. Abstract process safety analysis model

In this section, we present our protocol and methods used to perform safety analysis on IIGS systems. At the core of the protocol is our diagramming technique which is part of the Abstract Process Safety Analysis Model (APSAM).

In traditional digital control theory, the controllers (computer control systems) are generally composed of five classes of components Dunn (2003). These components, illustrated in Figure 2 are:

1. The *application* (process or plant), the physical entity that the control system monitors and controls.

[12] Software is said to be reliable if it behaves according to its specification requirement with few failures.

2. The *sensors*, convert the application's measured/observed physical properties into corresponding electrical signals that will be inputs for the computer system.
3. The *effectors*, convert electrical signals from the computer's outputs to corresponding physical actions that control an application's functions.
4. The *operator* the human(s) who monitors or activates the computer system in real-time (or near real-time).
5. The *computer/controller*, composition of software and hardware, uses the sensors and the effectors to monitor and control the application.

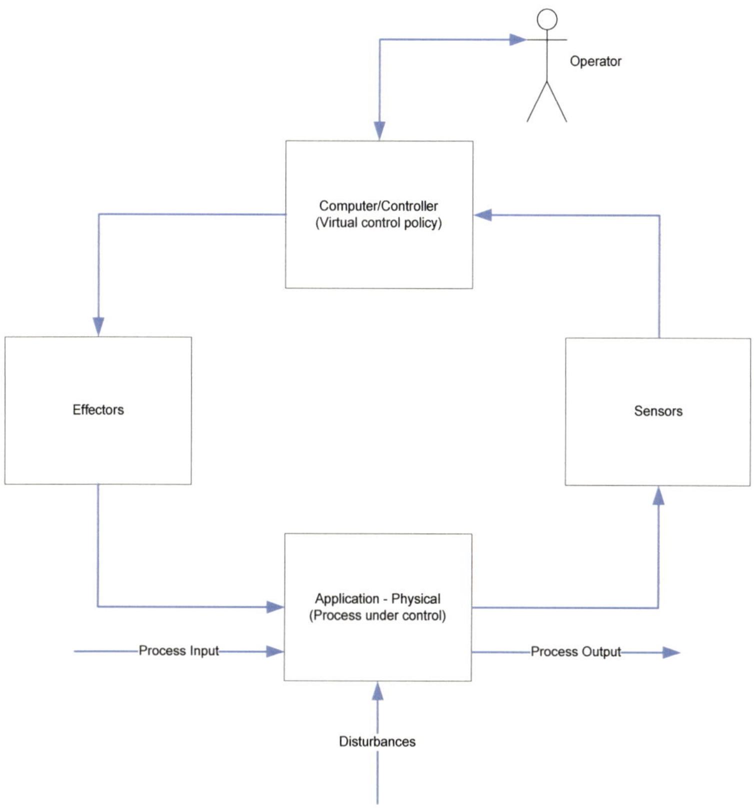


Fig. 2. Traditional Digital Control System Components

A simple control system view of the guidance phase of an IIGS system is presented in Figure 3[13]. There are several elements that make this representation different from traditional digital control theory as displayed in Figures 2. Some of the five components listed above change between the physical and virtual realms. The *controller* is external to the *computer*. The process under control (*application*) is in a virtual environment. The controlled variable is the accurate placement of surgical instruments in a human body. The surgeon, as the controller,

[13] This control system model was elaborated early in the research to represent a class of problems; it does not represent any specific system. It is presented here because it was the initial idea behind the research.

has limited observability[14] of the controlled variable in the physical domain. The observable behavior is the calculated position of surgical instrument models superimposed on the virtual environment. What is more interesting is that some of the views provided by the system are not there in the physical realm. The surgeon controls the calculated position of the instruments in a computer generated model. The *effectors* are an interactive system involving surgeon, display and surgical instruments. This is the inverse of what is normally considered a classical digital control problem, where the controller implements a control strategy through a series of specification functions and the process' observable behavior is in the physical environment.

The model of Figure 3 only represents the guidance phase of IIGS and must be augmented to include other phases, input variables, noise and disturbances. This will give us a system centric view of the safety problem.

One important aspect of this process control model is that it is independent of the software architecture of a particular system. Another added benefit of using process control diagrams in representing a virtual process is that the physical and conceptual (virtual) components, such as software supported processes and protocols, can both be represented in the same abstraction and be analyzed as part of a complete system. This visual representation of all components is critical to the complete description and analysis of the system. It allows for a more complete hazard analysis that is not compartmentalized. Contributing factors to accuracy errors, as well as the propagation of these errors through the system, will be more visible.

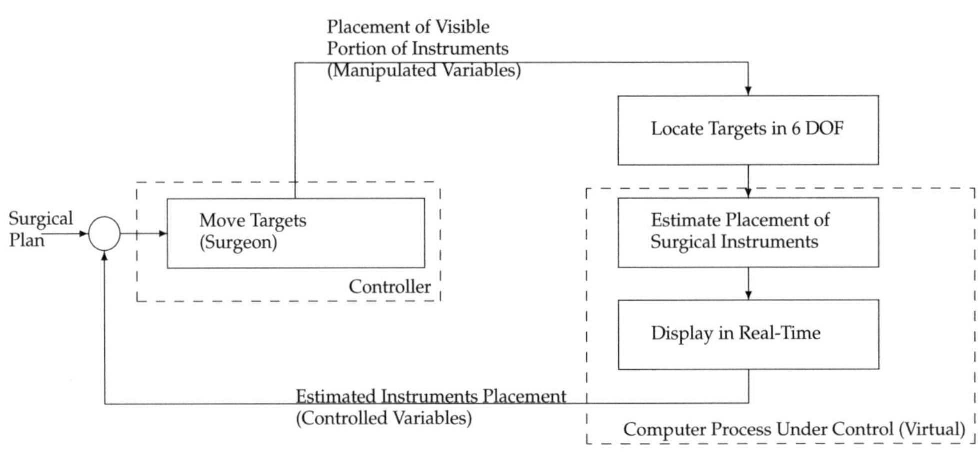


Fig. 3. Process Control View of Interactive Image-Guided Surgery

### 5.1 Process control model structure diagram

In this subsection we discuss the modeling diagram used as part of the Abstract Process Safety Analysis Model. The structure diagram is used to model the process of IIGS and will be used to guide the safety analysis performed at the lower layers of the architecture.

[14] For some procedures, the surgeon will not be able to observe the end of instruments and must rely on the computer model. In other cases, the surgeon can observe some aspects of the physical instruments and provide coarser placement in the absence of the computer model, but with reduced accuracy. Observability and controllability in the later case affect the ability to maximize surgical outcome.

The structure diagram is also used to display the current status of the system analysis based on the collation of safety analysis information. Each element of the Process Control Model Structure Diagram is to be coloured with the status information and the safety risk will be recorded numerically with each symbol on the structure diagram.

We first highlight the diagrammatic considerations that are sufficient to describe and substantiate our approach and to model the structure of IIGS systems as Process Control Models. We then introduce the syntax and notation used to model the structure of Process Control Models such as IIGS systems.

### 5.2 Diagrammatic modeling

In simple cases, a diagrammatic representation can model an idea to fully meet a given purpose; studying spatial relations, modeling the relationships in an organization or a system's structure (i.e. the command relationship in an organization or the floor plan of an office). For such simple cases, one item on the diagram fully represents a sufficient abstraction of this item from the physical world. For the case where the entire abstraction of the system can be represented on a diagram, we intend to capture, represent and analyze structure only. For this kind of analysis, we simply need to draw a diagram with components having recognizable and meaningful symbols (notation), rules for connecting the symbols (syntax) and appropriate naming labels or markings. There is no need for further meaning (semantics). We say that these diagrams have "*shallow semantics*"[15] because the entire design or idea is conveyed in one level of abstraction and no further semantics are required.

We use shallow semantics to convey the idea of representing the physical and virtual characteristics of a system on a single layer diagram of components and connectors. By comparison, deep semantics conveys the idea of adding layers to the model and adding meaning to describe the safety properties of the system being analyzed.

Process control modeling is the kind of problem domain that requires precise syntax and deep semantics. If we want to model the process control of a hydraulic turret in a missile defence system, and analyze it for safety we need to augment the turret's structure diagram with safety analysis techniques such as Failure Mode Effect Analysis (FMEA) or Fault Tree Analysis (FTA) IEC (1985; 1990); Leveson (1995). In a simplistic way, the structure diagram then describes the structure of physical components of the model such as hoses, valves, transducers, flow direction and pressure. The structure diagram is only part of the entire model. When we augment the structure diagram with mathematical models, analytical methods and information we further increase the semantics of the analysis.

The approach that we have taken to model IIGS systems to conduct safety analysis reflects the approach taken in process control modeling such as the one described in the paragraph above.

### 5.3 Design of the APSAM syntactic types

In this section, we describe the notation and syntax that will be used to create the APSAM structure diagram.

[15] Here we define shallow semantics. The expression has been used in various context but no reference could be found as a source to provide a definition.

### 5.3.1 Types

Syntactic types represent the different classes of components and connectors on a diagram and help to distinguish between elements in a system Dean & Cordy (1995). Syntactic types are similar to abstract data types in programming languages. They have shallow semantics and must be further detailed during instantiation as typed nodes Dean & Cordy (1995) onto the Process Control Model structure diagram (subsection 5.3.4).

### 5.3.2 Component types

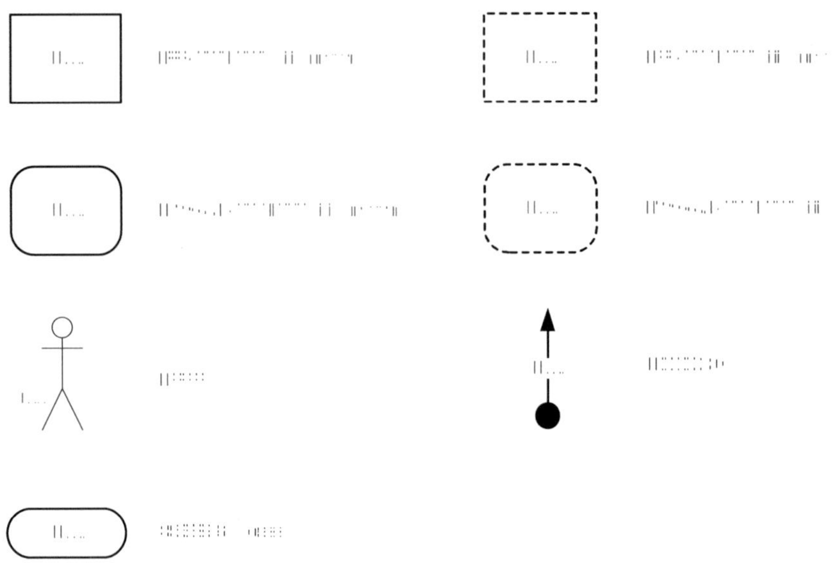

Fig. 4. Notation Types for Components.

The set of Types for components is displayed in Figure 4.

- Real-Time Physical Processes are those processes that change the physical environment and which have observe-and-react timing requirements that suffer from latency which can affect overall system performance and/or surgical outcome. Such processes include the movement of effectors, changes to model data and direct observation of the physical environment.
- Real-Time Virtual Processes are processes that change the virtual environment, may be subject to latency effects and may also contribute to these effects by means of computation delays.
- Near Real-Time Physical Processes must provide good quality of service in response time, but these processes can be interrupted without jeopardizing system outcome. It should be understood that the interruption should not be excessive to the point where the person in the loop forgets where he was in the process of transformation. Near Real-Time processes could have been called quality of service time as well because they closely characterize the timing requirements.

- Near Real-Time Virtual Processes must provide a good quality of service in response time to the person in the loop. These processes produce the input necessary to the conduct of the Real-Time processes (both virtual and physical).
- Sensors provide estimates of physical data for use by the virtual environment. They increase the visibility onto the physical world provided by the virtual environment. Effectors are physical components that are moved or used in the physical environment. Digital models of effectors are created to show their location in the virtual environment. We use the same syntactic type to represent sensors and effectors since labels can provide enough characterization without adding to the notation. Prostheses are also modeled using this syntactic type.
- Disturbances are unwanted input to the system that may change physical and virtual processes. They can cause deviation from the control policy as well as reduce visibility and controllability in the system. Disturbances can come from various sources including but not limited to: electronic noise, errors in images or digitization, motion artifacts, light noise (infrared camera interference), obscuration, etc...
- Person is any human participant in the process. Only those people who are directly involved in the process and can affect safety issues should be modeled.
- Labels are used to identify all components and provide a role for the component as part of the system.

### 5.3.3 Connector types

The set of types for connectors is displayed in Figure 5.

- The interface connector represents the unidirectional interface between two components. The interface may be physical or a flow of information. The flow of information is in the form of an analog or digital stream and the information is not retained or saved between the two components, it is not persistent. If one of the components is a process and it stops, the stream of information is interrupted.
- The information flow with memory is a unidirectional connector that has the responsibility to transfer data between components and provide persistence between successive executions of the processes. The round end of the connector is at the source of the information transfer. The arrow is at the sink end. There is no need to identify on the structure diagram where the information is persistent. This can happen at the source, sink, at both ends or in the middle. The importance of this connector is to highlight limitations and requirements for freshness of information, security, mishandling, misplacement, stable storage, recovery, duplication, bandwidth, coherence and transport. The issues listed here are unique to this connector because of possible time lag affecting information flow with memory.
- The interactive connector identifies the interfaces in the system that require continuous flow of information. It has significant symbiotic relationships between components.
- The summation point is a junction for connectors. The summation point is the only element on the APSAM structure diagram that is not part of the safety analysis. Its only purpose is to help clarify the diagram.
- Labels are used to identify the interface or relationship between components.

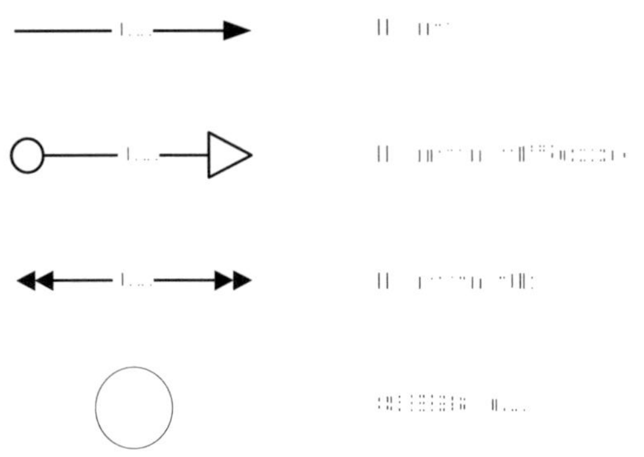

Fig. 5. Notation Types for Connectors.

An important distinction to be made is for the Disturbance component type. In classical process control modeling (Figure 2) input variables, set points and disturbances are normally represented as arrows that come from nowhere and point to where they induced an effect. When we developed the notation we wanted to differentiate between a connector that represents a flow of information and one that represents a disturbance, which is an unwanted manifestation representing uncontrollable effects that come from the environment. Our choice was to show such phenomena as a black dot representing the environment with an arrow to attach to the model at the point of induction. Disturbances can connect to components to show that the effect is specific or internal to the component, or to connectors to represent that the disturbance influences the flow of information or signal between components. Disturbances that can occur at the interface between the connector and the component are attached to the connector.

### 5.3.4 Process control model structure diagram

The Process Control Model Structure Diagram, or simply structure diagram, is a concept for the safety analysis expert to instantiate syntactic types to model system structure and behavior Dean & Cordy (1995). The modeler is responsible for providing each instantiated type with an identity in the form of a label.

Connectors are instantiated as first class objects in the model Shaw & Garlan (1996). Connectors as first class objects convey the idea that they not only show relationships on a diagram between two components, but that they have deeper semantics similar to that of components. The analyst uses connectors to represent relationships between components covering all meaningful system interfaces. Some interfaces need not be represented as they have no impact on the safety analysis. These interfaces could be represented on a separate view for completeness.

## 6. Results

We present some of the most interesting or significant findings of the application of the safety analysis protocol. The findings that were generated during the iterative elaboration of the analysis methods, design and the related research activities were key to the development of the protocol and conceptual architecture as well as in the identification of information requirements and analysis forms.

The APSAM structure diagram we elaborated for our orthopedic systems contains 28 Components and 29 Connectors, each was validated by computer system specialists that designed parts of the IIGS systems that were used during the analysis.

After the APSAM structure diagram was completed a System Hazard Analysis (SHA) Sha (1999) was performed for each component and connector. SHA analysis identified 57 Composite Hazards. Each of the hazard was identified with the system expert that validated the hazard. 33 of the composite hazards were identified to have propagation effects. The propagation effects were also described as part of the analysis and are recorded in an integral database. The Fault Tree Analysis (FTA) IEC (1990) that followed the SHA identified 139 Hazardous conditions (leaves). 49 of the FTA leaves were mitigated by competent human intervention. The analysis revealed only 7 uncontrolled or unresolved conditions. These uncontrolled or unresolved conditions did not imply that the system is unsafe but the experts believe that there is a need to further investigate these hazardous conditions. As part of the analysis we identified 31 Safeguard requirements; most were already are current practice but were not documented.

The findings below were elicited from various sources. They stem from direct observation during surgeries and observed surgical gestures of the physicians while using the IIGS systems for the surgeries; some of which are discussed in this section. Other findings came from the professional judgment and observations of the attending physicians during surgeries which were recorded.

The physicians would often address the clinical research scientist who operated the computers during the surgery on the operation of the system, limitations and improvements. Interviews with computer system specialists and a clinical research scientist were used to get the more technical information. The safety analysis protocol and the prototype of the architecture as well as the Process Control Model Structure Diagram were used to guide and record the iterative elicitation of hazards and their underlying hazardous conditions.

The most important finding is that there is a requirement for further research to evaluate the person machine interfaces in the system to better present information and reduce the loss of situational awareness. There are four different kinds of information that can be presented to the surgeon: Anatomic and morphologic using visualization of medical images, visual tracking, medical plans that show desired corrections and implants, and technical data which provides accuracy, measurements, depth, applied force and the like. Surgeons sometimes temporarily lose situational awareness during computer-guided surgery. This loss of situational awareness can occur if the presentation of the view is different from the normal physical views. Loss of situational awareness can also occur if the virtual surgical site is not the one the surgeon recognizes from the plan. In some cases the temporary loss in situational awareness can be caused if the image was not rotated in the right direction or the right plane by the computer operator. Zooming errors can also cause delays. Through all the surgeries that were witnessed for this research, the surgeons regained situational awareness in less than a minute. However, the temporary confusion could lead to longer procedures or loss of confidence in the tool in general clinical practice.

Complete identification of single points of failure is also very important. In some safety critical systems, if you cannot eliminate or mitigate single points of failure, your system is deemed unsafe and you must redesign or add redundant systems Dunn (2003). For IIGS we can allow the presence of single points of failure or degradation[16] in the system as long as competent human intervention can be used to mitigate the risk. That requires that there is visibility (or observability) of the failure. For example if a system fails to register, it represents a hazard, but the likelihood of occurrence is low and criticality is low because the surgeon can detect this condition in the large majority of cases and bail out of using the system.

Another important finding that quickly came to the forefront is that our system level approach encouraged thinking in terms of component and interface modifications to introduce safeguards or risk reduction mechanisms for introduced and attendant hazards. This system level approach makes visible potential hazards and ways to remove or mitigate those hazards.

By analyzing the leaves of the FTA trees we found that there are three main mitigation methods that can be applied to IIGS systems:

- Competent Human Intervention: Competent human intervention was very useful in providing mitigation information for hazardous conditions where the surgeon can use empirical geometric rules to decide if the procedure is still within operating ranges. The idea to create the state-based representation of competent human intervention came from observations in the operating room during several surgeries.
- Phantom Tests: The use of tests with phantoms can be used as a mitigation factor where lack of accuracy or spatial fidelity constitute a hazard. However, motion artifacts and the resulting propagation effects cannot be mitigated with phantom tests. Motion artifacts need to be further investigated to quantify their effects on IIGS. Articulated cadavers could be used to simulate tensing and patient movements during imaging. The movements could be measured mechanically and the effects on motion artifacts quantified on the resulting images.
- Code Inspections: Fagan style code inspection or some more agile inspection methods can be used to review parameters and transformation in the code of the IIGS systems. Pair programming or peer review could be used if the resources are not available. The calibration criteria for tracking cameras are set by programmers as are parameter files, marker types, lens models, interface packing routines, cable types and many other settings. The processing of tracking raw data from the 3-D cameras can also lead to inaccuracies. These settings, calibration data and calculations using the data to provide the registration and guidance information are not visible to the operator or the surgeon. Code and data inspections can be useful to ensure correct values are used.

## 7. Conclusion and future work

The research aimed at improving several attributes while performing safety analysis for IIGS systems. The safety analysis using the prototype implementation of the protocol provided us with the ability to validate traceability and visibility attributes. The notation used with the prototype helped us demonstrate the expressiveness of the APSAM. The maintainability

[16] We use failure to indicate that the system cannot be used and degradation if the system can be used in a degraded mode with concurrence from the surgeon.

attribute is validated by the integration of the safety analysis methods under a single high-level abstraction, the APSAM structure diagram and a repository that enforces relational integrity. Maintainability was identified as one of the main benefits of the protocol and its supporting conceptual architecture.

Finally the validation of the IIGS APSAM for orthopedic surgery with domain experts using the prototype helps us support the conclusion that the completeness of the safety analysis has been increased from what it would have been using the baseline methods for comparison described in Section 4.

We can also support the conclusion that the scale of rigor provided by the APSAM and its safety analysis protocol provides the necessary due care for safety analysis for such systems where competent human intervention is present. The traceability and visibility of the hazards and their resolution should be sufficient to obtain Food and Drugs Administration market clearance for like systems. The level of the analysis also provides for efficient use of domain experts.

Future research is required to apply the process control model including APSAM to other interactive systems where the operator or expert makes control decisions based on a virtual representation of the environment. Much work needs to be done to quantify system latency and its effects on safety. This quantification of latency is key when systems that warn surgeons of impending surgical errors like the one proposed by Luz et al. (2010) are considered.

Recently a specification for an extension to the Unified Modeling Language called the Systems Modeling Language or SysML was published under control of the Object Management Group Team (2006). The intent of the document is to retain the main structure and components of UML 2.0 and to perform system engineering domain modeling. Much of SysML makes use of new stereotypes but some interesting extensions have been proposed because UML was too restrictive to represent some system engineering concepts. Safety has been considered as part of this proposed standard to specify safety under stereotyped classes for requirements. There are no other syntactic elements or semantics to further model these system safety requirement classes or to drive and track a system safety analysis. The use of SysML is likely to become a standard for system engineering modeling similar to the use of UML 2.0 to model software. An interesting future research direction would be to propose an extension to SysML based on APSAM and implemented on Eclipse.

The generic notation and syntax, as well as the protocol, that have been produced as part of this research are not limited to IIGS systems. Trying the model in other safety critical system domains that have abstract interactive processes and person in the loop is certainly possible and should be investigated. Any system that provides estimated information for decision making in a critical environment could benefit from an analysis conducted with the APSAM and its protocol.

## 8. References

*Assessment and Management of Cancer Risks from Radiological and Chemical Hazards* (1998). *Report H39-428/1998E*, Health Canada, Atomic Energy Control Board and Ontario Ministery of Environment and Energy.

Ayache, N., Cinquin, P., Cohen, I., Cohen, L., Leitner, F. & Monga, O. (1996). Segmentation of complex three-dimensional medical objects: A challenge and a requirement for computer-assisted surgery planning and performance, *in* R. H. Taylor, S. Lavallée, B. G. C. & R. Mösges (eds), *Computer-Integrated Surgery - Technology and Clinical Applications*, MIT Press, Cambridge, Massachusetts, collection of new and reedited papers. 4, pp. 59–74.

Birkfellner, W., Watzinger, F., Wanschitz, F., Ewers, R. & Bergmann, H. (1998). Calibration of tracking systems in a surgical environment, *IEEE Transactions on Medical Imaging* 17(5): 737–742.

Breeuwer, M. et al. (1998). EASI Project - Improving the effectiveness and quality of image-guided surgery, *IEEE Transactions on Information Technology in Biomedicine* 2(3): 156–168.

Choi, J. J., Cleary, K., Zeng, J., Gary, K., Freedman, M., Watson, V., Lindisch, D. & Mun, S. K. (2000). I-SPINE: A software package for advances in image-guided and minimally invasive spine procedures, *Proceedings of SPIE - The International Society for Optical Engineering, 28th AIPR Workshop: 3D Visualization for Data Exploration and Decision Making, Oct 13-Oct 15 1999, Washington, DC, USA*, Vol. 3905, SPIE; AIPR Executive Committee Publisher: Society of Photo-Optical Instrumentation Engineers, Bellingham, WA, USA, Society of Photo-Optical Instrumentation Engineers, Bellingham, WA, USA, pp. 242–247.

Chudleigh, M., Berridge, C., May, R., Butler, J. & Poole, I. (1995). SADLI project: Safety critical software research in the medical diagnostic domain, *Computing & Control Engineering Journal* 6(5): 211–215.

Dean, D., Kamath, J., Duerk, J. L. & Ganz, E. (1998). Validation of object-induced MR distortion correction for frameless stereotactic neurosurgery, *IEEE Transactions on Medical Imaging* 17(5): 810–816.

Dean, T. R. & Cordy, J. R. (1995). A syntactic theory of software architecture, *IEEE Transactions on Software Engineering* 21(4): 302–313.

Dunn, W. R. (2003). Designing safety-critical computer systems, *IEEE Computer* 36(11): 40–46.

Elliott, L., Mojdehbakhsh, R. & Tsai, W.-T. (1994). Process for developing safe software, *Proceedings of the 1994 IEEE 7th Symposium on Computer-Based Medical Systems, Jun 11-12 1994, Winston-Salem, NC, USA*, IEEE Symposium on Computer-Based Medical Systems, IEEE Computer Society, IEEE, Los Alamitos, CA, USA, pp. 241–246.

Fei, B., Ng, W. S., Chauhan, S. & Kwoh, C. K. (2001). The safety issues of medical robotics, *Reliability Engineering and System Safety* 73(2): 183–192.

Fitzpatrick, M. J., West, J. B. & Maurer, Jr, C. R. (1998). Predicting error in rigid-body point-based registration, *IEEE Transactions on Medical Imaging* 17(5): 694–702.

Fries, R. C., Pienkowski, P. J. & Jorgens, III, J. (1996). Safe, effective, and reliable software design and development, *Biomedical Instrumentation & Technology* 30(2): 136–149. Publisher: Assoc for the Advancement of Medical Instrumentation, Arlington, VA, USA.

Galloway, Jr, R. L., Maciunas, R. J., Bass, W. & Carpini, W. (1994). Optical localization for interactive, image-guided neurosurgery, *Proceedings of SPIE - The International Society for Optical Engineering, Medical Imaging 1994: Image Capture, Formatting, and Display, Feb 13-14 1994, Newport Beach, CA, USA*, Vol. 2164, pp. 137–145.

Gary, K., Ibáñez, L., Aylward, S., Gobbi, D., Blake, B. M. & Cleary, K. (2006). Coping with defective software in medical devices, *IEEE Computer* 39(4): 40–45.

Gauldie, D. R. (2002). *Calibration and registration with 3d a-mode ultrasound*, Masters thesis, Queen's University, Kingston, Ont.

Gowen, L. D. (1994). Specifying and verifying safety-critical software systems, *Proceedings of the 1994 IEEE 7th Symposium on Computer-Based Medical Systems, Jun 11-12 1994, Winston-Salem, NC, USA*, IEEE Symposium on Computer-Based Medical Systems, IEEE Computer Society, IEEE, Los Alamitos, CA, USA, pp. 235–240.

Gowen, L. D. (1995). Summary of the '94 CBMS symposium's software safety workshop, *Proceedings of the 8th IEEE Symposium on Computer-Based Medical Systems, Jun 9-10 1995, Lubbock, TX, USA*, IEEE Symposium on Computer-Based Medical Systems, IEEE; SPIE, IEEE, Los Alamitos, CA, USA, pp. 330–337.

Gowen, L. D. & Collofello, J. S. (1994). Assessing traditional verification's effectiveness on safety-critical software systems, *Journal of Systems and Software* 26(2): 103–115.

Gowen, L. D. & Yap, M. Y. (1993). Traditional software development's effects on safety, *Proceedings of the 6th Annual IEEE Symposium on Computer-Based Medical Systems, Jun 13-16 1993, Ann Arbor, MI, USA*, IEEE Symposium on Computer-Based Medical Systems, pp. 58–63.

Halang, W. A., Sniezek, M. & Colnaric, M. (1998). Computerized controllers for safety critical medical applications, *International Journal of Medical Informatics* 49(2): 139–155.

Herrmann, D. S. (1995). Preview of IEC safety requirements for programmable electronic medical systems, *Medical Device and Diagnostic Industry* 17(6): 4pp.

Hindus, L. (2001). Medical visualization realities now: Less fantastic voyages through the body, *Advanced Imaging* 16(2): 42, 44, 50.

IEC (1985). *IEC 60812:1985 International Electrotechnical Commission - Analysis techniques for system reliability - Procedures for Failure Mode and Effects Analysis (FMEA)*, first edn.

IEC (1990). *IEC 61025:1990 International Electrotechnical Commission - Fault Tree Analysis - FTA*, first edn.

Jiang, Z., Miao, S., Zamorano, L., Li, Q., Gong, J. & Diaz, F. (1998). Technology and human errors in image-guided surgeries, *Proceedings of Surgical-Assist Systems, Jan 25-28 1998, San Jose, CA*, Vol. 3262 of *Proceedings of SPIE - The International Society for Optical Engineering*, IBOS; SPIE, The International Society for Optical Engineering, Bellingham, WA, USA, pp. 78–84.

Jones, P. L., Jorgens, III, J., Taylor, Jr, A. R. & Weber, M. (2002). Risk management in the design of medical device software systems, *Biomedical Instrumentation and Technology* 36(4): 237–266.

Knight, J. C. (1990). Issues of software reliability in medical systems, *Proceedings of the Third Annual IEEE Symposium on Computer-Based Medical Systems, Jun 3-6 1990, Chapel Hill, NC, USA*, IEEE Computer Soc; IEEE Engineering in Medicine & Biology Soc; IEEE Eastern North Carolina Section; Univ of North Carolina; North Carolina State Univ; et al; Research Triangle Institue, pp. 153–160.

Lavallé, S. (1996). Registration for computer-integrated surgery: Methodology, state of the art, *in* R. H. Taylor, S. Lavallée, B. G. C. & R. Mösges (eds), *Computer-Integrated Surgery - Technology and Clinical Applications*, MIT Press, Cambridge, Massachusetts, collection of new and reedited papers. 32, pp. 77–97.

Lavallé, S., Troccaz, J., Sautot, P., Mazier, B., Cinquin, P., Merloz, P. & Chirossel, J.-P. (1996). Computer-assisted spinal surgery using anatomy-based registration, *in* R. H. Taylor, S. Lavallée, B. G. C. & R. Mösges (eds), *Computer-Integrated Surgery - Technology and Clinical Applications*, MIT Press, Cambridge, Massachusetts, collection of new and reedited papers. 32, pp. 425–449.

Leffingwell, D. A. & Norman, B. (1993). Software quality in medical devices: a top-down approach, *Proceedings of the 6th Annual IEEE Symposium on Computer-Based Medical Systems, Jun 13-16 1993, Ann Arbor, MI, USA*, IEEE Symposium on Computer-Based Medical Systems, pp. 307–311.

Leveson, N. (1995). *Safeware: System Safety and Computers*, Addison Wesley, Boston.

Likert, F. (1932). A technique for measurement of attitudes, *Archives of Psychology* (140).

Loesh, R. E., Gosnell, A. B., Wyskida, R. M., Johannes, J. D. & Benoist, T. F. (1999). Engineering approach to critical software certification, *Proceedings of the 1999 32nd Annual Hawaii International Conference on System Sciences, HICSS-32, Jan 5-8 1999, Maui, HI, USA*, IEEE, IEEE Comp Soc, Los Alamitos, CA, USA, p. 282.

Lorensen, W. & Cline, H. (1987). Marching cubes: A high resolution 3d surface construction algorithm, *Computer Graphics* 21(4): 163–169.

Luz, M., Mueller, S., Strauss, G., Dietz, A., Meixensberger, J. & Manzey, D. (2010). Automation in surgery: The impact of navigated-control assistance on the performance, workload and situation awareness of surgeons, *Proceedings of the Human Factors and Ergonomics Society, 54th Human Factors and Ergonomics Society Annual Meeting 2010, HFES 2010, September 27, 2010 - October 1, 2010*, Vol. 2 of *Human Factors and Ergonomics Society Annual Meeting*, pp. 889–893.

Mojdehbakhsh, R., Tsai, W.-T. & Kirani, S. (1994). Retrofitting software safety in an implantable medical device, *IEEE Software* 11(1): 41–50.

Mösges, R. & Lavallée, S. (1996). Multimodal information for computer-integrated surgery, *in* R. H. Taylor, S. Lavallée, B. G. C. & R. Mösges (eds), *Computer-Integrated Surgery - Technology and Clinical Applications*, MIT Press, Cambridge, Massachusetts, collection of new and reedited papers. 1, pp. 5–19.

Murthy, S. (1995). Retrospective validation of medical device software, *Medical Device and Diagnostic Industry* 17(5): 7pp. Publisher: Canon Communications Inc, Santa Monica, CA, USA.

on Radiological Protection, I. C. (ed.) (1960-Present). *Annals of the ICRP*, Elsevier.

Patel, K. C., Duerk, J. L., Zhang, Q., Chung, Y.-C., Williams, M., Kaczynski, K., Wendt, M. & Lewin, J. S. (1998). Methods for providing probe position and temperature information on MR images during interventional procedures, *IEEE Transactions on Medical Imaging* 17(5): 794–802.

Peters, T. (2001). Image-guided surgery and therapy: Current status and future directions, *Proceedings of SPIE - The International Society for Optical Engineering, Medical Imaging 2001: Visualization, Display, and Image-Guided Procedures, Feb 18-20 2001, San Diego, CA*, Vol. 4319, pp. 1–12.

Pieper, S., McKenna, M., Chen, D. & McDowall, I. E. (1994). Computer animation for minimally invasive surgery: Computer system requirements and preferred implementations, *Proceedings of SPIE - The International Society for Optical Engineering, Stereoscopic Displays and Virtual Reality Systems, Feb 8-10 1994, San Jose, CA, USA*, Vol. 2177, IS&T - Soc for Imaging Science and Technology, Springfield, VA USA; SPIE - Int Soc for Opt Engineering, Bellingham, WA USA, Society of Photo-Optical Instrumentation Engineers, Bellingham, WA, USA, pp. 401–408.

Profio, A. E. (1979). *Radiation Shielding and Dosimetry*, Wiley, New York.

Radau, P. E., Slomka, P. J., Julin, P., Svensson, L. & Wahlund, L.-O. (2000). Automated segmentation and registration technique for HMPAO-SPECT imaging of Alzheimer's patients, *Proceedings of SPIE - The International Society for Optical Engineering, Medical*

*Imaging 2000: Image Processing, Feb 14-Feb 17 2000, San Diego, CA, USA*, Vol. 3979, Society of Photo-Optical Instrumentation Engineers, Bellingham, WA, USA, pp. 372–384.

Robb, R. (1996). VR assisted surgery planning, *IEEE Engineering in Medicine and Biology* 15(2): 60–69.

Schneider, P. & Hines, M. L. (1990). Classification of medical software, *Proceedings of the 1990 Symposium on Applied Computing, Apr 5-6 1990, Fayetteville, AR, USA*, IEEE Computer Soc; Arkansas Soc for Computer & Information Technology (ASCIT); ACM, IEEE, Piscataway, NJ, USA, pp. 20–27.

Sha, L. (1999). High assurance bio-medical device control, *Proceedings, v2, 1999, Proceedings of the 1999 IEEE Engineering in Medicine and Biology 21st Annual Conference and the 1999 Fall Meeting of the Biomedical Engineering Society (1st Joint BMES / EMBS), Oct 13-Oct 16 1999, Atlanta, GA, USA*, Annual International Conference of the IEEE Engineering in Medicine and Biology, p. 879.

Shaw, M. & Garlan, D. (1996). *Software Architecture: Perspectives on an Emerging Discipline*, Prentice Hall, Upper Saddle River, New Jersey.

Starreveld, Y., Gobbi, D., Finnis, K. & Peters, T. (2001). Software components for medical image visualization and surgical planning, *Proceedings of SPIE - The International Society for Optical Engineering, Medical Imaging 2001: Visualization, Display, and Image-Guided Procedures, Feb 18-20 2001, San Diego, CA*, Vol. 4319, pp. 546–556.

Taylor, R. H., Lavallée, S., C., B. G. & Mösges, R. (eds) (1996). *Computer-Integrated Surgery - Technology and Clinical Applications*, MIT Press, Cambridge, Massachusetts.

Team, S. M. (2006). Systems modeling language sysml specification draft, *Technical Report OMG Document ad/2006-03-01 Version 1.0*, Object Management Group.

Tenforde, T. S. (ed.) (1979). *Magnetic Field Effect on Biological Systems: Based on the Proceedings of Biomagnetic Effects Wrokshop held at Lawrence Berkeley Laboratory, University of California, on April 6-7, 1978*, Plenum Press, New York.

Udupa, J. (2001). Three-dimensional rendering in medicine: Some common misconceptions, *Proceedings of SPIE - The International Society for Optical Engineering, Medical Imaging 2001: Visualization, Display, and Image-Guided Procedures, Feb 18-20 2001, San Diego, CA*, Vol. 4319, pp. 660–670.

Udupa, J. K. & Gonçalves, R. J. (1996). Imaging transforms for volume visualization, *in* R. H. Taylor, S. Lavallée, B. G. C. & R. Mösges (eds), *Computer-Integrated Surgery - Technology and Clinical Applications*, MIT Press, Cambridge, Massachusetts, collection of new and reedited papers. 3, pp. 33–57.

Udupi, V., Raghavendra, A. & Inamdar, H. (2001). Computer vision method for biomedical image analysis, *IETE Technical Review (Institution of Electronics and Telecommunication Engineers, India)* 18(5): 365–373.

van der Weide, R., Zuiderveld, K. J., Bakker, C. J., Hoogenboom, T., van Vaals, J. J. & Viergever, M. A. (1998). Image guidance of endovascular interventions on a clinical MR scanner, *IEEE Transactions on Medical Imaging* 17(5): 779–785.

Verbeeck, R., Michiels, J., Nuttin, B., Knauth, M., Vandermeulen, D., Suetens, P., Marchal, G. & Gybels, J. (1995). Protocol for the clinical functionality assessment of a workstation for stereotactic neurosurgery, *IEEE Transactions on Medical Imaging* 14(3): 577–586.

Viergever, M. A. (1998). Image guidance of therapy, *IEEE Transactions on Medical Imaging* 17(5): 669–671.

Zamorano, L., Jiang, Z. & Kadi, A. M. (1994). Computer-assisted neurosurgery system: Wayne Sate University hardware and software configuration, *Computerized Medical Imaging and Graphics* 18(4): 257–271.

Zoroofi, R., Nishii, T., Sato, Y., Sugano, N., Yoshikawa, H. & Tamura, S. (2001). Segmentation of avascular necrosis of the femoral head using 3-D MR images, *Computerized Medical Imaging and Graphics* 25(6): 511–521.